D1175884

SURGERY
OF THE

Paranasal
Sinuses

SURGERY
OF THE

Paranasal
Sinuses

SECOND EDITION

Andrew Blitzer, MD, DDS

Professor of Clinical Otolaryngology and Vice Chairman
College of Physicians and Surgeons
Professor of Clinical Dentistry
School of Dental and Oral Surgery
Columbia University
Director, Division of Head and Neck Surgery
Columbia-Presbyterian Medical Center
New York, New York

William Lawson, MD, DDS

Professor of Otolaryngology
Mt. Sinai School of Medicine
Chief of Otolaryngology
Bronx Veterans Administration Hospital
New York, New York

William H. Friedman, MD, FACS

Chief of Otolaryngology
Deaconess Hospital
Director, Park Central Institute
St. Louis, Missouri

W.B. SAUNDERS COMPANY
Harcourt Brace Jovanovich, Inc.
Philadelphia ■ London ■ Toronto ■ Montreal ■ Sydney ■ Tokyo

W. B. SAUNDERS COMPANY
Harcourt Brace Jovanovich, Inc.

The Curtis Center
Independence Square West
Philadelphia, PA 19106

Library of Congress Cataloging-in-Publication Data

Surgery of the paranasal sinuses / [edited by] Andrew Blitzer,
William Lawson, William H. Friedman.—2nd ed.

p.   cm.

Includes bibliographical references and index.

1. Paranasal sinuses—Surgery.   I. Blitzer, Andrew.
    II. Lawson, William,   III. Friedman, William
    H. (William Hersh),

[DNLM: 1. Paranasal Sinuses—surgery.   WV 340 S961]

RF421.S87 1991   617.5′23—dc20

DNLM/DLC

for Library of Congress   91–14117

ISBN 0–7216–3583–0   CIP

Editor: Jennifer Mitchell
Designer: Dorothy Chattin
Production Manager: Ken Neimeister
Manuscript Editor: Wynette Kommer
Illustration Coordinator: Lisa Lambert
Indexer: Susan Thomas

SURGERY OF THE PARANASAL SINUSES   ISBN 0–7216–3583–0

Printed in the United States of America.

Last digit is the print number: 9   8   7   6   5   4   3   2   1

CONTRIBUTORS

Carol R. Archer, MD
Professor of Radiology, St. Louis University School of Medicine, St. Louis, Missouri; Chief, Section of Neuroradiology, St. Louis University Hospital, St. Louis, Missouri
Embolization of Tumors and Vascular Malformations

Eric E. Awwad, MD
Assistant Professor of Radiology, St. Louis University School of Medicine, St. Louis, Missouri; St. Louis University Hospital, St. Louis, Missouri
Embolization of Tumors and Vascular Malformations

Soly Baredes, MD
Associate Professor of Surgery, Director, Division of Head and Neck Surgery, Section of Otolaryngology—Head and Neck Surgery, New Jersey Medical School, Newark, New Jersey; Chief, Section of Otolaryngology, East Orange Veterans Administration Hospital, East Orange, New Jersey
Total Maxillectomy

John G. Batsakis, MD
Pathologist and Professor, Ruth Leggett Jones Chair of Pathology, University of Texas System Cancer Center, Houston, Texas; Head, Department of Pathology, MD Anderson Hospital and Tumor Institute, Houston, Texas
Pathology

Hugh F. Biller, MD
Professor and Chairman, Department of Otolaryngology, Mt. Sinai School of Medicine, New York, New York; Attending Otolaryngologist, Mt. Sinai Hospital, New York, New York
Lateral Rhinotomy
Orbital Decompression

Andrew Blitzer, MD, DDS
Professor of Clinical Otolaryngology and Vice Chairman, College of Physicians and Surgeons, Columbia University, New York, New York; Director, Division of Head and Neck Surgery, Columbia-Presbyterian Medical Center, New York, New York
Sphenoid Sinus
Surgery for Infection and Benign Disease of the Maxillary Sinus

Craniofacial Resection
Intracranial Complications of Disease of the Paranasal Sinuses

Peter W. Carmel, MD, DMedSci
Professor of Clinical Neurological Surgery, College of Physicians and Surgeons, Columbia University, New York, New York; Chief, Division of Pediatric Neurological Surgery, Columbia-Presbyterian Medical Center, New York, New York
Sphenoid Sinus
Cerebrospinal Fluid Rhinorrhea
Intracranial Complications of Disease of the Paranasal Sinuses

Hyun T. Cho, MD
Assistant Clinical Professor of Otolaryngology, College of Physicians and Surgeons, Columbia University, New York, New York; Chief, Otolaryngology, Beth Israel Medical Center, New York, New York
Total Maxillectomy

William C. Cooper, MD
Professor of Clinical Ophthalmology, Cornell University Medical College, New York, New York; Attending Ophthalmologist, The New York Hospital, New York, New York
Dacryocystorhinostomy

Blair Fearon, MD, FRCS(C), FACS, FAAP
Professor Emeritus, Department of Otolaryngology, Faculty of Medicine, University of Toronto, Toronto, Ontario, Canada; Senior Surgeon, Department of Otolaryngology, Hospital for Sick Children, Toronto, Ontario, Canada
Sinusitis in Infants and Children

Saul Frenkiel, MDCM, FRCS(C)
Associate Professor, Department of Otolaryngology, McGill University, Montreal, Quebec, Canada
Pathogenesis and Treatment of Nasal Polyps

William H. Friedman, MD, FACS
Chief, Department of Otolaryngology, Deaconess Hospital, St. Louis, Missouri
Ethmoid Sinus
Surgery of the Pterygopalatine Fossa

N. David Greyson, MD, FRCP(C)
Associate Professor of Radiology, University of Toronto, Toronto, Ontario, Canada; Director, Department of Nuclear Medicine, St. Michael's Hospital, Toronto, Ontario, Canada
Radionuclide Scanning

Donald F.N. Harrison, MD, PhD, FRCS
Professor of Laryngology and Otolaryngology, Institute of Laryngology and Otolaryngology, University of London, London England; Chairman and Senior Surgeon, Royal National E.N.T. Hospital, London, England
Transorbital Approach to the Ethmoid Sinus—The Patterson Procedure

Anthony F. Jahn, MD
Professor and Chief, Section of Otolaryngology—Head and Neck Surgery, University of Medicine and Dentistry of New Jersey, Newark, New Jersey; Chief of Otolaryngology, United Hospitals of Newark, Newark, New Jersey
General Principles

Eugene B. Kern, MD
Professor of Otorhinolaryngology, Mayo Medical School, Rochester, Minnesota; Consultant, Department of Otorhinolaryngology, Mayo Clinic and Mayo Foundation, Rochester, Minnesota
Physiology of the Human Nose

Wayne M. Koch, MD
Assistant Professor of Otolaryngology, Johns Hopkins University School of Medicine, Baltimore, Maryland
The Midfacial Degloving Approach to the Paranasal Sinuses and Skull Base

Arnold Komisar, MD, DDS, FACS
Clinical Associate Professor of Otorhinolaryngology, Cornell University Medical College, New York, New York; Director of Resident Education, Department of Otolaryngology, Lenox Hill Hospital, Manhattan Eye, Ear, Nose and Throat Affiliated Residency Program, New York, New York
Cerebrospinal Fluid Rhinorrhea

William Lawson, MD, DDS
Professor of Otolaryngology, Mt. Sinai School of Medicine, New York, New York; Chief of Otolaryngology, Bronx Veterans Administration Hospital, New York, New York
Frontal Sinus
Lateral Rhinotomy
Craniofacial Resection
Rhinologic Manifestations of Acquired Immunodeficiency Syndrome
Orbital Complications of Sinusitis

Howard L. Levine, MD
Head, Section of Nasal and Sinus Disorders, Department of Otolaryngology and Communicative Disorders, Cleveland Clinic Foundation, Cleveland, Ohio
Lasers and Rhinosinusology

Louis J. Loscalzo, DMD
Clinical Professor, Columbia University School of Dental and Oral Surgery, New York, New York; Chief, Oral-Maxillofacial Surgery, VA Medical Center, Bronx, New York
Management of Dental Disease and Oral Antral Fistula

Frank E. Lucente, MD
Chairman, Department of Otolaryngology, State University of New York—Health Science Center at Brooklyn, Brooklyn, New York; Chairman, Department of Otolaryngology, Long Island College Hospital, Brooklyn, New York; Chairman, Department of Otolaryngology, University Hospital at Brooklyn, Brooklyn, New York
Orbital Decompression
Rhinologic Manifestations of Acquired Immunodeficiency Syndrome

Thomas V. McCaffrey, MD, PhD
Associate Professor of Otorhinolaryngology, Mayo Medical School, Rochester, Minnesota; Consultant, Department of Otorhinolaryngology and of Physiology and Biophysics, Mayo Clinic and Mayo Foundation, Rochester, Minnesota
Physiology of the Human Nose

Beverly Denise McMillin, MD
Otolaryngologist, Private Practice, Lakeland, Florida; Staff Surgeon, Lakeland Regional Medical Center, Lakeland, Florida
Sinusitis in Infants and Children

Lawrence Z. Meiteles, MD
Chief Resident, Department of Otolaryngology, New York Eye and Ear Infirmary, New York Medical College, New York, New York
Rhinologic Manifestations of Acquired Immunodeficiency Syndrome

Kambiz T. Moazed, MD
Assistant Clinical Attending, College of Physicians and Surgeons, Columbia University, New York, New York; Chief of Oculoplastic and Orbital Surgery, Harlem Hospital Center, New York, New York
Dacryocystorhinostomy

Letty Moss-Salentijn, DDS, PhD
Professor of Anatomy and Cell Biology, Columbia University School of Dental and Oral Surgery, New York, New York; Director, Graduate Program on Dental Science, School of Dental and Oral Surgery, Columbia University, New York, New York
Anatomy and Embryology

H. Bryan Neel, III, MD, PhD
Professor of Otolaryngology and Associate Professor of Microbiology, Mayo Medical School, Rochester, Minnesota; Chairman Emeritus, Department of Otorhinolaryngology, Mayo Clinic and Mayo Foundation, Rochester, Minnesota
Juvenile Angiofibroma

Harold C. Neu, MD, FACP
Professor of Medicine and Pharmacology, College of Physicians and Surgeons, Columbia University, New York, New York; Chief, Division of Infectious Diseases, Columbia-Presbyterian Medical Center, New York, New York
Infectious Diseases of the Sinuses

Arnold M. Noyek, MD, FRCS(C), FACS
Professor of Otolaryngology and Radiology, University of Toronto, Toronto, Ontario, Canada; Otolaryngologist-in-Chief, Mt. Sinai Hospital, Toronto, Ontario, Canada
Radionuclide Scanning

P. Perry Phillips, MD
Chief Resident Associate in Otorhinolaryngology, Mayo School of Medicine, Rochester, Minnesota
Physiology of the Human Nose

Kalmon D. Post, MD
Professor of Neurological Surgery and Vice Chairman, College of Physicians and Surgeons, Columbia University, New York, New York; Vice Chairman, Department of Neurological Surgery, Columbia-Presbyterian Medical Center, New York, New York
Sphenoid Sinus
Craniofacial Resection

John C. Price, MD
Associate Professor of Otolaryngology—Head and Neck Surgery, Johns Hopkins University School of Medicine, Baltimore, Maryland
The Midfacial Degloving Approach to the Paranasal Sinuses and Skull Base

James J. Sciubba, DMD, PhD
Professor of Oral Pathology, State University of New York, Stony Brook, Stony Brook, New York; Chairman, Department of Dentistry, Long Island Jewish Medical Center, New Hyde Park, New York
Pathology

Gary Y. Shaw, MD
Assistant Professor, Department of Otolaryngology—Head and Neck Surgery, Louisiana State University, Shreveport, Louisiana
Ancillary Nasal Procedures

Peter Small, MDCM, FRCP(C), FACP
Associate Professor, Department of Medicine, McGill University, Montreal, Quebec; Chief, Division of Allergy and Clinical Immunology, Sir Mortimer B. Davis Jewish General Hospital, Montreal, Quebec, Canada
Pathogenesis and Treatment of Nasal Polyps

Howard W. Smith, MD, DMD
Clinical Professor Otolaryngology, College of Physicians and Surgeons, Columbia University, New York, New York; Attending, Columbia-Presbyterian Medical Center, New York, New York
Paranasal Sinus Trauma

Max L. Som, MD*
Emeritus Professor of Otolaryngology, Mt. Sinai School of Medicine, City University of New York, New York, New York; Director Emeritus, Head and Neck Division, Department of Surgery, Beth Israel Medical Center, New York, New York; Formerly, Attending Otolaryngologist, Mt. Sinai Medical Center, New York, New York
Total Maxillectomy

Peter M. Som, MD
Professor of Radiology and Otolaryngology, Chief, Head and Neck Radiology Section, Mt. Sinai School of Medicine, City University of New York, New York, New York; Attending Radiologist, Mt. Sinai Hospital, New York, New York
Radiology: Basic Concepts, Conventional Films, Computed Tomography and Magnetic Resonance Imaging

James A. Stankiewicz, MD
Professor and Vice Chairman, Department of Otolaryngology and Head and Neck Surgery, Loyola University Medical School, Maywood, Illinois; Attending Physician, Loyola University Medical Center, Maywood, Illinois
Endoscopic Nasal and Sinus Surgery

Bruce Sterman, MD
Facial Plastic and Reconstructive Surgery Fellow, Park Central Institute, St. Louis, Missouri
Lasers and Rhinosinusology

Fred J. Stucker, MD, FACS
Professor and Chairman, Department of Otolaryngology—Head and Neck Surgery, Louisiana State University School of Medicine, Shreveport, Louisiana
Ancillary Nasal Procedures

Eiji Yanagisawa, MD, FACS
Clinical Professor of Otolaryngology, Yale University School of Medicine, New Haven, Connecticut; Attending Otolaryngologist, Yale–New Haven Medical Center and Hospital of St. Raphael, New Haven, Connecticut
Paranasal Sinus Trauma

---

*Deceased

PREFACE

The authors undertook the writing of a second edition of *Surgery of the Paranasal Sinuses* to address the modern technological advances in imaging and instrumentation. Since the publication of the first edition of this book, advances in computed tomography, magnetic resonance imaging, radionuclide imaging, and endoscopic evaluation and surgery have revolutionized many aspects of surgery of the paranasal sinuses.

The goal of the second edition is to expand the knowledge of the clinician in the areas of the physiology and pathophysiology of nasal and paranasal sinus conditions. Older techniques and new methods of examination and evaluation of the nose and sinuses are reviewed, including an extensive review of computed tomography and magnetic resonance imaging. The second edition also presents for each paranasal sinus a comprehensive guide to the pathology, evaluation, decision making, and surgical techniques applicable to that sinus. The indications, intraoperative problems, limitations, complications and results are included in each chapter. Updated descriptions are included for specialized procedures including surgery for juvenile angiofibroma, endocrine exophthalmos, dacryocystorhinostomy, oral antral fistula, cerebrospinal rhinorrhea, craniofacial resection, and sinus fractures. Management of pediatric sinus disease, orbital complications, and intracranial complications is well described.

New chapters address endoscopic sinus surgery, with a description of techniques, indications, limitations, instrumentation, and complications. Laser sinus surgery is also discussed. The infectious diseases of the sinuses and antibiotic management have been added, as well as a chapter on the rhinologic manifestations of AIDS. There are also new chapters of facial degloving approaches to the midface, angiography and embolization, the transorbital approach to the ethmoid, and ancillary nasal procedures.

This book should continue to enhance the comprehensive knowledge of sinus surgery for the otolaryngologist, ophthalmologist, dental and oral surgeon, neurosurgeon, pediatrician, and infectious disease specialist.

We would like to thank the many contributors who have shared their expertise and experience with our readers, producing a volume of quality and completeness.

We would also like to thank our editor, Jennifer Mitchell, and the entire Saunders staff for the advice, effort, and encouragement they have given us throughout the preparation of this second edition.

Lastly we hope that our readers will find this second edition an invaluable adjunct to their practices. The first edition was the first comprehensive book dedicated solely to diseases and treatment of the paranasal sinuses. Currently there are many books available about many aspects of sinus surgery. We hope that in the second edition, *Surgery of the Paranasal Sinuses* continues to be *the* comprehensive text of sinus disease and surgery and will aid our readers in planning appropriate treatment for their patients.

ANDREW BLITZER
WILLIAM LAWSON
WILLIAM H. FRIEDMAN

CONTENTS

*Deceased

CHAPTER 1

ANATOMY AND EMBRYOLOGY

Letty Moss-Salentijn, DDS, PhD

The complexity of the three dimensional relationships of human paranasal sinuses is not easily grasped from anatomic descriptions. It is probably better understood by an appreciation of the embryology of the nasal region and the nasal frame. This chapter presents a succinct anatomic description of the paranasal sinuses, using a developmental approach.

EMBRYOLOGY OF THE NASAL FRAME

The developmental embryology of the structures surrounding the nasal cavities occurs in a sequence that may be divided arbitrarily into three distinct, consecutive stages: preskeletal, chondrocranial, and osteogenetic.

THE PRESKELETAL STAGE

Immediately following the closure of the anterior neuropore, the anterior pole of the forebrain is covered by a relatively thin layer of mesenchyme and an outer layer of ectoderm. This is the periprosencephalon, the future frontonasal region of the face. During further development, this mesenchyme will differentiate into the cartilages, bones, and connective tissues of much of the upper face.

There is now general agreement that the mesenchyme of the periprosencephalon is almost entirely of neural crest origin, derived from the midbrain area, and is not mesodermal.

Previously, such a statement could be made with assurance for nonmammalian species only. Recent experimental data on the development and fate of mammalian neural crest, acquired with the aid of in vitro culture of mammalian embryos and sophisticated labeling techniques of cell membranes, indicate that there is a general vertebrate pattern of behavior for neural crest cells and that earlier findings on nonmammalian species apply to mammals as well.[1-6] The cephalic neural crest cells are rather unique, compared with the neural crest cells in the trunk, in that their derivatives include most connective tissue structures, including bones, cartilages, and teeth, in facial and periprosencephalic regions. This unique ability to form connective tissue derivatives extends to the level of the fifth somite. Neural crest cells from the somite levels contribute to the aorticopulmonary and conotruncal septa of the developing heart.[7] The common neural crest origin of facial and cardiac connective tissues underlies the frequent co-incidence of congenital malformations in the face and heart.

Recent studies on bird chimeras have shown that the neural folds surrounding the prosencephalic neural plate give rise to the ectoderm of the nasal cavity and the nasal placode.[8]

A neural crest origin of the mesenchyme, and possibly of some ectoderm, in the frontonasal region of the human face has implications both for the development of craniofacial malformations in this region and for some still unspecified biochemical characteristics of the derived tissues.[9, 10] These problems are beyond the scope of this chapter.

The ectoderm in the frontonasal region undergoes localized thickening in the 24- to 26-day-old human embryo. Within a few days these thickenings become well-established nasal placodes. This is the first event in the development of the olfactory regions of the nasal mucosa. Although the placodes initially have a convex external surface, the unequal forward growth of the surrounding parts of the frontonasal swelling soon transforms this surface to a concave nasal groove. This groove is well established when the embryo is 32 to 33 days old. The surrounding parts of the frontonasal swelling, which are responsible for this transformation, are the medial nasal swelling at the medial side of the nasal placode and the lateral nasal swelling at the lateral side of the nasal placode. A third swelling, the maxillary swelling, is an outgrowth from the mandibular arch and is located at the inferolateral border of the placode (Fig. 1–1).

The three swellings are superficially separated from each other, by shallow depressions. As the swellings continue to grow forward and downward (relative to the position of the nasal

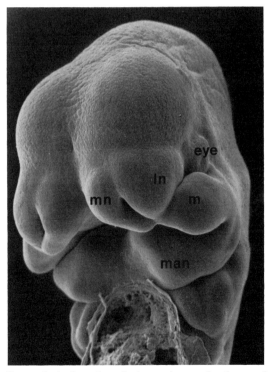

Figure 1–1. Scanning electron micrograph of normal primary palate development in a mammal (mouse). The nasal groove is visible between lateral and medial nasal swellings. The deep groove between maxillary and lateral nasal swellings will give rise to the nasolacrimal duct.

ln, lateral nasal swelling; *mn*, medial nasal swelling; *m*, maxillary swelling; *man*, mandibular arch. (Courtesy of Dr. K. Sulik, University of North Carolina.)

placodes), the epithelial linings of medial and lateral nasal swellings fuse inferiorly. As a result, the nasal groove becomes a blind-ending tube or pit.

The floor of the nasal pit is formed by the fused medial and lateral nasal swellings and, further anteriorly, by the fused medial nasal and maxillary swellings. The epithelial seam in the contact plane is variously called nasal fin or epithelial plate of Hochstetter. This is a relatively restricted band of epithelium. Once it has become interposed between the outgrowing facial swellings, it is disrupted anteriorly owing to the growth of the surrounding tissues. Posteriorly, this epithelial band persists for a limited period of time in the floor of the nasal pit. As it is further reduced in the vertical dimension, it becomes the oronasal membrane. The majority of the epithelial cells in this membrane remain viable, with only a few cells undergoing degeneration, resulting in cleavage spaces in the membrane. Between 42 and 44 days, the oronasal membrane ruptures completely. Surviving epithelial cells are incorporated in adjacent epithelia of the primary oral and nasal cavities.

The rupture of the oronasal membrane in the posterior floor of the nasal pit transforms this blind-ending cavity into a primary nasal cavity, which communicates via the newly formed opening (or primary choana) with the primary oral cavity.

During the forward and downward growth of the various facial swellings, each swelling also increases its dimensions in a mediolateral direction. Thus, during the transformation of the nasal groove into the primary nasal cavity, the depressions between maxillary and lateral nasal swellings are accentuated, both on the lateral (outside) surface and on the medial (inside) surface of the lateral wall of the primary nasal cavity. The groove on the outside surface is transformed into the nasolacrimal duct by the interposition of surface epithelium between the outgrowing maxillary and lateral nasal swellings and the loss of contact between this epithelium and the surface epithelium. The groove on the inside surface will develop into the inferior meatus of the nasal cavity.

The establishment of the primary nasal cavity, as it is described so far, appears to be centered on the olfactory region of the nose and the organization of the olfactory nerve. This process is completed by 42 to 45 days of developmental age.[11–16]

In the subsequent stages, the respiratory region of the nasal cavity develops during the further downward and forward growth of the midfacial complex.

THE CHONDROCRANIAL STAGE

Early in this stage, the definitive nasal cavities form, and a cartilaginous frame begins to provide primary skeletal protection and support of the nasal region.

Completion of Nasal Cavity Formation. During the seventh week and early eighth week of human embryonic development, the entire midfacial region continues its forward and downward growth. As a result, the primary choanae are enlarged in an anteroposterior direction, along with the nasal cavities. A large anterior segment of the choanal openings must be covered secondarily by a pair of palatal processes.

The palatal processes are outgrowths from the oral surfaces of the maxillary swellings. Initially, these processes have a predominantly vertical orientation as they grow downward alongside the developing tongue. Approximately in the middle of the eighth week the palatal processes assume a horizontal position. The mechanism underlying this change in orientation remains partially unresolved, but the dominant factor appears to be the greatly increased volume of extracellular matrix, particularly proteoglycans, synthesized by the mesenchymal cells of the palatal processes. The precise timing of this event (and all other developmental events) is subject to individual variations, and possibly also to sexual and racial ones.

The epithelial surfaces on the medial edges of the palatal processes and on the lower border of the nasal septum face each other and are about to fuse. Cell surface adhesion increases. Epithelial necrosis and basement membrane disruptions also increase, allowing fusion and subsequent epithelial breakdown between palatal processes and primary palate anteriorly and palatal processes and nasal septum posteriorly.

By the end of the eighth week, fusion has occurred in the future hard palate. The soft palate is completed by the end of the 12th week. At that time the definitive nasal cavity is established in the human fetus.[14, 17–23]

The Cartilaginous Nasal Frame. During the sixth week of development the mesenchyme of the medial and lateral nasal swellings undergoes localized condensation. In the earliest stages, several separate condensations may be identified:

1. *Trabeculae cranii.* Two strips of condensed mesenchyme run anteroposteriorly within the primitive nasal septum (formed by the two medial nasal swellings). These condensations possibly are vestiges of the trabeculae cranii of the chondrocranium.

2. *Tectal condensations.* Precartilaginous condensations arch dorsally around the primitive nares, within the medial and lateral nasal swellings.

3. *Paranasal condensations.* A third pair of precartilaginous condensations is present farther posteriorly, in the lateral nasal swellings.

Additional mesenchymal condensations may be found for the alar cartilage (just anterior to the tectal cartilage) and for the anterior paraseptal cartilage (bilaterally along the ventral border of the precartilaginous condensations in the primitive nasal septum). Occasionally, an additional posterior paraseptal cartilage may be present, but this is not common in humans.

The distinctiveness of separate mesenchymal condensations is soon lost. In a 6-week-old human embryo, the condensed mesenchyme forms a continuous capsule around the primary nasal cavities, except ventrally; a nasal floor is lacking in the human chondrocranium.

Fleetingly, independent chondrification centers appear within the condensed mesenchyme. These early cartilages are found in three locations: the central part of the nasal septum, the central parts of the tectal condensations, and the central parts of the paranasal condensations. Chondrification spreads rapidly from these centers throughout the condensed mesenchyme, and toward the end of the embryonic period proper the nasal septum (mesethmoid) and the nasal capsule (ectethmoid) are fully chondrified.

The *mesethmoid* is formed largely by the trabeculae cranii condensations and by contributions of tectal cartilage condensations (the fused medial parts). Superiorly, the mesethmoid is connected to the ectethmoid in front of the crista galli (a midline structure on the dorsal edge of the mesethmoid). Posterior to this point, the roof of the ethmoid region is still wide open during the embryonic period because the cribriform plate is not completed until the end of the third month of development. The most caudal part of the ectethmoid itself is not yet fully extended and is not completely continuous with the mesethmoid either.

At the end of the embryonic period proper, the *ectethmoid* is composed of a relatively thin plate of cartilage with some depressions and eminences on its outer surface. Some landmarks are found along the lines of fusion between the different ectethmoid components. One of these is the epiphanial foramen. This foramen is present only during the fetal and early postnatal periods. It is located on the fusion line between the tectal and paranasal cartilages. Through this foramen passes the external nasal branch of the anterior ethmoid nerve.

Farther laterally, the anterior edge of the paranasal cartilage partially overlaps the posterior edge of the tectal cartilage. Thus, the latter projects from the inner surface of the nasal capsular wall and gives rise to a curved ridge, representing an extremely rudimentary concha nasalis (agger nasi and uncinate process).

Posteriorly, the ala orbitalis (future lesser wing of the sphenoid) is connected with the ectethmoid by the lamina orbitonasalis, a cartilaginous plate running anteromedial to the optic foramen (Fig. 1–2). The posterior edge of the paranasal cartilage overlaps the anterolateral edge of this lamina, which results in the latter projecting into the nasal cavity as the first ethmoturbinal or middle concha.

Finally, the inferior border of the ectethmoid cartilage is curved slightly medially, extending into a mucosal fold on the lateral wall of the nasal cavity. This structure represents the developing maxilloturbinal or inferior concha.

The simple, relatively smooth internal surface of the ectethmoid at the beginning of the fetal period rapidly becomes increasingly complex during the second trimester of prenatal development. Additional conchae are formed. The number of conchae present prenatally may even exceed that found postnatally. During the development of the conchae the nasal mucosa folds first; only subsequently do the cartilages of the conchae form in the centers of the mucosal folds.

On the external surface of the ectethmoid

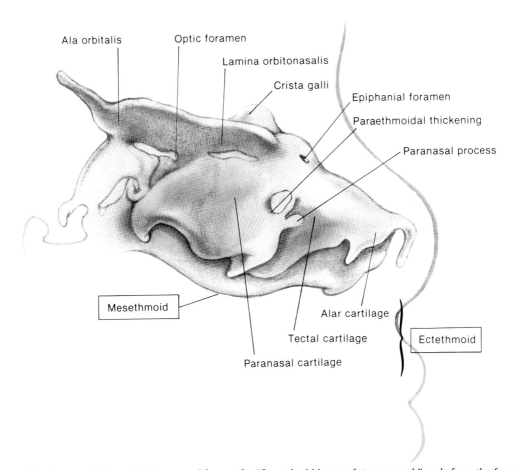

Figure 1–2. Diagram of the cartilaginous nasal frame of a 10-week-old human fetus, seen obliquely from the front and right side. The components of the nasal capsule (ectethmoid) and the nasal septum (mesethmoid) are shown. The cartilaginous ala orbitalis is the future lesser wing of the sphenoid. (See text.) (Redrawn after Bersch and Reinbach.[25])

some additional structures become apparent during the third month of development (Fig. 1–3). Three distinct cartilaginous extensions start protruding from a lateral prominence of the paranasal cartilage. All three are spatially related to the nasolacrimal duct. Two of these, the superior and inferior paraethmoid cartilages, are located medial to the duct, at the future site of the lacrimal bone. The third extension, the paranasal process, is located slightly lower and more laterally. It curves laterally around the nasolacrimal duct and is incorporated in the maxilla during further development.

When the human fetus is 12 weeks of age, the cartilaginous frame is well developed. Only minor modifications, such as the further growth and development of the ethmoturbinals, are yet to take place.[24–30]

OSTEOGENETIC STAGE

At the periphery of the cartilaginous nasal frame, several intramembranously forming bones appear between 7 and 10 weeks of developmental age (Fig. 1–4). Maxillary and premaxillary ossification centers appear early in the

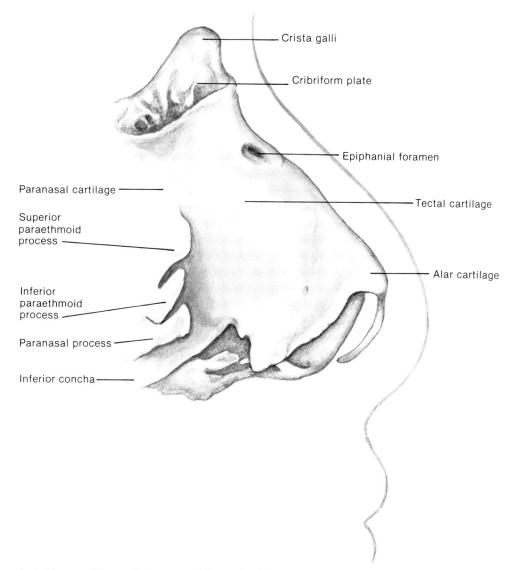

Figure 1–3. Diagram of the cartilaginous nasal frame of a 12-week-old human fetus (seen from the right side). On the outside surface of the paranasal cartilage, three distinct cartilaginous processes have developed: the superior and inferior paraethmoid processes and the paranasal process. The former two are located medial to the nasolacrimal duct; the latter is located lateral to it. The cribriform plate is undergoing chondrification at this stage. (Redrawn after Grube and Reinbach.[26])

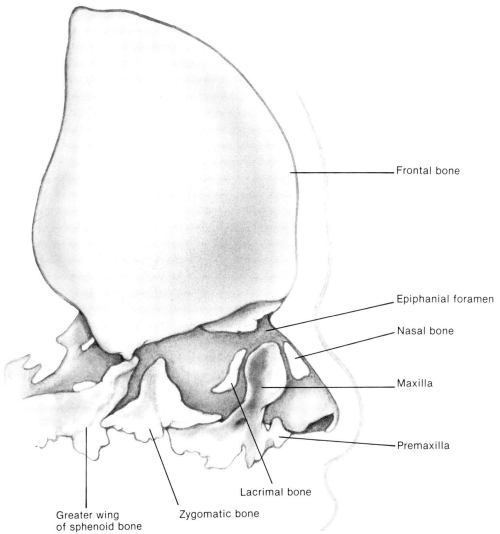

Frontal bone

Epiphanial foramen

Nasal bone

Maxilla

Premaxilla

Lacrimal bone

Greater wing
of sphenoid bone

Zygomatic bone

Figure 1–4. Diagram of the nasal frame, both cartilaginous and osseous, of a 12-week-old human fetus (seen from the right side). The cartilaginous components are darkly shaded. Lightly shaded are the intramembranously forming bones. (Redrawn after Grube and Reinbach.[26])

eighth week. By the end of the eighth week ossification centers are also present for vomer, frontal, zygomatic, and palatine bones. Nasal and lacrimal bones appear slightly later, generally during the ninth and tenth weeks of development.

Although the frontal bone overlaps the cartilage of the nasal frame to a minimal extent only, maxilla, premaxilla, vomer, lacrimal, and nasal bones cover much of the external surfaces of the ectethmoid and the lower surface of the mesethmoid.

Toward the end of the third fetal month, the membrane bones have expanded so far that the presumptive sites of the sutures are clearly recognizable. At this time the osseous frame, acting somewhat as an external scaffolding, begins to assume some of the supportive and protective roles of the cartilaginous frame,[24-28] hence the designation *osteogenetic stage*. Intramembranous ossification continues, whereas endochondral ossification of parts of the cartilaginous nasal frame will begin in the fifth fetal month.

Intramembranously Forming Bones. A brief description follows of the early development of the bones that constitute the skeletal frame around the nasal cavities and are important for the later developing paranasal sinuses.

Frontal Bone. This initially paired bone begins ossifying at the end of the eighth or the beginning of the ninth week of development. The ossification centers appear in the centers of the squamous regions, at the sites of the future frontal tuberosities. By the end of the tenth week, the bone is composed of an orbital and a squamous part. By the 12th week, the squamous part has frontal and temporal facies. The metopic suture between the two frontal bones begins closure in the second year of life. The process of closure usually is completed by the eighth year, at which time the suture may be obliterated completely.

Maxilla and Premaxilla. Individual ossification centers form during the late seventh and early eighth week of embryonic development in the maxillary and premaxillary regions. These separate ossification centers rapidly fuse into a single maxillary bone complex. At the end of the embryonic period proper, the bone has a frontal and a zygomatic process. At 10 weeks and 12 weeks, a developing alveolar process is visible, as well as a palatine process.

The frontal process of the maxilla covers the nasolacrimal duct and part of the external surface of the nasal capsule, specifically the most posterior part of the tectal cartilage and the anterior tip of the paranasal process. As early as the 12th week of development the latter is covered with a layer of perichondral bone. During subsequent development the paranasal process is incorporated in the expanding maxilla and loses the connection at its base with the ethmoid complex.

Palatine Bone. The palatine bone starts ossifying at the end of the eighth embryonic week. A single ossification center appears in the center of the future perpendicular lamina. From this center the ossification spreads. At 10 and 12 weeks a horizontal lamina is present. During subsequent fetal development, the orbital, sphenoid, and pyramidal processes are formed.

Nasal Bone. The nasal bone develops at the beginning of the third fetal month as a trapezoidal, thin plate of bone, covering the posterodorsal surface of the tectal cartilage just anterior to the epiphanial foramen. This foramen is covered gradually by the expanding nasal bone during the second trimester of prenatal development and persists until the surrounding cartilage is resorbed postnatally.

Lacrimal Bone. The lacrimal bone develops in the middle of the third fetal month as a thin plate of bone, covering both paraethmoid processes of the paranasal cartilage, but located medial to the corresponding segment of the nasolacrimal duct. By the 12th week a sharp angle is present in the bone plate, establishing a lateral (or orbital) surface and a facial surface, which will participate in the formation of the lacrimal fossa.

Vomer. The vomer is the only intramembranously forming bone that covers part of the surface of the mesethmoid. It forms toward the end of the eighth week of development as two separate, slender strips of bone, running parallel to each other anteroposteriorly along the lower border of the nasal septum. By the tenth week these two strips of bone have united below the lower border of the nasal septum (see Fig. 1–9).

The vomer, as it thus cups around the base of the cartilaginous nasal septum, expands in a predominantly upward direction until its upper edge meets the endochondral ossification front of the perpendicular plate of the ethmoid at the age of 5 to 6 years. A cartilage remnant remains between the two laminae of the vomer at least until adolescence.[25–27, 31–35, 42]

Endochondrally Forming Bones. The development of the paranasal sinuses involves three bones that form largely by endochondral ossification: sphenoid, ethmoid, and inferior nasal concha. The ethmoid and inferior nasal concha develop by endochondral ossification of components of the mesethmoid and ectethmoid. The sphenoid bone forms almost entirely independently, posterior to the skeleton of the nasal frame.

Sphenoid. From a number of separate chondrification centers a single cartilaginous mass is established by the end of the seventh week of embryonic development. Several components of the future sphenoid bone are recognizable: presphenoid and basisphenoid, sella turcica (surrounding the developing hypophysis), base of the greater wing, and the lesser wing (ala orbitalis), which is connected with the nasal capsule by a cartilaginous plate, the lamina orbitonasalis (see Fig. 1–2).

During fetal life, the sphenoid cartilage mass is continuous anteriorly with the cartilage of the mesethmoid (nasal septum) and posteriorly with the cartilage model of the future basioccipital bone.

The ossification of the sphenoid complex is complicated, involving up to 19 separate ossification centers. Although the larger part of the sphenoid bone ossifies endochondrally, additional intramembranous ossification centers develop for the pterygoid plates and major parts of the greater wings. The intramembranously formed bone components fuse with the endochondrally formed ones during late fetal and early postnatal life.

Endochondral ossification begins in the basisphenoid during the fourth fetal month and in the presphenoid during the fifth fetal month. By the end of the seventh fetal month, the basisphenoid and presphenoid ossification centers fuse, although large remnants of the intervening synchondroses may remain for several months.

Anterior to the presphenoid cartilage is the posterior cupola of the cartilaginous nasal capsule. During the fifth fetal month this part of the nasal capsule undergoes ossification medially (in its paraseptal wall), and during the seventh and eighth month it ossifies in the lateral wall. Between these two endochondral ossification centers, a third, intramembranous center arises, which fuses with the two earlier centers toward the end of the fetal period. The resulting thin, bony shell is the sphenoid concha or ossicle of Bertin. It fuses with the sphenoid bone between the third and ninth years of life.

The initial development of the sphenoidal sinus takes place in the space between this concha and the body of the sphenoid bone.[36–41]

Ethmoid. The ossification of the ethmoid begins during the fifth or sixth fetal month. At that time an endochondral ossification center appears in the wall of the ectethmoid at the site of the future lamina papyracea. During the seventh and eighth fetal months, endochondral ossification extends into the ethmoturbinals, where it is completed by the end of the eighth month. At birth, the cribriform plate, crista galli, and nasal septum are still completely cartilaginous.

Shortly after birth, two ossification centers develop: one for the perpendicular plate of the ethmoid, in the mesethmoid; and another for the rostrum sphenoidale, along the anterior surface of the sphenoid. The process of endochondral ossification spreads forward and downward from these centers. The sphenoid ossification is completed by 1 year of age. The ossification of the perpendicular plate proceeds in a downward and forward direction toward the vomer between birth and 5 years. The latter, an intramembranously formed bone, supports the lower part of the mesethmoid cartilage in a central vomerine groove. When the ossification front reaches the superior edges of this vomerine groove, ossification starts at the contact points, first unilaterally and later bilaterally. Eventually, this ossification results in a fusion between the left and right edges of the vomerine bone, transforming the vomerine groove into a canal and leaving part of the lower mesethmoid cartilage as a remnant in the vomerine canal. The vomerine canal persists through adult life, despite extensive remodeling and thinning of the vomer.[42] After the upper edges of the vomer and the ossification front of the perpendicular plate have come into contact, ossification of the latter proceeds at a considerably lower rate until about age 10 years.

The ossification of cribriform plate and crista galli occurs postnatally and continues for at least 6 years after birth. Between ethmoid and sphenoid a synchondrosis persists until puberty.

Inferior Concha. The inferior concha has two separate ossification centers (some investigators report a single center), which appear between the fifth and seventh months of fetal life. A bony layer forms at the periphery of the cartilaginous scroll. The enclosed cartilage calcifies and is subsequently resorbed, leaving a double bony lamella. The separate ossification centers meet by the eighth fetal month. During the ossification process, the inferior concha is detached from the ectethmoid and becomes an independent bony structure.[30, 34, 37, 43]

Cartilaginous Remnants of the Nasal Frame. Parts of the original nasal frame persist as cartilage structures postnatally. The anterior mesethmoid persists as the nasal septal cartilage and is continuous with the lateral nasal cartilage (the latter corresponding roughly with the embryonic tectal cartilage).

Late during fetal life the future lateral nasal and greater alar cartilages separate. This separation starts laterally and reaches the medial border shortly before birth. Thus, these two cartilages start as separate mesenchymal condensations in the embryo and chondrify as one single, continuous mass. This exists during most of the fetal period, only to become separate once again in the neonate, connected merely by a fibrous attachment that may contain some accessory cartilages.

Components of the cartilaginous nasal frame that are covered directly by membrane bones during development are resorbed and not replaced. This applies to the cartilage that is covered by lacrimal bones, nasal bones, and vomer particularly. The loss of these cartilages generally occurs postnatally.[37, 44–46]

ANATOMY OF THE NASAL FRAME

This section focuses on the osteology of the lateral nasal walls; the midline structure of the nasal frame will not be discussed further.

A central core of bones—sphenoid, ethmoid, and inferior nasal concha—is formed predominantly by endochondral ossification. The cartilage models of these bones were part of the embryonic chondrocranium. Peripheral to this core is a series of intramembranously formed bones: maxilla, frontal, nasal, lacrimal, and palatine bones. These bones overlap the endochondrally formed bones, and they also may overlap each other to some degree in areas of sutures and around the nasolacrimal duct, which is located between the maxilla and lacrimal bone.

The layered nature of the lateral bony wall of the nasal cavity allows consideration of the various layers sequentially to clarify their spatial relationships (Figs. 1–5 and 1–6). In the neonate, the nasal and orbital floors are located at about the same vertical level, and the lateral nasal wall serves as the medial orbital wall. In the adult, in contrast, only the upper half of the lateral nasal wall forms the medial orbital wall. Correspondingly, the nasal floor is at a lower level than the orbital floor. These changes reflect a greater increase in vertical height, specifically of the respiratory regions, during postnatal growth. One result of these changes is that the maxilla, which contributes minimally to the lateral nasal wall in the fetus and neonate, becomes a prominent component of the lateral nasal wall in the adult.

The *maxilla* is the most peripheral bone of the adult lateral nasal wall (Fig. 1–5A). The medial surface of the maxilla is incomplete, owing to the presence of a large maxillary hiatus, which gives bony access to the maxillary sinus. The aperture of the hiatus is reduced by the presence of palatine and lacrimal bones and the inferior concha, which articulate with the medial surfaces of the maxilla and partially cover the hiatus (Fig. 1–5A,B,C).

The *palatine bone* is composed of a perpendicular plate and a maxillary process. The perpendicular plate, when placed in articulation with the medial surface of the maxilla, covers the posterior part of the maxillary hiatus, thus reducing its size to some extent. On the medial surface of the perpendicular plate a conchal crest is present, where the inferior nasal concha articulates with the palatine bone.

The horizontal process of the palatine bone articulates with the palatine process of the maxilla to form the bony palate, the osseous floor of the nasal cavity. The palatine bone articulates with the medial pterygoid plate of the sphenoid posteriorly and with the body of the sphenoid bone posterosuperiorly. The sphenopalatine foramen is formed at the latter site of articulation (Figs. 1–5 and 1–6B).

When the *lacrimal bone* is placed in articulation with the maxilla, its descending process is located medial to the maxilla, converting the lacrimal groove on the latter's medial surface into the upper part of the bony nasolacrimal canal (Fig. 1–5B).

When the *inferior nasal concha* is added, it articulates with the conchal crests on the medial surfaces of the maxilla and the palatine bone. The maxillary process on the lateral aspect of the concha covers part of the maxillary hiatus and thus becomes part of the incomplete medial bony wall of the maxillary sinus. The lacrimal process of the inferior nasal concha articulates with the descending process of the lacrimal bone, thus completing the lower part of the bony nasolacrimal canal (Fig. 1–5C). A third, often delicate, ethmoid process protrudes from the upper surface of the inferior nasal concha. It articulates with the uncinate process of the ethmoid bone.

The ethmoid labyrinth of the *ethmoid bone* is located between lateral and medial plates of the ethmoid. The lateral or orbital plate forms the medial orbital wall. The medial plate forms the upper half of the lateral wall of the nasal cavity in the adult (Fig. 1–6A). The medial plate is not smooth. Two or three thin, scrolled bone plates project from its surface, forming middle, superior, and, when present, supreme nasal conchae. Below each concha a meatus of similar designation is present.

Most of the volume of the ethmoid is occupied by the ethmoid sinuses, which comprise the ethmoid labyrinth. The sinuses are separated from each other by delicate bone plates (Fig. 1–7). At some sites, particularly at the superior and anterior aspects of the ethmoid, the sinuses extend beyond the ethmoid bone into adjacent skeletal and nonskeletal territories. As a result, surface openings may be seen in the disarticulated ethmoid, which give access to the ethmoid sinuses. However, the only apertures of these sinuses are in the middle and superior (and supreme) meatus.

The middle concha scrolls over two additional components of the ethmoid bone: the ethmoid bulla and the uncinate process. These structures are suspended on the medial side of

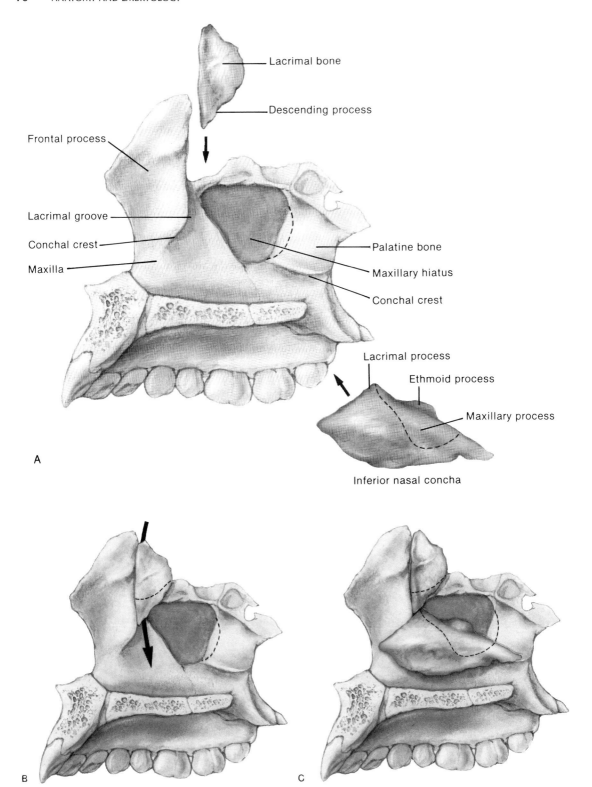

Figure 1–5. Osteology of the right lateral nasal wall (outer layer), medial view.

A, Maxilla and palatine bone are articulated. Bone is sectioned near the midline. The lacrimal bone and the inferior nasal concha are still disarticulated and shown in medial view.

B, The lacrimal bone is placed in articulation with the maxilla. The arrow runs inside the upper half of the bony nasolacrimal canal, which is formed by the articulation of maxilla and lacrimal bone.

C, The inferior nasal concha is placed in articulation with the maxilla, lacrimal bone, and palatine bone. As a result, the bony nasolacrimal canal is completed, and the opening of the maxillary hiatus is further reduced.

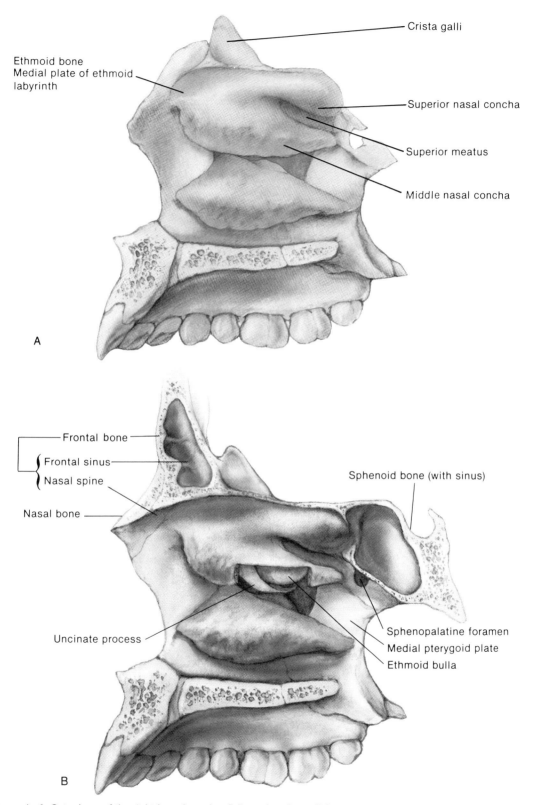

Figure 1–6. Osteology of the right lateral nasal wall (inner layer), medial view.

A, When the ethmoid is articulated with the bones of the outer nasal wall, most of the maxillary hiatus is covered. The perpendicular plate of the ethmoid is not shown in this diagram.

B, Frontal, nasal, and sphenoid bones complete the lateral nasal wall, as well as the piriform aperture anteriorly and the posterior nasal aperture posteriorly.

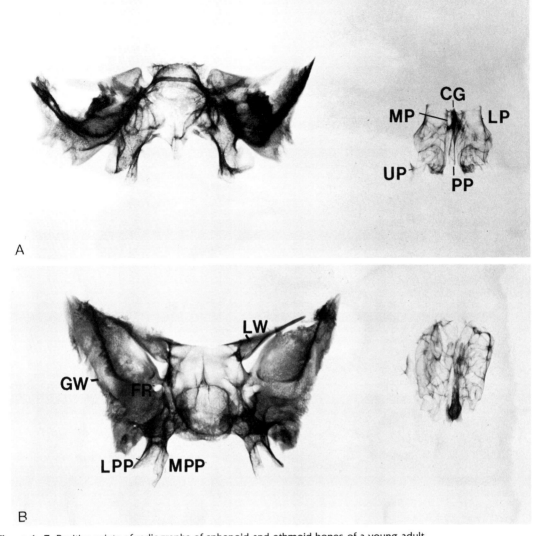

Figure 1–7. Positive prints of radiographs of sphenoid and ethmoid bones of a young adult.

A, Anteroposterior projection. In the ethmoid bone (right), thin bony plates separate the ethmoid sinuses. The curved outlines of the middle conchae are well visualized in this projection. The uncinate process is present on one side of this bone only; its counterpart probably was lost during the preparation of the bone. *CG,* Crista galli; *LP,* lateral plate of ethmoid; *MP,* medial plate of ethmoid; *PP,* perpendicular plate; *UP,* uncinate process.

B, Superoinferior projection. In the sphenoid bone (left), the sphenoid sinuses extend to a position just below the sella turcica. *FR,* Foramen rotundum; *GW,* greater wing; *LW,* lesser wing; *LPP,* lateral pterygoid plate; *MPP,* medial pterygoid plate.

the maxillary hiatus, further reducing the size of the C-shaped bony opening (Fig. 1–6*B*).

The ethmoid bulla is a bulging, bony structure, its convex surface facing medially. It is pneumatized centrally by one or more ethmoid sinuses. The uncinate process is a delicate bony bar that runs below the bulla, curving downward, posteriorly, and slightly laterally. Anteriorly, the process is continuous with the rest of the ethmoid bone. Its upper edge is usually not attached to the bulla; a narrow bony slit may be present between the two structures.

Posteriorly, the uncinate process runs freely toward the ethmoid process of the inferior nasal concha, with which it articulates.

The nasal frame is completed by the frontal and nasal bones anterosuperiorly and the sphenoid bone posterosuperiorly.

The adult *frontal bones* are fused together in the midline. They articulate with the ethmoid at the latter's superior surface, immediately above the labyrinth; with the frontal process of the maxilla and the nasal and lacrimal bones; and posteriorly, with the lesser wing of the sphenoid. Their articulation with the zygomatic bones is of limited interest here.

The frontal bones have a central nasal spine, which articulates with the perpendicular plate of the ethmoid and supports, in part, the nasal bones (Fig. 1–6B). Bony access into the frontal sinuses is at the inferior aspect of the frontal bones, near their most anterior points of articulation with the ethmoid, on either side of the nasal spine.

The *sphenoid bone* completes the bony posterior nasal aperture and the sphenopalatine foramen (Fig. 1–6B). The sphenoid body articulates anterosuperiorly with the cribriform plate of the ethmoid, anteriorly and centrally with the perpendicular plate of the ethmoid (sphenoid crest), and anterolaterally with the posterior aspect of the ethmoid labyrinth. On each side of the sphenoid crest a bony aperture of the paired, sphenoid sinuses is present. The lower, anterior wall of each sinus is composed of a thin, curved platelet of bone, the sphenoid concha. In a dry, disarticulated bone, this concha is usually lost, and the bony aperture of the sinus is correspondingly larger.

The medial pterygoid plate of the sphenoid forms the lateral border of the posterior nasal aperture, as it articulates with the medial and posterior aspects of the perpendicular plate of the palatine bone.[28, 35, 47–50]

EMBRYOLOGY OF PARANASAL SINUSES

The initial development of the paranasal sinuses takes place early in fetal life. With the exception of the sphenoid sinus, the paranasal sinuses begin their development as pockets of the nasal epithelium, which expand into concavities of the cartilaginous nasal capsule (ectethmoid). This process of *primary pneumatization* is followed by *secondary pneumatization,* by which these epithelially lined pockets expand into the skeletal elements of the nasal frame. Much of the secondary pneumatization takes place postnatally. Only the ethmoid sinuses are well developed at birth.[51] The development of the sphenoid sinus differs slightly in that it involves an initial constriction of the posterosuperior portion of the sphenoethmoid recess by the development of the sphenoid concha (see later). Secondary pneumatization follows.

The nasal epithelium that is involved in the formation of maxillary, frontal, and ethmoid sinuses originates in a relatively restricted area, which is derived embryologically from the nasal surface of the lateral nasal swelling present in the preskeletal stage.

Primary pneumatization occurs during the chondrocranial stage. In this stage the nasal mucosa develops several folds and depressions. The folds anticipate the cartilaginous projections on the medial surface of the nasal capsule: conchae, uncinate process, and ethmoid bulla. The depressions between the folds of the nasal mucosa are the sites where the sinus rudiments develop. These sites are the superior and, if present, supreme meatus; and the middle meatus with frontal recess, frontal furrows, suprabullar, bullar, and infrabullar furrows and the ethmoid infundibulum (Fig. 1–8).

As the nasal capsule undergoes chondrification, the cartilage forms around the sinus rudiments, thus establishing cartilaginous concavities. The sites of initial sinus rudiment formation (or of initial constriction in the case of the sphenoid sinus) are preserved in the adult as the locations of the sinus ostia.

MAXILLARY SINUS

The maxillary sinus is the first to develop during human fetal life.

Primary Pneumatization. Evidence of primary pneumatization is present in fetuses of 65 to 70 days' developmental age. Generally a single pocket of nasal mucosa develops as the rudiment of the maxillary sinus. It has been speculated that two rudiments may form and fuse farther distally. This is based on the occasional presence of an accessory ostium of the maxillary sinus. However, there is no embryologic support for this speculation.

The site of initial development, which will be the location of the future ostium, is on the inferolateral surface of the ethmoid infundibulum. The infundibulum is a blind recess between two parts of the future ethmoid bone: the uncinate process and the ethmoid bulla. During the first half of the third fetal month, the uncinate process consists of a slender, cartilaginous bar, which curves downward, dorsally, and laterally from its anteriorly located point of continuity with the ectethmoid. The ethmoid bulla chondrifies later, toward the end of the third fetal month, as a thickening of the lateral wall of the middle meatus, just above the uncinate process. A narrow, slitlike opening between these two mucosa-covered structures,

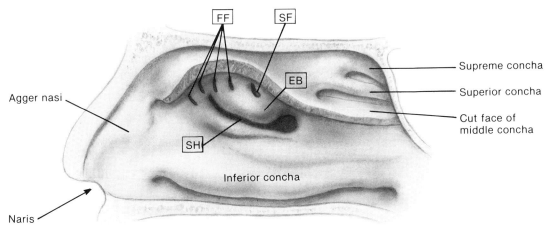

Figure 1–8. Diagram of the right lateral nasal wall of a neonate. The bones of the nasal wall are covered with nasal mucosa. The middle concha has been removed to show details of the middle meatus. Some sites of primary pneumatization are indicated. *EB*, ethmoid bulla; *FF*, frontal furrows; *SF*, suprabullar furrow; *SH*, semilunar hiatus (providing access to the ethmoid infundibulum). (Redrawn after Schaeffer.[28])

the semilunar hiatus, provides access to the ethmoid infundibulum. The depth of the infundibulum and the width of the semilunar hiatus are variable, dependent on the spatial relationships and the relative sizes of uncinate process and ethmoid bulla. In the adult the ethmoid infundibulum may be 4 to 12 mm deep.

Until late in the fourth fetal month the developing maxillary sinus remains internal to the nasal capsule (ectethmoid) as a shallow, oblong pocket at the inferolateral surface of the ethmoid infundibulum. This pocket is associated with a relatively large number of glandular primordia, which protrude from the epithelium into the surrounding mesenchyme (Fig. 1–9B). Although these glandular primordia have been held responsible by some for the invasive properties of the future sinus mucosa, this is unlikely, and the significance of their large numbers at this stage is not understood.

Secondary Pneumatization. During the fifth fetal month, endochondral transformation of the cartilaginous nasal frame begins. The cartilage of the nasal capsule between inferior and middle nasal conchae undergoes erosion. This erosion results in the separation of the inferior nasal concha (which now develops into a separate bone) from the remaining ethmoid complex.

The shallow primordium of the maxillary sinus grows beyond the nasal capsule into the spongy bone of the maxilla, which is developing external to it. Prenatally the process of secondary pneumatization proceeds slowly. At birth the sinus is still only an oblong groove on the medial side of the maxilla, just above the tooth germ of the first deciduous molar. Its shape is ovoid but subject to individual variation. The average dimensions range from 7.5 to 10 mm in anteroposterior length, 3.5 to 5 mm in height, and 3 to 3.5 mm in width.

Postnatally, the maxillary sinus increases in all dimensions. The sinus expands laterally to a position below the orbit, but not yet beyond the location of the infraorbital canal, by the end of the first year. During the second year the sinus expands farther laterally underneath the infraorbital canal. From this stage on, a bony ridge, representing the wall of the infraorbital canal, is present on the roof surface of the sinus.

Anteroposteriorly, the sinus expands to a position above the first permanent molar tooth germ by the middle of the second year. The anteroposterior growth of the sinus corresponds closely with the anteroposterior growth of the midface and is not completed until the eruption of the third permanent molar.

The growth in height of the sinus is best reflected by the changes in the relative position of the sinus floor. In young children, the sinus floor is about 4 mm above the level of the nasal floor. At the age of 8 years, the sinus floor is generally at the same level as the nasal floor. In time, the level of the sinus floor may become situated 1 to 5.5 mm below the level of the nasal floor, and the sinus lumen may become accessible through the inferior meatus (Fig. 1–10). However, this relationship is variable. In as much as half the adult population, either the floors of both cavities are at the same level or the sinus floor is slightly below the level of the nasal floor.[52, 53]

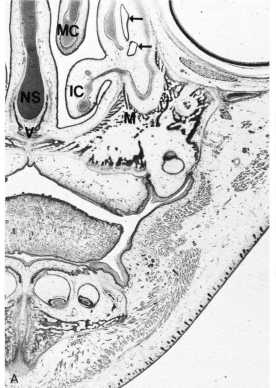

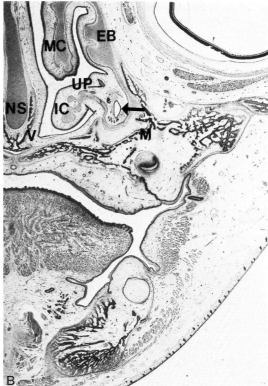

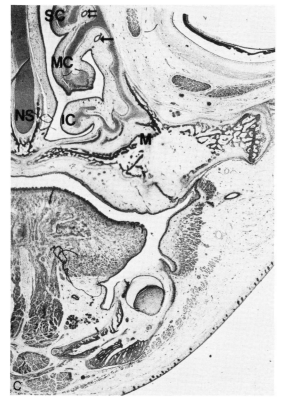

Figure 1–9. Three coronal (frontal) sections through the head of a 5-month-old human fetus. The photomicrographs are arranged in an anteroposterior sequence, with A the most anterior. *EB,* Ethmoid bulla; *IC,* inferior concha; *MC,* middle concha; *SC,* superior concha; *M,* maxilla; *NS,* nasal septum; *UP,* uncinate process; *V,* vomer.

A, Rudiments of anterior ethmoid sinuses in the middle meatus *(arrows).*

B, Rudiment of the maxillary sinus (with many glandular primordia) *(arrow).* The continuity between the ethmoid infundibulum and the sinus rudiment is not seen here. The proximal part of the infundibulum (between *EB* and *UP*) is not visible.

C, Rudiments of anterior *(arrow)* and posterior *(double arrow)* ethmoid sinuses in the middle meatus and superior meatus. (From the Applebaum photocollection.)

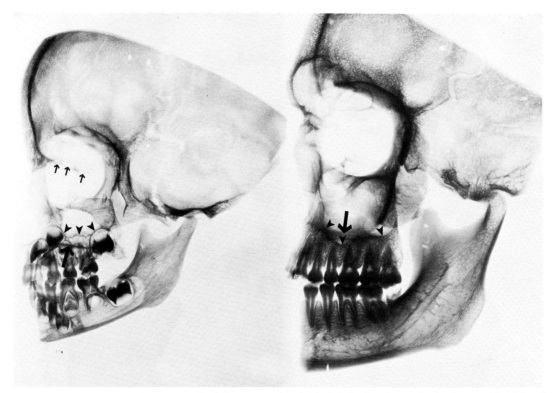

Figure 1–10. Positive print of a radiograph of the prepared and dried skulls (hemisected) of a 6-year-old child and a young adult.

In the child's skull (left), the floor of the maxillary sinus *(arrowheads)* is closely applied to the apical ends of the still-developing teeth of the permanent dentition. The sinus floor is located several millimeters above the level of the floor of the nasal fossa *(large arrow)*. The small arrows point to the sites of early secondary pneumatization in the orbital part of the frontal bone.

In the adult's skull (right), the sinus floor *(arrowheads)* is located below the level of the floor of the nasal fossa *(large arrow)*. In the adult, the frontal sinus is well developed.

Three growth spurt periods have been recognized in the development of the maxillary sinus: from birth to 2.5 years, from 7.5 to 10 years, and from 12 to 14 years. These growth spurts correspond closely with the eruption patterns of deciduous and permanent dentitions, which allow further pneumatization of the body of the maxilla. During adolescence, the sinus expands to fill the body of the maxilla and the maxillary part of the zygomatic bone. After 15 to 18 years, only minor shape modifications take place.

The ovoid shape of the maxillary sinus at birth is maintained until the eruption of the permanent molar teeth, when the adult pyramidal shape develops, with the base of the pyramid facing the lateral nasal wall and the apex extending toward the zygomatic bone. The shape of the maxillary sinus is subject to considerable individual variation. The average adult measurements range from 32 to 34 mm in anteroposterior length, 28 to 33 mm in height, and 23 to 25 mm in width. The volume of an adult sinus ranges from 8.5 to 15 ml.[28, 30, 36, 38, 51, 54–58]

Frontal and Ethmoid Sinuses. During the fourth fetal month, the middle meatus extends anteriorly and upward to form a blind-ending frontal recess. In the fifth fetal month, the surface of the middle meatus is no longer smooth, owing to the presence of the ethmoid bulla, the uncinate process, and the intervening semilunar hiatus, which gives access to the ethmoid infundibulum. Several additional furrows may be present in the mucosa of the middle meatus: suprabullar, bullar, and infrabullar furrows and up to four frontal furrows. At these furrows, the development of the anterior ethmoid sinuses, and occasionally the frontal sinus as well, begins.

Frontal and ethmoid sinuses develop at a later time, but in the same way as the maxillary sinus. The frontal sinus initially develops as a nasal mucosa pocket in or near the frontal recess of the middle meatus. The ethmoid sinuses develop from multiple sites in the middle meatus (to become anterior ethmoid cells) and the superior and, if present, supreme meatus (to become posterior ethmoid cells).

Pneumatization of the Frontal Sinus.

The primary pneumatization of the frontal sinus occurs during the fourth to fifth fetal month. At that time a pocket is formed in the nasal mucosa, which later will continue its development into the frontal bone. This initial pocket may develop at several different sites, but most frequently at the wall of the frontal recess, one of the frontal furrows, or the anteriormost extension of the ethmoid infundibulum. On the basis of these initial sites of development, the frontal sinus may be considered as one of the anterior ethmoid sinuses, separate and distinct only by its secondary pneumatization of the frontal bone.

Prenatally, the frontal sinus does not expand much further. Secondary pneumatization occurs postnatally, generally starting between the ages of 6 months and 2 years. At that time the sinus expands beyond the cartilage of the nasal capsule, which then erodes. Initially, the secondary pneumatization occurs laterally, into the orbital part of the frontal bone. During the second year of life, pneumatization also occurs in a vertical direction, with the top of the sinus reaching the midvertical height of the orbit at 4 years of age, reaching the level of the superior orbital rim at 8 years of age, and growing into the frontal squama at 10 years of age. Left and right frontal sinuses develop independently. The frontal sinuses continue their growth at a slow rate into adolescence, when they reach their final shape. Some further enlargement may occur until age 40 years.

The development of the frontal sinus may be affected by the expansion of neighboring anterior ethmoid cells. Occasionally, one or more of these cells begin pneumatizing the frontal bone and may supplant, partially or completely, the primary frontal sinus outgrowth. The sinus that is first present in such a case may encroach on the lumen of the second sinus by forming a bulbous projection (bulla frontalis) in the wall of the latter, larger sinus. In such cases a thin plate of bone separates the mucosa of the two sinuses.

The growth of the surrounding anterior ethmoid cells also may encroach on the proximal part of the frontal sinus, compressing it into a nasofrontal duct. This usually does not affect a frontal sinus, which develops directly from the wall of the frontal recess and has a distinct ostium. A frontal sinus that develops from the ethmoid infundibulum or one of the frontal furrows, however, may have its drainage pathway restricted into a nasofrontal duct. The diameter of this duct depends largely on the degree of encroachment by the surrounding ethmoid cells.

Pneumatization of the Ethmoid Sinuses.

Primary pneumatization of the ethmoid sinuses takes place during the fourth to fifth fetal month. The great majority of these sinuses develop from the middle meatus as anterior ethmoid cells, and a minority develop from the superior (and supreme) meatus as posterior ethmoid cells.

During primary pneumatization, the rudiments of the ethmoid sinuses consist of dimple-like depressions of the nasal mucosa, which are cupped in concavities of the nasal capsule (see Fig. 1–9A,C). These depressions may originate from any of the mucosal furrows in the middle meatus and along the mucosa of the superior meatus, which itself is no more than a furrow at that time. The depressions gradually deepen and become globular air cells. These grow in diameter until they abut, leaving only a thin honeycomb of bone between them. The ethmoid sinuses are well developed at birth. During the second year the air cells may grow beyond the confines of the ethmoid bone into the surrounding bones: frontal, maxilla, lacrimal, and sphenoid.

The growth of the ethmoid sinuses is variable. Continued growth will occur, which is proportional with further cranial growth, including a period of active growth during the early years of puberty. The labyrinth attains its final form by age 12 to 14 years. Some further enlargement may take place in early adulthood.

The fully formed ethmoid labyrinth has a pyramidal shape, with its base facing posteriorly. Anteroposteriorly, it is 40 to 50 mm long, 25 to 30 mm high, 5 mm wide anteriorly, and 15 mm wide posteriorly. The combined volume of the ethmoid cells ranges from 1 to 6 ml.

Ethmoid sinuses are grouped into anterior and posterior cells, based on their initial sites of pneumatization and the subsequent locations of their ostia. The ethmoid cells may be characterized further on the basis of the skeletal elements they pneumatize. Thus it is possible to define groups of cells as remaining within the ethmoid and extending beyond the ethmoid. Ethmoid cells that remain within the ethmoid include conchal, bullar, infundibular, and frontal recess cells. Among those that extend beyond the ethmoid are agger cells (anterior ethmoid cells that pneumatize the agger nasi on the medial surface of the frontal process of the maxilla), frontal sinus cells (anterior ethmoid cells that pneumatize the frontal bone), anterior ethmoid cells that pneumatize the orbital roof (these must be differentiated clinically from a posterior extension of the frontal sinus), and extensions of posterior ethmoid cells (that form an accessory maxillary sinus), cells in the palatine bone and cells in the sphenoid bone.

The degree of variation of the ethmoid sinuses allows only the most general discussion. The boundaries of the ethmoid labyrinth are only partially skeletal: anteriorly, the frontal sinus; posteriorly, the sphenoid sinus; superiorly, the frontal sinus; inferiorly, the uncinate process; laterally, the orbital contents; and medially, the medial surfaces of the nasal conchae.[28, 36, 38, 51, 55–62]

SPHENOID SINUS

The development of the sphenoid sinus does not involve a process of primary pneumatization but rather the constriction of an existing part of the sphenoethmoid recess.

Initial Constriction. The sphenoethmoid recess deepens in a posterior direction during the third fetal month. During late third and early fourth fetal months the posterosuperior portion of the recess is separated incompletely from the nasal cavity by the development of a nasal mucosal fold, inferiorly based, which curves upward anterior to the body of the sphenoid. Within this fold a cartilaginous sphenoid concha forms, which by the fifth fetal month clearly encloses the sphenoid recess. Initially this concha is a separate skeletal element, but during its complicated course of ossification it becomes attached inferiorly to the sphenoid body. This occurs postnatally during the third to fifth years of life. Erosion also takes place in the superior and medial parts of the nasal capsule, which still separate the sphenoid recess from the sphenoid body.

Secondary Pneumatization. At birth the sphenoid sinus is no more than a recess, located between the sphenoid concha and the sphenoid body. This situation, with a location more nasal than sphenoid, persists until the age of 6 or 7 years. The concha itself may become pneumatized prior to this age.

However, the actual secondary pneumatization of the sphenoid sinus begins with the resorption of the sphenoid during the seventh year of age. The sinus expands into the presphenoid and later the basisphenoid parts of the sphenoid bone, with the sphenoid concha remaining as the anterior sinus wall. By the age of 8 to 10 years, a real sinus cavity may be demonstrable.

The rate at which the sphenoid sinus extends posteriorly varies greatly among individuals, but in the same individual the posterior extent of left and right sphenoid sinus is roughly similar. If it is not, pathology may be suspected. Initially, most expansion occurs in a posterolateral direction. This results in a thin lateral bony wall, which separates the sinus from the trigeminal nerve. Similarly, the early lateral extension brings the sinus floor over the nerve of the pterygoid canal (vidian nerve) as early as the age of 6 or 7 years. With an average expansion rate, the posterior sinus wall reaches a position below the anterior portion of the sella turcica by age 8 to 10 years, and completely below the sella, with only a thin bony plate intervening, by the 15th year.

The definitive form of the sinus is attained at puberty. The ostium of the sinus, at the site where the sphenoid recess retained its continuity with the nasal cavity and where the sphenoid concha did not form, is located high on the anterior sinus wall, just a few millimeters below the sphenoethmoid recess. The sinus may remain small or it may expand extensively, into greater and lesser wings, pterygoid plates, and, beyond the sphenoid bone, into palatine and basioccipital bones.

A sphenoid sinus may be classified by the variable degree of its posterior extension as (1) a *conchal* or fetal type of sinus, with minimal extension, which is relatively rare; (2) a *presellar* or juvenile type of sinus, extending posteriorly to the anterior sellar wall, which may be found in as many as 40 per cent of the adult population; and (3) a *postsphenoid* or adult type of sinus, extending below the sella or further, which occurs in up to 60 per cent of all adults. The combined volume of left and right sphenoid sinuses ranges generally from 2 to 6 ml, but cases of up to 12 ml have been reported.[28, 36, 38, 39, 51, 56, 59, 63, 64]

ANATOMY OF PARANASAL SINUSES

The paranasal sinuses are mucosa-lined diverticula of the nasal cavity, which remain in communication with this cavity. The sinus wall usually consists of a compact layer of bone, lined with endosteum. The endosteum is fused with the overlying mucosa. The latter is continuous with the nasal mucosa; histologically, the two mucosae resemble each other. The epithelial lining of the sinus mucosa consists of ciliated cells, basal cells, and mucous secretory (goblet) cells. Occasionally, infiltrating leukocytes and mast cells may be present. The turnover of the ciliated cells in the nasal mucosa is relatively rapid, and this is probably true for the sinus mucosa as well. The cilia of the epithelial cells move the mucous secretions of the sinus mucosa toward the nasal cavity through the sinus ostia.[65, 66]

There are certain commonalities in the vascularization and innervation of the paranasal sinuses (see Tables 1–1, 1–2, 1–3, and 1–4). The arterial supply generally is derived from two sources. The nasal mucosal vasculature consists of branches of blood vessels that supply the mucosa of the sinus ostium, specifically branches of the sphenopalatine artery and the anterior and posterior ethmoid arteries. These arterial branches are carried along with the expanding sinus mucosa during development. The osseous vasculature consists of branches of blood vessels that run through the tissues (mostly bone) surrounding the sinus. The venous and lymphatic drainage pathways tend to be pragmatic and primarily transosseous: toward the nearest major venous and lymphatic channels.

The innervation of the sinus mucosa is supplied largely by branches of the maxillary division of the trigeminal nerve, specifically the medial and lateral posterosuperior nasal nerves, which enter the nasal fossa through the sphenopalatine foramen. These branches carry afferent as well as autonomic fibers: postganglionic parasympathetic fibers from the pterygopalatine ganglion and postganglionic sympathetic fibers from the superior cervical ganglion. Both sympathetics and parasympathetics are carried to the pterygopalatine ganglion by the nerve of the pterygoid canal (vidian nerve).

Additional afferent innervation may be supplied by branches of the trigeminal nerve, which pass near the sinus wall through the tissues around the sinus.[35, 48]

Anatomically, the most important attributes of the paranasal sinuses are their relations with the surrounding structures and the sites of the sinus ostia.

MAXILLARY SINUS

Generally, a single maxillary sinus is present bilaterally. The sinus occupies the larger part of the body of the maxilla in the adult. There is a direct correlation between the dimensions of the maxilla and those of the sinus. The sinus extends below the orbit and over the roots of the maxillary molar and premolar teeth. An alveolar recess is present in about 50 per cent; a zygomatic recess in 40 per cent, whereas a palatine recess is only rarely found.

Anatomic Relations (Table 1–1). Superiorly, a bony ridge is usually present in the roof of the sinus. This is the bone around the infraorbital canal, which houses the infraorbital nerve and blood vessels. Dehiscences may be present in this bony wall, resulting in a direct contact between infraorbital structures and the sinus mucosa.

The apex, the most cephalic portion of the maxillary sinus, lies just lateral, at the level of the lowermost ethmoid cells. Because of this position it may be mistaken for an ethmoid cell in computed tomography scans.

Inferiorly, the sinus is closely related to the apices of the maxillary molar and premolar teeth, particularly the second premolar and the first and second permanent molars. The apices of these teeth often protrude slightly above the level of the sinus floor. They may remain separated from the sinus mucosa by a thin layer of

---

TABLE 1–1. Vascularization and Innervation of the Maxillary Sinus

Arterial Supply

Nasal Mucosal Vasculature
  Arteries of the middle meatus (branches of the sphenopalatine artery, which enters the nasal fossa via the sphenopalatine foramen)
  Ethmoid arteries (branches of the ophthalmic artery, which enter the nasal fossa via the cribriform plate)

Osseous Vasculature
  Possible contributions from branches of the infraorbital artery (posterior superior alveolar arteries, artery of the maxillary tuberosity, anterior superior alveolar arteries), facial artery, and palatine artery

Venous Drainage
The medial sinus wall drains via the sphenopalatine vein
The other sinus walls drain via the pterygomaxillary plexus

Lymphatic Drainage
Via collecting vessels in the middle meatal mucosa

Innervation
  Nasal mucosal nerves
    Contributions from the lateral posterior superior nasal branches of the maxillary nerve (V2)
    Additionally, branches from the superior alveolar nerves and infraorbital nerve

bone. Occasionally, when the sinus floor lies well below the level of the nasal floor, the bone is perforated and the dental apices are in direct contact with the mucosa.

Medially, a variable portion of the antral wall is composed of mucosa only. The height of the wall below the inferior concha, clinically an important dimension, is extremely variable, ranging from 12 to 23 mm.

Anteriorly, the sinus wall is closely applied to branches of the infraorbital nerve and blood vessels, which provide innervation and vascularization to the maxillary canine and incisor teeth and the surrounding periodontal tissues. The blood vessels and nerves may run directly below the sinus mucosa.

Posteriorly and laterally, the posterior superior alveolar nerves and blood vessels are present; they supply the maxillary premolars and molars, as well as the tissues surrounding those teeth. The neurovascular structures frequently lie in bone grooves. A single incomplete bone septum is found in about 30 per cent of the population. Multiple septa tend to be rare.

The medial part of the posterior maxillary sinus wall forms the anterior boundary of the pterygopalatine fossa.[51-53]

Ostium. The ostium of the maxillary sinus is located in the anterosuperior portion of the medial sinus wall. It opens onto the inferolateral wall of the ethmoid infundibulum. The depth of the infundibulum, 4 to 12 mm, is a fairly direct measure of the distance between the ostium of the maxillary sinus and the semilunar hiatus and is inversely related to the accessibility of the ostium from the nasal cavity.

The maxillary sinus occasionally has an accessory ostium, opening either into the infundibulum or directly onto the wall of the middle meatus, 5 to 10 mm above the superior border of the inferior nasal concha. An "accessory" maxillary sinus is a posterior ethmoid sinus with its ostium in the superior meatus.

FRONTAL SINUS

Usually a pair of frontal sinuses extends into the frontal bone. The two frontal sinuses are separated completely by a bony septum, which is located approximately in the midline. Bilateral asymmetry of the frontal sinuses is a frequent finding, and the septum between the two sinuses may deviate as a result. In the better-developed sinuses, the border may be scalloped with incomplete bony septa separating deep recesses of the sinus. As a result the sinus is compartmentalized.

Occasionally, accessory frontal sinuses are present; these are formed by the invasion into the frontal bone of adjacent anterior ethmoid sinuses. If an accessory frontal sinus is present before the definitive frontal sinus is fully expanded, a *bulla frontalis* in the wall of the frontal sinus may indicate the presence of the smaller, accessory sinus.

The orbital roof may be pneumatized either by a posterior extension of the inferior recess of the frontal sinus, or by an extension of a neighboring ethmoid cell. Clinically, the differentiation between these two possibilities is important.

Anatomic Relations (Table 1–2). The frontal sinus is bordered inferiorly by the orbit and the orbital contents, the anterior ethmoid sinuses (which may extend into the orbital part of the frontal bone), and the nasal cavity. The supratrochlear and supraorbital nerves and blood vessels lie immediately over the anterior wall of the frontal sinus, as do the orbicularis oculi and frontalis muscles. The frontal lobes of the brain are located posterosuperiorly to the frontal sinus.

Ostium. The ostium of the sinus is in the posteromedial part of the sinus floor, usually at the lowest point of that floor. The ostium may open directly into the frontal recess, resulting in a relatively unimpeded drainage of the sinus. However, the lumen of the ostium is often

TABLE 1–2. Vascularization and Innervation of the Frontal Sinus

Arterial Supply
Anterior ethmoid artery (a branch of the ophthalmic artery)
Arteries of the middle meatus (branches of the sphenopalatine artery)

Venous Drainage
Transosseous drainage into subcutaneous veins, orbital veins and intracranial veins

Lymphatic Drainage
Transosseous drainage into the lymphatic network of the nasal fossa and the meningeal lymphatics

Innervation
Mucosal
Lateral posterior superior nasal branches of the maxillary nerve (V2)
Anterior ethmoid nerve (a branch of the ophthalmic nerve, V1)
Additional branches of the supratrochlear nerve and supraorbital nerve (both branches of the ophthalmic nerve, V1)

narrowed by the expansive growth of the surrounding anterior ethmoid cells, or by the enlargement of the middle nasal concha.

If a distal segment of the frontal sinus is compressed during fetal development, this segment becomes the nasofrontal duct. The ease of drainage of the frontal sinus is directly related to the diameter of the ductal lumen and also to the directness of the nasofrontal duct. It is inversely related to the length of the duct; the drainage is generally least complicated with the presence of a simple ostium and the absence of a nasofrontal duct.

When a nasofrontal duct is present, its ostium frequently is located near the ethmoid infundibulum. This may result in the drainage products of the frontal sinus being channeled into the ethmoid infundibulum and on into the ostium of the maxillary sinus at the far end of the infundibulum.[51]

ETHMOID SINUSES

The number of ethmoid sinuses is variable; there may be two to eight anterior ethmoid sinuses and one to five posterior ethmoid sinuses on either side. On average, the labyrinth contains ten sinuses. The cells of the anterior ethmoid group tend to be smaller than those of the posterior group. The ostia of the anterior ethmoid sinuses are located in the middle meatus. This includes cells with ostia in the ethmoid infundibulum or bullar furrows. Ostia of most posterior ethmoid sinuses are located in the upper anterior recess of the superior meatus. A small number of posterior ethmoid sinuses may drain in the supreme meatus, if the latter is present.

Anatomic Relations (Table 1–3). Lateral to the ethmoid labyrinth are the orbital contents. These may be separated from the ethmoid sinus mucosa by the thin, bony lamina papyracea, but this is not always the case. Any natural dehiscences in the lamina papyracea could permit the spread of infection into the orbit. The nasal conchae generally form the medial boundary of the ethmoid sinuses. Posteriorly, the ethmoid labyrinth may be applied directly to the sphenoid sinus. Posterior cells may pneumatize the lesser wing of the sphenoid bone and may come to lie in close proximity to the optic nerve. The possibility of optic nerve damage during ethmoidectomy should be considered in such cases.

Anteriorly are the lacrimal bone, the frontal process of the maxilla, and the nasolacrimal

TABLE 1–3. Vascularization and Innervation of the Ethmoid Sinuses

Arterial Supply

Anterior Ethmoid Sinuses
  Arteries of the middle meatus (branches of the sphenopalatine artery)
  Anterior ethmoid artery (a branch of the ophthalmic artery)

Posterior Ethmoid Sinuses
  Arteries of the superior concha (branches of the sphenopalatine artery)
  Posterior ethmoid artery (a branch of the ophthalmic artery)

Venous Drainage
Cavernous sinus
Facial vein
Pterygomaxillary plexus

Lymphatic Drainage
Via transosseous routes into the lymphatic network of the nasal fossa and the meninges

Innervation
  Lateral posterior superior nasal branches of the maxillary nerve (V2)
  Anterior and posterior ethmoid nerves (branches of the ophthalmic nerve, V1)

duct. Anterior cells may abut and encroach upon neighboring sinuses, especially the frontal sinus. Although the ethmoid sinuses often extend beyond the anatomic boundaries of the ethmoid bone, other sinuses rarely extend into the ethmoid owing to the early pneumatization of the ethmoid sinuses.

Inferiorly, the superior and middle meatuses of the nasal cavity are found; at the superior surface of the ethmoid labyrinth are the ethmoid blood vessels and nerves, as well as portions of the frontal and sphenoid sinuses and the frontal lobes of the brain.

Ostia. As is true for all paranasal sinuses, the sites of the ostia reflect the sites of the initial, primary pneumatization. The diameters of the ostia are smaller than in any other paranasal sinuses: approximately 1 to 2 mm. The ostia of the anterior ethmoid sinuses are located at multiple sites in the bullar furrows, ethmoid infundibulum, and frontal furrows of the middle meatus. The ostia of the posterior ethmoid sinuses are found along the superior (and supreme) meatus.[51, 62, 67]

SPHENOID SINUS

The sphenoid sinus is a paired structure that is located predominantly in the sphenoid bone.

The two sinus cavities are separated by a complete bony septum, approximately 0.6 mm thick, located in the midsagittal plane. Some asymmetry in size and shape is nearly always present, but marked septal deviations are relatively rare.

The walls of the sphenoid sinus are irregular. Crescentic, bony septa partially separate recesses, producing incomplete compartmentalization of the sinus. There may be dehiscences in the bony sinus wall, especially laterally and superiorly, where it is only about 1 mm thick. Such dehiscences may result in direct contacts between the sinus mucosa and the overlying dura.

Anatomic Relations (Table 1–4). The sphenoid sinus is located in a central position in the skull. It is surrounded by several important anatomic structures. Superior to the sinus are the cerebral hypophysis, olfactory tract, frontal lobes of the brain, and an often extensive intercavernous venous network. Anterosuperiorly, the optic chiasm is present. Anteriorly, the anterior margin of the sphenoid bone forms a small segment of the posterior orbital wall. Owing to this anatomic relation, sphenoid sinus disease may cause orbital apex symptoms.

Inferiorly, the nasopharynx is present, as are the blood vessels and the nerve of the pterygoid canal, which run anteroposteriorly immediately below the sinus floor. These structures may be surrounded completely by the bony wall of the pterygoid canal, or they may lie directly underneath the mucosa of the sinus floor.

Posteriorly, a thick, bony wall separates the sinus from the basilar artery and the pons. Anteriorly, an incomplete bony wall separates the sinus mucosa from the nasal mucosa and from the posterior ethmoid sinuses. If the sphenoid sinus is large, it may extend over the pterygopalatine fossa with its contents, and it may be located directly posterior to the maxillary sinus.

Laterally, a thin, bony wall with occasional dehiscences separates the sphenoid sinus from Meckel's cave, the cavernous sinus, the internal carotid artery (which may leave a depression in the bony wall or even be in direct contact with the sinus mucosa), the abducens nerve (which similarly may be in direct contact with the sinus mucosa), and, along the lower border of the sinus, the maxillary division of the trigeminal nerve.

Ostium. The ostium of the sphenoid sinus is placed disadvantageously high in the anterior sinus wall. It may be as high as 14 mm above the level of the sinus floor. The sinus drains into the posteriormost portion of the sphenoethmoid recess, above the level of the highest nasal concha.[51, 67, 68]

CONCLUDING REMARKS

In the past, some attempt has been made to study the comparative anatomy of the paranasal sinuses in order to clarify their significance.[69, 70] Although the comparative anatomy of the lateral nasal wall is problematic, paranasal sinuses appear to make their first rudimentary appearance in amphibians. Reptiles and birds have distinct maxillary sinuses. The paranasal sinuses become particularly prominent in mammals.

It is interesting that paranasal sinuses are absent in small and aquatic animals. This fact might be an argument in favor of the suggestion that they serve to reduce the weight of the cranial skeleton, but other arguments have been advanced against this theory.[69]

The maxillary sinus appears to be most constantly present in vertebrates, but even in higher primates its presence apparently depends on dimensional and spatial relationships in the skull. The sinus tends to be absent when orbit and teeth encroach on its potential space.[71] The sphenoid sinus is the second most frequently present sinus in vertebrates. In hoofed animals, carnivores, and some of the anthropoid apes, the ethmoid sinuses are particularly prominent. The frontal sinus appears only in some

TABLE 1–4. Vascularization and Innervation of the Sphenoid Sinus

Arterial Supply
  Nasal Mucosal Arteries
    Ostial artery (a branch of the nasopalatine artery)
    Branches of the sphenopalatine artery

  Osseous Vasculature
    Branches of the internal carotid artery and artery of
      the pterygoid canal (vidian artery)

Venous Drainage
  Nasal veins
  Via transosseous routes into the sinuses surrounding the
    sella turcica, specifically cavernous and
    sphenoparietal sinuses

Lymphatic Drainage
Via the lymphatic networks of nasal fossa and meninges

Innervation
  Medial posterior superior nasal nerves (branches of the
    maxillary nerve, V2)
  Posterior ethmoid nerve (a branch of the ophthalmic
    nerve, V1)

anthropoids (gorilla and chimpanzee) and in humans.

If one analyzes the incidence of paranasal sinuses, it appears that their actual location may be of secondary significance, determined by the particular spatial relationships in the cranium. The embryology of the sinuses seems to indicate that these structures may be more than the "hole in the doughnut" passively pneumatizing the bones that surround the nasal cavity.

There is no consensus of opinion on the possible role(s) of paranasal sinuses. Their most likely role appears to be to aid in the retention of moisture through turbulence enhancement, which would serve to humidify the inhaled air.[72] Whatever the function of these structures, paranasal sinuses can be present only in those areas of the skull that remain statically and especially dynamically unloaded during masticatory function and are not involved in any load transmission.[73, 74] The development and the definitive anatomic relationships of the paranasal sinuses ultimately are determined within this operational constraint.

References

1. Hall BK: Chondrogenesis and osteogenesis of cranial neural crest cells. In Pratt RM, Christiansen RL (eds): Current Research Trends in Prenatal Craniofacial Development. New York, Elsevier North Holland, 1980, p 47.
2. Johnston MC, Noden DM, Hazelton RD, et al: Origins of avian ocular and periocular tissues. Exp Eye Res 29:27, 1979.
3. Noden DM: Origins and patterning of craniofacial mesenchymal tissues. J Craniofac Genet Dev Biol (Suppl 2):15, 1986.
4. LeDouarin N: The Neural Crest. Cambridge, Cambridge University Press, 1982.
5. Tan SS, Morriss-Kay GM: Analysis of cranial neural crest cell migration and early fates in postimplantation rat chimaeras. J Embryol Exp Morph 98:21, 1986.
6. Smits-van Prooije AE, Vermeij-Keers C, Dubbeldam JA, et al: The formation of mesoderm and mesectoderm in presomite rat embryos cultured in vitro, using WGA-Au as a marker. Anat Embryol 176:71, 1987.
7. Phillips MT, Kirby ML, Forbes G: Analysis of cranial neural crest distribution in the developing heart using quail-chick chimaeras. Circ Res 60:27, 1987.
8. Couly GF, LeDouarin NM: Mapping of the early neural primordium in quail-chick chimaeras. II. The prosencephalic neural plate and neural folds: Implications for the genesis of cephalic human congenital abnormalities. Dev Biol 120:198, 1987.
9. Chiakulas JJ: The specificity and differential fusion of cartilage derived from mesoderm and mesectoderm. J Exp Zool 136:287, 1959.
10. Fyfe DM, Hall BK: Lack of association between avian cartilages of different embryological origins when maintained in vitro. Am J Anat 154:485, 1979.
11. Bossy J: Development of olfactory and related structures in staged human embryos. Anat Embryol 161:225, 1980.
12. Gaare JD, Langman J: Fusion of nasal swellings in the mouse embryo. DNA synthesis and histological features. Anat Embryol 161:225, 1980.
13. O'Rahilly R: The timing and sequence of events in the development of the human digestive system and associated structures during the embryonic period proper. Anat Embryol 153:123, 1978.
14. O'Rahilly R, Boyden EA: The timing and sequence of events in the development of the human respiratory system during the embryonic period proper. Z Anat Entwickl Gesch 141:237, 1973.
15. Vermeij-Keers C: Transformations in the facial region of the human embryo. Adv Anat Embryol 46(5):1, 1972.
16. Hinrichsen K: The early development of morphology and patterns of the face in the human embryo. Adv Anat Embryol Cell Biol 98:1–79, 1985.
17. Burdi AR, Silvey RG: Sexual differences in closure of the human palatal shelves. Cleft Palate J 6:1, 1969.
18. Burdi AR, Silvey RG: The relation of sex-associated facial profile reversal and stages of human palatal closure. Teratology 2:297, 1969.
19. Iizuka T: Stage of the closure of the human palate. Okajimas Folia Anat Jpn 50:249, 1973.
20. Kraus BS, Kitamura H, Latham RA: Atlas of Developmental Anatomy of the Face; With Special Reference to Normal and Cleft Lip and Palate. New York, Harper and Row, 1966.
21. Mato M, Aikawa E, Katahira M: Further studies on cell reaction at the lower surface of the nasal septum of human embryos during fusion to the palate. Acta Anat 71:154, 1968.
22. Pratt RM, Christiansen RL (eds): Current Research Trends in Prenatal Craniofacial Development. New York, Elsevier North Holland, 1980.
23. Yokoh Y: Development of the palate in man. Acta Anat 68:1, 1967.
24. de Beer G: The Development of the Vertebrate Skull. Oxford, Clarendon Press, 1937.
25. Bersch W, Reinbach W: Das Primordialcranium eines menschlichen Embryo von 52 mm Sch.-St.-Länge. Zur Morphologie des Cranium älterer menschlicher Feten II. Z Anat Entwicklungsgesch 132:240, 1970.
26. Grube D, Reinbach W: Das Cranium eines menschlichen Embryo von 80 mm Sch.-St.-Länge. Zur Morphologie des Cranium älterer menschlicher Feten III. Anat Embryol 149:183, 1976.
27. Müller F, O'Rahilly R: The human chondrocranium at the end of the embryonic period proper, with particular reference to the nervous system. Am J Anat 159:33, 1980.
28. Schaeffer JP: The Nose, Paranasal Sinuses, Nasolacrimal Passageways, and Olfactory Organ in Man. A Genetic, Developmental, and Anatomico-physiological Consideration. Philadelphia, P Blakiston's Son & Company, 1920.
29. Slabý O: Die frühe Morphogenesis der Nasenkapsel beim Menschen. Acta Anat 42:105, 1960.
30. Vidić B: The morphogenesis of the lateral nasal wall in the early prenatal life of man. Am J Anat 130:121, 1971.
31. Melsen B: Histological analysis of the postnatal development of the nasal septum. Angle Orthod 47:83, 1977.
32. Melsen B, Melsen F, Moss ML: Postnatal development of the nasal septum studied on human autopsy material. In Carlson DS (ed): Craniofacial Biology. Ann Arbor, Center for Human Growth and Development, 1981.
33. O'Rahilly R, Gardner E: The initial appearance of ossification in staged human embryos. Am J Anat 134:291, 1972.
34. Schultz-Coulon H-J, Eckermeier L: Zum postnatalen

Wachstum der Nasenscheidewand. Acta Otolaryngol 82:131, 1976.

35. Williams PL, Warwick R: Gray's Anatomy. 36th ed. Philadelphia, WB Saunders, 1980.

36. Davis WB: Development and Anatomy of the Nasal Accessory Sinuses in Man. Philadelphia, WB Saunders, 1914.

37. Keibel F, Mall FP: Manual of Human Embryology. Vol I. Philadelphia, JB Lippincott, 1910.

38. Keith A: Human Embryology and Morphology. 6th ed. London, Edward Arnold & Company, 1948.

39. Kier EL, Rothman SLG: Radiologically significant anatomic variations of the developing sphenoid in humans. *In* Bosma JF (ed): Development of the Basicranium. Bethesda MD, DHEW Publ No (NIH) 76–989, 1976.

40. Kodama G: Developmental studies on the presphenoid in the human sphenoid bone. Okajimas Folia Anat Jpn 41:159, 1965.

41. Kodama G: Developmental studies on the body of the human sphenoid bone. Hokkaido J Med Sci 46:313, 1971.

42. Takahashi R: The formation of the nasal septum and the etiology of septal deformity. The concept of evolutionary paradox. Acta Otolaryngol (Suppl) 443:1,36, 1987.

43. Bertolini R, Herrling C: Die pränatale Entwicklung der Binde-und Stützgewebe in der unteren Nasenmuschel des Menschen. Z Mikrosk Anat Forsch 94:1009, 1980.

44. De Lara GS, Cuspinera De GE, Cardenas Ramirez L: Anatomical and functional account on the lateral nasal cartilages. Acta Anat 97:393, 1977.

45. Wen CI: Ontogeny and phylogeny of the nasal cartilages in primates. Carnegie Contrib Embryol 22:109, 1930.

46. Dion MC, Jafek BW, Tobin CE: The anatomy of the nose. External support. Arch Otolaryngol 104:145, 1978.

47. Anson BJ (ed): Morris' Human Anatomy. 12th ed. New York, McGraw-Hill, 1966.

48. Legent F, Perlemuter L, Vandenbrouck C: Cahiers d'Anatomie O.R.L. 2. Fosses Nasales, Pharynx. 2nd ed. Paris, Masson, 1976.

49. McMinn RMH, Hutchings RT, Logan BM: Color Atlas of Head and Neck Anatomy. Chicago, Yearbook Medical Publishers, 1981.

50. Pierce RH, Mainen MW, Bosma JF: The Cranium of the Newborn Infant. An Atlas of Tomography and Anatomical Sections. Bethesda MD, DHEW Publ No (NIH)78–788, 1978.

51. Som PM: CT of the paranasal sinuses (review article). Neuroradiology 27:189, 1985.

52. Hajniš K, Kustra T, Farkas LG, Feiglová B: Antrum Highmori. Biologica 1967:1, 1968.

53. Hajniš K: Die Ebene des Kieferhöhlenbodens und oroantrale Fisteln. Verh Anat Ges 80:743, 1986.

54. Cullen RL, Vidić B: The dimensions and shape of the human maxillary sinus in the perinatal period. Acta Anat 83:411, 1972.

55. Ritter FN: The Paranasal Sinuses. Anatomy and Surgical Technique. 2nd ed. St. Louis, CV Mosby, 1978.

56. Romanes GJ (ed): Cunningham's Textbook of Anatomy. 12th ed. Oxford, Oxford University Press, 1981.

57. Schumacher GH, Heyne HJ, Fanghänel R: Zur Anatomie der menschlichen Nasennebenhöhlen. 1. Räumliche Darstellungen. Anat Anz 130:132, 1972.

58. Schumacher GH, Heyne HJ, Fanghänel R: Zur Anatomie der menschlichen Nasennebenhöhlen. 2. Volumetrie. Anat Anz 130:143, 1972.

59. Sperber GH: Craniofacial Embryology. 3rd ed. Bristol, John Wright & Sons, 1981.

60. Van Alyea OE: Nasal Sinuses: Anatomic and Clinical Considerations. Baltimore, Williams & Wilkins, 1942.

61. Caffey J: Pediatric X-Ray Diagnosis. 7th ed. Chicago, Yearbook Medical Publishers, 1978.

62. Mattox DE, Delaney RG: Anatomy of the ethmoid sinus. Otolaryngol Clin North Am 18(1):3, 1985.

63. Hajniš K: Die Kapazität der Keilbeinhöhlen. Anat Anz 167:23, 1988.

64. Hajniš K: Grösse des Körpers und der Höhlen des Keilbeins. Anthropol 24:159, 1986.

65. Carson JL, Collier AM, Knowles MR, et al: Morphometric aspects of ciliary distribution and ciliogenesis in human nasal epithelium. Proc Natl Acad Sci USA 78:6996, 1981.

66. Thaete LG, Spicer SS, Spock A: Histology, ultrastructure and carbohydrate cytochemistry of surface and glandular epithelium of human nasal mucosa. Am J Anat 162:243, 1981.

67. Hesselink JR, New PFJ, Davis KR, et al: Computed tomography of the paranasal sinuses and face. Part I: Normal anatomy. J Comput Assist Tomogr 2:559, 1978.

68. Kapila A, Chakeres DW, Blanco E: The Meckel cave: Computed tomographic study. Radiology 152:425, 1984.

69. Negus V: The Comparative Anatomy and Physiology of the Nose and Paranasal Sinuses. Edinburgh, E. & S. Livingstone, 1958.

70. Stupka W: Die Missbildungen und Anomalien der Nase und des Nasenrachenraumes. Vienna, Julius Springer Verlag, 1938.

71. Lund VJ: The maxillary sinus in the higher primates. Acta Otolaryngol 105:163, 1988.

72. Franciscus RG, Trinkaus E: Nasal morphology and the emergence of *Homo erectus*. Am J Phys Anthrop 75:517, 1988.

73. Endo B: Experimental studies on the mechanical significance of the form of the human facial skeleton. J Fac Sci Univ Tokyo, Sec.V, III:1–106, 1966.

74. Endo B: Structure of the human facial skeleton from the viewpoint of statics. Proc 19th Jpn Natl Congr Appl Mech, 8–14, 1969.

CHAPTER 2

PHYSIOLOGY OF THE HUMAN NOSE

P. Perry Phillips, MD
Thomas V. McCaffrey, MD, PhD
Eugene B. Kern, MD

The nose is a puzzling yet remarkably efficient organ. It allows us to sample many scents that are critical to events in our lives. In many other species the effective functioning of the nose often means the difference between life and death. In humans, however, the nose has evolved with the rest of our body to suit the needs and tasks that confront us daily. The importance of olfaction in modern mankind's day-to-day survival is much lower than it was for our ancestors.

At present the act of respiration, with all its permutations, is likely the most important as well as the most extensively studied of nasal functions. Only through abnormalities in these complex tasks of olfaction do we begin to understand what constitutes the realm of nasal physiology. This chapter discusses the details of the normal function of the nose and sinuses. The methodology concerning the objective study of nasal airflow (rhinomanometry) is also presented.

OVERVIEW

We consider that there are three major functions of the nose: olfaction, respiration, and defense. Many additional minor functions of the nose exist: aiding and modifying voice production,[1] providing vocal resonance, serving as a secondary sex organ, and so on. Throughout time, however, the relative value of these functions has continued to fluctuate. Presently, the function of respiration seems to be the most important.

RESPIRATION

The act of respiration consists of a complex chain of physiologic events that eventually leads to the effective transfer of gases between a human being and the environment. Only with proper nasal function can the act of respiration take place efficiently. The nose has a crucial role in airflow, resistance, warming, and humidification of the inspired air. The normal resting adult breathes at a rate of 12 to 24 cycles per minute. This accounts for approximately 30 liters of airflow per minute, which enters the nose at a velocity of 45 miles per hour.[2] The character of the airflow through the nose is primarily turbulent,[3] which offers the advantage of prolonging air-mucosa contact time. This turbulent airflow begins at 0.3 to 0.5 liter of flow per second,[4] with the nose having more laminar flow characteristics below this flow rate. The path that airflow takes on its passage to the lungs is also dependent on tidal volume. In normal subjects who have a tidal volume below 35 liters per minute, most of the airflow is distributed through the nasal cavity, with the mouth contributing little to respiration.[5] With exertion and an increase in the airflow above this rate, breathing becomes more oronasal in character, and a larger percentage of airflow passes through the mouth. Thus a larger total volume of air not well warmed or humidified is passed to the lungs.

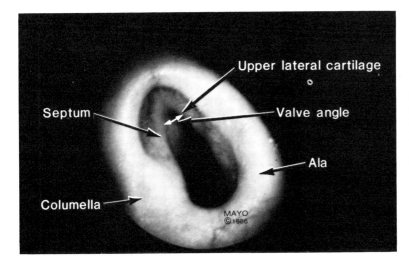

Figure 2-1. The nasal valve. (From Kasperbauer JL, Kern EB: Nasal valve physiology. Otolaryngol Clin North Am 20:699–719, 1987. By permission of Mayo Foundation.)

VALVES OF THE NOSE

To better control the passage of air, the nose is equipped with a series of high-resistance areas (valves). These valves act to modify the quantity of air that passes through the nose, as well as the direction of flow through its interior. The first valve that inspired air passes is the nasal valve, which was first described at the turn of the century by Mink.[6] Synonyms for this valve are the liminal valve, liminal chink, area 2, flow-limiting segment, limen vestibuli, and os internum. Its surface area is approximately 50 cm^2, and it is responsible for half the nasal resistance. Kasperbauer and Kern[6a] have described the anatomic components of the valve to include the nasal septum, upper lateral cartilage, head of the inferior turbinate, and floor of the nose (Fig. 2–1A,B). Studied in detail, it has been shown to be a cone-shaped, inverted teardrop area. The most important feature of the valve is the total surface area and not just the angle that the upper lateral cartilage and nasal septum form[7] (Fig. 2–2). The total area of this valve, determined by each of the aforementioned structures, is the most important flow-limiting segment in the nose.

As air passes through this constricting segment, the airflow accelerates and changes from a laminar type to a turbulent type of flow. This allows the nose to humidify, filter, and warm the inspired air more efficiently. It is the most important inflow regulator to the nose[8, 9] and has been demonstrated to be the site of maximal resistance to inspiratory airflow.[10, 11] Because of the small cross-sectional area in the valve re-

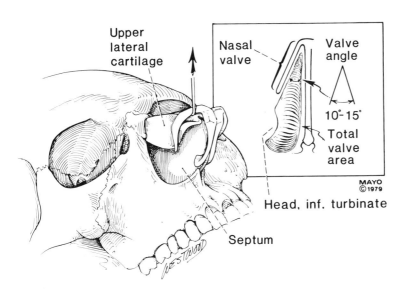

Figure 2-2. Diagram of the nasal valve area. (From Kern EB: Nasal septal reconstruction versus submucous resection. In Snow JB (ed): Controversy in Otolaryngology. Philadelphia, WB Saunders, 1980. By permission of Mayo Foundation.)

gion, even small deformities can lead to significant airflow obstruction. The most common pathology in this region is a deformity of the upper lateral cartilage in relation to the nasal septum.

The septal valve is formed by the relationship of the erectile turbinate tissues to the septum. Though less important as an inflow regulator than the nasal valve, the septal valve is very important in humidifying and warming the inspired air. It becomes more apparent with allergic or vasomotor conditions of the nose, when it can lead to significant nasal obstruction. When functioning in concert, the liminal and septal valves actively control the inflow and passage of air through the nose. Accordingly, they also function to adjust the modification of this air in preparation for alveolar ventilation.

ACCESSORY RESISTORS

Another important modifier of nasal resistance is the function of the dilator naris muscle. Through voluntary action of this muscle and flaring of the nasal ala, a 29 per cent decrease in nasal resistance has been shown.[12] Similar results have been noted in preterm infants in whom activation of the dilator naris muscles[13] accounted for a 23 per cent decrease in transnasal resistance. In addition, the dilator naris also plays an active role in response to both hypoxia and hypercapnia.[14] When either of these stimuli is present, the dilator naris contracts, leading to a dilated nasal ala and thus a decreased nasal resistance.

At high inspiratory flow rates, however, the negative intraluminal pressure overcomes the action of the dilator naris and the ala collapses.[8] In this situation the nasal ala functions as a Starling resistor and becomes the chief flow-limiting valve of the nose. The alar region then acts as an upstream flow-limiting segment that accounts for most of the resistance in the nose (Fig. 2–3). This is of minimal importance in the normal nose except when forced maximal inspiratory maneuvers are performed. In the previously traumatized (often operated) nose, however, this effect can lead to significant nasal obstruction at normal flow rates. Unfortunately, surgical correction of the collapsing ala is very difficult and fraught with failure.

MODIFICATION OF INSPIRED AIR

As air traverses the nasal passages, it is prepared for alveolar exchange by several

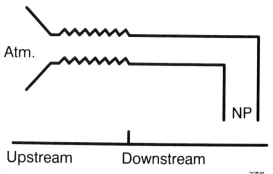

Figure 2–3. Representation of the caudal end of the nose acting as an upstream resistor and the posterior portion of the nose acting as a downstream resistor. *Atm.,* Atmosphere; *NP,* nasopharynx. (From Kasperbauer JL, Kern EB: Nasal valve physiology. Otolaryngol Clin North Am 20(4), 1987.)

means. First, despite varying environmental humidities, the nose functions to adjust precisely the inspired air to have a humidity of approximately 85 per cent.[15] This enhances the gas exchange at the alveolar level as well as preventing drying of the lower airways. In return, a large portion of the moisture taken from the nose during inspiration is returned to the nasal mucosa during exhalation.[16] This prevents overdrying of the nasal mucosa and thickening of the nasal secretions. Unfortunately, in climates with low humidity, the nose's ability to humidify the inspired air adequately is often exceeded, resulting in a dry, sticky throat and a sensation of postnasal drip owing to thickening of the normally thin, watery nasal mucus. This usually is treated effectively by increasing a patient's fluid intake and increasing the humidity of the home with a humidifier.

In addition to humidification, the nose also warms the inspired air to allow for proper respiratory function. The rich capillary beds that make up the side wall of the nose, along with their accompanying venous sinusoids, make an ideal surface for conduction of heat to the passing air. Together, the heat exchange and humidification functions of the nose work in harmony to ensure the efficient function of the entire respiratory system. Without these normal actions, the entire system becomes inefficient and places the patient at risk for many other problems.

RESISTANCE AND PULMONARY MECHANICS

The nose plays an important role in pulmonary mechanics. The upper airway with its conduits accounts for 50 to 70 per cent of total airway resistance.[17, 18] In addition, the resistance of the upper airway is much more variable than that of the lower airway. Upper airway resistance is important in maintaining the necessary resistance during changing environmental conditions. This resistance is required in pulmonary mechanics to allow the lungs to expand optimally for normal pulmonary venous return.

The resistance of the nose is measured by calculating the relationship of the pressure to transnasal flow rate:

$$\text{Rn (nasal resistance)} = \frac{\text{P (transnasal pressure difference)}}{\dot{V}\text{ (transnasal flow)}}$$

The units of resistance are expressed in centimeters of H_2O/liter/sec. This formula holds true, however, only when the Reynolds number is less than 2000 (Fig. 2–4). The actual resistance of the nose, however, does not obey this formula because the airflow through the nose is not laminar. The turbulence in the nose makes the airflow much more difficult to interpret (Fig. 2–5). An understanding of these principles enables better therapeutic decisions regarding airflow disorders.

FACTORS AFFECTING NASAL RESISTANCE

Among the many variables that affect nasal resistance, two of the most important are hypoxia and hypercapnia. Several investigators have shown direct correlation between hypoxia and hypercapnia and decreasing nasal resistance.[19, 20] The mechanism for this change in the nasal resistance is mediated through the vascular beds in the mucosa. By this mechanism the nose is able to maintain the optimal resistance for pulmonary function. Without continuously varying resistance, the essential actions of the nose, such as humidification, warming, and filtration, would be impaired, thus leading to less efficient respiration.

Exercise has been noted to decrease nasal

LAMINAR FLOW

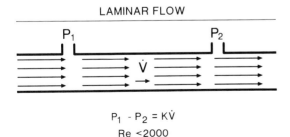

$$P_1 - P_2 = K\dot{V}$$

Re <2000

Figure 2–4. Laminar airflow and ideal gas behavior. P_1, pressure 1; P_2, pressure 2; $K\dot{V}$, Constant × flow. (From McCaffrey TV, Kern EB: Rhinomanometry. Facial Plastic Surgery 3(4), 1986.)

TURBULENT FLOW
Regular Conduit

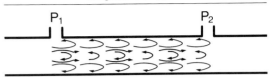

$$P_1 - P_2 = K\dot{V}^{1.75}$$

Re >2000

Figure 2–5. Turbulent airflow in the nose. (From McCaffrey TV, Kern EB: Rhinomanometry. Facial Plastic Surgery 3(4), 1986.)

resistance in normal individuals, as well as in those with obstructed noses.[21–23] (This has also been shown in patients with asthma and allergic rhinitis.[24]) The amount of decreased resistance in exercising patients is proportional to the intensity of the exercise performed. Following discontinuation of exercise, nasal resistance reverts to normal with a brief rebound effect (increased resistance compared with the pre-exercise state). Rhinosterometry in the postexercise state has documented mucosal decongestion.[25] The proper functioning of the nasal resistance system and its ability to adapt to changing stimuli during exercise allow individuals to achieve peak athletic performance.

Many other extrinsic stimuli affect the resistance of the nose. Inhaled cigarette smoke has been shown to increase the nasal resistance of young adult patients.[21] This is thought to be a protective function of the nose to prevent entry of smoke into the lungs. Another commonly used drug, ethanol, also has been shown to increase nasal resistance.[26] Though not usually significant, in the sleep apnea patient even occasional use of ethanol can markedly increase the severity of the disease. Other common chemicals such as ammonia also have been shown to increase nasal resistance.[27] Nonchemical stimuli also can have this effect: asymmetric pressure applied to one side of the body has been noted to result in an ipsilateral increase in nasal resistance. The mechanism for this congestion is via stimulation of pressure receptors on the pelvis, pectoral girdle, and thorax, not the effect of recumbency[28] or increasing venous pressure in the capillary beds of the nose. This phenomenon is commonly experienced upon arising from sleep, when the side of the nose ipsilateral to the dependent side of the body is congested.

Internal systemic derangements in the body also can be responsible for changes in nasal resistance. Pregnancy has been shown to be associated with severe congestion of the nose, along with increased viscosity of the nasal mucus. These changes seem to be correlated with the amount of circulating estrogen in the blood stream[29] and resolve promptly following the termination of the pregnancy. Similarly, hyperthyroidism has been known for a long time to cause chronic congestion of the nasal mucosa and increased viscosity of the nasal mucus. This then leads to increased nasal resistance and symptoms of nasal obstruction. Hypothyroidism also has been noted to produce changes in the mucous membranes of the nose. In hypothyroid patients, the mucosa is pale and boggy and has a greatly increased likelihood of infection.[30] The endocrine system has a significant effect on the nasal membranes and resistance.

Many pathologic conditions of the nose also cause increases in nasal resistance. Vasomotor rhinitis and allergic reactions are some of the most common causes of increased nasal resistance and nasal obstruction. These conditions generally act on both sides of the nose and when severe can lead to total nasal obstruction. Structural problems, such as septal deformities and adenoid hypertrophy, are also common causes of unilateral or bilateral increases in nasal resistance. When discovered, however, they are often correctable by surgery. In addition, air pollution, air temperature, humidity, and psychologic factors all play a role in nasal resistance and the perception of nasal airflow. These factors must be taken into account when evaluating any patient with nasal obstruction.

An interesting phenomenon is paradoxic nasal obstruction. This is usually seen in patients who have had a unilateral nasal obstruction over a period of years. They learn to eliminate the perception of obstruction in the blocked side of the nose and often live without any other symptoms. A problem arises, however, when these patients experience obstruction in the normal side of the nose, upon which they have become dependent for all nasal breathing. This is often the result of nasal cycling or nasal pathology such as allergic or vasomotor rhinitis. The paradox occurs when a patient complains of obstruction on the more "normal" side of the nose while experiencing few or no symptoms on the totally obstructed side. When this is due to a normally cycling nose, the patient complains of intermittent nasal obstruction that naturally cycles throughout the day. Rhinomanometry discloses a very high total nasal resistance when the normal side of the nose is congested. This also has been well documented with serial tomography and direct patient observation.[31] Amelioration of this problem requires patient education about the phenomenon and surgical correction of all the underlying structural pathology.

On the other hand, certain stimuli can cause a perception of decreased nasal resistance by altering the sensation of the nose through stimulation of the cold receptors in the mucosal lining. The patient experiences subjective feelings of increased nasal airflow. Examples of these stimuli include camphor, eucalyptus, and menthol. These ingredients are in many over-the-counter cold remedies but have no actual effect on the resistance of the nose.[32] Topical lidocaine in the nose produces a similar sensation of increased nasal patency but no objective change in airflow resistance.[33] Although almost every patient in one study had a sensation of increased airflow through the nose, none had a documented decrease in nasal resistance.[34]

In summary, many intrinsic and extrinsic stimuli affect nasal resistance as well as the sensation of nasal airflow. This fact underscores the importance of nasal airway resistance testing to determine the actual state of airflow through the nasal passages. Determination of nasal pathology and airflow status is impossible without objective testing because of the subjective nature of nasal breathing.

RHINOMANOMETRY

Rhinomanometry is a test in which resistance to nasal airflow is calculated by measuring the amount of air pressure and airflow through the nose during breathing. Nasal resistance can be calculated directly from the measurement of pressure divided by airflow. Unfortunately, the relationship of pressure and flow rate is not constant because of the everchanging turbulent airflow in the nose. Therefore, to determine nasal resistance, it is necessary to use the same nasal flow rate each time or to keep the pressure at which flow rates are measured constant at an arbitrary point.[35] This is the only way to obtain an accurate, reliable, reproducible calculation of nasal airway resistance.

The methods used to determine the change in pressures and flow rates through the nose are numerous; each has its advantages and disadvantages. In anterior nozzle rhinomanometry, nozzles are placed into the nasal vestibules to measure these changes (Fig. 2–6). Unfortunately, the placement of nozzles into the vestibule bypasses the nasal valve. This may accidentally open a deformity responsible for nasal obstruction. Eliminating the ability to measure accurately the resistance across the valve area is critical and renders this form of rhinomanometry much less valuable. Anterior mask rhino-

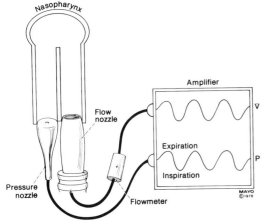

Figure 2–6. Anterior nozzle rhinomanometry. (From Kern EB: Rhinomanometry. Otolaryngology 2:1–8, 1979. By permission of Mayo Foundation.)

manometry is a similar method, except that the flowmeter nozzle is replaced by a mask that has a built-in flowmeter (Fig. 2–7). The mask covers the face and allows for measurements of flow and pressure across the region of the nasal valve. In this method a pressure transducer is placed into the nostril not being tested to measure the pressure in the patient's nasopharynx. This reading is then compared with the atmospheric pressure to determine the change in pressure. The flow rate is measured via the flowmeter in the mask. Accurate measurement of each nostril is obtained independently without using instrumentation in the nostril being examined. One limitation of these forms of rhinomanometry is the inability to determine the nasal resistance in patients with nasal septal perforations. When the septum is intact, however, measurement of unilateral nasal resistance

and calculation of bilateral nasal resistance can be performed accurately.

Posterior rhinomanometry requires the placement of a pressure transducer in the oral cavity to measure the nasopharyngeal pressure (Fig. 2–8). The flowmeter is again placed in the mask to avoid instrumentation of the valve region. With this method it is possible to measure transnasal pressure and airflow directly to calculate the total nasal resistance. This method, therefore, can be used to determine nasal resistance in patients with nasal septal perforations. The technique is difficult for some patients, with 10 to 25 per cent being unable to relax the oropharyngeal musculature adequately to allow accurate measurements. Posterior rhinomanometry is thus less attractive for routine clinical situations, though it remains a valuable tool for research.

Any of the foregoing methods can be performed in an active or passive fashion. Active rhinomanometry refers to the patient's active breathing to produce airflow through the nose. This is the most commonly used technique of rhinomanometry and is the easiest for patients to perform. It also requires less equipment and time to perform than passive rhinomanometry. In passive rhinomanometry, an external positive pressure device is used to produce airflow of a constant velocity and flow rate through the nose. This has the advantage of controlling the exact airflow but is not as physiologic as active rhinomanometry. It does, however, offer the benefit of constant flow rates, which are useful in some settings. Either method can yield excellent reproducible results to aid in the evaluation of patients with nasal obstruction.

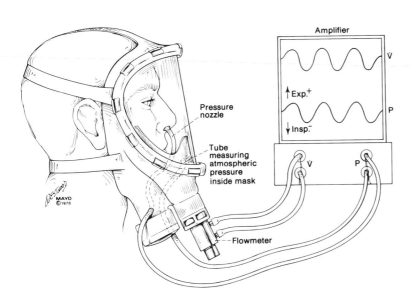

Figure 2–7. Anterior mask rhinomanometry (note that the flowmeter is in the mask and no longer in the nostril to be tested). (From Kern EB: Rhinomanometry. Otolaryngology 2:1–8, 1979. By permission of Mayo Foundation.)

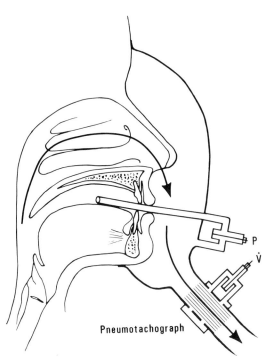

Pneumotachograph

Figure 2–8. Posterior rhinomanometry. (From McCaffrey TV, Kern EB: Rhinomanometry. Facial Plastic Surgery 3(4), 1986.)

Interpretation and Limitations of Rhinomanometry. Fortunately, the results of rhinomanometry correlate well with the severity of patients' symptoms. It has been well established that objective elevations in unilateral nasal resistance are associated with increased symptoms of nasal obstruction on that side of the nose.[36] Likewise, patients with bilateral nasal obstruction have been shown to have significantly higher nasal resistances compared with those with unilateral nasal obstruction. It also has been shown that rhinoscopic evidence of intranasal deformity was not an accurate predictor

of elevations in nasal resistance. Many patients in this study had normal nasal resistances (Fig. 2–9) despite the descriptions of intranasal pathology considered to account for significant obstruction. Normal nasal resistances also have been determined in a study of 80 normal patients without symptoms of nasal obstruction.[34] These patients underwent anterior mask rhinomanometry; their nasal resistances were reported at varying pressures and flows to help determine what constitutes abnormal nasal resistance. Therefore, a reliable, reproducible, objective test such as rhinomanometry has a role in the assessment of patients with nasal obstruction.

To perform meaningful rhinomanometry, one must follow a specific protocol to decongest the nose. First, the calculation of nasal resistance is performed on both sides of the nose prior to the use of any decongestants. The nasal passages are then sprayed with a 1 per cent phenylephrine spray, and 10 minutes are allowed for it to take effect. Nasal resistance is then measured again on both sides of the nose. Measurements before and after decongestion of the nose determine whether the obstruction is due to mucosal disease, structural (bony or cartilaginous) deformity, or a combination of both. With structural septal deformities there is very little change in the nasal resistance before and after use of phenylephrine (Fig. 2–10). Mucosal diseases such as allergic and vasomotor rhinitis, however, give a much different result (Fig. 2–11). The change in nasal resistance in these patients after use of phenylephrine often can be dramatic, with markedly elevated nasal resistances becoming quite normal. This finding often suggests that other studies and a trial of medical therapy may be indicated. Another common finding is partial correction of the nasal obstruction through decongestion,

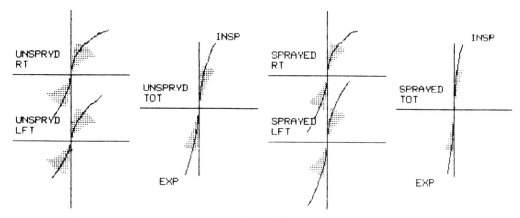

Figure 2–9. Normal nasal resistance on rhinomanography. *RT*, right; *LFT*, left; *TOT*, total; *EXP*, expiration; *INSP*, inspiration. (From McCaffrey TV, Kern EB: Rhinomanometry. Facial Plastic Surgery 3(4), 1986.)

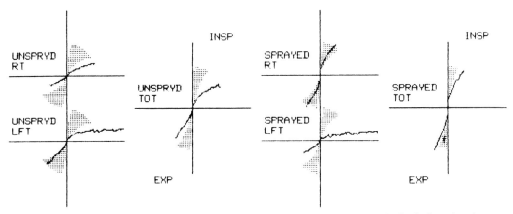

Figure 2–10. Structural nasal deformity causing increased left nasal resistance. Note the lack of effect that decongestion has on nasal resistance. (From McCaffrey TV, Kern EB: Rhinomanometry. Facial Plastic Surgery 3(4), 1986.)

though overall resistance remains elevated. This is commonly associated with mixed nasal obstruction in which there is a significant structural defect associated with mucous membrane pathology. Fortunately, rhinomanometry is of great use in the interpretation of these disorders and can be extremely helpful in guiding the choice of medical versus surgical therapy.

Rhinomanometry is also very helpful in the interpretation of nasal alae and nasal valve collapse. This abnormality is due to collapse at a critical negative pressure in this region and is very difficult to diagnose on physical examination. Fortunately, these abnormalities produce their own characteristic patterns on rhinomanometric examination that help distinguish them from other forms of nasal obstruction. When collapse does occur in this area, the valve/alae act as a Starling resistor, shutting off flow entirely. This results in a "shouldering effect" on the rhinomanogram with inspiration (Fig. 2–12). This finding, along with the positive Cottle test, helps the clinician to diagnose more ac-

curately a nasal valve collapse. Correction of this problem often requires the use of carefully designed cartilage grafts to prevent continuing collapse.

For daily clinical purposes in the practice of rhinology, anterior mask rhinomanometry seems to be best. It is simple, reliable, and easier to perform than posterior mask rhinomanometry. Posterior mask rhinomanometry, however, is still the most accurate method of rhinomanometry and is the method of choice in research investigation of the nasal airways. Both methods allow for the examination of nasal resistance without altering the nasal valve regions or alae, which is a distinct advantage over any form of nozzle rhinomanometry. This is very helpful in the preoperative assessment of patients with nasal obstruction, but it does not provide the diagnosis. It is merely a helpful adjunct in the armamentarium for the evaluation of nasal obstruction to aid in the management and selection of the most effective therapy possible for patients.

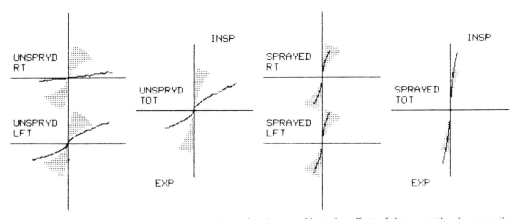

Figure 2–11. Mucosal pathology causing increased nasal resistance. Note the effect of decongestion in correcting the nasal resistance. (From McCaffrey TV, Kern EB: Rhinomanometry. Facial Plastic Surgery 3(4), 1986.)

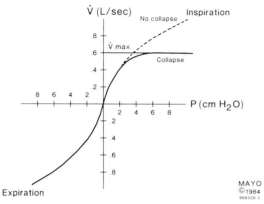

Figure 2–12. Rhinomanogram showing nasal valve collapse. Note the shouldering effect with the collapse above 0.6 liter/sec flow rate. (From MacKay IS: Facial Plastic Surgery Monograph. 3(4), 1986. By permission of Mayo Foundation.)

NASAL CYCLE

Another important phenomenon in the nose is the alternating congestion and decongestion of each side of the nose known as the nasal cycle. This cyclic engorgement and decongestion of the cavernous tissues in the nose has been documented by multiple investigators since early in this century.[37–42] This phenomenon has been observed in 80 per cent of patients and has been well documented by rhinomanometric studies[43] (Fig. 2–13). The cycle normally varies from 1 to 4 hours, though occasionally it may last up to 6 hours. The reason for its existence is not known. It is known that the action of the cycle depends on the presence of an intact nasal septum. The septum acts as a partition against which the congested side of the nose compresses during the nasal cycle. The pressure on the congesting tissues of the side wall of the nose allows feedback to occur, which eventually leads to decongestion. Without the nasal septum in place, the feedback mechanism is disturbed, and the cycle may be altered or even abolished. During the cycling of the nose, the total (binasal) resistance of the nose remains almost constant. Thus while one side of the nose is congested, the other side is reflexively decongested to maintain the normal airflow. This allows the patient to breathe normally at all times and to avoid the sensation of nasal obstruction. One theory postulates that the nasal cycle functions as a rheostat in the nostrils, which are essentially parallel resistors controlling the airflow. This allows for better control of the amount of airflow into the nasopharynx.[44, 45]

Several other stimuli also have been noted to affect the nasal cycle. Recumbency and asymmetric body pressure have been noted to alter the amplitude of the nasal cycle, but neither has an effect on total nasal resistance.[46] Light activity and periods of rest, however, have no effect on the nasal cycle or total nasal resistance. Interruption of the supraglottic airway, on the other hand, does alter the cycle. Patients who have undergone a laryngectomy or other interruption of the normal supraglottic airway have been shown to lose their nasal cycles.[47] Patients whose airway is eventually re-established have been shown to regain the normal rhythm of their nasal cycles. This suggests that the supraglottic airway and airflow have a role in the maintenance of the nasal cycle.

Some patients, however, have no nasal cycle (20 per cent). Such patients have been subdivided into three groups according to the amount of fluctuation that occurs in the nasal mucosa. The first group has no cycle and no evidence of fluctuation of the mucosa on either side of the nose. The second group has no cycle, but patients exhibit fluctuation on one side of the nose. The third group demonstrates fluctuations in the mucosa on both sides of the nose, but there is no cycle because there is no reversal of the dominantly congested side (the definition of the nasal cycle).[48] To date, however, no increase in nasal pathology associated with the noncycling nose has been documented.

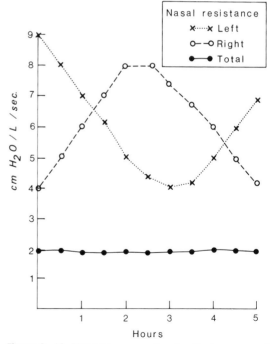

Figure 2–13. Rhinomanogram showing the human nasal cycle. Note the alternating congestion and decongestion on each side of the nose. (From McCaffrey TV, Kern EB: Rhinomanometry. Facial Plastic Surgery Monograph. 3(4), 1986.)

OLFACTION

The second function of the nose is olfaction. The surface area of the cribriform plate, where the olfactory center is located, is approximately 200 to 400 mm^2 in size.[49] In this region there are approximately 6 million receptor cells on each side of the nose. Though 12 million seems like a large number, it is small compared with the 50 million receptor cells in the rabbit's olfactory center.[50] The olfactory center contains four distinct cell populations. The olfactory *bipolar neuron* is a fusiform cell that is responsible for the detection of odors. This cell synapses in the olfactory bulb and sends its messages to the brain via the first cranial nerve. The *basal cell* in this area is essentially a resting cell waiting to become a bipolar neuron. The cycle of bipolar neurons dying and being replaced by the basal cells takes place over a 7-week period and is believed to be the only place in the body where special sensory neurons are replaced after they die.[51] The third type of cell is the *sustentacular cell*. It functions as a support cell to provide nutrients and protection for the surrounding bipolar neurons. The last cell in this region is the *microvillar cell*; its function is still a mystery. Some believe that there may be some olfactory role for this cell, but no conclusive evidence supporting or refuting this has been presented. When all these cells are working properly, the end result is the average human nose, which can distinguish among 4000 different odors. Noses, however, are quite insensitive compared with the visual system. For the nose to perceive a difference in odor, a 30 per cent change in intensity is required, whereas the human eye can detect changes as small as 1 per cent.

The theories concerning olfaction are controversial, and many questions remain unsettled. The molecular theory of olfaction suggests that stereospecific receptors on the bipolar neurons function to discriminate between odors.[52–54] When matched with their identical odor molecule, these receptors would then lead to depolarization of that cell and perception of that odor. Unfortunately, no evidence supports the existence of these receptors. Another popular theory is the temporal spatial theory suggested by Mozell.[55] He suggests that when the odor molecules arrive at the olfactory center they are separated out in a fashion similar to that of a chromatograph. By being separated in this specific manner the odor molecules would stimulate that specific area, leading to a discriminating sense of smell. A third theory of olfaction suggests that the actual chemical properties of the odor molecules are important in the perception of the odor. In this model, properties such as molecular volume, proton affinity, and the ability to donate protons are important in the perception of odor.[56] Another theory proposes the existence of pigment molecules analogous to those found in the eye, which are stimulated in a specific manner to yield discriminatory olfaction. However, no evidence at this time supports the presence of a pigmented molecule in the olfactory mucosa.[57] As in many areas of human physiology, the number of theories on a topic is usually proportional to how poorly we understand that topic.

The biochemical events that occur at the cellular level are more clearly understood than the overall theories on olfaction. However, there is still some disagreement on the ion responsible for depolarization of the bipolar neuron. In the model of the lamprey, it has been suggested that this ion is calcium.[58] Other evidence, however, points toward sodium and chloride as the ions responsible for depolarization.[59] Whichever ion functions in depolarization, the result is the formation of a generator potential that combines with other generator potentials to form an action potential. This in turn leads to firing of the first cranial nerve and central interpretation of olfaction. The central processing of this information takes place in the olfactory tubercle, prepiriform cortex, amygdaloid nucleus, and hypothalamus. When this signal has been processed and integrated, we experience the sensation of olfaction.

The olfactory mucosa, however, is not the only source of sensation for the perception of odors. The trigeminal nerve also participates via free nerve endings in its maxillary division that are sensitive to noxious stimuli. Common examples of these stimuli include hot peppers, ammonia, and other pungent chemicals in our environment. The amount of stimulation these fibers actually provide is small compared with the input from the cribriform region, but they add critical meaning to the odors we smell. These receptors are also particularly important in testing suspected malingerers. Patients feigning anosmia would deny that they are perceiving stimulation of the trigeminal nerve by means of ammonia. The truly anosmic patient with cribriform pathology would quickly respond in the affirmative when tested with ammonia. This is also a protective function of the nose, as most chemicals that stimulate the trigeminal nerve are toxic or unpleasant to humans.

PSYCHOLOGIC ASPECTS OF OLFACTION

Many factors other than the odor molecules and their reception at the level of the cribriform are important in the process of olfaction. The central processing and integration of these messages is the key to understanding how we actually perceive what we smell. Much of the research in this area has dealt with the role of hunger and how it modifies this perception. When one is hungry, the perception of a food odor becomes more pleasant, and this is directly related to the severity of the state of hunger the person is experiencing.[60] In this same state, however, nonfood odors do not create the same shift in the perception as do food odors.[61]

Another interesting phenomenon is the act of adaptation to environmental odors. This is the unconscious loss of the perception of an odor after one has been subjected to that odor for a prolonged period of time.[62] This generally occurs 1 to 5 minutes after becoming exposed to a new odor, and the threshold to perception of that odor becomes higher with prolonged exposure.[63] The mechanism of this adaptation has been demonstrated to occur at both a central[62] and a peripheral level.[64] Recovery from this adaptation also occurs quickly and generally requires several minutes in an environment that is devoid of the odor to which one has become adapted. When this phenomenon occurs between two different odors, it is referred to as cross-adaptation. An example of this is adaptation to the odor of substance 1 after being exposed to substance 2 for a period of time prior to exposure to substance one.

When mixing odors in this fashion, other phenomena also may occur. Usually the mixing of two odors results in a blend of the two odors, though occasionally a distinct new odor emerges that does not resemble either of the parent odors. Less commonly, these two odors can mask each other and no odor will be perceived. Between these extremes, many other combinations exist that magnify the complexity of the olfactory system and our perception of odors.

NASOSYSTEMIC REFLEXES

The nose is intimately involved with the rest of the body through a group of complex pathways. The nasocardiac and nasopulmonary pathways have been documented for many years[65] and are present in many lower species as well as humans. The afferent loop of this system is carried via fibers of the maxillary division of the trigeminal nerve. These nerve fibers then synapse in the main sensory, spinal tract, and mesencephalic nuclei of the brain stem. From here they ascend through the ipsilateral mesencephalic tract or contralateral trigeminal lemnisci to reach their central nervous system synapses. After processing, the efferent limb of this system is carried via the vagus nerve to its various end organs. Those most profoundly affected by this stimulation are the heart, lungs, and vascular system. The effects produced by stimulation of these reflexes include apnea, hypopnea, bradycardia, cardiac dysrhythmias, and decreases in the peripheral vascular resistance that result in hypotension. In humans, these reflexes have been well documented by a variety of studies. The relationships between the upper and lower respiratory tracts have been clearly established by Ogura.[66, 67] In the dog model, this relationship has been well demonstrated. When the nasal membranes of dogs were stimulated, pulmonary resistance increased in awake animals.[68] Humans demonstrate similar findings: obstruction of the nose revealed significant increases in pulmonary resistance, which reverted to normal following removal of this obstruction.[69]

Other work has demonstrated that the nose has an effect on the rhythmicity of nocturnal breathing. When the nose was anesthetized prior to sleep, the number of apneic episodes increased markedly during those hours.[70] A separate study linked increasing numbers of apneas during a night's sleep with intentional obstruction of the nose.[71] In other species such as the seal, these reflexes enable the animal to dive for extended periods of time. In humans, however, these reflexes appear to have no positive role in day-to-day living. Some investigators even suggest that they are dangerous to our well-being and may be etiologic in sudden crib deaths and the "sniffing deaths" associated with the inhalation of airplane glues.[65]

MUCOUS MEMBRANE FUNCTION: BLOOD VESSELS

To perform its previously described functions, the nose utilizes a complex system of blood vessels to maintain normal resistance. Three types of blood vessels are found here. The first are the small arteries and arterioles that make up the resistance vessels. The second are the fenestrated capillaries that function in the transport of high molecular weight solutes through the mucosa as exchange vessels. The last are the sinusoidal vessels—arteriovenous shunts that act to regulate the blood flow into different parts of the nose. Their basic function is that of a capacitance vessel. When stimulated by a sympathetic discharge, these sinusoidal vessels shunt the flow of blood into the capillary beds of the mucosa.[72] The effect of this shunting is the marked decongestion that is seen when sympathomimetics are sprayed into the nose. It has been shown that the alpha-adrenergic receptor causes this shunting.[73] This seems to be the most important receptor in the vascular control of resistance in the nose. In addition, the effects of hypoxia, hypercapnia, and exercise also are mediated by the alpha-adrenergic receptor.

In the cat model, adrenergic innervation also has been studied with electron microscopy and special stains.[74] The results show that both cholinergic and adrenergic receptors are present in the vascular smooth muscle nerve terminals. However, the preponderance of alpha-adrenergic terminals is in the fenestrated capillaries, whereas the cholinergic terminals are found in the glands of the nasal mucosa. Thus, as expected, sympathetic stimulation of the nose leads to vasoconstriction, while parasympathetic stimulation leads to congestion and production of nasal mucus. This effect of the cholinergic receptors can be blocked by the use of anticholinergic agents such as atropine.[75] This helps explain why antihistamines with their anticholinergic properties are helpful in the treatment of some patients with vasomotor rhinitis.

VASOACTIVE INTESTINAL POLYPEPTIDE

Evidence now points to the presence of a new neurotransmitter that may function in maintaining the resistance of the nose. This polypeptide molecule is known as vasoactive intestinal polypeptide (VIP). It has been shown to cause vasodilation in the nasal mucosa of the cat;[76] this effect is not blocked by atropine like that of the cholinergic receptors. Another study explored the effect of stimulation of the vidian nerve in sympathectomized cats: there was a vasodilatory response that corresponded to the rise in venous plasma VIP from these regions.[77] This response was not affected by the use of atropine to rule out the possibility of cholinergic

interference. Thus, these receptors all function in harmony to allow the nose to maintain the delicate balance of resistance and secretion.

SUBSTANCE P

Another neuropeptide, substance P, has been discovered in the nasal mucosa.[78] The role of this peptide, however, appears to be quite different from that of VIP. It seems to be important in the mediation of pain perception through polymodal pain receptors in the nose. In support of this theory, a number of stimuli, such as chemicals, pressure, infections, and other irritants, have been noted to produce its release from the nasal mucosa. Its effect has been blocked by the action of capsaicin, which desensitizes these receptors in the nose. This may play a role in the mediation of pain associated with nasal diseases. The importance of this substance in the mediation of sinus and nasal pain is only beginning to be discovered and much more research is needed.

DEFENSE MECHANISMS

The nose also functions in protection from airborne contagions as well as the foreign bodies that humans breathe. The most basic of these protective mechanisms is the sneeze reflex, which is stimulated by allergens, local irritants, autonomic discharges, and psychologic input. The most common are noxious, irritating stimuli to the nose.[79] The afferent limb of the sneeze reflex is mediated through the trigeminal pathways as described earlier. The efferent limb involves a complex coordination of the respiratory musculature and sphincters to produce a forceful expulsion of the irritant. Once they are expelled, the nose returns to its normal functions.

The most important role of the nose in defense is performed by the mucociliary blanket. This very complicated system is made up of the cilia of the pseudostratified columnar epithelium and the mucous blanket they propel. There are approximately 50 to 300 cilia on each of these cells, and they measure 8 microns in length by 3 microns in diameter.[80] They function with a two-component motion that propels the mucus through the nose. The first portion of the beat is known as the effective stroke and consists of a quick snapping motion in the direction of the mucous propulsion. The second

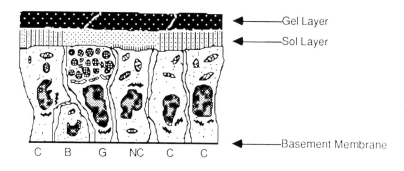

Figure 2–14. Nasal epithelium. *C,* Ciliated pseudostratified columnar cell; *B,* basal cell; *G,* goblet cell (mucous cell); *NC,* nonciliated columnar cell (microvillar).

component is the recovery stroke, which is a slower motion in the opposite direction that does not propel the mucus. The mechanics of ciliary motion have been studied, and the average beat frequency of the cilia in the nose is approximately 14.5 hertz.[81] This action of the cilia results in a mucociliary clearance time through the normal adult nose of 10 minutes.[82] However, a wide variety of factors affect the function of the cilia and mucociliary clearance. The temperature of the system, moisture in the nose, and the pH and viscosity of the mucus all play an essential role in the function of the system.

NASAL MUCUS

The mucous layer in the nose consists of two sheaths (Fig. 2–14). The outer sheath is a highly viscous fluid that rests on top of the cilia. This thick, sticky outer layer is ideal for trapping particulate matter and foreign bodies that enter the nose. The inner layer has a much lower viscosity, which makes it much more suitable for ciliary propulsion. This layer occupies the space between the outer mucous layer and the bottom of the cilia on the cell surfaces. The pH of the mucus is variable, usually in the 5.5 to 6.5 range. The more acidic the mucus, the

more gel-like it becomes, with more alkaline mucus becoming watery.

Nasal mucus is composed of 96 per cent water and 3 to 4 per cent glycoproteins.[83] The source of the mucus is primarily the posterior nose, with the anterior nose being much less significant in production.[84] The average amount of mucus produced every day is 10 to 30 ml per kg, which amounts to 600 to 1800 ml of mucus in a 60-kg individual. Important antibacterial and antiviral substances are also found in the mucus, including specific secretory antibodies (sIgA).[85] These play a key role in preventing the replication of viral particles in the nose. In addition, many nonspecific antibacterial and antiviral substances are present in the nose. Lysozyme, fatty acids, interferon, and other nonspecific enzymes also aid in the prevention of infection through the nose. When all these components are functioning properly, the health of the nose as well as that of the body is maintained.

The cilia of the nose prevent infection by continuously sweeping the trapped debris of the mucous blanket into the alimentary tract. Normally the cilia beat at a rate of 11.2 hertz and propel nasal mucus without difficulty.[86] This activity is easily assessed with a computed microphotometry system and is reported as a histogram of the beat spectrum (Fig. 2–15).

Figure 2–15. A normal cilia study. Mean frequency, 10.8 Hz.

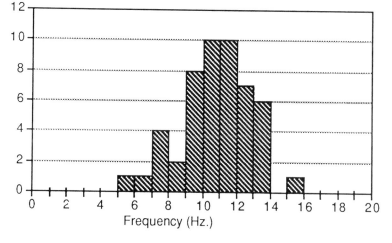

However, the cilia are subject to dysfunction from a wide variety of environmental toxins. It has been demonstrated in vitro that the effect of both *Pseudomonas aeruginosa* bacteria, *Haemophilus influenzae* bacteria, and their filtered supernatants have a cilioinhibitory effect when mixed with the cilia.[87] In a similar study it was shown that *H. influenzae* bacteria do indeed slow the activity of cilia but certain other bacteria, such as *Streptococcus pneumoniae* and *Branhamella catarrhalis*, do not impede ciliary function.[88] This suggests that some bacteria may be pathogenic, in part due to their ability to inhibit cilia. In addition, many noninfectious agents also have a cilioinhibitory effect. General anesthesia,[89] lidocaine in high doses,[90] and flunisolide[91] all have been shown to have a negative effect on the action of cilia. Tobacco does not decrease the ciliary beat frequency, though it does decrease the mucociliary transit time.[92] This is thought to be secondary to loss of the total number of ciliated cells owing to the toxicity of the smoke. The effect of many other toxins, as well as nasal medications, remains unknown.

PARANASAL SINUS FUNCTION

Perhaps the most puzzling area of the nose is its accessory sinuses. These organs have no clear-cut role, though many functions have been suggested. Some suggestions include respiration, vocalization, olfaction, and stasis; as thermal regulation and as dead space.[93] These enigmatic structures may exist to act as surge tanks similar to those of an automobile's hydraulic braking system, dampening the pressure surge in the nose during the act of breathing.[94] The change in the maxillary intrasinus pressure actually has been recorded during the respiratory cycle.[95, 96] Thus the theorized function of these surge tanks is to prevent the development of high pressures. The average PO_2 in the maxillary sinus is 117 mm Hg, with a patent natural ostia. However, obstruction of the ostia leads to a decrease in this value to 88 mm Hg.[97] When maxillary sinusitis is present, this level falls even further, to 75 mm Hg, which has prompted some to theorize that the low level may be in part the cause for the pain associated with acute sinusitis.[95] Unfortunately, no other clear-cut evidence has been presented to define the exact function of the paranasal sinuses.

References

1. Cottle MH: Concepts of nasal physiology as related to corrective nasal surgery. Arch Otolaryngol 72:27–36, 1960.
2. Naumann HH: On the physiology of the nasal cavity. *In* Conley J, Dickinson JT (eds): Plastic and Reconstructive Surgery of the Face and Neck. Proceedings of the First International Symposium. Vol 1: Aesthetic Surgery. New York, Grune & Stratton, 1983.
3. Dawes JDK, Prichard MML: Studies on the vascular arrangement of the nose. J Anat 87:311–322, 1953.
4. Proctor DF: Nasal physiology and defense of the lungs. Am Rev Respir Dis 115:97–129, 1977.
5. Niinimaa V, Cole P, Minz S, Shepard RJ: Oronasal distribution of respiratory airflow. Respir Physiol 43:69–75, 1981.
6. Mink PJ: Le nez comme voie respiratoire. Presse Otolaryngol (Belg) 481–496, 1903.
6a. Kasperbauer JL, Kern EB: Nasal valve physiology. Otolaryngol Clin North Am 20(4):699–719, 1987.
7. Haight JS, Cole P: The site and function of the nasal valve. Laryngoscope 93:49–55, 1983.
8. Bridger GP: Physiology of the nasal valve. Arch Otolaryngol 92:543–553, 1970.
9. Bridger GP, Proctor DR: Maximal nasal inspiratory flow and nasal resistance. Ann Otolaryngol 79:481–489, 1970.
10. Van Dischoeck HAE: Inspiratory nasal resistance. Acta Otol 30:431–439, 1942.
11. Van Dischoeck HAE: The part of the nasal valve in total nasal resistance. Rhinology 3:19–26, 1965.
12. Strohl KP, O'Cain CF, Slutsky AS: Alae nasi activation and nasal resistance in healthy subjects. J Appl Physiol 52:1432–1437, 1982.
13. Carlo WA, Martin RJ, Bruce EN, Strohl KP, Fanaroff AA: Ala nasi activation (nasal flaring) decreases nasal resistance in preterm infants. Pediatrics 72:338–343, 1983.
14. Brancatisano TP, Dodd DS, Engel LA: Respiratory physiology. 64:177–189, 1986.
15. Hair CE, Fischer MD, Preslar MJ: Humidification of air by nasal mucosa. Laryngoscope 79:375–381, 1969.
16. Cole P: Nasal turbinate function. Can J Otolaryngol 2:259–262, 1973.
17. Dewit G: The function of the nose in the aerodynamics of respiration. Rhinology 1:59–67, 1963.
18. Rohrer, Fritz Arch. F. D. ger Physiology #162 Oct. 1915.
19. Syabbalo NC, Bundgaard A, Entholm P, Schmidt A, Widdicombe JG: Measurement and regulation of nasal airflow resistance in man. Rhinology 24:87–101, 1986.
20. McCaffrey TV: Physiologic control of nasal airway resistance. Thesis to the Triologic Society, Sept 1987. Submitted for publication.
21. Mertz JS, McCaffrey TV, Kern EB: Role of nasal airway in regulation of airway resistance during hypercapnia and exercise. Otolaryngol Head Neck Surg 92:302–307, 1984.
22. Togawa K, Konno A, Hohino T, Nishihira S, Okamoto Y: Respiratory function during physical exercise in normal and obstructed noses. Arch Otol-Rhinol-Laryngol 232:1–10, 1981.
23. Olson LG, Strohl KP: The response of the nasal airway to exercise. Am Rev Respir Dis 135:356–359, 1987.
24. Syabbalo NC, Bundgaard A, Widdicombe JG: Effects of exercise on nasal airflow resistance in healthy subjects and in patients with asthma and rhinitis. Bull Eur Physiopathol 21:507–513, 1985.
25. Juto JE, Lundberg C: Methods for standardization of

nasal mucosal decongestion in man. Rhinology 21:361–368, 1983.

26. Robinson RW, White DP, Zwillich CW: Moderate alcohol ingestion increases upper airway resistance in normal subjects. Ann Otolaryngol 79:481–489, 1970.

27. McClean JA, Mathews KP, Solomon WR, Brayton PR, Bayne NK: Effect of ammonia on nasal resistance on atopic and non-atopic subjects. Ann Otol Rhinol Laryngol 88:228–234, 1979.

28. Haight JS, Cole P: Unilateral nasal resistance and asymmetrical body pressure. J Otolaryngol (Suppl) 16:1–31, 1986.

29. Taylor M: An experimental study of the influence of the endocrine system on nasal respiratory mucosa. J Laryngol 75:972–977, 1961.

30. Proetz AW: Further observations of the effects of thyroid insufficiency on the nasal mucosa. Laryngoscope 60:627–633, 1950.

31. Kern EB, Arbour P: The phenomenon of paradoxical nasal obstruction. Arch Otolaryngol 102:669–671, 1976.

32. Burrow A, Eccles R, Jones AS: The effect of camphor, eucalyptus, and menthol vapor on nasal resistance to airflow and nasal sensation. Acta Otol (Stockh) 96(1–2):157–161, 1983.

33. Jones AS, Lancer JM, Shone G, Stevens JC: The effect of lidocaine on nasal resistance and nasal sensation of airflow. Acta Otol (Stock) 101(3–4):328–30, 1986.

34. Pallanch JF, McCaffrey TV, Kern EB: Normal nasal resistance. Otolaryngol Head Neck Surg 93:778, 1985.

35. McCaffrey TV, Kern EB: Rhinomanometry. Facial Plastic Surg 3:4, 1986.

36. McCaffrey TV, Kern EB: Clinical evaluation of nasal obstruction. Arch Otol 105:542–545, 1979.

37. Connell JT: Reciprocal nasal congestion-decongestion reflex. Trans Am Acad Ophthalmol Otolaryngol 72:422–426, 1968.

38. Heetderks DR: Observations on the reactions of the normal nasal mucous membrane. Am J Med Sci 174:231–244, 1927.

39. Keunig J: Le cycle nasal. Int Rhinol 1:57, 1963.

40. Lillie HI: Some practical considerations of the physiology of the upper respiratory tract. J Iowa Med Soc 13:403–408, 1923.

41. Stoksted P: Rhythm of the turbinates. Rhinology 8:28–36, 1970.

42. Stoksted P: Rhinomanometric measurements for determination of the nasal cycle. Acta Otolaryngol(Suppl) 109:159–175, 1952.

43. Hasegawa M, Kern EB: The human nasal cycle. Mayo Clin Proc 52:28–34, 1977.

44. Williams HL: The history of rhinomanometry in North America. Rhinology 6:34–49, 1968.

45. Williams HL: A reconsideration of the relation of the mechanics of nasal airflow to the function of the nose in respiration. Rhinology 10:145–161, 1972.

46. Cole P, Haight JS: Posture and the nasal cycle. Ann Otol Rhinol Laryngol 95:233–237, 1986.

47. Havas TE, Cole P, Gullane PJ, Kassel R, Kamino D: The nasal cycle after laryngectomy. Acta Otol (Stockh) 103:11–16, 1987.

48. Kern EB: The non-cycle nose. Rhinology 19:59–74, 1981.

49. Jafek BW: Ultrastructure of human nasal mucosa. Laryngoscope 93:1576, 1983.

50. Allison AC, Warwick PTT: Quantitative observations of the olfactory system in the rabbit. Brain 72:186, 1949.

51. Graziadei PPC: Cell dynamics in olfactory mucosa. In The Ultrastructure of Sensory Organs. New York, Elsevier North-Holland Inc, 1986.

52. Moncrief RW: The chemical senses. London, Leonard Hill, 1967.

53. Beets MGJ: Olfactory response and molecular structure. In Beidler LM: Handbook of Sensory Physiology. Vol 4: Chemical Senses; Part 1: Olfaction.

54. Beets MGJ: Odor and stimulant structure. In Carterette EC and Friedman MP: Handbook of Perception. 2nd ed. Vol 6a: Tasting and Smelling. New York, Academic Press, 1978, pp 245–255.

55. Mozell DG: Electrophysiology of the olfactory system. Ann NY Acad Sci 116:380–428, 1964.

56. Laffort P, Patte F, Etcheto M: Olfactory coding on the basis of physiochemical properties. Ann NY Acad Sci 237:193–208, 1974.

57. Wright RH: Odor and molecular vibration, I–II. J Appl Chem 27:611, 1954.

58. Suzuki N: Effects of different ionic environments on the responses of single olfactory receptors in the lamprey. Comp Biochem Phys 61:461, 1978.

59. Takagi SF, Wyse FA, Kitamura H, Ito K: The roles of sodium and potassium ions in the generation of the electroolfactogram. J Gen Phys 51:552, 1968.

60. Cabanac M: Physiological role of pleasure. Science 173:1103, 1971.

61. Mower GD, Mair RG, Engen T: Influence of internal factors on the perceived intensity and pleasantness of olfactory and gustatory stimuli. In The Chemical Senses and Nutrition. New York, Academic Press, 1977.

62. Stuvier M: Biophysics of the sense of smell. Doctoral dissertation. Groningen, The Netherlands, Rijks University, 1958.

63. Zwardemaker H: Die psychologie des gerchs. Leipzig, Engelman, 1895.

64. Baylin F, Moulton DG: Adaptation and cross-adaptation to odor stimulation of olfactory receptors in the tiger salamander. J Gen Physiol 74:37, 1979.

65. Allison DJ: Dangerous reflexes of the nose. Lancet 2:909, 1977.

66. Ogura JH: Physiological relationships of the upper and lower airways. Ann Otol Rhinol Laryngol 79:495–498, 1970.

67. Ogura JH, Nelson JR, Dammkoehler R, et al: Experimental observations of the relationships between upper airway obstruction and primary function. Ann Otol Rhinol Laryngol 73:381–403, 1964.

68. Whicker JH, Kern EB: The nasopulmonary reflex in the awake animal. Ann Otol Rhinol Laryngol 82:355, 1973.

69. Wyllie JW III, Kern EB, O'Brien PC, Hyatt RE: Alteration of pulmonary function associated with artificial nasal obstruction. Surg Forum, Vol XXVII, 1976.

70. White DP, Cadieux RJ, Lombard RM, Bixler EO, Kales A, Zwillich CW: The effects of nasal anesthesia on breathing during sleep. Am Rev Respir Dis 132:172–175, 1985.

71. Olsen KD, Kern EB, Westbrook PR: Sleep and breathing disturbance secondary to nasal obstruction. Otolaryngol Head Neck Surg 89:804–810, 1981.

72. Anggard A: Capillary and shunt blood flow in the nasal mucosa of the cat. Acta Otolaryngol 78:418–422, 1974.

73. Dawes JDK, Prichard MML: Studies on vascular arrangements of the nose. J Anat 87:311–322, 1953.

74. Anggard A, Densert O: Adrenergic innervation of the nasal mucosa in cats. Acta Otol 87:232–241, 1974.

75. Anggard A: Parasympathetic control of blood circulation and secretion in the nasal mucosa. Rhinology 13:147–153, 1975.

76. Malm L, Sundler F, Uddman R: Effects of vasoactive intestinal polypeptide (VIP) on resistance and capacitance vessels in the nasal mucosa. In Uddman R (ed): Vasoactive Intestinal Polypeptide Distribution and Possible Role in the Upper Respiratory and Digestive Regions. University of Lund, Lund, Sweden, 1980.

77. Uddman R, Malm L, Fahrenkrug J: VIP increases in nasal blood during stimulation of the vidian nerve. *In* Uddman R (ed): VIP Distribution and Possible Role in the Upper Respiratory and Digestive Regions. University of Lund, Lund, Sweden, 1980.
78. Stammberger H, Wolf G: Headache and sinus disease: The endoscopic approach. Ann Otol Rhinol Laryngol (Suppl 134) 97:Pt. 2, 1988.
79. Stromberg BV: Sneezing: Its physiology and management. ENT Monthly 54:449–453, 1975.
80. Jazbi B, Sayegh FS: Skin and electroscaling and electron microscopy of the nasal mucosa. Otolaryngol Clin North Am 10:167–175, 1977.
81. Low PM, Luk CK, Dulfano MJ, Finch PJ: Ciliary beat frequency of human respiratory tract by different sampling techniques. Am Rev Respir Dis 130:497–498, 1984.
82. Passali D, BianchiniCiampoli M: Normal values of mucociliary transport time in young adults. Int J Pediatr ORL 9:151–156, 1986.
83. Malcolmson KG: Vasomotor activities of the nasal mucous membrane. J Otolaryngol 73:98, 1959.
84. Tos M: Mucous elements in the nose. Rhinology 14:155–162, 1976.
85. Taylor M: The origin and function of nasal mucus. Laryngoscope 84:612–636, 1974.
86. Phillips PP, McCaffrey TV, Kern EB: Measurement of nasal ciliary activity using computerized microphotometry. Otolaryngology H & W Surgery, Oct., 1990.
87. Wilson R, Roberts D, Cole P: Effect of bacterial products on ciliary function in vitro. Thorax 40:125–131, 1985.
88. Ferguson JL, McCaffrey TV, Kern EB, Martin WJ: The effects of sinus bacteria on human ciliated nasal epithelium in vitro. Otolaryngol Head Neck Surg 98:299–304, 1988.
89. Cavaliere F, Schiavello R, Masieri S, Passali D: Mucociliary transport in the nose during general and epidural anesthesia. Acta Anes (Belg) 34:33–39, 1983.
90. Rutland J, Griffin W, Cole PJ: An in vitro model for studying the effects of pharmacological agents on human ciliary beat frequency: The effects of lignocaine. Br J Clin Pharm 13:679–683, 1982.
91. Connell JT: Comparison of saccharin transit times after treatment with beclomethasone and flunisolide. Immunol Allergy Prac 6:58–62, 1984.
92. Stanley PJ, Wilson R, Greenstone MA, Macwilliam A, Cole PJ: Effect of cigarette smoking on nasal mucociliary clearance and ciliary beat frequency. Thorax 41:519–523, 1986.
93. Aust R, Drettner B: Oxygen tension in the human maxillary sinus under normal and pathologic conditions. Acta Otolaryngol 78:264–269, 1974.
94. Williams HL: Nasal physiology. *In* Paparella MM, Shumrick DA (eds): Otolaryngology. Philadelphia, WB Saunders, 1973, pp 329–346.
95. Drettner B: Pressure recordings in the maxillary sinus. Rhinology 3:13–18, 1965.
96. Drettner B: Pressures in the nose and sinuses during breathing. Proceedings of the 9th International Conference on Otorhinolaryngology, Mexico, 1969.
97. Aust R: Measurements of the ostial size and oxygen tension in the maxillary sinus. Rhinology 13:43–44, 1976.

CHAPTER 3

PATHOGENESIS AND TREATMENT OF NASAL POLYPS

Saul Frenkiel, MDCM, FRCS(C)
Peter Small, MDCM, FRCP(C), FACP

The formation of nasal polyps is part of a complex phenomenon manifested by a local mucosal disturbance. Clinically, it is a common disorder resulting in the edematous swelling of mucous membranes into the cavities of the nose and sinuses. Polyps are found in conjunction with a number of systemic diseases, including cystic fibrosis, asthma, and disorders of ciliary motility. They may accompany local conditions such as perennial rhinitis and chronic sinusitis. But despite the awareness of polyps for many centuries, the precise etiologic mechanism continues to be obscure, and treatment methods have remained equally basic.

In the medical sense, the term *polyp* refers to a tumor or growth. The word *polypus* (polypous) itself is of Greek derivation. It can be literally translated to mean "having many feet," and it thus becomes apt terminology for this nasal condition.

Polyps have been well recognized for more than 3000 years, with writings dating back to the Indian scriptures of 1000 B.C. Further accounts are attributed to Hippocrates (460–370 B.C.) and subsequently to the prominent physicians of Arabia.[1] These practitioners developed snarelike instruments for polyp removal and hot irons for cauterization. They also used a variety of odors, herbs, caustics, leaves, and vines to treat patients. Today, we continue to rely on snares, forceps, electrocautery and the everchanging pharmaceuticals.

INCIDENCE

Although the precise incidence in the general population is unknown, nasal polyps are seen frequently in otolaryngology practice and might represent the commonest benign intranasal tumor. Male patients outnumber female patients by a ratio of approximately two to one. They are seen in all age groups, indicative of the chronicity of the disease process and the propensity for recurrence after polypectomy (Fig. 3–1).

Certain conditions are associated with a higher incidence of nasal polyposis. Cystic fibrosis is the commonest cause in children, in which polyps occur in up to 20 per cent of cases.[2] Settipane and Chafee reported a frequency of 2.2 per cent in rhinitis patients and a 6.7 per cent incidence in the asthmatic group.[3] The frequency of nasal polyps in asthmatic patients who are also aspirin intolerant may be as high as 36 per cent, whereas the classic triad of asthma, aspirin sensitivity, and nasal polyps occurs in approximately 8 per cent of all polyp cases.[4, 5] Polyps also can be found in some rare conditions, such as Young's syndrome (sinopulmonary disease, azoospermia, nasal polyps) and Kartagener's syndrome (sinusitis, situs inversus, bronchiectasis).

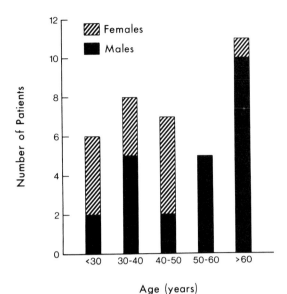

Figure 3–1. Age and sex distribution of patient series with nasal polyps. (From Frenkiel S, Small P, Rochon L, et al: Nasal polyposis—a multidisciplinary study. J Otolaryngol 11:275–278, 1982, with permission.)

THEORIES OF PATHOGENESIS

A number of theories about polyp formation have emerged through the years. Some are of historic interest only, whereas others tend to provide greater insight into the pathogenesis of this lesion. The theories can be divided into those that advocate a primary development and those that attribute polyp formation to be a secondary event.

NEOPLASTIC THEORY

As part of the neoplastic concept, polyps were given the terms *fibromas, fibrous polypi,* or *myxomatous fibroids.* These were differentiated from the usual "mucous polypi" thought to occur more posteriorly in the nose. The connective tissue hypothesis was further strengthened by evidence that certain metabolic processes resulted in accumulation of acid mucopolysaccharides, collagen, and elastic tissue.[6] The fibroblast was thought to be the active cell laying down the excessive ground substance, and this process of polyposis became known as "the polysaccharide nose."[7]

MECHANICAL THEORY

A mechanical theory of polyp formation was prevalent in older writings.[8] It was thought that in a situation of chronic inflammation the normal folds of mucous membrane became edematous and thinned-out, particularly in the ethmoid region where subepithelial tissues were more lax. Progressive mucosal expansion into the nasal chamber resulted from the forces of internal fluid expansion, external dependency, and the effects of gravity. A further sucking-out of weakened ethmoid mucosa into the valve area was thought to be caused by the Bernouilli phenomenon, which states that a negative pressure results when air passes through an area of relative constriction.

VASOMOTOR IMBALANCE

Theories emerged that implicated a vasomotor imbalance or an autonomic dysfunction of the nasal mucosa. The hypothesis was put into perspective by Bumstead and colleagues,[9] who found higher concentrations of biogenic amines (catecholamines, histamine, serotonin) in the stalks of polyps where nerve endings and blood vessels are more abundant. They proposed a model of polyp formation based on alpha-adrenergic receptor activation by vasoactive substances. The polypoid change was therefore caused by a situation of increased vascular permeability, edema, and leakage of fluid and cells into the submucosal tissues.

INFLAMMATORY THEORY

The mechanical and the vasomotor theories incorporate in part the principle of inflammation. Nasal polyposis frequently coexists with conditions such as chronic rhinitis and sinusitis. The inflammatory process is the cause of this hypertrophic mucosa noted within the nose and sinuses. Histologic evidence of phlebitis, lymphangitis, and appropriate cellular infiltrates gives further support for a local inflammatory pathogenesis.

ROLE OF INFECTION

It is thought that polyps of cystic fibrosis or the immotile cilia syndrome may develop from an associated susceptibility to infection. A viral etiology was proposed by work that demonstrated strongly positive complement-fixation tests to polyp antigen.[10] Bacterial cultures of nasal secretions rarely demonstrate pathogenic organisms in polyp patients. By virtue of their location, polyps will obstruct the ostia of sinuses, thus promoting infection as a secondary event. However, antibiotics do not cause polyps to disappear, which casts doubt on the role of infection as a primary factor in pathogenesis.

IMMUNOLOGIC THEORY

An allergic etiology was postulated by Kern and Schenk in 1933,[11] and the thrust of current research is directed toward implicating an IgE-mediated process. Support for the hypersensitivity mechanism comes from finding eosinophilia within nasal secretions of polyp patients and within polyp tissue. Further evidence is based on the presence of degranulating mast cells, increased levels of chemical mediators, and allergen-specific IgE within polyp tissue.

PATHOLOGY

GROSS CHARACTERISTICS

Nasal polyps are frequently bilateral and multiple, and they come in various sizes. They appear as smooth, grayish, glossy lesions hanging from a narrowed stalk (Fig. 3–2). In cases of chronicity, they may assume a reddish or more fleshy appearance, but this should not be mistaken for a hypertrophic or polypoid turbinate. Palpation demonstrates the soft, mobile, and insensitive nature of the polyp. They usually emanate from the middle turbinate, hiatus semilunaris, or mucosa of the ethmoidal air

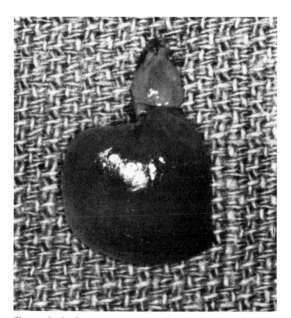

Figure 3–2. Gross appearance of an "edematous" polyp emanating from a narrowed mucosal stalk.

cells. Rarely they can project beyond the anterior nares or descend posteriorly into the choana. By virtue of their location within the middle meatus, they may cause obstruction of sinus ostia. In extreme cases, benign nasal polyposis can expand surrounding bone or cause bony destruction within the nose, sinuses, or orbits.

HISTOLOGY

The polyp surface is commonly of the typical respiratory type. Most sections show the pseudostratified columnar epithelium (Fig. 3–3A), although focal areas of squamous or goblet cell metaplasia and basement membrane thickening may be found (Fig. 3–3B,C). These latter changes indicate chronic irritation, repeated infection, or previous surgery. Polyp stroma contains variable degrees of cellular elements and edema fluid (Fig. 3–3D). There is a lack of blood vessels or nerve endings, except in the connecting stalk.

A traditional concept classified polyps as "allergic," based on eosinophilic predominance, or "inflammatory," related to a lymphoplasmocytic infiltrate. However, histologic studies have been unable to substantiate this concept of an allergic or nonallergic polyp. The eosinophil is the major cell in all specimens (Fig. 3–3E). Plasma cell counts generally mirror the eosinophilia, but in lesser numbers. Other components of the cellular infiltrate include neutrophils, lymphocytes, macrophages, and mast cells (Fig. 3–3F). In contrast, cystic fibrosis polyps have thinner basement membranes and lesser degrees of eosinophilia. Glandular cell hyperplasia with a preponderance of acid mucin within the surface mucous blanket is also found. In the Kartagener's and Young's syndromes, polyps lack the eosinophilia, and the neutrophil becomes the predominant cell.

EXFOLIATE CYTOLOGY

The gamut of cells found within polyps can appear in nasal secretions. The reference level for "significant eosinophilia" means a count of at least 10 per cent in representative samples of the smear. Significant eosinophilia is often found in secretions of both atopic and nonatopic polyp patients. This latter subgroup has been categorized as a syndrome of "eosinophilic nonallergic rhinitis"; patients have an increased incidence of aspirin intolerance and respond more favorably to local steroids.

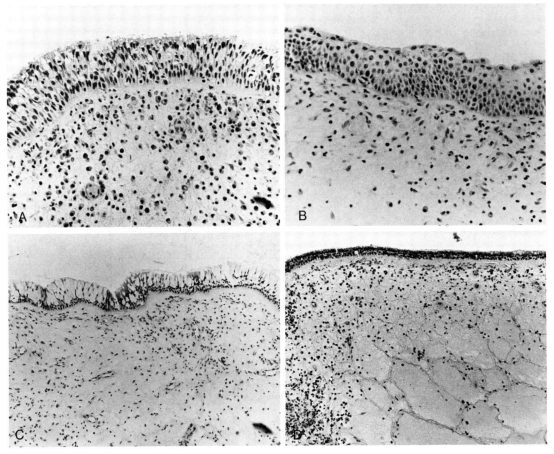

Figure 3–3. Polyp histopathology.
A, Typical respiratory-type surface epithelium of the pseudostratified columnar form.
B, Squamous metaplasia of epithelium.
C, Goblet cell metaplasia of epithelium.
D, Variable degrees of cellular infiltrates and edema fluid within polyp stroma.

ELECTRON MICROSCOPY

Ultrastructure preparations[12–14] reveal a respiratory type of epithelium that is ciliated and contains branching microvilli. These microvilli act to increase surface area but otherwise are of unknown significance. The stroma consists of electron-lucent material composed largely of mucopolysaccharides intertwined within a web of fibroblastic cytoplasmic processes. Free collagen of the immature variety admixed with coarser elastic fibers is an indication of active synthesis by the fibroblasts. Busuttil and colleagues[13] were unable to find ultrastructural evidence of microorganisms within the stroma. The most interesting cellular finding involves mast cell degranulation, a process indicative of the hypersensitivity reaction. Other ultrastructural changes involve swelling of blood vessel endothelial cells with emigration of inflammatory cells.

IMMUNOLOGIC STUDIES

THE HYPERSENSITIVITY MODEL

IgE-mediated reactions have long been considered important in at least a minority of patients with both seasonal or perennial rhinitis and nasal polyps. IgE antibody is produced by plasma cells found mainly at the mucosal surfaces of the nose, lung, and gastrointestinal tract. When stimulated by appropriate allergens, these cells will produce IgE locally, which can then be transported systemically and is found bound to mast cells or basophils throughout the body, in addition to being found in small amounts in the plasma compartment. Cell-bound IgE can interact specifically with allergens, leading to a series of biochemical events that results in production and release of a variety of mediators into the surrounding

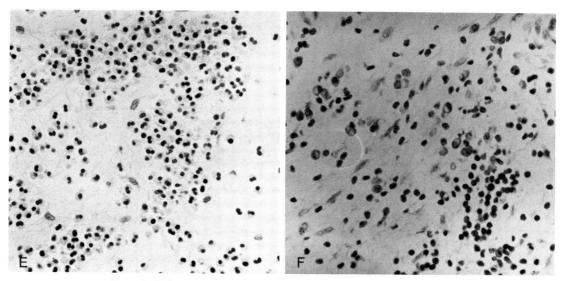

Figure 3–3 *Continued*
E, Numerous eosinophils as the predominant cell type within polyp tissue.
F, Mixture of plasma cells and lymphocytes within polyp.

tissue (Fig. 3–4). This classic early-phase allergic reaction generally occurs within minutes after the interaction between allergen and IgE molecules. The late phase of the allergic response has been documented in the lungs, skin, and nose and actually may be the more important phase of the IgE-mediated reaction clinically. It is marked by a secondary release of mediators from the mast cell in association with inflammatory cells, including lymphocytes,

Figure 3–4. Theoretical model of IgE-mediated mechanism leading to polyp formation.

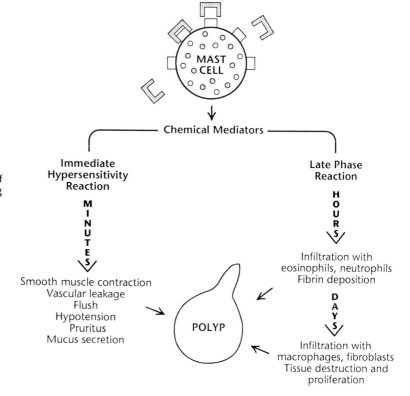

macrophages, and eosinophils. It occurs a number of hours after the early phase and often lasts for 1 or 2 days.

CHEMICAL MEDIATORS

The production and release of chemical mediators are critical in the pathogenesis of an IgE-mediated response. Both the early and late phases of this reaction are marked by a panoply of mediators that can be detected in both the local and systemic environments. These mediators include histamine, serotonin, leukotrienes, norepinephrine, kinins, TAME-esterase, and prostaglandins. Kaliner and colleagues reported the release of these mediators from nasal polyps after IgE sensitization.[15] Others have reported increased amounts of histamine in the nasal polyps, in addition to a variety of immunoglobulins.[9] These data suggest that mast cell releasability may play an important role in the formation of nasal polyps. However, since an IgE-mediated mechanism is only one form of mast cell activation, a number of other factors may have a part. Elevated levels of circulating immune complexes and decreased levels of serum complement have been noted in some patients with nasal polyps.[16] These are alternative ways of activating mast cells other than by IgE-mediated mechanisms.

LOCAL IgE PRODUCTION

It is generally considered that IgE is produced locally in mucosal tissue. Once produced, the antibody is transported throughout the body and can be found in a variety of tissues bound to mast cells or basophils. Based on this theory, skin testing and serum measurements of IgE are considered indicative of the presence of allergen-specific IgE. However, there are studies showing that local production may occur with no detection of these antibodies elsewhere.[17, 18] Some investigators have found higher concentrations of IgE in polyp tissue than in the serum and have demonstrated allergen-specific IgE in polyp sac fluid in the absence of elevated serum values.[19, 20] Despite this information, there is insufficient evidence to support the theory that local production of IgE may be pathogenic in the formation of polyp tissue in patients who do not have detectable IgE elsewhere.

IMMUNOFLUORESCENCE

The various immunoglobulins can be found within polyp tissue. By direct immunofluorescence, significant levels of IgE are demonstrable within most polyps (Fig. 3–5A) in association with lymphocytes and plasma cells.[21, 22] By comparison, there is a paucity of IgE in the surrounding nasal mucosa of polyp patients or within the mucosa of nonpolyp patients. IgA can be found intracellularly, but it is also present on polyp surfaces or within the secretions (Fig. 3–5B). Some polyps may contain significant IgM levels, possibly reflecting the predisposition of these patients to infection. The immunoglobulins IgG and IgD are rarely detected.

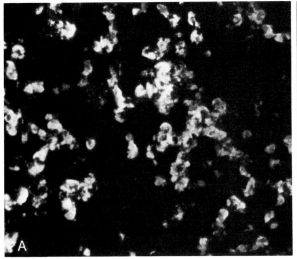 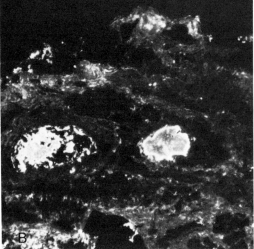

Figure 3–5. Direct immunofluorescence.
A, Significant pattern of IgE within polyp tissue.
B, Concentrations of IgA on polyp surface and within secretions.

ASSOCIATED DISEASES

BRONCHIAL ASTHMA

It is important to recognize that asthma is a common accompanying disease and may occur in approximately 50 per cent of polyp cases.[5, 20] All patients with nasal polyps should have a careful evaluation of their lower airways. Pulmonary function testing is necessary for most polyp patients, and a histamine challenge should be considered in those with suggestive symptomatology but inconclusive pulmonary function tests. Although it has been believed that nasal polypectomy may cause exacerbation of asthma over the long term, current evidence indicates that surgery will not adversely affect the lower airway.[5]

ASPIRIN INTOLERANCE

Although the incidence of severe aspirin intolerance marked by life-threatening bronchospasm is not common, its potential morbidity and mortality make it a serious concern for all patients. Urticaria and angioedema associated with aspirin intolerance are not usual in patients with nasal polyps. Some patients may be aspirin sensitive and develop bronchospasm but may not have detectable polyps. The mechanism of aspirin sensitivity is not well understood, although most evidence suggests a relationship to arachidonic acid metabolism. Aspirin inhibits cyclooxygenase pathway metabolism, and, by inhibiting this pathway, arachidonic acid metabolites may be shunted into the lipoxygenase pathway, leading to increased quantities of leukotrienes. Leukotrienes are known to induce bronchospasm in both animals and humans. This may account for certain patients being sensitive to all forms of nonsteroidal anti-inflammatory agents that have as a common characteristic their ability to inhibit the enzyme prostaglandin synthetase and subsequent prostaglandin formation.

The treatment of aspirin sensitivity is to avoid all nonsteroidal anti-inflammatory agents. Some investigators have attempted to desensitize patients to aspirin by administering small incremental doses beginning with minute amounts of aspirin. This desensitization procedure has been reported to be effective in controlling both asthma and nasal polyps, but it must be considered an experimental treatment at the present time.[23]

THE TRIAD

The triad of nasal polyps, asthma, and aspirin intolerance is an exceedingly important clinical syndrome and should be carefully assessed in all patients with nasal polyps. The relationship is more than casual and has been found to occur in approximately 8 per cent of all polyp cases.[5]

CILIARY DYSKINESIA

Primary ciliary dyskinesia is classically manifested in Kartagener's syndrome, an uncommon genetic condition inherited as an autosomal recessive trait. This syndrome is characterized by bronchiectasis, chronic sinusitis, and situs inversus. The ciliary abnormality usually involves the whole body, including the respiratory tract. The disorder involves an ultrastructural defect in which the dynein arms are missing, and the cilia remain completely immobile.

CYSTIC FIBROSIS

A diagnosis of nasal polyps in a young patient should immediately stimulate a consideration of cystic fibrosis. The basic abnormality involves obstruction of exocrine glands, with stagnation of secretions and distention of the duct system. Chronic sinusitis is often present, and polyps may occur in up to 20 per cent of cases. A sweat chloride test should be performed in such patients.

YOUNG'S SYNDROME

Young's syndrome consists of recurrent respiratory diseases, azoospermia, and nasal polyposis. Patients often have severe chronic sinusitis and associated bronchiectasis. Cystic fibrosis can be excluded because the patients have normal sweat chloride tests and pancreatic function. Their ciliary ultrastructure also is unaltered.

CLINICAL ASSESSMENT

HISTORY

Nasal obstruction, either partial or complete, is the commonest presentation, but its onset may be so gradual as to pass unnoticed by the patient. The obstructive complaints also may be described as a foreign body sensation or a valvelike flapping as air passes through the nose. Other symptoms include nasal congestion, watery rhinorrhea, hyposmia or anosmia, sneezing, itchy eyes, and cough. When present, pain is commonly described as an intranasal sensitivity or a discomfort over the bridge of the nose. Frontal headaches and deep facial pains may also occur. An associated acute rhinosinusitis will augment the pain and possibly cause a purulent rhinorrhea. Asthma, allergy, or both may be present in approximately 50 per cent of all polyp cases. Aspirin sensitivity may occur, and the family history can be positive for atopy. Polyp patients frequently have had previous nasal surgery, and they may have used a variety of vasoconstrictors, contributing to a rhinitis medicamentosa.

PHYSICAL EXAMINATION

Polyps are readily visible by speculum examination. Posterior rhinoscopy, either direct or indirect, may reveal choanal polyps or hypertrophied posterior turbinates. Commonly, a diffusely edematous mucosa with a watery secretion is evident. The inferior turbinates can swell, often assuming a polypoid appearance. The polyps themselves emanate from the middle meatus and ethmoid areas. They are readily mobile and are not painful to palpation. A single pendulous polyp at times may obscure the view of others beyond. Sinus tenderness is not a feature unless there is accompanying infection. When bony expansion is evident, the benign process becomes suspect.

INVESTIGATIONS

The basic immunologic assessment should include skin testing, after stopping antihistamines for at least 48 hours. Blood testing for specific IgE may be necessary in some cases. Providing fresh polyps at the time of surgery may help demonstrate specific IgE within the sac fluid. Nasal cytology to search for eosinophilia is sometimes helpful. Pulmonary function testing is important to exclude the presence of asthma, and children with polyps require a sweat chloride analysis to detect cystic fibrosis. When ciliary dyskinesia is suspected, a mucosal biopsy for ultrastructural analysis may be helpful.

The radiologic workup should include sinus roentgenograms and, occasionally, computed tomography (CT). The plain films can give evidence of diffuse mucosal disease, retention cysts, or air-fluid levels. Bony expansion or destruction, skull base involvement, or orbital pathology might be an indicator of a malignant process, and a CT scan is then essential. Coronal CT cuts would be useful for assessment of the middle meatus if endoscopic surgery is contemplated.

DIFFERENTIAL DIAGNOSIS

CHILDREN

Benign polyps may be confused with a number of childhood nasal masses. In infants, meningoceles or meningomyeloceles may project into the nose through defects in the cribriform plate. Benign neoplasms, such as hemangiomas, or malignancies, such as rhabdomyosarcomas, can appear in children. A diagnosis for consideration in preadolescent males is the juvenile nasopharyngeal angiofibroma, which frequently arises from the nasopharynx but can originate in the nose itself.

ADULTS

A nasal tumor that is unilateral and has a fleshy appearance should raise suspicion of pathology other than benign polyposis. The two important diagnostic considerations are inverting papilloma and squamous cell carcinoma.

ANTROCHOANAL POLYP

This unilateral benign lesion occurs at all ages. It represents a polypoid formation of antral mucosa that projects through the ostium into the middle meatus. Less commonly, the polyp may push through a bony opening in the posteromedial antral wall. Because of space availability or from ciliary flow patterns, the polyp proceeds toward the posterior choana and often descends into the nasopharynx. The flexible nasopharyngoscope is an ideal instrument to confirm the diagnosis. Treatment involves removing the mucosa of origin from within the antrum and subsequent delivery of the polyp through the nose or mouth.

MEDICAL MANAGEMENT

The medical approach to nasal polyps is quite similar to that of both allergic and nonallergic nasal disease. In the management of allergic disease, the three cornerstones of therapy include avoidance, pharmacotherapy, and immunotherapy.

AVOIDANCE

The patient should be instructed to avoid all possible stimuli that may lead to nasal polyp formation or enlargement. Allergic factors, such as dust, animals, and a variety of pollen allergens, can contribute to allergic disease. Other nonspecific factors, such as cigarette smoke, toxins, and a variety of chemical irritants and pollutants, also should be avoided. Patients should be cautioned against using nasal decongestant sprays, which may cause rebound congestion and polyp-like changes in the nasal mucosa.

PHARMACOTHERAPY

Antihistamines. A large number of antihistamines are available to treat both seasonal and perennial rhinitis, in addition to nasal polyps. The common feature of all these agents is that they competitively antagonize the peripheral end-organ effects of histamine. The fact that antihistamines only antagonize one of the many mediators released by mast cells limits their clinical effectiveness. A number of newer antihistamine agents, the H_2-antagonists, are nonsedating and are a more attractive treatment modality.[24] Unfortunately, these are not more effective clinically than the older antihistamines and, therefore, are not a major advancement in the treatment of nasal polyps.

Decongestants. The role of systemic nasal decongestants in the management of nasal polyps is not entirely clear. Topical vasoconstrictive agents should be avoided since there is a possibility of worsening the polyps.

Cromoglycates. Cromoglycates have been used in the treatment of allergic nasal disease for many years. Pathophysiologically, these drugs have an effect on both the early and late response of the IgE-mediated reaction. Therefore, they may be of value in treating nasal polyps, but their efficacy has yet to be demonstrated.

Steroids. Corticosteroids are effective agents in treating all forms of seasonal and perennial rhinitis, in addition to nasal polyps. The action of steroids is to alter the late-phase IgE-mediated reaction causing inhibition of the inflammatory response. Because of potentially dangerous side effects, caution is required, with systemic usage generally reserved for patients with severely obstructed upper airways and an unresponsive bronchospasm. In the solitary lesion or preoperative situation, steroids of low molecular weight may be injected directly into polyps, resulting in temporary shrinkage. Caution is again advised in view of the isolated reports of blindness resulting from similar turbinate injections. The mainstay of medical polyp management is via the topical agents. Local steroid sprays are effective over the long term in shrinking polyps and may help prevent recurrences postoperatively.

IMMUNOTHERAPY

Immunotherapy is effective in treating allergic rhinitis, but this has not been proved for patients with nasal polyps. Although a subpopulation of patients with nasal polyps does have IgE-mediated disease, it would appear that a place exists for immunotherapy. However, double-blind control studies have not been performed in patients with nasal polyps, and therefore it is impossible to recommend immunotherapy for nasal polyps based on data.

SURGICAL TREATMENT

INDICATIONS

Surgical intervention should be reserved for patients with ongoing severe nasal obstruction after medical measures have failed. Polypectomy also may be considered to relieve a conductive anosmia, to control pain from ostial obstruction, or to deal with sinus complications.

POLYP REMOVAL

Polyp removal can be performed with the patient on an ambulatory basis, using agents to provide both local anesthesia and vasoconstriction. Large polyps are best removed with a wire snare tightened gradually about the pedicle and pulled upon slowly so as to avulse a portion of surrounding mucosa. Smaller polyps, or those more posteriorly located, require removal with a biting forceps. It is important to do at least a partial ethmoidectomy in conjunction with the polypectomy. Although slight bleeding may ensue for several hours, a postoperative pack is rarely necessary.

ANCILLARY PROCEDURES

Other procedures may be required, either to facilitate the polypectomy or to deal with associated pathology. For example, a grossly deviated septum or a localized spur may make the polyps inaccessible for instrumentation. It would be judicious to perform a septoplasty as part of the overall surgical treatment, but this should be discussed with the patient first. Surgery to hypertrophied inferior turbinates also may help establish a better nasal airway. Some type of turbinate reduction or electrocauterization would be required in selected cases.

The radiographic assessment might indicate more severe sinus involvement by the polypoid process, in which case a Caldwell-Luc procedure or sphenoidectomy might be considered. The external ethmoidectomy approach is not advised for benign polyposis.

NEWER TECHNIQUES

The techniques of cryosurgery to necrose polyps and the laser, which emulsifies the tissue, can be substituted for the traditional polypectomy. These procedures may avoid some blood loss but are limited in performing an adequate ethmoidectomy. The present trend is toward the use of telescopic instrumentation, which has an advantage in removal of polyps from the middle meatus where they obstruct the sinus ostia. However, caution is required in the case of a repeat polypectomy, when normal anatomic landmarks may be obscured.

References

1. Vancil ME: A historical survey of treatments for nasal polyposis. Laryngoscope 79:435–445, 1969.
2. Tos M, Mogensen C, Thomsen J: Nasal polyps in cystic fibrosis. J Laryngol Otol 91:827–835, 1977.
3. Settipane GA, Chafee FH: Nasal polyps in asthma and rhinitis. J Allergy Clin Immunol 59:17–21, 1977.
4. Settipane GA: Nasal polyps: Epidemiology, pathology, immunology and treatment. Am J Rhinol 1:119–126, 1987.
5. Frenkiel S, Small P, Rochon L, Cohen C, Darragh D, Black M: Nasal polyposis—a multidisciplinary study. J Otolaryngol 11:275–278, 1982.
6. Dolowitz DA, Hecker HC: Hyperplastic respiratory mucosa and nasal polyposis. Ann Allergy 24:555–558, 1966.
7. Smith MP: Dysfunction of carbohydrate metabolism as an element in the set of factors resulting in the polysaccharide nose and nasal polyps. Laryngoscope 81:636–644, 1971.
8. Gleason EB: Manual of Diseases of Nose, Throat and Ear. 4th ed. Philadelphia, WB Saunders, 1920, pp 124–127.
9. Bumstead RM, El-Ackad T, Smith JM, Brody MJ: Histamine, norepinephrine and serotonin content of nasal polyps. Laryngoscope 89:832–843, 1979.
10. Weille F: Further experiments in the viral theory of nasal polyp etiology. Ann Allergy 24:549–551, 1966.
11. Kern RA, Schenck HP: Allergy a constant factor in the etiology of so-called mucous nasal polyps. J Allergy 4:485–497, 1933.
12. Busuttil A, More AR, McSeveney D: Branching microvilli of the nasal respiratory epithelium. Arch Otolaryngol 104:260–262, 1978.
13. Busuttil A, More AR, McSeveney D: Ultrastructure of the stroma of nasal polyps. Arch Otolaryngol 102:589–595, 1976.
14. Drake-Lee AB, Barker THW, Thurley KW: Nasal polyps. J Laryngol Otol 98:285–292, 1984.
15. Kaliner M, Wasserman SI, Austen KF: Immunologic release of chemical mediators from human nasal polyps. N Engl J Med 289:277–281, 1973.
16. Small P, Frenkiel S, Black M: Multifactorial etiology of nasal polyps. Ann Otol Rhinol Laryngol 81:41–58, 1972.
17. Small P, Barrett D, Frenkiel S, Rochon L, Cohen C, Black M: Measurement of antigen-specific IgE in nasal secretions of patients with perennial rhinitis. Ann Allergy 55:68–71, 1985.
18. Huggins KG, Brostoff J: Local production of specific IgE antibodies in allergic rhinitis patients with negative skin tests. Lancet 2:148–150, 1975.
19. Small P, Barrett D, Frenkiel S, Rochon L, Cohen C, Black M: Local specific IgE production in nasal polyps associated with negative skin tests and serum RAST. Ann Allergy 55:736–739, 1985.
20. Frenkiel S, Chagnon F, Small P, Rochon L, Cohen C, Black M: The immunological basis of nasal polyp formation. J Otolaryngol 14:89–91, 1985.
21. Jones E, Frenkiel S, Small P, Rochon L: Immunopathological characteristics of nasal polyps. J Otolaryngol 16:19–22, 1987.
22. Whiteside TL, Rabin BS, Zetterberg J: The presence of IgE on the surface of lymphocytes in nasal polyps. J Allergy Clin Immunol 55:186–194, 1975.
23. Stevenson DD, Pleskow WW, Simon RA, Mathison DA, Lumry WR, Schatz M, Zeiger RS: Aspirin-sensitive rhinosinusitis asthma: A double-blind crossover study of treatment with aspirin. J Allergy Clin Immunol 73:500–507, 1984.
24. Drouin MA: H1 antihistamines: Perspective on the use of conventional and new agents. Ann Allergy 55:747–752, 1985.

CHAPTER 4

RADIOLOGY: BASIC CONCEPTS, CONVENTIONAL FILMS, COMPUTED TOMOGRAPHY AND MAGNETIC RESONANCE IMAGING

Peter M. Som, MD

This chapter presents a working approach to paranasal sinus imaging. It is designed to give the clinician a basis on which the conventional films, computed tomography (CT), and magnetic resonance imaging (MRI) can be analyzed and correlated with the clinical findings. The final aim is to localize and map the pathology accurately and to suggest a diagnosis so that proper treatment planning can be initiated. This approach to film analysis will allow the clinician to know when to utilize CT or MRI, when to suspect hidden pathology, when to question a histologic diagnosis, and how to detect recurrent disease.

PLAIN FILMS

The basic conventional film examination of the paranasal sinuses can vary. Among the projections utilized are posteroanterior (PA), Caldwell, Waters, lateral, submentovertex, and Rhese.[1, 2] The PA view projects the tops of the petrous pyramids at the level of the superior orbital margin (Fig. 4–1). For the Caldwell view, the chin is lifted enough to depress the posteriorly placed petrous pyramids so that they are projected over the lower third of the orbits (Fig. 4–2). The Waters view elevates the chin even more, so that the petrous pyramids are projected just below the maxillary sinuses (Fig. 4–3). The submentovertex projection is essentially a base view looking at the sinuses from below (Fig. 4–4). The lateral projection is a direct lateral view (Fig. 4–5). The Rhese view is an oblique projection similar to an optic canal view (Fig. 4–6); it allows evaluation of the frontal sinuses, the posterior ethmoids, the anterior antral wall, and portions of the orbital floor.

COMPUTED TOMOGRAPHY

The standard CT sinonasal examination is performed in the axial projection, which is essentially a modified base view. The scans are most often taken in a plane parallel to the infraorbital meatal line. Direct coronal scans also can be obtained in some patients by placing them either in a supine hanging head position with a bolus support under the shoulders, or in a prone position with the chin extended. The scan plane often has to be modified from a

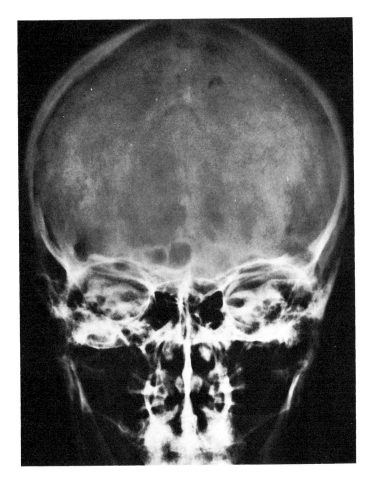

Figure 4–1. Posterior anterior (PA) view. The petrous pyramids are projected through the orbits. Although this projection provides a direct view of the nasal cavity and ethmoid sinuses, the superimposition of the skull base structures limits its usefulness for evaluation of the sinonasal cavities.

Figure 4–2. Caldwell view. The petrous pyramids are projected over the lower orbits. This provides the best plain film view of the ethmoid sinuses, frontal sinuses, and nasal fossae. The maxillary sinuses are obscured. Only the posterior lamina papyracea are seen (arrow).

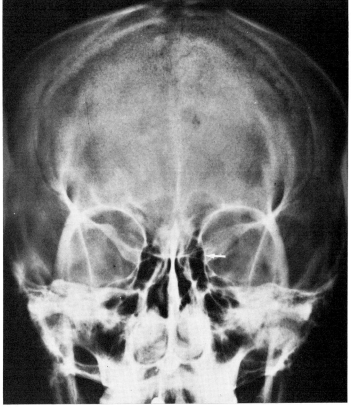

Figure 4–3. Waters view. The petrous pyramids are projected below the maxillary sinuses. This gives the best plain film view of the antra. The infraorbital canal (curved arrow) and the zygomatic recess (straight arrow) are well seen. The anterolateral sinus wall (arrowhead) is the most reliable region to evaluate mucosal thickening.

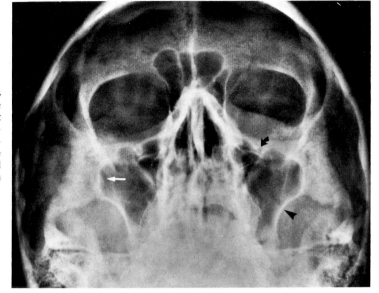

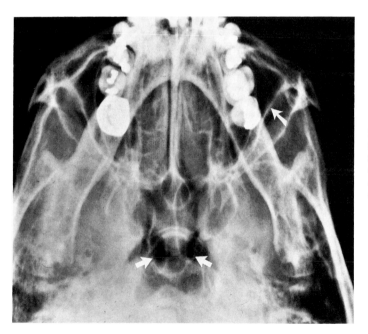

Figure 4–4. Submentovertex view. The slightly curved posterolateral antral wall is seen (angled arrow). The nasal cavity structures are projected on the ethmoid sinus and calvarium, obscuring detail. The sphenoid sinus (short arrows) is partially obscured by the soft palate.

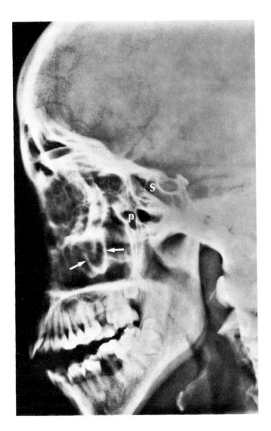

Figure 4–5. Lateral view. The sphenoid sinus (s) is partially obscured by the floor of the middle cranial fossae. The right and left ethmoid and maxillary sinuses are superimposed on each other. The zygomatic antral recesses are each seen as a V-shaped bone line (arrows). The frontal sinuses are only visualized in the midline portion of the sinuses. The pterygoid fossae are also visualized (p).

Figure 4–6. Rhese view. This oblique view shows the optic canal on end (arrowhead). The frontal sinuses (F) are seen and the posterior ethmoid sinuses (E) are partially projected on the opposite ethmoid cells. The anterior antral wall (arrow) and portions of the orbital floor on the opposite side are also seen.

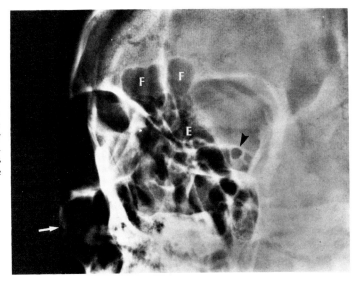

direct coronal plane because of the patient's inability to fully extend the chin or the limitations of the scanner's gantry angles, or because of image degradation artifacts from tooth fillings. As a result, the coronal scans are often modified coronals that are from 60 to 80 degrees off the axial scan plane. The standard examination consists of 5-mm-thick contiguous scans that extend from the top of the frontal sinuses caudally to the maxillary teeth. Coronal scans are usually obtained through the area of interest.[3, 4] If the osteomeatal complex is being studied, coronal thin-section, 1- to 2-mm-thick scans are performed through the area[5] (Fig. 4–7).

If the examination is being used to map inflammatory disease, noncontrast scans can provide this information. However, if the CT scan is being used to differentiate inflammatory disease from tumor, intravenous contrast agents should be utilized. Such postcontrast studies allow variations in contrast accumulation to help distinguish tumor from inflammatory disease, as well as to increase the modality's sensitivity of detecting any intracranial disease extension. The major strength of CT is its ability to directly image the bone and resolve alterations in bone matrix as well as focal areas of fracture or erosion.[3, 4]

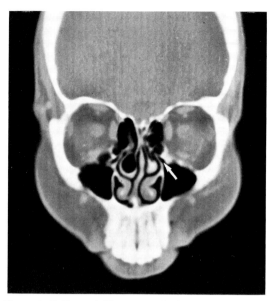

Figure 4–7. Coronal CT scan reveals the maxillary sinuses and on the left, a clear picture of the osteomeatal complex. The arrow lies in the left infundibulum. Incidentally noted is a concha bullosa in the right nasal fossa.

MAGNETIC RESONANCE IMAGING

If MRI is used, the standard examination is performed in a transverse (axial) plane, similar to that used in the CT study. However, MRI scanners also can obtain direct coronal or sagittal scans without having to reposition the patient. This multiplanar ability is a great advantage of MRI and allows better evaluation of such regions as the orbital floor and the floor of the anterior cranial fossa. In addition, the degradation artifacts caused by tooth amalgams produce only a local alteration (black spot) in the scan rather than the more generalized and severe image artifacts found in CT scans. The MRI studies usually are obtained as 5-mm-thick scans with a 1-mm interscan gap.

The complex nature of MRI physics, a discussion of which is beyond the scope of this chapter, allows the imager to alter certain critical variables to produce three basic types of images. The variables are the TR, or time to repetition, and the TE, or time to echo. Most often spin echo (SE) sequences are used, al-

though inversion recovery and short FLIP angle gradient echo pulse sequences are also employed. In the most common SE sequences, if the TR (300 to 700 msec) and TE (20 to 40 msec) are short, the image produced is called T_1-weighted (T_1W). These images have the best resolution and are best for mapping the anatomy. If the TR (1500 to 3500 msec) and TE (80 to 150 msec) are long, the image produced is called T_2W. These images have a poorer signal-to-noise ratio than the T_1W images and thus appear coarser. However, the T_2W studies are the best for detecting inherent differences in tissue MRI characteristics. Thus in general, pathology and normal anatomy, and infection and tumor, are best distinguished on T_2W sequences. If the TR is long and the TE is short, the images are said to be either balanced, mixed, or proton dense. These studies combine some of the better detail of the T_1W studies with some of the tissue specificity of T_2W scans.

Other variables that affect the image quality and scan time include the matrix size, the number of excitations, the number of methods used to suppress flow and motion artifacts, the slice thickness, and the field of view. As each variable is maximized to produce the best possible MRI picture, the examination time increases. As a result, in the practical world, compromises in image quality are often made in order to improve patient put-through time.

In addition, since on MRI the bone is visualized only by its absence of signal, focal bony defects and matrix alterations are poorly, if at all, identified.

The use of paramagnetic contrast agents for extracranial disease is a topic that presently has few significant clinical trials on which to base any solid conclusions. The initial impression with Magnevist gadolinium DTPA is that it may improve the identification of some tumor boundaries, but in the sinonasal cavities it may not provide a significant advantage over the routine SE T_1W and T_2W studies. In addition, Magnevist is an extra expense to the patient, and it may add slightly to the examination time, since both noncontrast and postcontrast studies must be obtained.

ANATOMY

Because the frontal sinuses develop independently from anterior ethmoid cells (see Chapter 1), there usually is some degree of asymmetry between the left and right sides.[7] This may be reflected radiographically as a mild deviation of the intersinus septum to one side, as unilateral hypoplasia or aplasia, or as rare bilateral aplasia. Careful film review can differentiate an absent sinus from a completely clouded or airless sinus. If all the routine paranasal sinus films are studied carefully, some roentgen evidence of a sinus margin will be seen on at least one view when the sinus is present and completely opacified. The key is to identify a portion of the sinus margin. If no sinus margin is seen, the sinus is most probably aplastic, and a CT scan can be performed to verify this impression.

At birth, the frontal sinuses cannot be radiographically identified. By age 4 years, they usually are at a level of one half the vertical height of the orbit. By age 8 years, they have ascended to the level of the superior orbital rim and after age 10 years, they pneumatize the vertical plate of the frontal bone above the orbits.[8] The smaller the sinus, the more difficult it is to evaluate radiographically. Although no general statement can be made concerning the etiology of the sinus size, if bilateral hypoplasia is seen in a young patient age 8 years or older, the possibility of mucoviscidosis should be considered, especially if there is a clinical history of chronic sinusitis.

Regardless of the sinus size, all frontal sinuses share certain common roentgen findings (Fig. 4–8).[1, 9] The first is that they are more radiolucent than the adjacent frontal bone. This is because the adjacent calvarium has bone in its inner table, in its outer table, and in the

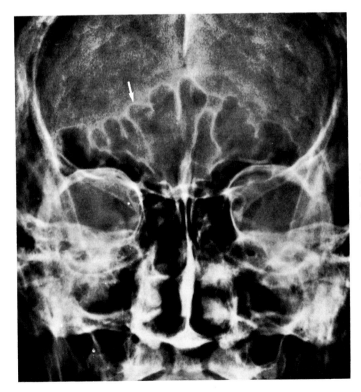

Figure 4–8. Caldwell view. The thin white mucoperiosteal line of the frontal sinus is seen (arrow). Note the scalloped margin and the septae that project into the sinus cavity. The orbital contours are preserved.

diplöe or middle table, whereas the frontal sinus develops in the diplöe, replacing the bone density with the lower radiodensity of mucosa and air. Thus only the inner and outer tables attenuate the x-rays over the sinus cavities, and the sinuses appear radiolucent compared with the adjacent bone. This point cannot be stressed too often, and mild degrees of sinus opacification may be the major plain film findings of frontal sinus disease. Conversely, if the frontal sinus radiodensity is greater than that of the adjacent frontal bone, a bone-producing or fibro-osseous lesion is probably present.

Second, normally a thin white mucoperiosteal line separates the sinus from the adjacent bone. When this line is not seen, deossification from an acute inflammatory process or, rarely, destruction by a tumor may be present. If the thin white line is seen as a thick, unsharp zone of sclerosis, chronic infection has been present.

Third, if the sinuses are moderately well developed, they will have scalloped margins that create septa that can extend well into the sinus cavity. If a mucocele or other slow-growing tumor process is present in the sinus, as it expands it will erode the septa and smooth out the sinus margins. This results in a rounded or ovoid sinus shape, which is abnormal for a moderate-to-large frontal sinus.

If the sinuses are hypoplastic, they never

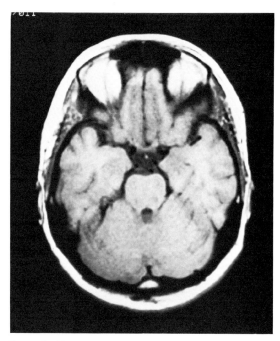

Figure 4–10. Transverse T₁W MRI scan reveals the frontal sinuses to be normal. The bone and the sinus air give little if any signal, so that they are not well distinguished and minimal bone abnormalities can be missed. The intracranial structures are better seen than on CT.

develop the scalloped margins and septa. This makes them more difficult to evaluate radiographically. In addition, the small sinuses contain less air and often appear somewhat clouded when compared with well-developed sinuses.

Fourth, no matter what the sinus size is, it will never violate the adjacent superomedial orbital contour. Any erosion, depression, or flattening of the orbital roundness indicates a frontal sinus process and statistically suggests a mucocele.

Last, the intersinus septum may be far to the left or right at its peripheral sinus margin; however, it almost always lies in the midline at its frontoethmoid base. Thus, deviation of the lower portion of the intersinus septum far to one side suggests that an expansile process is present on the opposite side, even if there is no other radiographic visualization of the process.

Two of the best applications of sectional imaging are the evaluation of the integrity of the curved posterior frontal sinus wall and the detection of any intracranial extension of frontal sinus disease (Figs. 4–9 and 4–10).[3, 10] The routine lateral paranasal sinus plain film only detects the anterior and posterior frontal sinus walls in the midline. The majority of these curved bones are not seen. The axial scan plane best illustrates this area, and CT best visualizes

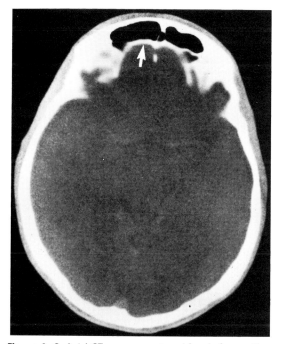

Figure 4–9. Axial CT scan seen at a wide window setting clearly reveals the frontal sinuses. The curved anterior and posterior (arrow) sinus walls are well seen. This is the best CT view to separate the frontal sinuses from the anterior cranial fossae.

the bone. The CT scans should be viewed at wide window settings to detect subtle bone changes best and best distinguish an aplastic sinus from a totally opacified sinus.

If intracranial spread of frontal sinus disease is suspected, MRI is the modality of choice. This reflects the better soft tissue definition when compared with CT. However, a focal fracture or erosion may be visualized only on CT studies. The radiologist can best suggest which modality to use in a specific case after consulation with the clinician.

The ethmoid sinuses are the only sinuses radiographically visualized at birth. There are 3 to 15 cells in each ethmoid, and the posterior cells tend to be larger.[11] The ethmoid complex itself is wider posteriorly near the orbital apex than it is anteriorly near the nose. This results in the medial orbital walls, or ethmoid lamina papyracea, lying obliquely oriented to a direct frontal x-ray beam. Because bone must present an edge en face to the incident radiation beam to be visualized on conventional films, the lamina papyracea is incompletely seen on these films. What appears to be the entire medial orbital wall on a frontal or Caldwell view (see Fig. 4–2) is, in fact, only the most posterior margin of the medial wall. Thus a mucocele or tumor of the middle or anterior ethmoid cells may be difficult or impossible to visualize on conventional films. In addition, on conventional films the ethmoid cells are superimposed on each other in every projection, and this prevents a precise localization of pathology.

Sectional imaging is clearly the best way for evaluating the ethmoid sinuses (Figs. 4–11 through 4–15). Both CT and MRI display the relationship of the ethmoid cells to one another and to the anterior cranial fossa, nasal fossae, sphenoid sinuses, maxillary sinuses, and orbits. In the axial plane, two normal areas may cause diagnostic problems. The first occurs at the caudal ethmoid level where the ovoid or circular-appearing apices of the maxillary sinuses may be confused with ethmoid cells. The second problem occurs at the cranial ethmoid level where the midline structures of the anterior cranial fossa may simulate an upper nasal fossa mass. If the crista galli is visualized in the axial plane, the scan level is cranial to the nasal fossa. This area can be best appreciated on coronal scans.[4]

The maxillary sinuses are affected most often by inflammatory diseases, tumors, and trauma. As such, they always should be carefully scrutinized. Traditionally, the best evaluation by conventional films utilizes the Waters view (see Figs. 4–3 and 4–16). However, only the anterior antral roof and the anterolateral sinus margin can be clearly seen. A small defect in the medial wall can be easily overlooked because the entire medial wall is projected on itself. In

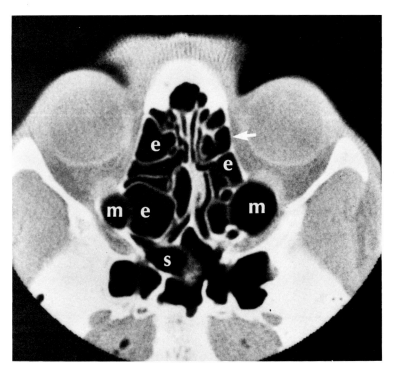

Figure 4–11. Axial CT scan reveals the lamina papyracea (arrow) and ethmoid cells (e) to be well seen. The apices of the maxillary sinuses (m), and the sphenoid sinus (s), are also clearly identified and should not be confused with the ethmoid cells.

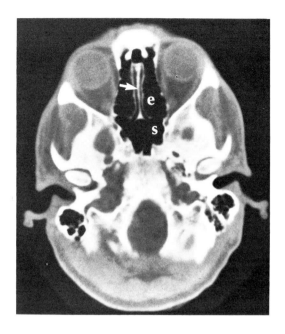

Figure 4–12. Axial CT scan reveals the upper nasal septum (arrow) to be outlined by air in each of the olfactory recesses of the nasal fossae. The ethmoid (e) and sphenoid sinuses (s) are well seen.

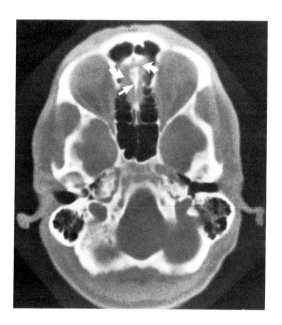

Figure 4–13. Axial CT scan just cephalad to that shown in Figure 4–12. The crista galli (straight arrow) identifies the scan as being intracranial in the midline region and not through the level of the upper nasal fossae. The normal midline soft tissues of the anterior cranial fossae (curved arrows) are seen.

Figure 4–14. Coronal CT scan better reveals the anatomic relationships seen in the axial scan in Figure 4–13. The crista galli (large arrowhead) rests on the cribiform plate (long arrow). The ethmoid (e) sinuses are well seen, as is the nasal septum (N). The cranial margin of the middle turbinate (small arrowheads) is also seen. This projection should be utilized if intracranial extension from sinonasal cavities or orbit is suspected or if extension of an antral tumor into the orbit is considered.

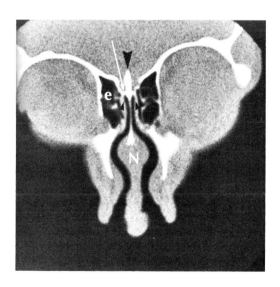

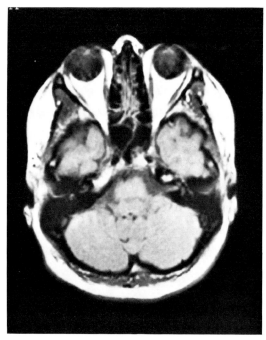

Figure 4–15. Transverse T₁W MRI scan through the ethmoid sinuses reveals the ethmoid and sphenoid sinuses to be well seen. The brighter signal outlining the ethmoid cells is minimal mucosal thickening and not bone, which would give no signal.

addition, the majority of the posterolateral wall is poorly seen on conventional films.

On CT, all the sinus margins are well visualized, and this modality is the best method of evaluating the bony sinus walls (Fig. 4–17).[3, 4, 10] The sinus mucosa and the soft tissues adjacent to the sinuses can be well visualized by either CT or MRI (Figs. 4–18, 4–19, 4–20). Since these soft tissues cannot be properly evaluated on conventional films, imaging must be performed to visualize the presence of any extra sinus disease.[3–5, 10, 12]

Normal sinus mucosa is so thin that it is not seen on plain films, CT, or MRI scans. Only when this mucosa is abnormally thickened can it be visualized on these studies. An often-made mistake on plain films is to diagnose localized antral mucosal thickening in the region of the zygomatic recess. The hazy appearance often seen in the area of this recess is because there is less air and thicker surrounding bone here than in the other portions of the antrum. True mucosal thickening is seen best along the lower lateral antral wall.[4]

When the maxillary sinuses are imaged, a region in the medial antral wall may cause an error in diagnosis. This area is the portion of this wall that is composed only of mucosa. It is just cranial to the inferior turbinate and should not be mistaken for an area of bone erosion on CT or MRI.[13] Comparison with the opposite antrum is the best way of avoiding this error.

The routine plain sinus films occasionally can pose diagnostic problems as adjacent normal structures are projected on the maxillary sinus cavities (Figs. 4–16 and 4–21). These include the infraorbital canals, the superior orbital fissures, the anterior margins of the middle cranial fossae, and the soft tissues of the lip or cheek on frontal films and the mandibular coronoid processes on lateral films.[14–18]

The sphenoid sinuses are truly the "silent" sinuses on conventional films. Regardless of the projection, they are partially obscured by overlying soft tissue structures and the bones of the skull base, sinuses, and calvarium.

Again, only sectional imaging displays the sinus walls, sinus cavity, soft tissues under the skull base, nasopharynx, and the adjacent intracranial structures of the cavernous sinuses, pituitary fossa and anterior and middle cranial fossae (Fig. 4–15 and Figs. 4–22 through 4–26).

Anteriorly, the sphenoid sinus roof is the

Text continued on page 65

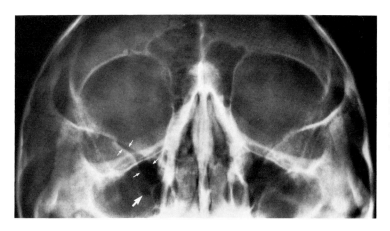

Figure 4–16. Waters view reveals the superior orbital fissures (small arrows) to be projected over the antra and orbital floors. The foramen rotundum (large arrow) is projected in the antra.

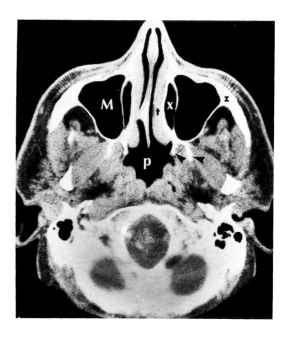

Figure 4–17. Axial CT scan reveals the maxillary sinuses (M), inferior turbinates (t), and meatus (x). The pharynx (p), parapharyngeal space structures, pterygoid plates (arrowheads), and infratemporal fossae are also seen. z = zygoma.

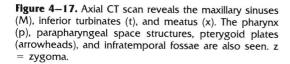

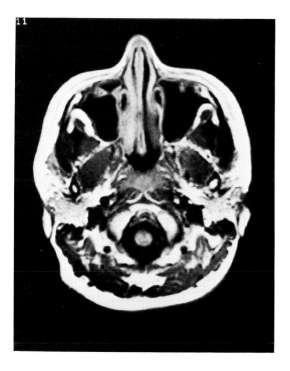

Figure 4–18. Transverse T_1W MRI scan reveals the same anatomy as in Figure 4–17. Note the better definition on magnetic resonance imaging of the muscles and fat planes.

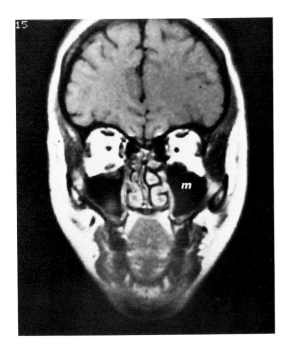

Figure 4–19. Coronal T₁W MRI scan reveals the maxillary sinuses (m) and nicely shows their relationship to the orbits.

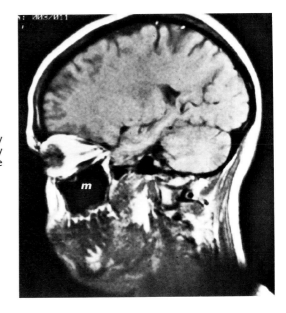

Figure 4–20. Sagittal T₁W MRI scan reveals the maxillary sinus (m), the orbital floor and orbit. This projection is very helpful in evaluating the spread of antral disease into the orbit.

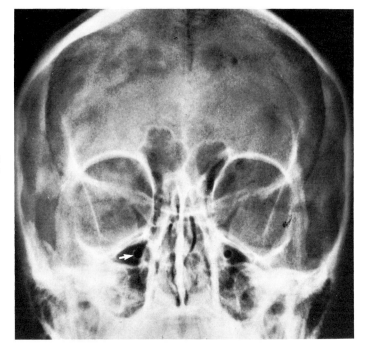

Figure 4–21. Caldwell view reveals the foramen rotundum (arrow) to be projected through the upper medial antrum.

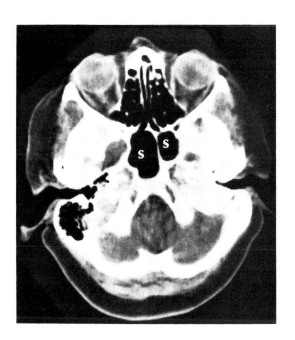

Figure 4–22. Axial CT scan reveals the sphenoid sinuses (s) and nicely displays their relationship to the remaining skull base and ethmoid sinuses.

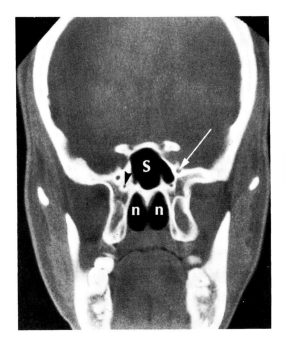

Figure 4–23. Coronal CT scan reveals the sphenoid sinus (S) and its relationship to the anterior cranial fossa above, the orbital apex anteriorly, and the posterior nasal fossae (n). The foramen rotundum (long arrow) and vidian canal (arrowhead) are also well seen.

Figure 4–24. Coronal CT scan posterior to that shown in Figure 4–23 reveals the sphenoid sinus (S) and its relationship to the sella turcica superiorly, the cavernous sinuses (c) laterally, and the roof of the nasopharynx (N) inferiorly.

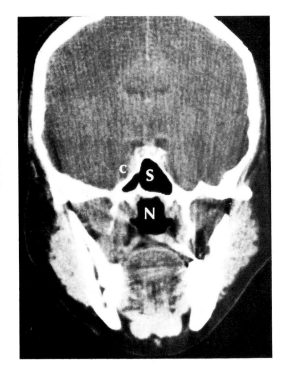

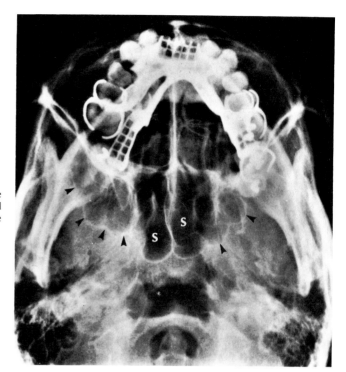

Figure 4–25. Submentovertex view reveals the main sphenoid sinus cavities *(S)* and the lateral recesses that are pneumatizing the floor of the middle cranial fossae *(arrowheads).*

planum sphenoidale, which separates the sinus from the anterior cranial fossa. The lateral walls are in relationship to the orbital apices, and the sinus floor relates to the posterior nares. More posteriorly, the sinus roof is the floor of the sella turcica, and the lateral walls relate to the cavernous sinuses. The floor is the roof of the nasopharynx.

About one half of the sphenoid sinuses have lateral recesses.[19] These can extend into the lesser sphenoid wings as pneumatization of the anterior clinoid processes, into the greater sphenoid wings, either in the floor of the middle cranial fossae or the posterior orbital walls, or down into the pterygoid processes. Each of these areas has a classic roentgen appearance, and familiarity with them will avoid needless confusion with suspected pathology.

PATHOLOGY

The most common diseases that involve the sinonasal cavities are inflammatory in nature. Whether bacterial, viral, or allergic in etiology, these diseases share the common findings of submucosal edema and increased sinonasal secretions. Because the interstitial fluids and secretions are composed primarily of water, these inflammatory diseases are characterized on MRI by the signal intensities of water, which are a low (dark) T_1W signal intensity and a high (bright) T_2W signal intensity. This is the most accurate way of establishing the inflammatory nature of the processes[12] (Fig. 4–27).

On CT, the thickened mucosa (which will enhance on postcontrast scans in a patient with active infection) and submucosal edema can be seen. On plain films only the thickened mucosa is appreciated[3, 4] (Figs. 4–28 and 4–29).

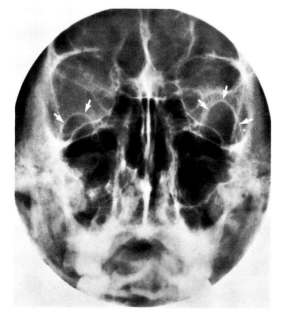

Figure 4–26. Modified Waters view reveals bilateral sphenoid sinus recesses *(arrows)* in the greater sphenoid wings in the posterior orbital walls.

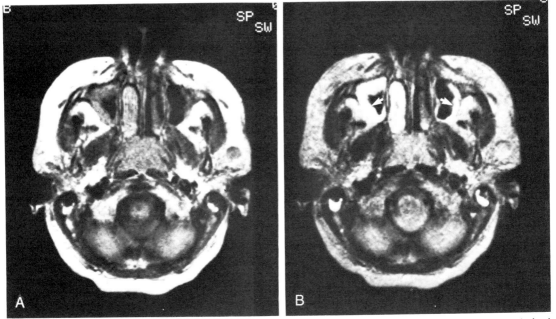

Figure 4–27. Transverse spin echo mixed image *(A)* and T$_2$W image *(B)* MRI scans reveal mucosal thickening in both maxillary sinuses (arrows). In (A), the signal intensity is low-to-intermediate while in (B) it is bright (high). These findings indicate inflammatory tissue.

The mucosal disease can vary from focal mucosal thickening to diffuse polypoid mucosal thickening to obliteration of the sinus cavity by a varying combination of thickened mucosa and entrapped secretions.

It must be noted that the mere presence of minimal mucosal thickening does not necessarily mean that these changes are responsible for the patient's complaints, since such mucosal thickening may represent acute, subacute, chronic, or fibrotic changes. It is the postcontrast CT enhancement and the MRI signal intensities that help differentiate these conditions.

The bacterial diseases develop secondary to the obstruction of a sinus ostium. Thus, they tend initially to involve only one sinus (usually the antrum) or only adjacent unilateral sinuses (Fig. 4–30). Pansinusitis can occur but is usually a latter stage in the disease evolution. By comparison, allergic disease is a systemic process and tends initially to cause mucosal disease in all the sinonasal cavities[1] (Fig. 4–31).

A pansinusitis with swelling of the nasal turbinates and associated nasal polyposis most often suggests an allergic process; however, allergy and infection can coexist so that their distinction is often a moot academic point.

Air-fluid levels are rarely seen in allergic disease. The presence of an air-fluid level most often suggests an acute bacterial sinusitis. If plain films are made, the patient must be erect

to allow visualization of the air-fluid level (Fig. 4–32). If the patient is either supine or prone, the fluid will layer out along the dependent wall and the sinus will look uniformly opaque on the x-ray film. On CT and MRI, the air-fluid levels are imaged directly because the patient is usually supine and the scan plane is axial (Figs. 4–33 and 4–34).

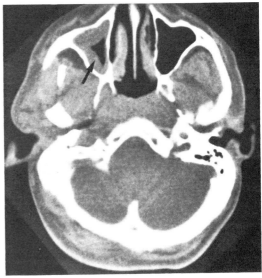

Figure 4–28. Axial noncontrast CT scan reveals uniform mucosal thickening in the right antrum (arrow). There is no bone destruction. These are the typical CT findings of inflammatory disease.

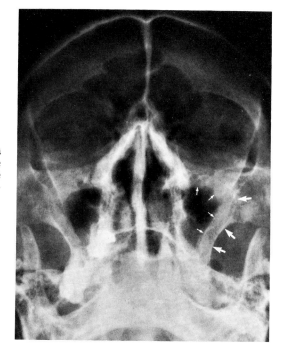

Figure 4–29. Waters view reveals thickened antral mucosa lying between the sinus bony margin (large arrows) and the sinus air (small arrows). Similar changes are present in the right antrum. These are typical plain film findings of inflammatory disease.

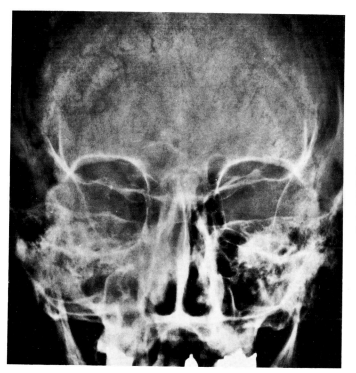

Figure 4–30. Caldwell view reveals opacification of the right frontal, ethmoid, and maxillary sinuses. There are also increased soft tissues in the right nasal cavity. The left-sided sinuses and nasal fossa are normal. This appearance is suggestive more of bacterial sinusitis (with or without a nasal mass) than it is of allergic disease.

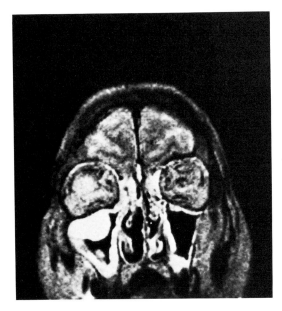

Figure 4–31. Coronal T$_2$W MRI scan reveals bilateral mucosal inflammatory disease in the ethmoid and maxillary sinuses. This appearance is consistent with either a panbacterial sinusitis or allergic disease.

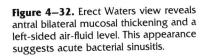

Figure 4–32. Erect Waters view reveals antral bilateral mucosal thickening and a left-sided air-fluid level. This appearance suggests acute bacterial sinusitis.

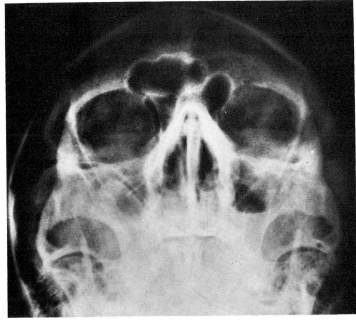

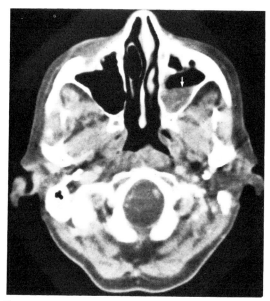

Figure 4–33. Axial CT scan reveals an air-fluid level in the left antrum (arrow).

The most common cause of an air-fluid level is acute bacterial sinusitis. The second most common cause is the result of antral lavage. At least 3 to 4 days are required after an antral washing for the saline to drain from the sinus. Any roentgenogram taken within that 3- to 4-

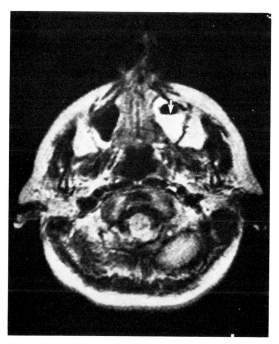

Figure 4–34. Transverse T_2W MRI scan reveals a left antral air-fluid level (arrow) with some mucosal thickening.

day period probably will reveal an air-saline level and not give the therapeutic follow-up information that the clinician wants. It is safest to obtain the postlavage film about 1 week after the procedure. Other causes of air-fluid levels include trauma, with or without an associated sinus wall fracture; barotrauma; and blood dyscrasias, such as von Willebrand's disease, which tend to bleed at mucosal surfaces.[4]

The plain film finding of a totally opacified antrum in a patient who has signs and symptoms of an acute upper respiratory infection most often reflects only the presence of mucosal thickening and entrapped secretions (Fig. 4–35).

With conservative medical treatment, most patients clinically improve within several days, and the assumption is that the opacified antrum also will clear on routine films. However, only 80 per cent of such sinuses actually have improved on follow-up studies. In the remaining 20 per cent of the patients, some underlying sinus disease is present that causes the sinus to remain opacified.[20] In such cases, sectional imaging should be performed to identify this pathology. The differential diagnosis of these lesions includes a large retention cyst or polyp, an antrochoanal polyp, a mucocele, an obstructing nasal mass, or rarely a tumor. All these conditions require sectional imaging for mapping and surgery for attempted cure. This approach can avoid unnecessary recurrent episodes of acute infection and clinical delays in resolving the underlying pathology. This is especially important if a tumor is present.

Since both retention cysts and polyps are filled with fluid (water), they have the T_1 and T_2 MRI signal characteristics of inflammation: namely, low T_1W and high T_2W signal intensities[12] (Fig. 4–36). On CT, only the polypoid configuration of the masses can be identified, and their attenuation (density) can vary from that of mucoid secretions (less than muscle, but higher than fat) to that of muscle (Fig. 4–37). It must be noted that the mere presence of a small retention cyst or polyp does not necessarily mean that it is related to the patient's complaints. Such cysts or polyps are seen as incidental findings on paranasal sinus examinations in 10 per cent of people.[21]

If the sinus is expanded, a mucocele is most probably present, since this is the most common expansile process of any paranasal sinus[22, 23] (Fig. 4–38). Most mucoceles have a mucoid attenuation on CT and the signal intensities of water on MRI. However, if the mucocele has been present long enough, the mucous glycoproteins become concentrated, the free water

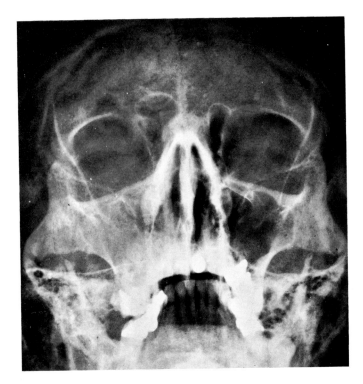

Figure 4–35. Erect Waters view reveals an airless, completely opacified right antrum. If this appearance remains 1 to 2 weeks after symptoms have resolved, imaging should be performed.

is absorbed, and the MRI signal characteristics can vary (Fig. 4–39). The T_1W signal becomes progressively brighter while the T_2W signal remains bright. Eventually, if the secretions become desiccated, both the T_1W and T_2W signals are dark. Thus, the varied MRI appearance of a mucocele can roughly date where in the evolution of this process the secretions are.

The response of bone to an adjacent lesion can provide information about the nature of the

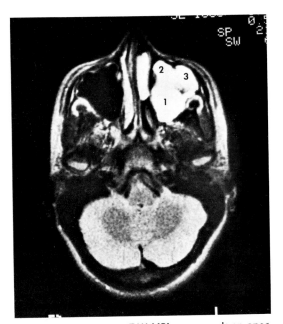

Figure 4–36. Transverse T_2W MRI scan reveals an opacified left antrum that is filled with at least three (1,2,3,) distinct polyps or retention cysts. The high T_2W signal suggests the presence of an inflammatory process.

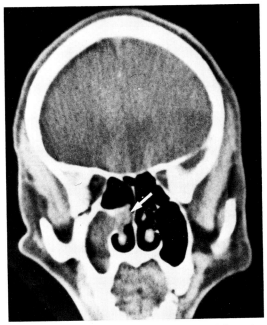

Figure 4–37. Coronal CT scan reveals a right antrochoanal polyp that fills the sinus cavity and extends into the nasal cavity (arrow).

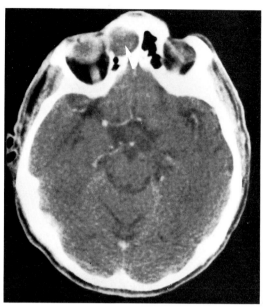

Figure 4–38. Axial postcontrast CT scan reveals an expansile right frontal sinus mass *(arrow)*. This mass has an attenuation between that of muscle and that of fat and has the typical CT appearance of a mucocele.

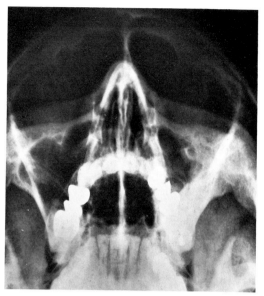

Figure 4–40. Waters view reveals a thickened, sclerotic left lateral antral wall and sinus roof. Some reaction also extends into the zygoma. This represents the bony response to chronic sinusitis and can be seen with or without the presence of coexistent active infection.

pathologic process. Primarily, three types of changes can occur in the bones of the sinonasal area. First, they can become thickened and sclerotic; second, they can be aggressively destroyed; and third, they can be remodeled or displaced away from the lesion. In certain instances, various combinations of these responses occur. The roentgen analysis of these changes often can suggest the diagnosis.

Thickened, dense, or sclerotic bone almost always indicates that chronic infection has been present. It does not reveal whether or not active infection is coexistent. This type of bony response often can be seen in the margins of the frontal sinuses or in the walls of the sphenoid or maxillary sinuses (Figs. 4–40 and 4–41).

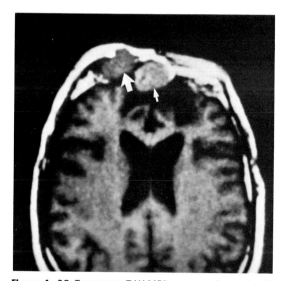

Figure 4–39. Transverse T_1W MRI scan reveals two frontal mucoceles *(arrows)* in this patient who had prior severe frontal trauma. One mucocele has a low signal intensity *(larger arrow)* while the other has an intermediate signal intensity.

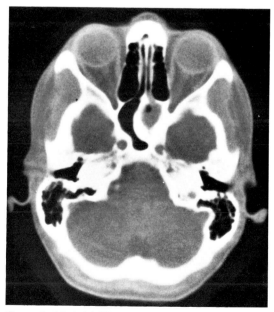

Figure 4–41. Axial CT scan reveals soft tissue disease in the left sphenoid sinus, with thickened and sclerotic bone surrounding this sinus. This CT appearance represents the response to a chronic infection, which in this patient was caused by aspergillosis.

MRI can identify the presence of any related inflammatory disease, as previously described, but may be unable to detect any subtle bony changes.

Rarely, an anaplastic carcinoma can cause a sclerotic bone response. However, the MRI appearance of the carcinoma is different from that of the inflammatory diseases; the carcinoma has low-to-intermediate signal intensities on all imaging sequences.

A thickened, sclerotic bone also can occur in response to prior irradiation. This may, in fact, reflect a low-grade osteitis.

In the walls of the sphenoid or rarely the ethmoid sinuses, a hyperostotic bone reaction occasionally can be seen in response to an adjacent intracranial meningioma. Contrast-enhanced CT scans and MRI scans will detect the size and precise location of these tumors.

Dense and thickened bone also can be seen in both fibrous dysplasia and ossifying fibroma, which can affect any of the facial bones. This bone reponse, however, is different from that of the chronic infections. The fibro-osseous lesions expand the middle table or diploë, pushing the inner and outer cortices apart (Figs. 4–42). On tomograms, and especially on CT scans, the mixed fibro-osseous nature of the process can be easily appreciated in the diploë (Fig. 4–43). These lesions can involve the facial bones without any other osseous involvement.

Paget's disease rarely can also cause a thickened, dense bone; however, this occurs only after the calvarium has first been involved.

Thus, a skull film will reveal pagetoid changes in the calvarium that suggest the diagnosis.[12]

Lastly, metastatic disease to the head is rarely a purely blastic event. Usually the metastases are lytic or mixed lytic and blastic. Metastatic prostate, however, can give pure sclerotic metatasis to the facial bones, which may be impossible to differentiate radiographically from Paget's disease (Fig. 4–44).

Although most of these osseous changes can be identified on MRI studies, they are more easily diagnosed and accurately differentiated on CT scans (Fig. 4–45). This ability to resolve such fine bony detail is the primary strength of CT in the sinonasal cavities.

Aggressive bone destruction means that the bone is destroyed without being displaced. It is the result of a disease process that permeates the bone and destroys it before any reparative bone can be laid down. The most common cause of this type of bone response is squamous cell carcinoma, which accounts for about 80 per cent of all the sinonasal malignancies. The expected roentgen appearance of this tumor is a soft tissue mass with adjacent aggressive bone destruction (Figs. 4–46, 4–47, 4–48). Most of the other causes of this type of bone destruction are a few aggressive sarcomas and metastatic lesions.

On CT, if an aggressive-appearing lesion enhances significantly with contrast, a malignant fibrous histiocytoma or angiosarcoma is the most likely diagnosis, as most of the other tumors enhance little if at all.

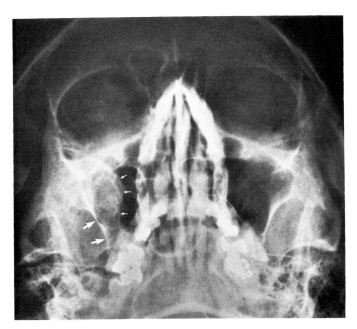

Figure 4–42. Waters view reveals thickening of the right lateral antral wall. The process has widened the bone and left the outer (large arrows) and inner (small arrows) cortical surfaces intact. This could be a case of fibrous dysplasia, but it proved to be an ossifying fibroma.

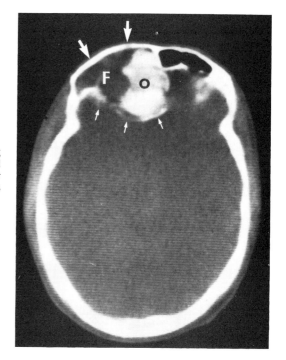

Figure 4–43. Axial CT scan reveals a large mass widening the right frontal bone. The mass has both osseous (O) and fibrous (F) material, and the inner (small arrows) and outer (large arrows) cortices remain intact. This patient had fibrous dysplasia.

Only with CT or MRI can the true size of the tumor be seen and the extrasinus extension evaluated. Since this is critical to the decision of whether or not a curative or palliative approach to the patient will be taken, sectional imaging must be performed on all patients with sinonasal tumors.

Aggressive bone destruction can occur in conjunction with areas of thickened sclerotic bone. When this is seen, an infection with osteomyelitis is usually the cause. Most of these cases result from fungal infections or highly aggressive or neglected bacterial infections.

Bone remodeling reflects an active process in which, as the bone is being destroyed on one side, new bone is being laid down on the other side. This is reflected radiographically as a bowing or displacement of the bone away from

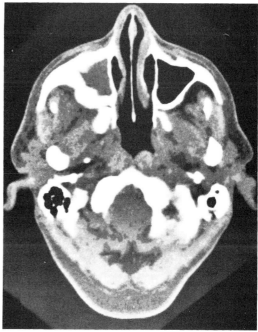

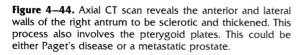

Figure 4–44. Axial CT scan reveals the anterior and lateral walls of the right antrum to be sclerotic and thickened. This process also involves the pterygoid plates. This could be either Paget's disease or a metastatic prostate.

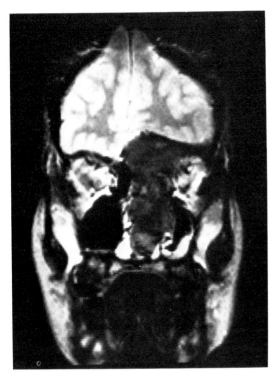

Figure 4–45. Coronal T₁W MRI scan reveals an expansile mass in the left nasal fossa, ethmoid sinuses, and medial orbit. The upper cortex is elevated, and the mass has a slightly nonhomogeneous low-signal intensity. The CT ground-glass bony appearance should make the diagnosis of fibrous dysplasia easier with CT than it is with MR.

the tumor. This process indicates that the growth of the causative lesion is slow enough to allow remodeling, but a conclusion about the biologic behavior of the lesion cannot be made. Although polyps are the most common expansile lesions of the nasal cavity and mucoceles are the most common expansile lesions of any paranasal sinus, several uncommon malignancies can cause bone remodeling to occur. These include fibrosarcomas, esthesioneuroblastomas,

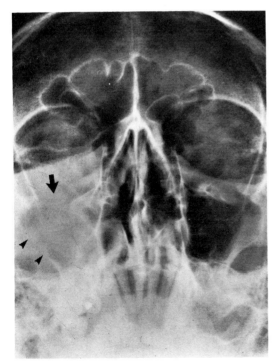

Figure 4–46. Waters view reveals a soft tissue mass in the right antrum and cheek, with destruction of the antral roof (arrow) and lateral wall (arrowheads). This is the typical aggressive, bone-destroying appearance of squamous cell carcinoma.

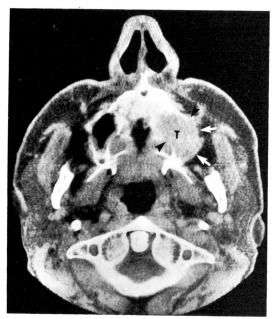

Figure 4–47. Axial CT scan reveals a mass in the left antrum *(T)* that has aggressively destroyed portions of the left hard palate and alveolus *(arrowheads)*. This squamous cell carcinoma also extends into the adjacent soft tissues *(arrows)*.

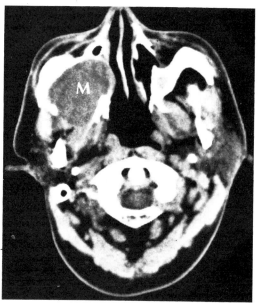

Figure 4–49. Axial CT scan reveals a primarily expansile right antral mass *(M)*. This adenoid cystic carcinoma has also destroyed localized portions of the posterolateral and medial antral walls.

histiocytic lymphomas, most adenocarcinomas, most adenocystic carcinomas, most melanosarcomas, some embryonal rhabdomyosarcomas, and most extramedullary plasmacytomas (Figs. 4–49, 4–50). On a rare occasion other tumors

may also cause some bone remodeling; however, this group of neoplasms accounts for the vast majority of the lesions.

Although as a group these tumors have a

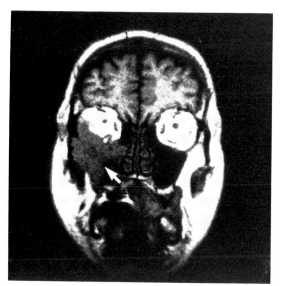

Figure 4–48. Coronal T$_1$W MRI scan reveals a destructive right antral mass *(arrow)* that has eroded up into the lateral right orbit. This mass had low-to-intermediate signal intensity on both T$_1$W and T$_2$W MRI scans.

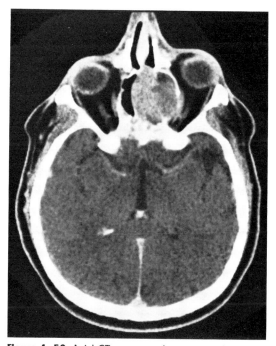

Figure 4–50. Axial CT scan reveals an expansile mass in the left ethmoid sinuses and nasal fossa. This minor salivary gland tumor has primarily remodeled the ethmoid bone, although focal areas of erosion are present.

more benign imaging appearance with regard to their bony changes than does squamous cell carcinoma, some of these latter neoplasms have a worse 5-year prognosis than the more aggressive-appearing squamous cell carcinoma.[24, 25]

Thus, although the degree of biologic aggressiveness cannot be ascertained, the observation of bone remodeling can be very useful in certain instances. If a histologic diagnosis of anaplastic carcinoma is made and some bone remodeling is present, two main diagnostic possibilities should be considered. First, the diagnosis is wrong and one of the tumors that can be histologically confused with anaplastic carcinoma is really present. These include esthesioneuroblastoma, embryonal rhabdomyosarcoma, melanosarcoma, plasmacytoma, and histiocytic lymphoma. All these tumors can be differentiated by electron microscopy and histochemical testing. Second, an anaplastic carcinoma is present with an associated mucocele, large retention cyst, or polyp. Such a circumstance usually can be diagnosed by CT or MRI scanning.[24, 25]

To avoid a wrong histologic diagnosis, it is best to obtain electron microscopy and histochemical testing on all small cell or anaplastic tumors.

One of the main benefits of MRI is its ability to distinguish about 95 per cent of all sinonasal tumors from inflammatory disease. It can accomplish this because these tumors are highly cellular and have little water content. Therefore, they do not have the signal characteristics of water. Instead, they have low-to-intermediate signal intensities on both T_1W and T_2W images. This means that on T_2W images, about 95 per cent of sinonasal tumors will not be bright whereas the inflammatory lesions will be bright (Fig. 4–51). This allows a more accurate mapping of the true tumor margins than can be accomplished on CT.[12]

The few tumors that have bright T_2W signal intensities are almost exclusively minor salivary gland neoplasms with areas of cystic change and seromucinous products.

When the radiologist's findings are compared with the clinician's evaluation, it will be noted that pain is a prominent feature of most sinonasal infections. Tumors, on the other hand, almost never present clinically with pain. Only the uncommon adenoid-cystic carcinoma with perineural invasion may present with pain as a complaint. Rather, patients with tumors usually complain of symptoms related to the tumor mass itself, such as nasal stuffiness, diplopia, facial asymmetry, change in voice quality, and so on.

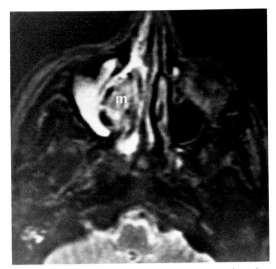

Figure 4–51. Transverse T_2W MRI scan reveals a low signal intensity mass (m) in the right nasal fossa that has obstructed inflammatory secretion around it in the anterior and posterior nasal cavity and in the right antrum. Such a degree of distinction between this melanoma and the inflammatory tissues is usually not possible on CT.

POSTOPERATIVE CHANGES

One of the more difficult problems confronting the radiologist is detecting the presence of recurrent malignancy after operative intervention. The main obstacle is in differentiating postoperative fibrosis and granulation tissue from early recurrent tumor. On plain films this is virtually impossible because the major landmarks for evaluating disease, the sinus walls, have been surgically removed. By the time a soft tissue mass becomes large enough to be identified on conventional films, the recurrence would be clinically obvious and probably hopelessly advanced.

CT and MRI scanning can be applied to this problem with good results. Today, the radiologist can detect subclinical recurrences reliably and guide the surgeon to a suspicious area for a directed biopsy.[26]

In a planned regimen, a baseline scan should be obtained 6 to 8 weeks postoperatively. This time interval usually is sufficient to allow resolution of most postoperative hemorrhage and edema. This baseline scan is essentially the new normal study for the patient, and it is the study with which all follow-up scans can be compared. Routine follow-up scans should then be obtained at 4- to 6-month intervals for at least 3 years. In this way, an early recurrence can be detected during the greatest at-risk time interval.

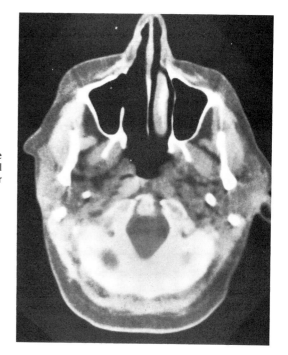

Figure 4–52. Axial CT scan reveals the normal postoperative appearance after a right partial maxillectomy and lateral rhinotomy. The anteromedial bony walls and the right inferior turbinate have been removed.

The normal postoperative CT scan has sharply defined areas of missing bone. No isolated nonsurgical areas of focal bone destruction or sites of destruction with irregular bony margins should be present. A knowledge of the exact surgery allows the radiologist to know precisely what areas of absent bone to expect (Fig. 4–52). More importantly, the postoperative cavity is smooth. No focal mucosal nodularity or irregularity is seen.

As in the normal nonoperated patient, areas of remaining normal sinus mucosa are not seen on the postoperative scans. If radiation fibrosis or sinusitis is present, the mucosa is thickened,

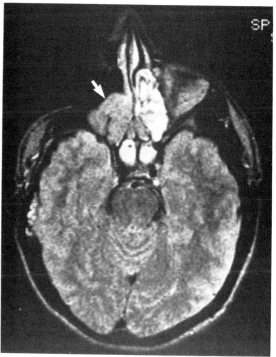

Figure 4–53. Axial CT scan reveals recurrent squamous cell carcinoma (arrow) in a patient who has had a prior partial left maxillectomy.

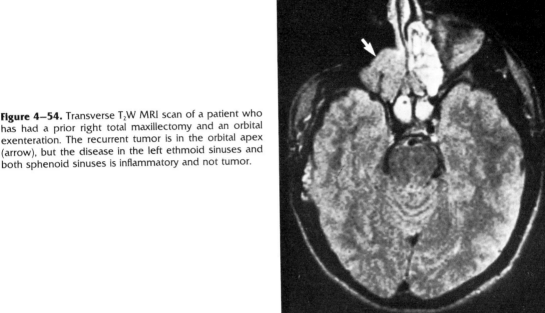

Figure 4–54. Transverse T₂W MRI scan of a patient who has had a prior right total maxillectomy and an orbital exenteration. The recurrent tumor is in the orbital apex (arrow), but the disease in the left ethmoid sinuses and both sphenoid sinuses is inflammatory and not tumor.

usually in a smooth manner, with no areas of focal nodularity being present. Even if a split-thickness skin graft has been applied to a post-operative maxillary sinus, no focal masses are to be expected. Any such areas of focal irregularity or abnormal thickening of the soft tissues in a postoperative antrum must be considered as a tumor recurrence until proved otherwise[2, 6] (Fig. 4–53).

On MRI, areas of inflammation can be distinguished from most recurrent tumor by observing the T₂W signal intensities (Fig. 4–54). However, granulation tissue also has low-to-intermediate signal intensities on all imaging sequences and, as such, cannot be differentiated from recurrent tumor.[12] Nevertheless, early tumor recurrences have been detected with a greater frequency than by clinical examination alone, and any high-risk areas can be identified by the radiologist so that the surgeon can perform a directed (rather than blind) biopsy.

The same general observations apply to the other paranasal sinuses and the nasal fossae.

The hope of this approach is to detect local tumor recurrence early enough so that more of the patients can be salvaged. It is only reasonable to expect that, as imaging techniques continue to improve and as surgeons and radiologists continue to build a dialogue, more accurate and detailed information can allow the best possible treatment decisions to be made.

References

1. Dodd GD, Jing BS: Radiology of the Nose, Paranasal Sinuses and Nasopharynx. Baltimore, Williams & Wilkins, 1977.
2. Merrill V: Atlas of Roentgenographic Positions. 3rd ed. St. Louis, CV Mosby, 1967.
3. Hasso AN, Vignaud J: Normal anatomy of the paranasal sinuses, nasal cavity and facial bones. In Newton TH, Hasso AN, Dillon WP (eds): Modern Neuroradiology. Vol 3: Computed Tomography of the Head and Neck. New York, Raven Press, 1988, pp 6.1–6.18.
4. Som PM: The paranasal sinuses. In Bergeron RT, Osborn AG, Som PM (eds): Head and Neck Imaging, Excluding the Brain. St. Louis, CV Mosby, 1984, pp 1–142.
5. Lloyd GAS, Lund VJ, Phelps PD, Howard DJ: Magnetic resonance imaging in the evaluation of nose and paranasal sinus disease. Br J Radiol 60:957–968, 1987.
6. Zinreich SJ, Kennedy DW, Rosenbaum AE, Gayler BW, Kumar AJ, Stammberger H: Paranasal sinuses: CT imaging requirements for endoscopic surgery. Radiology 163:769, 1987.
7. Van Alyea OE: Nasal Sinuses: Anatomic and Clinical Consideration. Baltimore, Williams & Wilkins, 1942.
8. Caffey J: Pediatric X-ray Diagnosis. 5th ed. Chicago, Year Book Medical Publishers, 1967.
9. Zizmor J, Noyek A: Radiology of the nose and paranasal sinuses. Otolaryngology 1:1043, 1973.
10. Mancuso AA, Hanafee WN: Computed Tomography of the Head and Neck. Baltimore, Williams & Wilkins, 1982.
11. Ritter FN: The Paranasal Sinuses; Anatomy and Surgical Technique. St. Louis, CV Mosby, 1973.
12. Som PM, Shapiro MD, Biller HF, Sasaki C, Lawson W: Sinonasal tumors and inflammatory tissues: Differentiation with MR imaging. Radiology 167:803–808, 1988.

13. Alberti PW: Applied surgical anatomy of the maxillary sinus. Otolaryngol Clin North Am 9(1):49, 1976.
14. Yanagisawa E, Smith HW, Thaler S: Radiographic anatomy of the paranasal sinuses. II. Lateral view. Arch Otolaryngol 87:196, 1968.
15. Yanagisawa E, Smith HW, Merrill RA: Radiographic anatomy of the paranasal sinuses. III. Submentovertical view. Arch Otolaryngol 87:299, 1968.
16. Yanagisawa E, Smith HW: Radiographic anatomy of the paranasal sinuses. IV. Caldwell view. Arch Otolaryngol 87:311, 1968.
17. Yanagisawa E, Smith HW: Normal radiographic anatomy of the paranasal sinuses. Otolaryngol Clin North Am 6:429, 1973.
18. Yanagisawa E, Smith HW: Radiographic anatomy of the paranasal sinuses. Otoloaryngol Clin North Am 9:55, 1976.
19. Etter LE: Atlas of Roentgen Anatomy of the Skull. Springfield, Ill, Charles C Thomas, 1955.
20. Eichel BS: The medical and surgical approach in management of the unilateral opacified antrum. Laryngoscope 87:737–750, 1977.
21. Fascenelli FW: Maxillary sinus abnormalities: Radiographic evidence in an asymptomatic population. Arch Otol Laryngol 90:190–193, 1969.
22. Som PM, Shugar JMA: Antral mucoceles—a new look. J Comput Assist Tomogr 4:484, 1980.
23. Som PM, Shugar JMA: The CT classification of ethmoid mucoceles. J Comput Assist Tomogr 4:199, 1980.
24. Som PM, Shugar JMA: The significance of bone expansion associated with the diagnosis of malignant tumors of the paranasal sinuses. Radiology 136:97, 1980.
25. Som PM, Shugar JMA: When to question the diagnosis of anaplastic carcinoma. Mt. Sinai J Med 48:239, 1981.
26. Som PM, Shugar JMA, Biller HF: The early detection of antral malignancy in the post maxillectomy patient. Radiology 143:509, 1982.

CHAPTER 5

RADIONUCLIDE SCANNING*

Arnold M. Noyek, MD, FRCS(C), FACS
N. David Greyson, MD, FRCP(C)

The air-containing, mucosa-lined and bone-confined paranasal sinuses remain clinically inaccessible to the rhinologist's inspecting eye and palpating hand. The clinician has come to depend, therefore, on the anatomic information obtained by conventional and advanced x-ray studies for the diagnosis of paranasal sinus disease.[1-3] Over the past three quarters of a century, and especially in the last decade, improved morphologic information concerning the paranasal sinuses in health and disease has evolved by the rational use of conventional plain films, complex motion tomography, xeroradiography and, ultimately, current generation computed tomography (CT) scanning and magnetic resonance imaging (MRI). The interface between air and soft tissue, and between soft tissue and bone lends itself ideally to the gray scale imaging of conventional radiography; computed tomography (CT) extends the gray scale anatomic information still further. The sophistication of these morphologic modalities has been indicated in the preceding chapter. This chapter demonstrates the physiologic imaging that can result from the innovative use of radionuclide scanning of the paranasal sinuses. In many instances, the correlation of anatomic imaging studies with these physiologic imaging studies will result in improved diagnosis and hence better treatment for the patient.

The clinician not only looks to the radiologist/imager for help in extending the physical examination through diagnostic imaging but also seeks assistance in solving a variety of clinical problems. These problems may involve either qualitative or quantitative diagnosis. The search for a qualitative diagnosis may yield a specific diagnosis (such as fracture) or a group disorder diagnosis (such as cystic lesion, bone destructive lesion, vascular lesion). More often the questions are quantitative—does disease exist (including occult disease)? Is overt disease local or systemic? Can mass disease be quantified in three-dimensional terms, and does it transgress regional boundaries (intraorbital extension, intracranial extension)? Are there specific anatomic or physiologic deficits (such as airway obstruction or cerebrospinal fluid leak)?

The physiologic imaging potential of radionuclide scans has areas of obvious application to some of these problems. The bone scan may permit the recognition of primarily osteoblastic or reactively osteoblastic (to bone destruction) disease in a qualitative sense. Similarly, flow phase radionuclide studies may identify vascular lesions, again in a qualitative sense. In quantitative terms, radionuclide bone scanning may permit the identification of systemic disease as it affects the entire bony organ system. Combined with gallium scanning,[4] radionuclide bone scans allow quantification of osteomyelitis and its response to treatment.[5] Finally, the sophisticated correlative use of radionuclide scans permits the understanding of abnormalities of a structural nature, detected by conventional films, tomography and CT; for example, the opacified or thick-walled sinus can be quantified as housing active or burned out disease. Radionuclide scans may thus augment diagnos-

*Supported by the Saul A. Silverman Foundation, Toronto, Ontario, Canada.

tic information and lead to more directed diagnostic studies or eliminate the need for other studies in some instances.

The major advances in radionuclide scanning, which have particular relevance to the study of paranasal sinus disease, have come about since the use of the modern bone scan. Radioactive technetium ^{99m}Tc agents were first introduced in 1971.[6] Concurrently, there have been technologic advances in the gamma camera recording of radiation photon emissions. Detail of the history and evolution of radionuclide scanning is provided elsewhere.[7, 8]

Although the bone scan is the obvious physiologic imaging modality for study of the paranasal sinuses and related viscerocranial and neurocranial structures,[9] other radionuclide scans utilizing preferentially the same safe gamma-emitting technetium tag, or other radioactive labels such as gallium citrate ^{67}Ga, are included in the diagnostic armamentarium. These radionuclide scans (bone scan, gallium scan, and, less commonly, brain scan and CSF scan) utilize the gamma camera detection of photon emissions from safe radioactively tagged substrates and permit the recording of essentially physiologic diagnostic images of organ systems. These are emission phenomena, as opposed to the transmission image recording of conventional radiology and CT scanners.

However, as physiologic changes precede morphologic changes, the clinical application of these radionuclide scans, in a general philosophic sense, becomes readily apparent. The diagnostic imaging of the distribution, accumulation, and excretion of homeopathic amounts of specific radiopharmaceuticals can be applied to a variety of paranasal sinus disorders, as discussed later.

The bone scan is the prototypic study for the physiologic assessment of the paranasal sinuses and related bony visceral facial skeleton and related neurocranium. The classic triphasic scan, as recorded in the ^{99m}Tc methylene diphosphonate bone scan,[10] allows the sequential recording of flow phase, blood pool phase and delayed images (both local sinus views and whole body images). The flow and blood pool phase images provide soft tissue diagnostic information; the delayed phase images provide input as to bone metabolism itself, as the technetium phosphate analogue is ultimately incorporated into the bony skeleton.

These radionuclide scans are highly sensitive.[9, 11] Detected abnormalities (which offer a visual gray scale image or a computed quantified image) always reflect an alteration in function that can be frequently documented by sophisticated clinical radiologic interpretation. However, these findings, though highly sensitive, are nonspecific; they often require other morphologic studies (by conventional x-ray beam or biopsy) for ultimate diagnostic understanding. Further, these radionuclide scans are less well suited to discrete anatomic imaging; they permit the detection of relatively superficial photon emission phenomena (for which the maxillary, ethmoid, and frontal sinuses are well positioned and the sphenoid sinus reasonably well positioned). A resolution capability of current gamma cameras defines lesions of 0.5- to 1-cm dimension.

Although details are provided elsewhere,[12–17] two important principles are enumerated here—one concerning imaging potential and one concerning patient safety. Physiologic changes precede morphologic changes in disease processes; this includes the evolution of soft tissue and bone disease. The bone scan has particular application in its delayed phase to the detection of bone changes well in advance of their detection by conventional and advanced anatomic radiologic studies (conventional radiology and CT scanning). Bone destruction requires a 30 to 50 per cent osteolysis or demineralization before the conventional x-ray beam can detect this change on radiograph. The delayed bone scan may manifest bone lysis or osteonecrosis as a photon-deficient area; however, its real significance lies in the detection of the almost universal osteoblastic reparative response about an area of bone destruction. The bone scan, therefore, can detect increases in bone deposition by a factor of approximately 5 per cent, whereas the conventional x-ray beam cannot detect these changes until there has been a 10 to 30 per cent hypermineralization.

Even though complex motion tomography and computed tomography better reveal established bone mineralization, they do not reflect the level of metabolic activity of the osteoclasts and osteoblasts to achieve that net effect. The bone scan thus images specific osteoblastic activity in the demonstration of the early evolution of disease, as physiologic changes predate structural changes by days or weeks. Even in primary osteoblastic disease itself, such as osteoblastic tumors or fracture healing, the bone scan again detects these findings well in advance of conventional studies. In general, all radionuclide scans have the potential to demonstrate the precursor physiologic changes.

As for patient safety, the radionuclide scans, in the main, depend on safe gamma-emitting radionuclides. The images are readily obtained. Even an ill patient can simply lie on a stretcher and be positioned appropriately under the gamma camera. The bone scan, for example, requires a single intravenous injection of a radionuclide bolus (usually 15 mCi of ^{99m}Tc methylene diphosphate in the adult). This is followed by soft tissue imaging over the first several minutes, with the patient being placed in standard sinus positions (Waters, Caldwell, right and left anterior oblique, right and left lateral views). In approximately 2 to 3 hours the same sinus views are repeated with or without whole body imaging, depending upon the clinical situation.

A bone scan provides the same radiation exposure as a set of conventional sinus radiographs; it is relatively noninvasive, as technetium ^{99m}Tc is not a naturally occurring element and hence there is no biologic sensitivity to it. The bone scan can be carried out in children and can be conducted repetitively if necessary, in accordance with clinical discretion. The main restriction is in the avoidance of radionuclide scanning in the pregnant, or possibly pregnant, patient or nursing mother.

The triphasic scan concept deserves further description. The bone scan will be described, though the triphasic concept applies to the sodium pertechnetate images of brain scan and salivary scan. In fact, the triphasic scan concept applies to any radionuclide imaging in which there is an early soft tissue and a delayed organ system image. After the initial intravenous injection of the bone scan agent in an antecubital vein, anterior gamma camera images of the head and neck are recorded sequentially, at 3-second intervals. Only one position may be recorded for this flow phase study, which in essence provides a low resolution angiogram. The Waters view is best for studying possible vascular abnormality involving the maxillary antra; a Caldwell or anterior view is best for frontal sinus lesions. A lateral view may be elected for envisioning the region of the sphenoid sinus. In any event, the radionuclide bolus enters the right side of the heart, passes through the lungs to the left ventricle, and makes its first transit passage into the carotid circulation and into the head and neck. Initial images of photon emissions record a low resolution carotid angiogram; this examination will detect a relatively superficial hypervascular abnormality if it has sufficient vascularity, is greater than 1 cm in diameter, and is not obscured by related normal vascular images. As the sequential images are recorded, the sagittal sinus fills and the internal jugular veins fill and drain.

Within the first 1 to 3 minutes, the soft tissue images of the blood pool phase are next recorded. This results as the radionuclide bolus has now diffused itself homogeneously throughout the vascular compartment and has made several serial passages through the entire circulatory system. This pool phase (an equilibration image) then allows the detection of hyperemia or oligemia in the plane of the sinus studied. Thus the hyperemia of an acute inflammatory process, vascular tumor, or healing fracture may be detected. Again, these images are highly sensitive but nonspecific: the image must be placed in clinical context for true physiologic recognition.

After approximately 1.5 to 3 hours, the bone scan agent has been incorporated as the radioactively tagged substrate itself has become chemically fixed into the bony skeleton. Fifty per cent of the radionuclide bolus is excreted in the urinary system and 50 per cent of the radionuclide substrate enters the bony skeleton; it has only a 6-hour half-life, so optimal imaging must be obtained, as indicated, prior to its decay. The axial skeleton takes up approximately twice the substrate that the peripheral skeleton does. Hence the paranasal sinuses, orbits, and skull vault can be clearly identified. However, there is a more intense triangular area of photon emission from the midmaxillary central area, a constant phenomenon that probably reflects this increased axial uptake of the skull base, as well as vascular factors; these emissions are augmented by the unattenuated emission of radiation photons through the air-containing nasal passages.[18] The normal triphasic bone scan is depicted in Figure 5–1. The normal triphasic brain scan is imaged, for comparison, in Figure 5–2, after intravenous injection of 15 mCi of sodium pertechnetate in the adult.

The ^{67}Ga scan is not recorded in triphasic display. Gallium images are recorded preferentially by local sinus or whole body views 48 hours after intravenous injection of approximately 3 mCi of the radionuclide in the adult. When combined with sequential bone scans (as for diagnosis and evaluation of osteomyelitis), the bone scan is performed initially, followed by gallium injection at conclusion of the delayed bone scan. The patient returns in 48 hours for the gallium imaging.

^{67}Ga is primarily a tumor-seeking agent but has avidity for sepsis as well. It localizes in acute inflammation within an actively dividing granulocyte population but not in intrasinus extramucosal pus, which lacks a blood supply to carry in the tracer. Acute uncomplicated

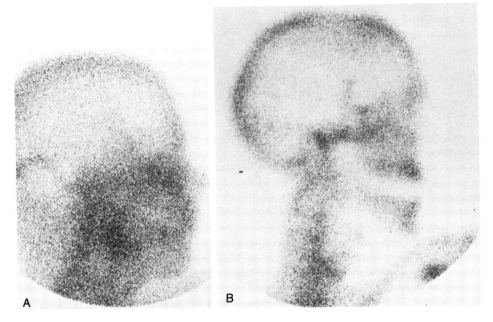

Figure 5–1. Normal bone scan.

A, The pool phase image.

B, The delayed phase image recorded 2 hours after injection. Note the normal bony uptake of the skull vault and facial skeleton. The midfacial structures are well identified, as are the mandible and cervical spine.

purulent sinusitis may therefore give a cool to warm image. Infective osteomyelitis, however, provides intense photon emission from the bone-infecting septic insult rather than from the osteoblastic bony reaction to the insult. Bone reaction is best imaged by a bone scan, not by gallium. As soon as treatment is effective, the gallium scan reverts to normal uptake.[5]

Tumor uptake varies from neoplasm to neoplasm but is most consistently demonstrated by lymphoma and melanoma. Sometimes there is discrepancy in uptake of gallium by the primary and secondary tumor.

[67]Ga has a biologic half-life of 78 hours. The radiation exposure with radiogallium scanning to the head and neck is less than with conventional sinus radiographs; however, the whole body exposure is roughly equivalent to that from an abdominal or lumbar spine series. There are no side effects otherwise.

CLINICAL APPLICATIONS

The various radionuclide scans have greater and lesser areas of application.[9, 11] Some scans are of proven diagnostic value, others are only of supplemental, adjunctive, or even marginal merit. However, all aid in understanding the physiologic correlates with morphologic changes in disease of the paranasal sinuses. A representative group of these disorders is discussed here.

INFLAMMATION

Acute sinusitis[19] is rarely imaged by bone scan unless acute osteomyelitis is a diagnostic consideration. However, the bone scan images in acute purulent sinusitis provide interesting physiologic recordings; there is a positive blood pool phase response from the sinus in question, reflecting the hyperemia of the inflammatory process. This is best seen in the earliest blood pool images recorded. In the delayed phase, there may be some marginal bone response, but it does not have the intensity of that in osteomyelitis. The range of minimal (Fig. 5–3) to maximal (Fig. 5–4) bone scan response, which one might anticipate without raising a diagnosis of osteomyelitis, is demonstrated. The variation in the delayed phase response depends on vascular and other local factors, but there is always an increase in hyperemia of the bone about an acutely inflamed sinus, which subsequently leads to increased deposition of the bone scan agent. In chronic purulent sinusitis (Fig. 5–5), a variable marginal osteoblastic delayed-phase bone response is detected; usually no blood pool phase soft tissue activity is de-

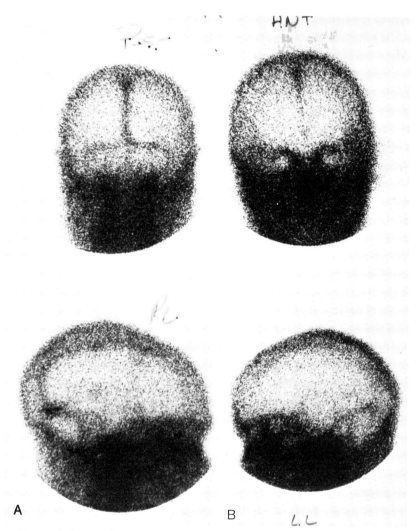

Figure 5–2. A sodium pertechnetate brain scan in the adult following injection of 15 mCi of the radionuclide bolus intravenously in an antecubital vein.

A, The pool phase images.

B, The delayed phase images. Note that the normal delayed-phase brain scan image is similar in distribution to the normal blood pool image; this occurs because the radioactively tagged pharmaceutical remains within the vascular compartment and does not pass through the blood-brain barrier. The radionuclide does not localize in bone, as does the tagged phosphate anion.

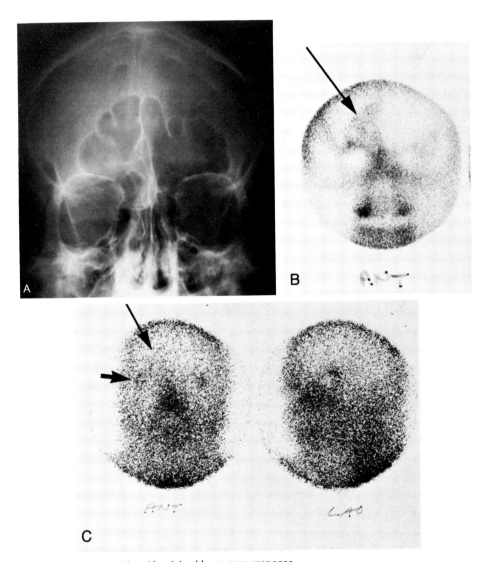

Figure 5–3. Acute frontal sinusitis, with minimal bone scan response.

  A, A Caldwell view demonstrates an opacified right frontal sinus. The left frontal sinus is aerated.

  B, The delayed phase of the bone scan demonstrates the minimal but definite increased bone uptake in the region of the right frontal sinus, in conjunction with the general increase in vascularity to the region of the right frontal sinus due to the inflammatory process. The arrow demonstrates the configuration of the right frontal sinus; it points to its roof. Compare this with the conventional Caldwell view image.

  C, A gallium citrate (^{67}Ga) scan demonstrates the usual minimal gallium uptake in conjunction with the acute sinusitis, as opposed to that with osteomyelitis. The upper arrow demonstrates the configuration of the right frontal sinus, contrasted with the absolutely photon-deficient left frontal sinus region. Note the normal uptake in the two lacrimal glands by the radionuclide; the short arrow points to the right lacrimal gland.

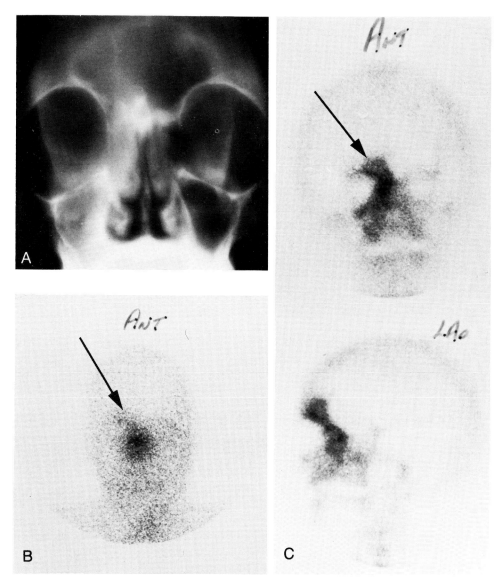

Figure 5–4. Acute frontal, ethmoid, and maxillary sinusitis with maximal bone scan response without osteomyelitis. The patient is a 29-year-old man.

A, An anteroposterior (AP) tomogram confirms the conventional plain film findings.

B, The pool phase demonstrates the hyperemia of the inflammatory reaction on bone scan. The arrow demonstrates the localization of radionuclide in the right frontal sinus on anterior (Caldwell) view.

C, The delayed phase of the bone scan demonstrates bony uptake in the region of the right frontal sinus (arrow), right ethmoid sinus and right maxillary antrum along its superior and medial walls. The intensity of the bone scan response is insufficient to warrant a diagnosis of osteomyelitis.

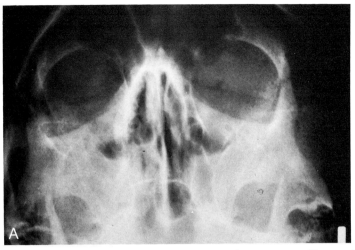
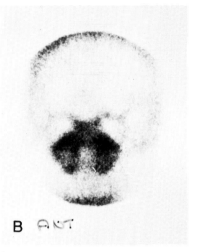

Figure 5–5. Chronic purulent bimaxillary sinusitis. The patient is a 40-year-old woman.
 A, A Waters view demonstrates opacification of both maxillary antra with small air-fluid levels superomedially in each instance.
 B, The delayed phase of the bone scan demonstrates the reactive response to the chronic purulent sinusitis. The imaging is compatible with a marked reactive osteitis but not osteomyelitis.

tected unless an acute clinical episode of infection is present. Chronic noninvasive fungal sinus infection incites only an indolent minimal adjacent bone reaction (Fig. 5–6).

Chronic polypoid sinusitis produces no significant soft tissue response and, perhaps, only a minimal osteoblastic response in the affected paranasal sinus walls (Fig. 5–7). Chronic bony thickening of the sinus walls usually reflects an inactive osteitis, and the bone scan will record this clinically insignificant bony event. However, if chronic polypoid sinusitis produces expansion of the paranasal sinuses (for example, with hypertelorism), the displacement of the bony paranasal sinus walls incites a marked osteoblastic response. All these images can be understood in appropriate clinical context.

The major role of bone scanning in sinusitis is the detection of acute and chronic osteomyelitis. In acute osteomyelitis (Fig. 5–8), there is focal or diffuse bone lysis in relation to the affected paranasal sinus. Morphologic changes may not be recorded on conventional or advanced x-ray study for several days or even a week or more. However, within 24 hours of the insult, the constant osteoblastic response is recognizable on bone scan as an intense hot bony reaction on delayed phase.[5a] Morphologic studies should be used to detect the presence of other complications, such as brain abscess. In acute osteomyelitis, the lytic lesion itself may be detected as a photon deficient area; however, it is the marginal osteoblastic response that is diagnostic. A ^{67}Ga scan will yield positive results

and will image the infective focus. When treatment is successful, the gallium scan will promptly revert to normal, indicating that the insult has been withdrawn. The bone scan will continue to reflect the reaction to the insult; its blood pool phase will become quiescent as the inflammatory component to the lesion regresses; however, its delayed bony responses will gradually resolve over a period of perhaps 6 to 18 or even 24 months, as in the healing of any bone lesion.

In acute flare-ups of chronic osteomyelitis (Figs. 5–9 and 5–10), the blood pool phase of the bone scan will reflect the hyperemia of the inflammatory lesion, as with acute osteomyelitis. The delayed phase of the bone scan remains intensely hot, as most chronic osteomyelitis is dramatically osteoblastic on conventional radiologic study. The gallium scan can again be used to image the acute insult before and after treatment.

Radionuclide scans have application in the detection of other complications of acute purulent sinusitis. In oroantral fistula, the bone scan may allow the localization of the inflammatory process to the fistula site; this is important when the maxillary antral walls are thickened, the sinus is opacified, and chronic osteomyelitis may be present. Similarly, the bone scan may give useful physiologic information in unusual inflammatory diseases, such as inflammatory pseudotumor; here the vascularity may be so intense as to produce a positive flow phase examination, as well as a positive blood pool

Text continued on page 94

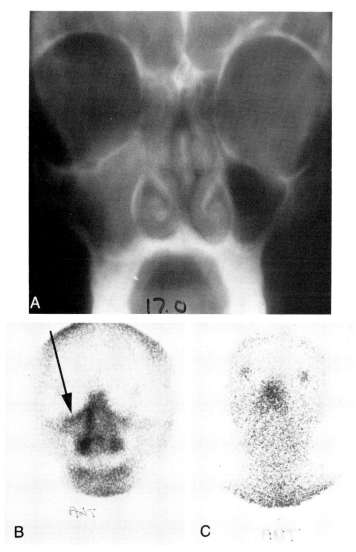

Figure 5–6. A chronic fungus infection (aspergillosis) of the right maxillary sinus, in which a large fungus ball was found at surgery, is depicted in a woman aged 25 years.

A, An AP tomogram demonstrates soft tissue density within the right maxillary sinus, primarily in relation to the medial wall and superiorly. There is no bone destruction.

B, The delayed phase of the bone scan demonstrates some osteoblastic thickening of the right maxillary sinus walls, especially medially, in relation to the fungus ball. There is some osteoblastic reaction of the right orbital floor (arrow).

C, Results of the gallium scan are normal.

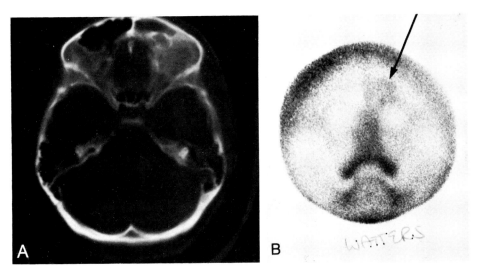

Figure 5–7. Chronic polypoid frontal sinusitis.

A, A computed tomography (CT) scan demonstrates opacification of the left frontal sinus, caused by polypoid mucosa; no bone destruction or displacement exists.

B, The delayed phase of the bone scan indicates a minimal response about the left frontal sinus to the mucosal polypoid hypertrophy. The arrow indicates the superior limit of the left frontal sinus on Waters view.

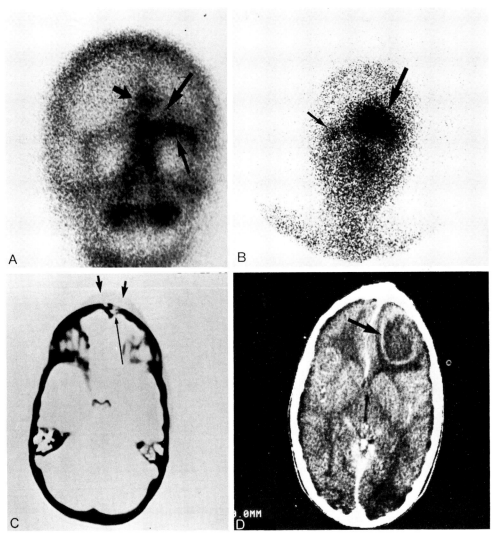

Figure 5–8 *See legend on opposite page*

90

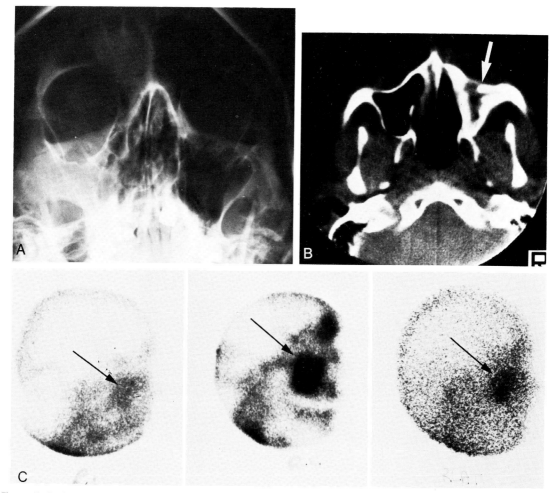

Figure 5–9. Chronic osteomyelitis of maxillary sinus.

A, A Waters view demonstrates opacification of the right maxillary sinus in a 26-year-old man with chronic osteomyelitis and recurrent acute bouts of infection. The patient had previous dental extraction, as well as right Caldwell-Luc surgery. The right orbital floor appears to be sagging.

B, A CT scan in axial display demonstrates bony thickening of the right maxillary sinus *(arrow).* The maxillary sinus is filled with soft tissue/fluid in its small central cavity; its morphologic nature is uncertain from the CT scan. There is an apparent area of reduced bone density and thickness anteriorly in the maxillary sinus; this may reflect the site of the previous Caldwell-Luc antrotomy.

C, Sequential bone and gallium scans are demonstrated in lateral display. *Left,* a right lateral view of the pool phase of a bone scan. The arrow indicates the hyperemia of the inflammatory process at the mucosal level (the insult). *Middle,* the osteoblastic response of the bony walls of the maxillary sinus to the chronic active osteomyelitis (reaction to the insult). Note that the right frontal sinus has an increased response on the lateral view in delayed phase but does not image as osteomyelitis on the pool phase or the gallium scan. The arrow demonstrates the same maxillary sinus bone response as in the left picture. *Right,* the gallium uptake by the inflammatory lesion *(arrow);* this again indicates the insult. Examination of the bone scan in pool and delayed phase, and the gallium scan in correlation, allows understanding of the diagnosis of osteomyelitis and permits determination of the success or failure of treatment.

Figure 5–8. Acute osteomyelitis, frontal sinus. A 12-year-old boy with an acute left frontal sinusitis and tender swelling of the overlying forehead.

A, The anterior view of a delayed bone scan demonstrates the marginal osteoblastic response to acute osteomyelitis. The medial response is demonstrated by the short arrow; the response of the orbital roof to the osteomyelitis of the left frontal sinus is demonstrated by the lower arrow. The upper right arrow indicates the central photon-deficient area caused by bone lysis.

B, A gallium citrate ⁶⁷Ga scan images the infective insult of the acute osteomyelitis *(large arrow);* this matches exactly the photon deficient lytic area of the bone scan. The small arrow indicates the normal uptake in the right lacrimal gland. An anterior view is shown.

C, A CT scan in axial display demonstrates the morphologic adjunctive information to the radionuclide studies. The soft tissue swelling of the forehead anteriorly is seen in axial display *(short black arrows).* A dehiscence in the posterior wall of the left frontal sinus is indicated by the thin black arrow on this reverse image CT display.

D, A CT scan, 3 cm above the axial cut shown in *C,* demonstrates the vascular ring sign *(arrow)* of a brain abscess; the CT study is contrast enhanced.

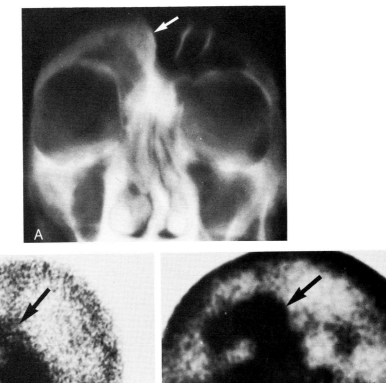

Figure 5–10. Chronic osteoblastic osteomyelitis, frontal sinus.

A, An AP tomogram demonstrates a densely osteoblastic and thickened right frontal sinus (arrow) in a 62-year-old man with active chronic osteoblastic osteomyelitis. Note the uninvolved left frontal sinus, which remains aerated; its normal scalloped appearance is preserved.

B, The pool phase of the technetium phosphate bone scan demonstrates an intense hyperemia (arrow), indicating that the bone morphology shown on conventional radiography actually has a marked underlying vascular basis. The medial aspect of the right frontal sinus, which is demonstrated by arrow on the conventional x-ray film, is indicated by a matching arrow in the pool phase image.

C, The delayed phase bone scan demonstrates the osteoblastic response in identical anterior imaging relationship (arrow). Again the arrow matches the preceding two arrows in anatomic localization. There is some osteoblastic reaction in the right maxillary sinus, but the pool phase suggests that it is not active. Treatment was directed only toward the frontal sinus osteomyelitis, with success.

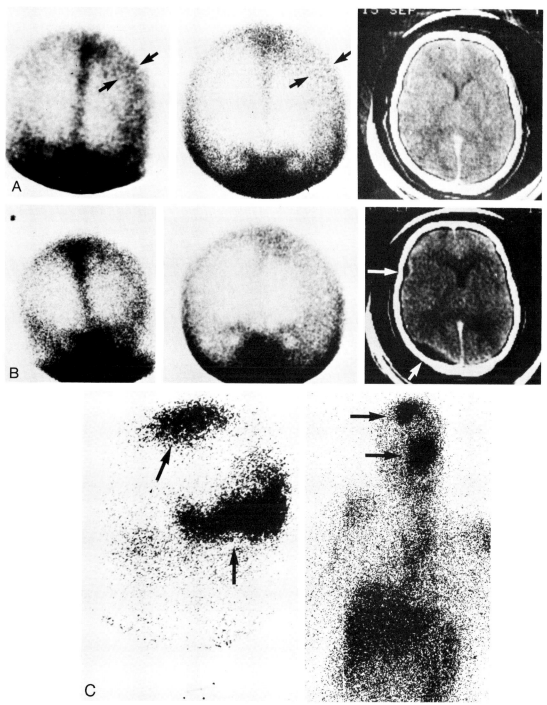

Figure 5–11. Rhinogenic brain abscess. An 18-year-old woman developed an acute left maxillary sinusitis following a dental extraction. She subsequently developed signs of intracranial infection.

A, A composite photograph illustrates a brain scan, utilizing sodium pertechnetate, in pool phase *(left)* and delayed phase *(center)*. A CT scan carried out at the same time demonstrates the apparently normal brain findings. The pool phase of the brain scan demonstrates a hyperemia involving the entire left extradural space from vertex to skull base *(between arrows)*. The same abnormality is shown in the same dimension on the delayed phase image *(between arrows)*. Radionuclide scan findings predate CT findings.

B, The pool phase *(left)* and delayed phase *(center)* of the brain scan, imaged 5 days after A, show the same physiologic responses to the extradural abscess. However, the CT scan *(right)*, demonstrated at approximately the same level as in A, shows two abscess cavities. These abscess cavities are in communication.

C, A gallium citrate ^{67}Ga scan (the same time as B) shows the functional activity of the infective focus along the vertex *(upper arrow)* and about the skull base *(lower arrow)* in left anterior oblique display. The right picture demonstrates an anterior view of the upper half of the body, with similar arrows.

phase and delayed-phase study. The diagnostic images are highly sensitive, but again not specific.

In rhinogenic brain abscess, the brain scan findings may indicate the presence of extradural empyema or localized brain abscess well in advance of morphologic localization by CT scan (Fig. 5–11).

FRACTURES

Radionuclide bone scans provide some useful information in fractures involving the paranasal sinuses (midthird facial fractures). However, the diagnostic information is not important in the detection of complications of midfacial fractures (such as nonunion), whereas it plays a major role in revealing such problems in mandibular fractures.

The physiologic imaging recorded on the radionuclide scan is of both clinical and academic interest. Within 12 hours of facial fracture, a hyperemia of repair can be detected in the blood pool phase of the bone scan, which demonstrates the physiologic organization of soft tissue in preparation for fracture healing. This may or may not be detected on bone scan,

depending on the size of the fracture and its resolution by gamma camera. However, frequently the exact morphology of the fracture can be recognized. For example, the most common isolated fracture to involve the paranasal sinuses, the tripod fracture (Fig. 5–12), often can be recognized in all three of its fracture lines. Radionuclide imaging, by bone scan, can show the second most common isolated fracture of the paranasal sinuses, the blow-out fracture of the orbital floor. After 12 hours and certainly by 3 days, the delayed phase image should demonstrate the osteoblastic response of a given fracture at its various sites in previously healthy bone.

The major role of bone scanning, in midfacial fractures, is the detection of multiple isolated fractures. A single isolated fracture is best imaged by conventional radiology.[20] Complex maxillofacial fractures (with possible intraorbital and intracranial extension) are best imaged by sophisticated CT.[21] However, the bone scan has value in the detection of multiple, isolated facial fractures in the stable but difficult-to-evaluate patient in whom clinical examination fails to discern clearly possible fracture sites.[9] Similarly, such patients with possible systemic fractures should be imaged by bone scans to detect

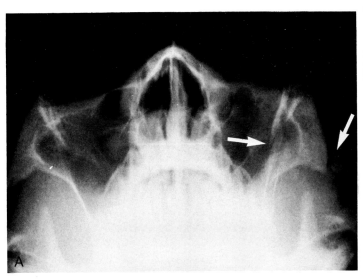 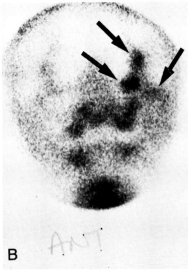

Figure 5–12. Zygomatic fracture.
A, A Waters view demonstrates a zygomatic fracture, with some medial displacement. There is an obvious fracture involving the inferolateral wall of the left maxillary antrum (left arrow). Note the fracture line in the zygomatic arch (right arrow). The zygomaticofrontal suture is not seen in this view.
B, The delayed bone scan demonstrates the classic tripod fracture. The delayed bone scan, in usual views, demonstrates the three fracture lines, hence the term tripod fracture. The uppermost arrow on Waters view demonstrates the zygomaticofrontal fracture. The medially placed arrow demonstrates the fracture involving the inferior orbital rim; it extends to the inferolateral aspect of the maxillary antrum (increased bone uptake in this area, not arrowed). The zygomatic arch fracture is indicated by the lateral arrow. This is a small bony fracture, and a reduced photon emission is therefore recorded compared with that from the other two fracture sites.

multiple skeletal fractures in their general management.[9] Stress injuries to the facial buttresses can be shown on bone scan; the zygomatico-frontal suture line often responds to facial injury, even in the absence of overt fracture(s).

CYSTS

Cysts of the paranasal sinuses can be classified as innocent, non–bone-destructive cysts and symptomatic bone-destructive cysts.[22] Conventional radiologic studies usually can make this distinction, and the surgical significance of bone destruction is apparent. However, when morphologic studies fail to indicate whether bone destruction is truly present, the bone scan may clarify the issue. The non–bone-destructive cysts are the innocent mucous retention and serous cysts;[23] they require no treatment beyond reassurance. The bone-destructive cysts can arise either intrinsic or extrinsic to the paranasal sinuses. The most common intrinsic bone-destructive cyst is the mucocele;[24] its bone scan imaging features are shown in Figure 5–13. The bone scan is of particular value in demonstrating the bone-destructive nature of the lesion when radiologic studies are equivocal. The bone destruction of a dentigerous cyst is shown in Figure 5–14; this cystic lesion is less aggressive than the mucocele, and the bone scan reflects this finding. A congenital fissural cyst, which is not actively enlarging, can be seen on scan. The radiologic correlation demonstrates the true nature of the lesion and also records that it is not actively destroying bone; the delayed bone scan shows a photon-deficient rather than a hot photon-emitting area.

BENIGN TUMORS

A variety of benign tumors of the paranasal sinuses can be imaged with several of the radionuclide bone scans, providing a variety of physiologic images.[22, 23, 25] Some images are of clinical significance; others are of pathologic interest.

The inverting papilloma should be imaged by bone scan to demonstrate bone destruction, if that is in its biologic nature. Inverting papilloma may be non–bone destructive or bone destructive; if it changes to a bone-destructive lesion, a concern should be raised regarding the possibility of the evolution of squamous cell carcinoma. If radionuclide bone scanning is carried out in cases of inverting papilloma, a whole body delayed scan can rule out systemic bony metastases (Fig. 5–15).

Of the mesenchymal tumors, osteoma involving the paranasal sinuses (especially the frontal sinus) lends itself to bone scan examination. The classic site of origin of the frontal sinus osteoma is the junction between the membranous bone of the skull vault and the enchondral bone of the skull base. The bone scan can be utilized to demonstrate the biologic activity of these osteomas, which are usually asymptomatic. The bone scan can indicate whether the osteoma, often detected on routine sinus or skull radiographs, is physiologically active and hence whether surgical treatment should be initiated. A very active osteoma with bone destruction is depicted in Figure 5–16; it has a hot blood pool phase, indicating its hyperemia, as well as a hot delayed phase, indicating the biologic accumulation of bony metabolites. This osteoma should be contrasted with the routine indolent frontal osteoma depicted in Figure 5–17; here there is only minimal bone scan response on delayed phase. Surgery, therefore, was not advised.

Another mesenchymal tumor, an ossifying capillary hemangioma,[26] is depicted in Figure 5–18. Here the vascular nature of the hemangioma is demonstrated by the flow phase of the bone scan. The hemangiomatous nature of the tumor is demonstrated on the blood pool phase; the delayed phase demonstrates two ossific components of the tumor—the intratumor ossification of the hemangioma and the marginal intense osteoblastic response about the tumor.

Meningioma, which usually has an intracranial origin, may extend into the paranasal sinuses. When it does, it has a classic radionuclide scan image (Fig. 5–19). It is positive on brain scan and bone scan, reflecting the dual tissue activity both within and about the tumor. The brain scan is positive in pool phase (it is a hyperemic tumor) and delayed phase (reflecting the altered blood-brain barrier of the tumor itself). The bone scan is positive in blood pool phase (again because of its hyperemia) and in delayed phase. The delayed bone scan response can reflect both intratumor ossification and the constant osteoblastic response about the tumor. If the tumor is of usual vascularity, the flow phase of both brain and bone scans may be positive, as a screening angiogram (see later). The positive brain scan/bone scan result is virtually diagnostic of meningioma.

Sometimes unique biologic information can be obtained concerning intrasinus tumors. The subtle bone-destructive nature of a tumor can

Text continued on page 103

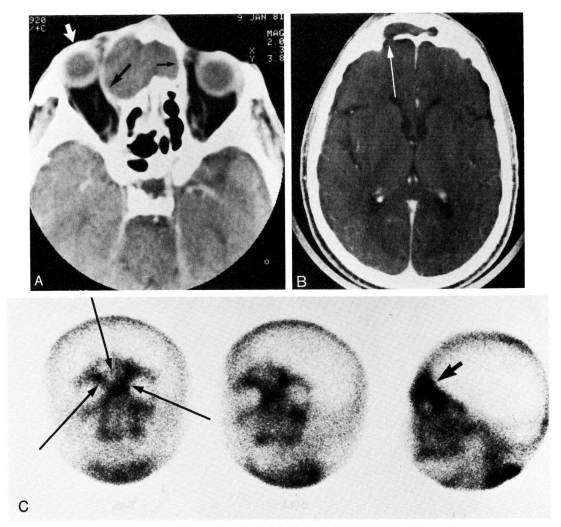

Figure 5–13. Frontal sinus mucocele, with intraorbital and dural extension.

A, A CT scan in axial display demonstrates a large frontal sinus mucocele encroaching on the right orbit *(heavy black arrow)* producing proptosis of the right globe *(white arrow).* The mucocele also extends toward the medial wall of the left orbit *(thin black arrow).*

B, A higher axial CT cut demonstrates a dehiscence in the posterior wall of the right frontal sinus *(white arrow).*

C, A bone scan in delayed phase, in usual views, demonstrates the mucocele as a photon-deficient area *(left, upper arrow).* The two lower oblique arrows demonstrate the osteoblastic response as the mucocele encroaches on the superomedial aspect of each orbit. In left lateral display *(right),* the dense osteoblastic response of the posterior wall of the frontal sinus is indicated by the arrow. The marked osteoblastic response of the posterior wall of the frontal sinus suggests the lesion is pushing in this area and perhaps relates to the ultimate production of a defect in the posterior sinus wall.

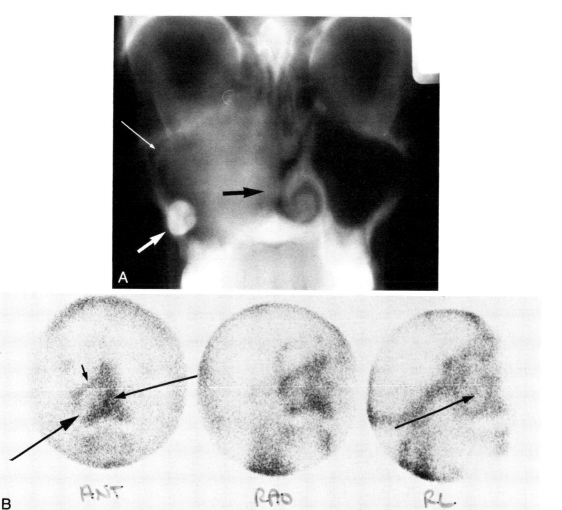

Figure 5–14. Dentigerous cyst, maxillary sinus. The patient is a 32-year-old man.

A, An AP tomogram demonstrates opacification and expansion of the right maxillary sinus. It encroaches on the right nasal cavity (black arrow). The crown of a tooth is evident laterally (heavy white arrow). The small residual aerated maxillary antral space superolaterally (thin arrow) demonstrates the extrinsic encroachment of this cystic lesion on the sinus cavity; only this normal residual remains.

B, The delayed phase of the bone scan in anterior, right anterior oblique and right lateral views is shown. In the anterior (Waters) view (left), the tiny arrow indicates the osteoblastic response of the right maxillary antral roof. The medially placed long arrow demonstrates the osteoblastic response to the cystic lesion encroaching on the nasal cavity. The heavier long arrow demonstrates a photon deficient area in the inferolateral wall of the maxillary sinus, reflecting an area of bone destruction. In the right lateral view (right), the cystic lesion appears as a photon-deficient cold area (arrow).

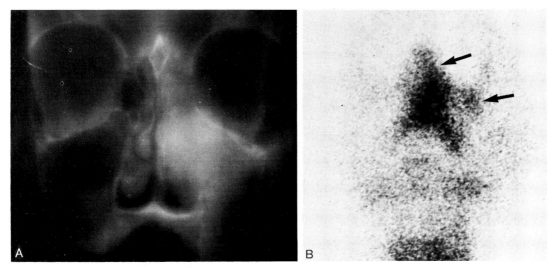

Figure 5–15. Inverting papilloma, maxillary sinus.

A, An AP tomogram demonstrates opacification of the left maxillary sinus and ethmoid labyrinth owing to inverting papilloma. There is no clear evidence of bone destruction radiologically.

B, A delayed phase bone scan, in Waters view, demonstrates the usual central nasomaxillary increase in uptake. However, there is some increase in the left ethmoid area (upper arrow), as well as in the superolateral aspect of the left maxillary sinus (lower arrow). These findings indicate an inciting osteoblastic response, presumably from focal bone destruction.

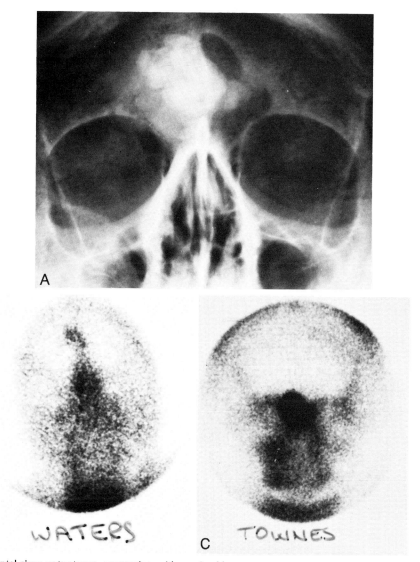

Figure 5–16. Frontal sinus osteotoma, aggressive, with maximal bone response.

A, A Waters view demonstrates a mixed cancellous-cortical osteoma of the right frontal sinus. It extends into the left frontal sinus. The superolateral margin of the right frontal sinus has lost its definition.

B, The blood pool phase of a bone scan demonstrates a marked hyperemia in this osteoma.

C, The delayed phase of the same bone scan indicates the tremendous osteoblastic activity of the bone lesion and reflects its aggressive biologic behavior. The patient had a palpable mass eroding through the anterior wall of the frontal sinus, as confirmed at surgery.

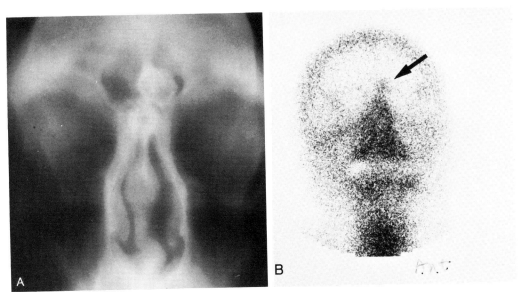

Figure 5–17. Frontal sinus osteoma, with minimal biologic activity.

A, An AP tomogram demonstrates a mixed cortical-cancellous osteoma occupying the left frontal sinus.

B, The minimal bone scan activity of the osteoma is well shown on Waters view *(black arrow).* No surgery was suggested.

Figure 5–18. Ossifying capillary hemangioma, maxillary sinus.

A, An axial CT scan demonstrates a destructive expansile lesion occupying the entire left maxillary sinus and encroaching on the left infratemporal fossa, as well as the nasal cavity. The mass has a marginating osteoblastic response and has areas of bone density within it.

B, A coronal CT cut demonstrates the mass lesion with its nasal encroachment. Its displacement of the intraorbital structures can also be appreciated.

C, A lateral view of an angiogram, in capillary phase, demonstrates the vascular blush of hemangioma. A capillary hemangioma, with ossification, was confirmed at surgery.

D, A composite image of a bone scan in flow phase *(left),* pool phase *(middle),* and delayed phase *(right),* all in anterior view, is shown. The flow phase demonstrates, as a screening angiogram, the hypervascular nature of the tumor mass. The pool phase image demonstrates its intrinsic hyperemia. The delayed phase shows a marked osteoblastic response involving the left maxillary sinus and left ethmoid labyrinth; the bone response is due to both intrinsic intratumor ossification and extrinsic marginal osteoblastic response in attempted physiologic confinement. (From Freeman J.L., Shemen L.J., Alberti F.W., et al: Ossifying capillary hemangioma. Otolaryngol 10(6):481, 1981.)

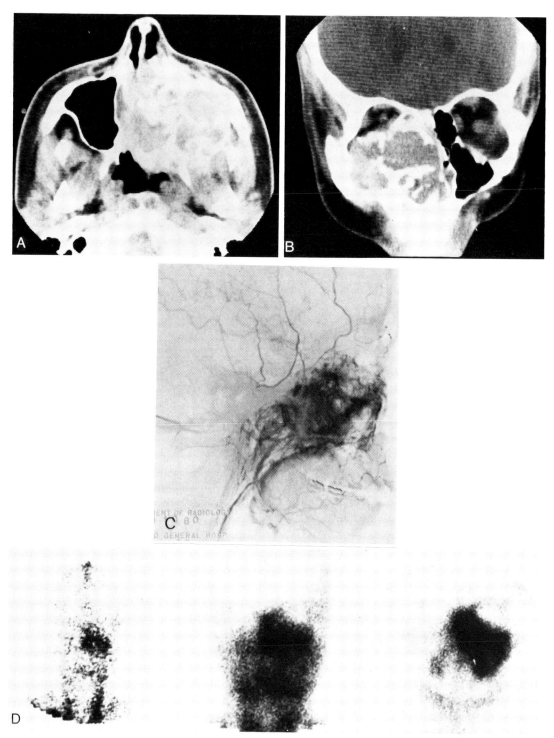

Figure 5–18 *See legend on opposite page*

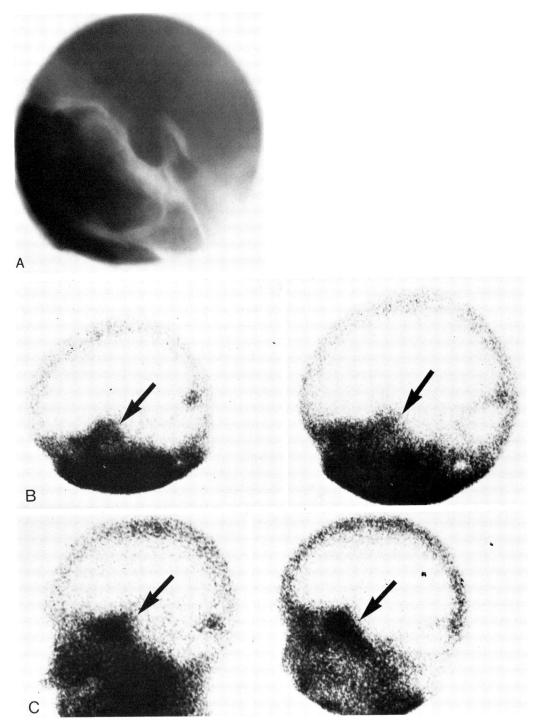

Figure 5–19. Sphenoid sinus meningioma.

   A, A lateral view of the sphenoid sinus demonstrates an osteoblastic mass occupying the upper half of the sphenoid sinus in relation to the sellar floor.

   B, Left lateral brain scan views, in pool phase *(left)* and delayed phase *(right)* demonstrate the physiologic activity of the meningioma, which arises intracranially. The hyperemic nature of the tumor is shown on the left *(arrow);* the altered blood-brain barrier due to tumor is shown on the right *(arrow).*

   C, Left lateral views of a bone scan, again in pool phase *(left)* and delayed phase *(right).* The arrows in each instance indicate the hyperemia *(left)* and the bone inductive response *(right).* This imaging pattern is classic of meningioma. Note the hypervascular effect on the blood pool phase as the vascularity of the tumor overshadows the altered blood-brain barrier effect on brain scan, and delayed bone response on these images.

be recognized on the bone scan. The functioning nature of a tumor, diagnostic of oncocytoma, was recognized on the hot delayed salivary scan,[27] the image being recorded at 3.5 hours in standard sinus views.

MALIGNANT TUMORS

Bone scans have selective usefulness in malignant tumors of the paranasal sinuses; gallium scans have special application, though infrequently utilized.

The bone scan response of a massive carcinoma of the maxillary and ethmoid sinuses is shown in Figure 5–20; the bone scan may quantify the extent of the disease, but this is much more reliably evaluated by axial and coronal CT scan.[28] In sclerosing carcinoma, whether of the paranasal sinuses or nasopharynx (Fig. 5–21) or metastatic from the prostate gland, the bone scan may add an interesting correlation. In carcinoma, when major resectional procedures are envisioned, the bone scan may prove cost-effective in the detection of

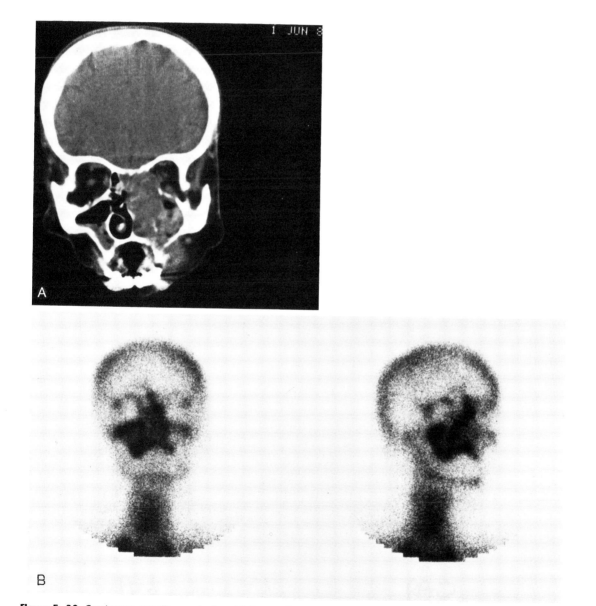

Figure 5–20. Carcinoma, maxillary and ethmoid sinus with intraorbital invasion.
 A, Coronal CT scan demonstrates a carcinoma of the right maxillary and ethmoid sinuses, extending into the adjacent orbit.
 B, An anterior view of the delayed phase of a bone scan reflects the morphologic activity noted in A.

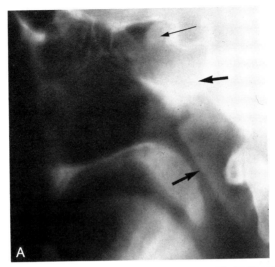

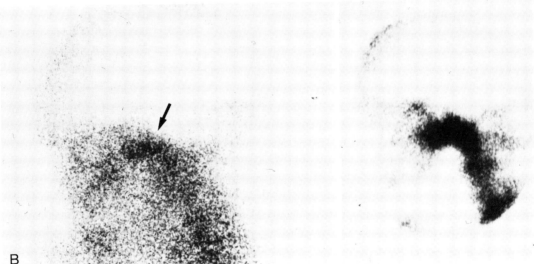

Figure 5–21. Sclerosing carcinoma of the nasopharynx.

A, A lateral complex motion tomographic cut demonstrates a soft tissue mass in the nasopharynx (lowest arrow) in midline; this almost occludes the postnasal airway. The middle arrow demonstrates marked sclerosis in the adjacent skull base, especially in the region of the floor of the sphenoid sinus. The upper arrow demonstrates a soft tissue mass within the sphenoid sinus, extending to its roof. This represents soft tissue extension of the nasopharyngeal carcinoma.

B, A bone scan in pool phase (left) and delayed phase (right) demonstrates the radionuclide correlation with the conventional study. There is a significant hyperemia in the skull base and sphenoid sinus region (arrow). The dense osteoblastic activity in response to the tumor is indicated in the delayed-phase image. Lateral views are shown to match the lateral tomogram in A. A total body delayed phase image (not shown) did not indicate systemic body metastases.

systemic bony metastases or subclinical local bone invasion.

In osteogenic sarcoma, the bone scan may reflect both the osteolytic and osteoblastic nature of the tumor (Fig. 5–22). It may also detect the presence of functioning metastases.

A malignant schwannoma is shown in Figure 5–23. This vascular tumor was correctly identified by bone scan as involving only the lower half of the right maxillary sinus; the blood pool phase reflected the hyperemia of the tumor and the delayed phase recognized the vertical dimension of the tumor. The entire maxillary sinus was opacified on conventional radiograph and on CT scan, and the tumor was thought to extend to the floor of the orbit. The true tumor delineation, which was detected by radionuclide bone scan, was confirmed at surgery, allowing partial maxillectomy to be performed with preservation of the orbital floor.

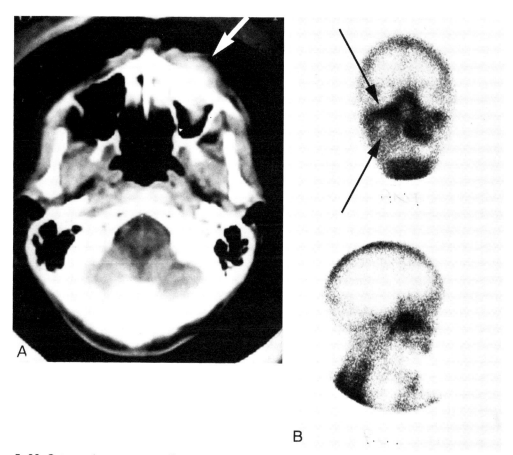

Figure 5–22. Osteogenic sarcoma, maxillary sinus.

A, An axial CT scan demonstrates an osteogenic sarcoma of the right maxillary sinus. Internally it encroaches on the sinus lumen; externally it raises an elevated knobby mass (arrow).

B, A bone scan, in delayed phase, is shown in anterior view (*top*) and right lateral view (*bottom*). The tumor has a varying osteoblastic and osteolytic response, as is commonly seen in osteogenic sarcoma. The upper arrow demonstrates an osteoblastic response in the region of the orbital floor; the lower arrow indicates a photon deficient area of osteolysis involving the inferior portion of the maxillary sinus.

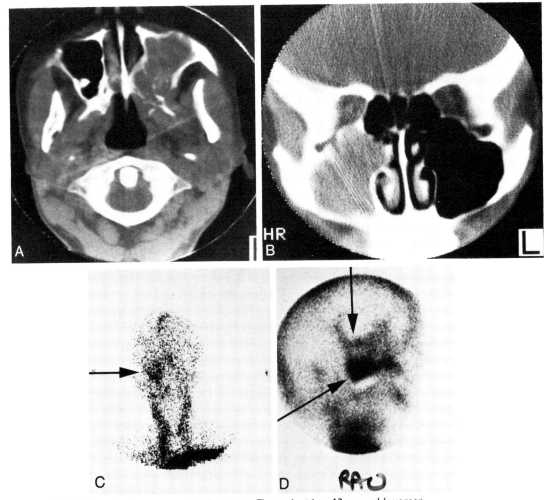

Figure 5–23. Malignant schwannoma, maxillary sinus. The patient is a 42-year-old woman.

A, An axial CT cut demonstrates opacification of the right maxillary sinus and displacement of its medial wall into the nasal cavity posteriorly. The posterior wall of the maxillary sinus is fragmented on this inferiorly placed antral cut, as the tumor extends into the pterygoid fossa.

B, A coronal CT cut shows an opacified right maxillary sinus. The orbital floor appears intact on this view, but the tumor is suggested as completely filling the vertical dimension of the maxillary sinus.

C, The flow phase of a bone scan demonstrates the vascular nature of the tumor (arrow).

D, The delayed phase of the bone scan demonstrates the localization of the tumor in the lower half of the maxillary sinus. The right anterior oblique view demonstrates the dimension of the osteoblastic response to the tumor (lower arrow); the intact orbital floor is imaged by the upper arrow; there is a definite area of noninvolvement inferior to the obviously intact orbital floor. This was confirmed at surgery in which partial maxillectomy could be successfully carried out.

In systemic lymphoma,[29] with paranasal sinus and nasopharyngeal involvement, the bone scan and gallium scan can be used to stage the lymphomatous process (Fig. 5–24). In extramedullary plasmacytoma of the maxillary sinus, the bone scan correlates the pathophysiology of this vascular, bone-destructive tumor with the morphologic conventional radiologic studies. The main role of the bone scan is to detect systemic foci of multiple myeloma.

As a result of advances in gamma camera technology, most contemporary departments of nuclear medicine are now equipped with at least one SPECT (single photon emission computed tomographic) camera. This is essentially similar to a conventional gamma camera, except that the detector head is mounted so that it can rotate 360 degrees around the patient, acquiring up to 128 images in different angular projections. These multiple images are reconstructed into a tomographic format using mathematical "back projection" formulas similar to those of

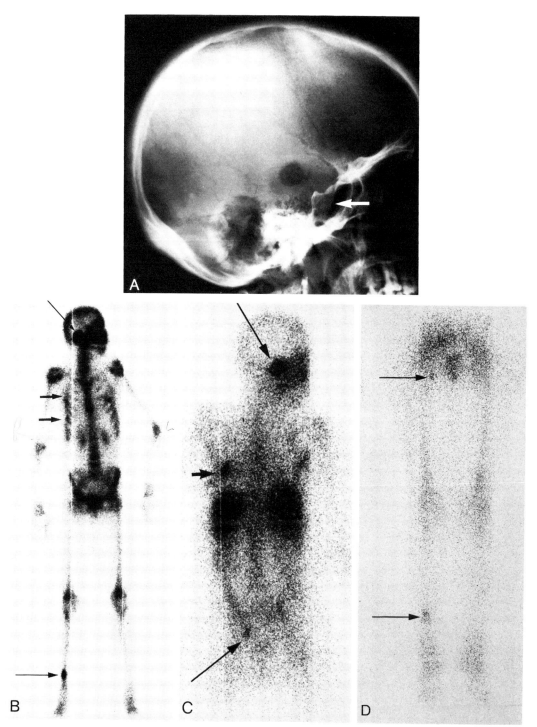

Figure 5–24. Histiocytic lymphoma, sphenoid sinus and systemic foci.

A, A lateral radiograph of the skull demonstrates a soft tissue mass, a histiocytic lymphoma, within the upper and posterior half of the sphenoid sinus (arrow). The anterior portion of the sinus remains aerated. There are a lytic, punched-out lesion of the temporal squama and bone destruction within the mastoid air cells.

B, A delayed bone scan, in whole body image, demonstrates the systemic nature of the lymphoma. The upper arrow indicates the skull base involvement. The two middle black arrows show involvement of the rib cage. The lowest arrow points to a focus of bony lymphoma involving the tibia.

C, A gallium scan demonstrates the presence of systemic lymphoma, correlating with the bone scan images. The uppermost arrow indicates the skull base focus; the middle arrow shows rib involvement. The lowest arrow indicates soft tissue involvement of lymphoma; the inguinal node mass is imaged.

D, The lower extremities are imaged on gallium scan, again indicating the inguinal lymph node involvement (upper arrow) and the tibial involvement (lower arrow). The gallium scan obviously can image both soft tissue and bony involvement; the bone scan obviously images only the bony involvement.

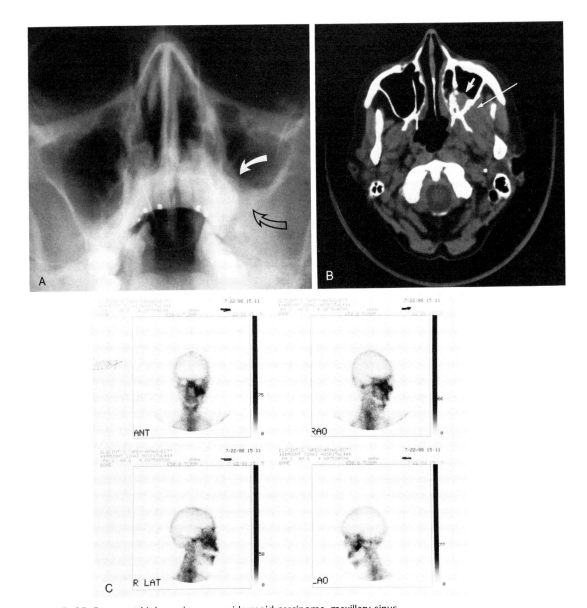

Figure 5—25. Recurrent high-grade mucoepidermoid carcinoma, maxillary sinus.

A, A Waters view indicates a soft tissue mass (white arrow) in the lower third of the left maxillary sinus in a 64-year-old woman with left midfacial pain 4 years following resection of the alveolus (black arrow) for a high-grade mucoepidermoid carcinoma.

B, Axial CT demonstrates a soft tissue mass posteriorly (thick arrow) within the left maxillary sinus. The adjacent bone is thickened medially and laterally and is fragmented medially. The long thin arrow indicates effacement of adjacent fat planes beyond the posterolateral maxillary sinus wall.

C, Planar images in an MDP bone scan show areas of increased uptake but do not allow localization.

CT and MRI. Tomographic sections in coronal, sagittal, axial, or oblique projections may be displayed.

SPECT images[30, 31] provide improved lesion detection by eliminating superfluous activity from adjacent structures. This results in better contrast between the lesion and background than in planar images.[32] More precise anatomic localization is possible because of enhanced depth perception. The applications of this technology to paranasal sinus imaging lie in the early detection of bone erosive disease, by a more sensitive demonstration of osteoblastic response. This also has application in the extra-sinus extension of bone erosive disease (Fig. 5–25), and in the evaluation of the adjacent skull base (Fig. 5–26).

POSTSURGERY

The bone scan is useful in determining the status of the paranasal sinuses following surgery.[9] This is particularly valuable after Caldwell-Luc surgery of the maxillary sinus when clinical considerations raise the possibility of recurrent disease versus normal healing status. There is a great variation in the normal healing pattern after Caldwell-Luc surgery, depending on the nature of the surgery and the radical or conservative approach of the operator. On the conventional x-ray study, the maxillary sinus may be normal, partially opacified or even ossified following Caldwell-Luc surgery.[29, 30]

A volume effect due to increased bone in an ossified but quiescent maxillary sinus is shown in Figure 5–27. A healing maxillary sinus 14 months following Caldwell-Luc surgery can be seen at the site of the anterior antrotomy. However, the periosteum that was stripped from the posterior wall of the maxillary sinus at surgery has occasioned a bony response in this area, which is still reactive. The bone scan findings in this case do not indicate active disease. However, if there is infection within the maxillary sinus following surgery, soft tissue inflammation can be detected by the positive blood pool phase of the bone scan, reflecting hyperemia. If osteomyelitis has occurred, the bone scan findings may be as depicted in Figure 5–9. Sometimes local injuries provide curious but correlative diagnostic images; a patient underwent an antral lavage in which the trochar was obviously introduced beneath the periosteum of the posterior wall of the maxillary sinus and intense pain was produced; the still healing reaction to this traumatic event can be seen 3 months later in the delayed bone scan.

Postoperative bone scanning is of value in following tumor patients, in some instances. Osteotomies can continue to heal for 12 to 18 to 24 months postsurgery, as can fractures. However, a quiet bone scan that becomes active may reflect the presence of recurrent tumor.

The bone scan is also useful in determining the success of bone grafts to the midfacial skeleton.[9] Following iliac bone graft to the nasal dorsum (if the graft is large enough to image by

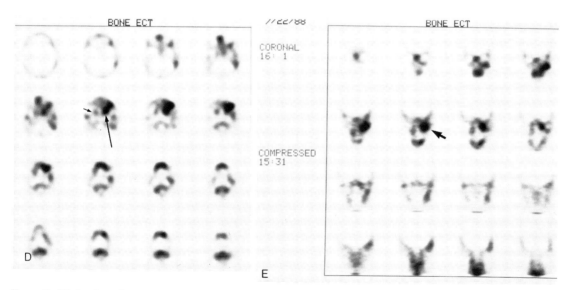

Figure 5–25 Continued
   D, Axial SPECT shows osteoblastic reaction extending through the posterior wall of the left maxillary sinus to pterygoid plates (long arrow). Compare this with the normal right pterygoid plates (short arrow).
   E, Coronal SPECT demonstrates tumor extension to the skull base (arrow).

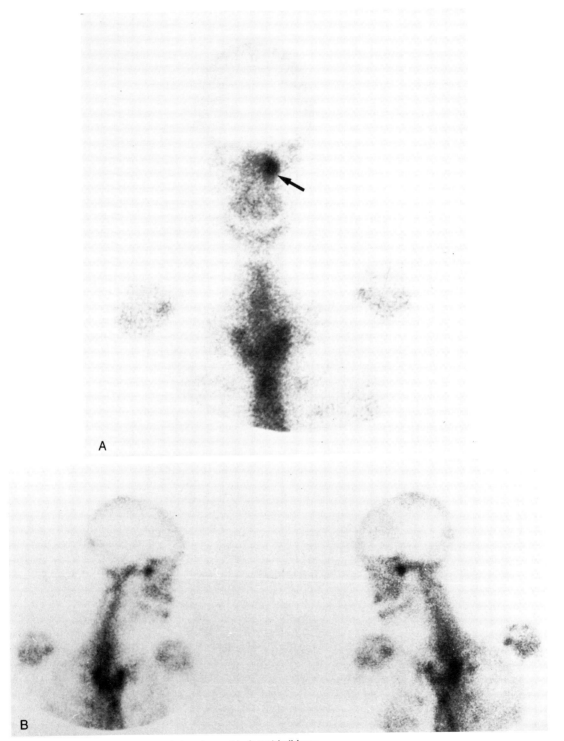

Figure 5–26. Osteoblastic metastasis to pterygoid plates/skull base.

A, Planar anterior image of an MDP bone scan (delayed-phase) demonstrates an area of increased activity *(arrow)* in the plane of the ethmoid labyrinth.

B, Right and left lateral planar images indicate a focal "hot spot."

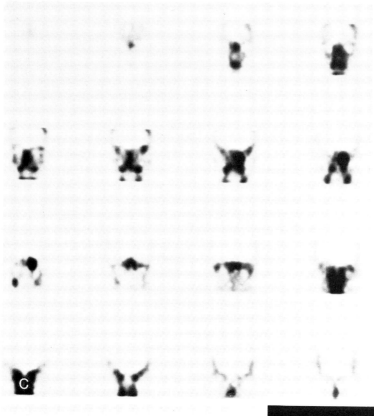

Figure 5–26 *Continued*

C, Serial coronal SPECT images provide an overview coronal tomographic display of the skull base.

D, A coronal SPECT bone scan image, during the same study, allows the localization of this intense osteoblastic activity to the junction of the pterygoid plates with the skull base (thick arrow). A lesser focus of uptake, due to dental infection, is seen in the right upper alveolus (hollow arrow). The long thin arrow indicates the inferior aspect of the left medial and lateral pterygoid plates. The "hot" focus at the base of the pterygoid plates is due to metastatic malignant melanoma in this patient complaining of deep-seated facial pain, thought initially to be "sinusitis."

E, An axial CT scan demonstrates the osteoblastosis (arrow) resulting from this metastasis within the left pterygoid plates.

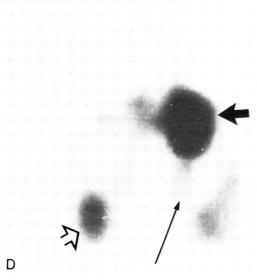

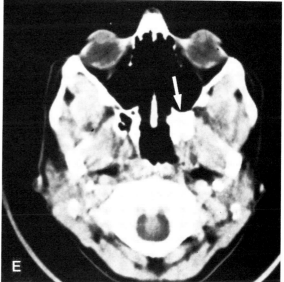

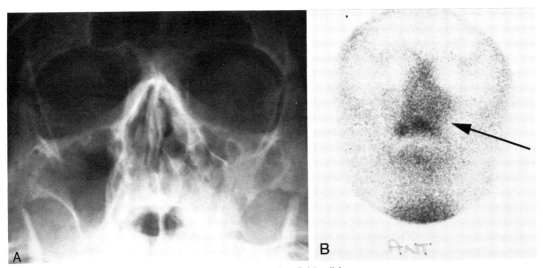

Figure 5—27. Asymptomatic ossification of maxillary sinus, after Caldwell-Luc surgery.

A, A Waters view demonstrates irregular opacification and increased density of the left maxillary sinus. The patient had undergone left Caldwell-Luc surgery 26 years previously. As occasionally occurs, the floor of the orbit is now depressed on this side. The nature of the morphologic change within the maxillary sinus is uncertain from the conventional Waters view.

B, A bone scan, anterior view in delayed phase, demonstrates an increase in bone density in the plane of the left maxillary sinus (arrow). However, this is not biologically active bone, compared with the rest of the bone on the facial skeleton; this is simply an increase in bone, obliterating in large measure the left maxillary sinus. This volume effect accounts for the radionuclide image shown.

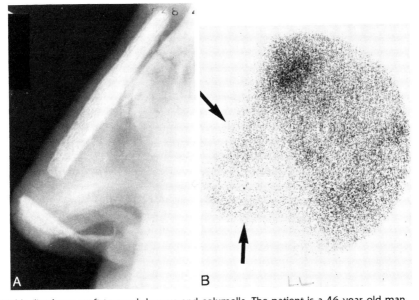

Figure 5—28. Viable iliac bone graft to nasal dorsum and columella. The patient is a 46-year-old man.

A, A lateral radiograph demonstrates the position of an iliac bone graft to the nasal dorsum, as well as a smaller iliac bone graft positioned as a columellar strut. The procedure has been carried out for nasal collapse.

B, A magnified image of the delayed bone scan, in left lateral view, demonstrates the osteogenic activity of the nasal dorsal bone graft (upper arrow) and the columellar graft (lower arrow) on the fourth postoperative day. These grafts survived, and the patient had an excellent surgical result.

gamma camera), a viable bone graft may demonstrate an osteogenic response from approximately the third postoperative day (Fig. 5–28). It may even be possible to image the hyperemia of the restored microcirculation on blood pool phase image sometime later. Thereafter, the healing of the bone graft will reflect the same process as facial fracture healing.

SYSTEMIC BONE DISEASE

Fibrous dysplasia, which can offer a variety of conventional radiographic findings, can be studied by radionuclide bone scan. The conventional radiologic studies may demonstrate a soft tissue mass, a mixed pattern or a dense sclerosis.[25] However, the bone scan will demonstrate the hyperemia of the soft tissue and the intense bone reaction of the osteoblastic lesion itself. In fibrous dysplasia, the bone scan will demonstrate the monostotic or regional nature of the disease or the occasional systemic bone involvement (often in conjunction with endocrine syndromes such as Albright's syndrome). Although fibrous dysplasia is thought to be an abnormality in bone maturation,[35] it may continue into adult years and its biologic activity

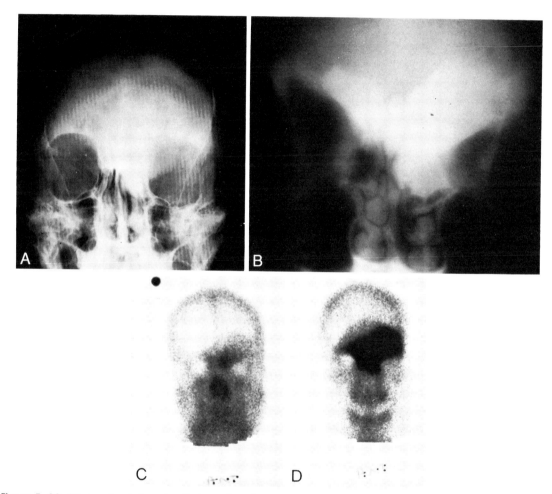

Figure 5–29. Fibrous dysplasia, sclerotic type, frontal sinus. The patient is a 37-year-old man whose disease was thought to have been latent; the radionuclide images, however, indicate a continued biologic activity of the disease process.

A, A Caldwell view demonstrates the dense hyperostosis of fibrous dysplasia involving the left frontal bone primarily. The adjacent bones are involved across suture lines. The fibrous dysplasia encroaches on the left orbit, producing a small volume orbit.

B, An AP tomogram defines the configuration of the anatomic abnormality to better advantage, especially its involvement of the anterior cranial fossa floor.

C, The pool phase of the bone scan indicates the tremendous hyperemia of what might be judged morphologically to be a quiescent lesion.

D, The delayed phase of the bone scan demonstrates the intense incorporation of phosphate anion into the bony lesion, reflecting its continued metabolic activity.

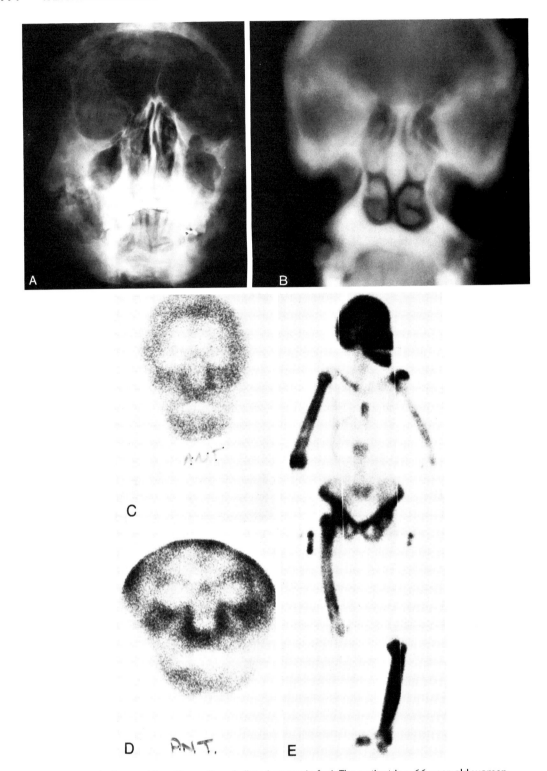

Figure 5–30. Paget's disease, bimaxillary, other skull and systemic foci. The patient is a 66-year-old woman.

A, A Waters view demonstrates the typical cotton wool skull appearance of Paget's disease. Both maxillary sinuses are of small volume owing to thickened bony walls with Paget's disease. The radiographic findings are classic.

B, An AP tomogram better defines the morphologic changes seen on the conventional film in *A.*

C, A bone scan, in pool phase, demonstrates the hyperemia of the Paget's bony lesions.

D, The bone scan in delayed phase indicates the osteogenic activity of the Paget's lesions.

E, The whole body view demonstrates the systemic distribution of Paget's disease in this patient. The softened, thickened, typically deformed long bones are imaged; the skull reaction is intense.

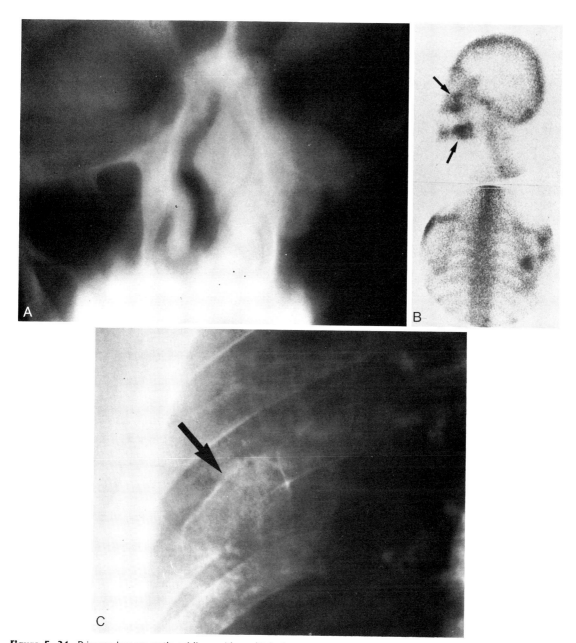

Figure 5–31. Primary hyperparathyroidism with multiple brown tumors involving maxillary sinus, mandible and ribs. The patient is a 55-year-old man who had multiple bony tumor masses and hypercalcemia; a primary carcinoma of a parathyroid gland was ultimately discovered and successfully resected. The brown tumors continued to heal on bone scan over a number of years.

A, An AP tomogram defines a brown tumor occupying the anterior aspect of the left maxillary sinus in its superomedial angle. The relationship of the mass to the bony orbital floor is clearly defined; bone definition is lost medially.

B, A delayed phase bone scan demonstrates the osteoblastic reparative response about the brown tumor in the upper portion of the left maxillary sinus *(upper arrow)*; the lower arrow indicates a brown tumor of the body of the mandible on the left, again with the same physiologic characteristics. A posterior view of the thorax demonstrates rib involvement.

C, A conventional radiograph details the expansile nature of the brown tumor as it involves a rib and expands its cortices *(arrow)*.

may be recognized by both the positive blood pool phase and delayed phase images (Fig. 5–29). The flow phase is usually positive as well.

Paget's disease[9] lends itself ideally to bone scan imaging (Fig. 5–30). The vascular nature of the lesions, with expanded capillary bed, may be recognized on the flow phase screening examination. The actual hyperemia of the Paget's focus is almost always seen, when the disease is active, on the blood pool phase. The delayed phase mirrors the bone response in Paget's disease of the local lesion; the bone is often expanded and typically pagetoid, even at gamma camera resolution. Systemic foci are easily recognized as Paget's disease; this study

may often avoid biopsy diagnosis in lesions that might otherwise seem obscure.

Primary hyperparathyroidism is another systemic bone disease that can be easily recognized on bone scan (Fig. 5–31). The individual expansile bone scan lesions (the brown tumors) are imaged with sensitivity but not with specificity. The systemic lesions may be recognized by conventional radiographs, which have been utilized to study hot anatomic areas in accordance with bone scan findings; the reparative osteoblastic response provides the positive bone scan image and the intense response of the delayed image continues into the healing phase of the disease.

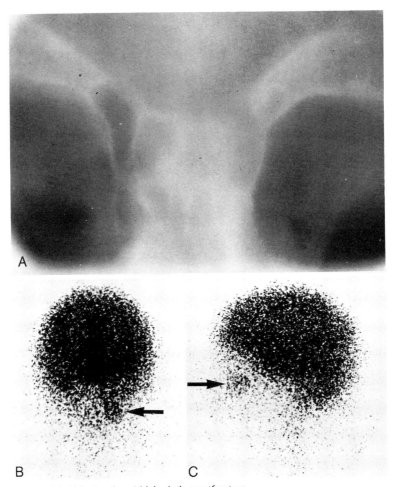

Figure 5–32. Cerebrospinal fluid leak, ethmoid labyrinth, postfracture.

  A, A conventional AP tomogram demonstrates opacification of the left ethmoid labyrinth in a 7-year-old child who experienced intermittent CSF rhinorrhea following a suspected anterior fossa floor fracture. The conventional images failed to localize the site of the presumed CSF leak.

  B, An anterior view of a DTPA CSF scan, tagged with technetium ^{99m}Tc imaged at 24 hours, indicates the lateralization of the CSF leak (arrow) in anterior display.

  C, Lateral image, recorded also at 24 hours, demonstrates the relative position of the CSF leak in anteroposterior dimension (arrow).

VASCULAR LESIONS

As indicated previously, the flow phase of the bone scan (and the flow phase of the brain scan, for that matter) may be utilized to detect primary vascular abnormalities such as hemangiomas, arteriovenous malformations, and vascular tumors. Venous obstruction also can be detected in the late flow phase of the bone scan; this may be useful in the evaluation of internal jugular venous obstruction prior to the initiation of functional neck dissection.

Wegener's granulomatosis with destruction of the nasal septum has been detected on the flow phase of the bone scan; here the vasculitis is reflected as increased vascularity. There is insufficient experience to say whether this is a constant finding; perhaps the vasculitis could lead to a hypovascular lesion as well.

CEREBROSPINAL FLUID LEAK

Cerebrospinal fluid (CSF) leak can be identified, if imaged during the phase of active leakage, by the radioactive tagging of diethylenetriaminepentaacetic acid with ^{99m}Tc or ^{111}indium. The radioactively tagged DPTA is injected intrathecally into the lumbar subarachnoid space and imaged in relation to the skull base and paranasal sinuses at 1, 6, and 24 hours during active CSF leak. This technique may demonstrate the site and side of CSF rhinorrhea (Fig. 5–32). However, radionuclide scans now play a lesser clinical role in CSF rhinorrhea; CSF leak preferentially should be imaged during activity by CT scan, in prone position, 1 hour after intrathecal injection of metrizamide. Coronal cuts should be obtained, and careful preview featuring and thin slice selection should allow exact localization of the fistula site.

References

1. Zizmor J, Noyek AM: The radiologic diagnosis of maxillary sinus disease. Otolaryngol Clin North Am 9(1):93, 1976.
2. Wortzman G, Holgate RC: Special radiological techniques in maxillary sinus disease. Otolaryngol Clin North Am 9(1):117, 1976.
3. Noyek AM, Holgate RC, Wortzman G, et al: Sophisticated radiology in otolaryngology. II. Diagnostic imaging: Non-roentgenographic (non-x-ray) modalities. J Otolaryngol 6(Suppl 3):95, 1977.
4. Lisbona R, Rosenthall L: Observations on the sequential use of ^{99m}Tc phosphate complex and ^{67}Ga. Radiology 123:123, 1977.
5. Noyek AM, Kirsh JC, Greyson ND, et al: The clinical significance of radionuclide bone and gallium scanning in osteomyelitis of the head and neck. Laryngoscope 94:(Suppl 34), 1984.
6. Subramanian G, McAfee JG: A new complex of ^{99m}Tc for skeletal imaging. Radiology 99:192, 1971.
7. Brucer M: A history of bone scanning. II. The second generation: Sr-85, Sr-87m and F-18. III. The third generation: Tc-labelled phosphate. Vignettes Nucl Med 82:1, 1976.
8. Brucer M: A history of bone scanning. IV. Obligatory indications, qualified indications and non-indications. Vignettes Nucl Med 83:1, 1976.
9. Noyek AM: Bone scanning in otolaryngology. Laryngoscope 89(Suppl 18), 1979.
10. Subramanian G, et al: ^{99m}Tc-MDP (methylene diphosphonate): A superior agent for skeletal imaging. J Nucl Med 14:640, 1973.
11. Greyson ND, Noyek AM: Nuclear medicine in otolaryngological diagnosis. Otolaryngol Clin North Am 11(2):541, 1978.
12. Charkes ND: Bone scanning: Principles, technique and interpretation. Radiol Clin North Am 8(2): 259, 1970.
13. Charkes ND, Valantine G, Kravitz B: Interpretation of the normal ^{99m}Tc polyphosphate rectilinear bone scan. Radiology 107(3):563, 1973.
14. Merrick MV: Review article: Bone scanning. Br J Radiol 48:327, 1975.
15. Wagner HJ Jr.: Principles of Nuclear Medicine. Philadelphia, WB Saunders, 1968.
16. Blahd WH: Nuclear Medicine. 2nd ed. New York, McGraw-Hill, 1971.
17. Baum S, Bramlet R: Basic Nuclear Medicine. New York, Appleton-Century-Crofts, 1970.
18. Houle S: St. Michael's Hospital, Toronto. Personal communication.
19. Zizmor J, Noyek AM: Inflammatory diseases of the paranasal sinuses. Otolaryngol Clin North Am 6(2):459, 1973.
20. Zizmor J, Noyek AM: Fractures of the paranasal sinuses. Otolaryngol Clin North Am 6(2):473, 1973.
21. Noyek AM, Kassel EE, Wortzman G, et al: Sophisticated CT in complex maxillofacial trauma. Laryngoscope 92:(Suppl 27), 1982.
22. Zizmor J, Noyek AM: Cysts, benign tumors and malignant tumors of the paranasal sinuses. Otolaryngol Clin North Am 6(2):487, 1973.
23. Zizmor J, Noyek AM: Cysts and benign tumors of the paranasal sinuses. Semin Roentgenol 3(2):172, 1968.
24. Zizmor J, Noyek AM, Chapnik JS: Mucocele of the paranasal sinuses. J Otolaryngol 3(Suppl 1), 1974.
25. Zizmor J, Noyek AM: Calcifying and osteoblastic tumors of the paranasal sinuses. J Otolaryngol 6(Suppl 3):22, 1977.
26. Freeman JL, Shemen LJ, Alberti FW, et al: Ossifying capillary hemangioma of the maxillary and ethmoid sinuses—a case report. J Otolaryngol 10(6):481, 1982.
27. Noyek AM, Greyson ND, Cooter N, Shapiro BJ: Radionuclide salivary scan imaging of maxillary sinus oncocytoma. J Otolaryngol 11(1):17, 1982.
28. Noyek AM, Wortzman G, Holgate RC, et al: The radiologic diagnosis of malignant tumors of the paranasal sinuses and related structures. J Otolaryngol 6(5):399, 1977.
29. Noyek AM, Zizmor J: Lymphoma and leukemia of the upper airway and orbit. Semin Roentgenol 15(3):251, 1980.
30. Katzberg RW, O'Mara RE, Tallents RH, et al: Radionuclide skeletal imaging and single photon emission

computed tomography in suspected internal derangements of the temporomandibular joint. J Oral Maxillofac Surg 42:782, 1984.
31. Collier BD, Hellman RS Jr, Krasnow AZ: Bone SPECT.
Semin Nucl Med 17:247, 1987.
32. Israel O, Jerushalmi J, Frankel A, Kuten A, Front D:
Normal and abnormal single photon emission computed
tomography of the skull: Comparison with planar scintigraphy. J Nucl Med 29:1341, 1988.

33. Zizmor J, Noyek AM: The radiologic diagnosis of postsurgical disease of the sinuses and mastoids. Otolaryngol Clin North Am 7:251, 1974.
34. Noyek AM, Zizmor J: Radiology of the maxillary sinus
after Caldwell-Luc surgery. Otolaryngol Clin North
Am 9(1):135, 1976.
35. Van Nostrand AWP: Pathologic aspects of osseous and
fibro-osseous lesions of the maxillary sinus. Otolaryngol
Clin North Am 9(1):35, 1976.

CHAPTER 6

PATHOLOGY

John G. Batsakis, MD
James J. Sciubba, DMD, PhD

Pathologic conditions that involve the paranasal sinuses may be simplistically divided into non-neoplastic and neoplastic lesions. In terms of general morbidity and incidence, the non-neoplastic diseases far outnumber malignancies.

INFLAMMATORY AND NON–NEOPLASTIC DISEASES

Inflammatory disorders of the paranasal sinuses are encompassed by the descriptive, yet not etiologically based, term of *sinusitis*, of which there are acute and chronic forms. The inflammatory diseases can be divided into those resulting from infectious agents (bacterial, fungal, viral, parasitic) and those associated with noninfectious diseases (allergy, barotrauma, exposure to chemicals or other nonmicrobial agents, sarcoidosis, and disorders with an unknown or unproved basis, such as Wegener's granulomatosis and vascular diseases).

Because of the anatomic and functional relationship of the paranasal sinuses and the nasal cavity,[1–8] many of the inflammatory processes of the sinuses result from extension of an intranasal disease. The maxillary sinus is additionally vulnerable to direct spread from infection about the roots of teeth, especially the first and second molars.

SINUSITIS

The surgical pathologist rarely sees tissue from a totally acute sinusitis, which is usually a short-course disease unless complicated.

Chronic sinusitis, resulting from either a persistence of an acute inflammatory process or repeated attacks of acute sinusitis, more often provides indication for surgical intervention and tissue removal.

Van Nostrand and Goodman[9] classify sinusitis into two major groups—hypertrophic (or polypoid) and atrophic (or sclerosing). Histomorphologic changes in the hypertrophic type result in considerable thickening of the sinus mucosal lining. Unless there is squamous metaplasia, the regenerative pseudostratified columnar epithelium may contain a marked increase in goblet cells or a decrease in these cells. There may also be a reactive hyperplasia and hypertrophy of the seromucinous glands. The lamina propria is thickened, and its vessels manifest perivascular fibrosis and thickening of their walls. Lymphocytes and plasma cells are the dominant inflammatory cells; their density may be marked and at times may be associated with prominent germinal centers—so-called lymphofollicular sinusitis. Variable numbers of eosinophils and histiocytes may be present. The basement membrane is also thickened and often hyalinized. Foci of dystrophic calcification may also be present. Mucosal ulcers may be in evidence or indicated by patches of squamous metaplasia. Depending on the degree of hemorrhage, metaplasia and necrosis, variable numbers of foreign body giant cells may be found.

The thickened mucosa is frequently thrown up into irregular polypoid projections or folds—so-called polypoid hypertrophy or polyps.

The atrophic form of sinusitis consists of a scarred lamina propria either denuded or covered by metaplastic squamous epithelia. In addition to the change in the mucosal cells, the most striking feature is dense collagenized connective tissue, associated with vascular sclerosis.

Both atrophic and hypertrophic forms may coexist in a given chronic sinusitis or be independent of each other. On occasion, nasal polyps and progressive sinusitis are causes of bone destruction in the nasal cavity and sinuses.

POLYPS

An inflammatory basis is also ascribed to the commonly occurring nasal and paranasal polyps (Fig. 6–1), but their pathogenesis is elusive. Allergy, atopy, infection, and vasomotor impairment have all been proposed as factors in the development of these lesions.[1] A classification of nasal polyps according to a predominant cellular infiltrate is not reliable.[1] Eosinophilia varies from patient to patient regardless of the atopic state, and the degree of eosinophilia may depend only on recent contact with an allergen. Except for some tenuous light microscopic findings, neither routine light nor electron microscopic examinations have been helpful in elucidating the pathogenesis of nasal polyps.[1]

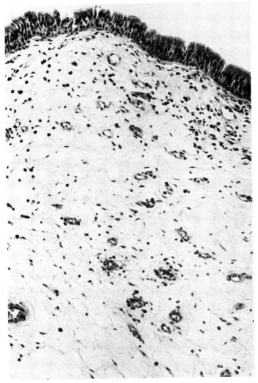

Figure 6–1. Nasal polyp manifesting a moderately vascularized and edematous stroma.

The relationship among nasal polyps, paranasal sinus disease, and cystic fibrosis requires underscoring. So too does the association of polyps with Kartagener's syndrome.[10]

CYSTIC FIBROSIS

Cystic fibrosis, a disease with its principal impact on the exocrine glands of multiple organ systems, is the most common autosomal-recessive disease of Caucasians, affecting 1 in every 1600 to 2500 live births. Geneticists consider the disease to be the most lethal inherited disease of whites.[1]

The clinical hallmarks of cystic fibrosis are chronic suppurative, staphylococcal, or pseudomonal lung disease, pancreatic insufficiency, and abnormally salty sweat. For indisputable diagnosis, evidence of all three should be present. Each of the principal clinical manifestations varies in degree and severity. The great majority of patients have sweat chloride concentrations above 60 mmol/L, varying between 60 and 120 mmol/L, but a few have levels between 50 and 60 mmol/L.

The clinical manifestations of cystic fibrosis result from a basic metabolic defect, which is associated with changes in the physical character of macromolecule-containing exocrine gland excretions and in the electrolyte content of serous secretions.[11–13] This is reflected in an increase is sweat sodium and chloride concentrations and a deficiency in pancreatic enzymes. The exocrine secretions aggregate to block ducts or tubes, producing secondary and even tertiary pathologic changes in the involved organs, with subsequent variable alterations in function.

The otolaryngologic aspects of cystic fibrosis are dominated by involvement of the paranasal sinuses, delayed development of the frontal sinuses and panopacification, and a high incidence of nasal polyposis.

Patients with cystic fibrosis almost never have normal sinus x-ray examination results. Over 99 per cent of patients demonstrate a panopacification of the sinuses, but less than 1 per cent have clinical signs and symptoms of a sinus infection.[14] The combination of panopacification without appreciable signs and symptoms of sinusitis in a child should always lead to suspicion of cystic fibrosis. When sinus infection is superimposed, it is almost always severe and requires operative intervention because of the tenacity of the mucus.

Despite the extraordinary prevalence of upper respiratory allergy and infection in children, nasal polyposis is rare. When it is found in a child, the possibility of cystic fibrosis should always be considered. Most cases of nasal polyposis in children occur in patients known to have cystic fibrosis, but there are reports of the polyps having preceded the diagnosis.[1, 14] Some evidence exists that the incidence of nasal polyps in affected children is decreasing, at least to lower levels than when aerosol antibiotic use was more widespread.[14] This association raises the question of synergistic action with environmental factors.

Patients with nasal obstruction caused by the polyps are quite markedly benefited by surgical removal of the polyps. As a group, however, the patients manifest recurrences, which are often multiple.

Rhinoscopy may show only a mild congestion of the nasal mucosa, clear mucoid secretions, or mucopurulent material. The polyps are usually bilateral, in the middle meatus, and bulky and multiple. They are grossly and microscopically indistinguishable from inflammatory nasal polyps of adults.

Even though the mucosa of the middle ear and the eustachian tube is a respiratory type and in direct continuity with the mucosa of the upper respiratory tract, otologic manifestations in cystic fibrosis are not marked. There is no greater incidence of a conductive or sensorineural hearing loss when compared with that in normal age-adjusted population.[15] Secretory otitis media and acute suppurative otitis media are also uncommon.

KARTAGENER'S SYNDROME

Cilia of the respiratory tract manifest a metachronal rhythm, with the direction of the beat always the axis. Among the several factors affecting the frequency and coordination of the beat are the concentrations of adenosine triphosphate (ATP) and calcium and magnesium, temperature, viscosity, and dynein. Dynein molecules are important components of the microtubules of the cilia in that they exhibit adenosine triphosphatase (ATPase) activity. The energy for the basic motion of cilia is derived from dynein breaking down ATP. Absence or deficiency of the ATPase activity of dynein has been proposed as the primary defect in the autosomal-recessive Kartagener's syndrome.[16] The immobile cilia retard the drainage and clearance of paranasal sinus and nasal mucus. Abnormal (compound and mega) cilia found in subjects with the syndrome may be acquired or also part of the fundamental defect, but microtubular changes are always present.

ANTRAL CHOANAL POLYP

The antral choanal polyp occurs much less often than the benign inflammatory or allergic polyp, but it exhibits certain characteristics that make it distinctive.[1] The antral choanal polyp is the most common polyp in children; however, it constitutes less than 4 per cent of nasal polyps removed from *all* patients.

By definition, an antral choanal polyp is a mucosal polyp protruding from a choana. It may be clinically apparent in the nasopharynx (hence its synonyms: nasoantral polyp, benign nasopharyngeal polyp, postnasal polyp, recurring polyp, choanal polyp, retronasal polyp).

The antral choanal polyp typically and classically arises from the lateral wall of the maxillary antrum. Only rarely has an origin other than the maxillary sinus been reported, e.g., sphenochoanal polyps and some from the ethmoid air cells.[17, 18] Patients with antral choanal polyps invariably have antral and often associated ethmoid opacification.[17, 18] Contralateral sinus mucosal thickening is an inconsistent finding. In the study by Schramm and Effron,[19] over half of their pediatric patients with antral choanal polyps were found to have maxillary sinusitis at the time of surgery.

The role of sinusitis points to an inflammatory basis for these polyps. Indeed, a history of allergy is rarely elicited from these patients. The lesion is typically solitary and unilateral, and there are, as a rule, no other polypoid changes or polyps in the nose.

On clinical inspection, the antral choanal polyp is smooth, rounded, and gray or bluish. By posterior rhinoscopy, it may be seen either projecting from a choana or completely filling the nasopharynx. It may drop below the level of the soft palate into the oropharynx. The polyp gains entrance to the nasal fossa by way of an ostium (usually a large accessory ostium), and the polyp will generally manifest a pedicle, which passes from the polyp anteriorly into the middle meatus.

Except for gross and clinical features, there is little to distinguish the antral choanal polyp from other inflammatory polyps of the sinonasal tract. The mucosal surface, unless ulcerated or metaplastic, is a respiratory-type epithelium. Because of the normally fewer numbers of mucoserous glands in the sinuses, the polyp is usually also sparsely populated by these structures. The polyp's stroma is usually myxoid but has a tendency to be fibrovascular. Variable densities of inflammatory cells are found, and these tend to be more concentrated near the mucosal surface.

These polyps manifest two other characteristics of either clinical or histopathologic diagnostic importance. Avulsion alone carries with it a recurrence rate of up to 25 per cent; thus a Caldwell-Luc procedure is necessary.[1, 17, 18] Unfamiliarity with the secondary alterations that may occur in the polyps accounts for varying degrees of misinterpretation of diagnosis. Perhaps more so than with any other sinonasal polyp, the antral choanal polyp is subject to secondary stromal alterations. These take the form of prominent fibrovascularity, neovascularization and thrombosis, and the appearance of atypical stromal cells (Fig. 6–2). The vascularized form may simulate an angiofibroma or other vascular lesion and the atypical cells may be misconstrued as components of sarcoma.[1, 20]

Stromal atypia in nasal polyps is not restricted to choanal polyps, but the combination of the patient's age, solitary mass, and the atypical cells may result in disastrous misdiagnosis. The atypical cells are often numerous, large pleomorphic histiocytes or facultative fibroblasts that may be dispersed or tend to be aggregated about fibrovascular or occlusive-vascular areas of the polyp. The pleomorphic spindle cells have prominent nuclei, often with large nucleoli, and ill-defined cell membranes. The cytoplasm of the cells often has a foamy character. Although these cells may be histologically alarming, no distinct pattern of definable supporting tissue malignancy is present.[1, 20]

FUNGAL DISEASES

Space does not allow discussion of clinicopathologic correlates with specific fungal disorders of the sinuses, and we will use aspergillosis as an example only.

Aspergillosis. This is the most common fungal infection of the paranasal sinuses. It has invasive and noninvasive forms, is caused by any of the several species of the *Aspergillus*, and usually develops in patients who are otherwise healthy.

Invasive aspergillosis mimics a malignancy, produces a mass in the orbit, nose or cheek, and occasionally extends to the skin. It can involve the ethmoid or maxillary sinus or both. Bone destruction is usually evident.

Noninvasive primary aspergillosis of the paranasal sinuses is more common. It produces symptoms of chronic sinusitis and differs from a chronic bacterial sinusitis in being more resistant to conservative management. Any sinus can be the site, but the maxillary sinus is involved most frequently. Opacification of the sinus without bone destruction is seen radiographically.

In the noninvasive form of aspergillosis, the sinus mucosa is thick and edematous. An aggregate of greasy, necrotic material may be present and the mucosa is diffusely infiltrated by acute and chronic inflammatory cells. Masses of hyphae (fungus balls) are separate from or on the surface of the epithelium. Fruiting bodies can also be found. In general, a granulomatous or giant cell reaction and/or fibrosis is not present.

Invasive aspergillosis, on the other hand, is associated with a granulomatous inflammatory process (giant cells, lymphocytes, plasma cells, and fibrosis). Some granulomas manifest microabscesses or necrosis, and fungal hyphae are found in the center of granulomas in giant cells

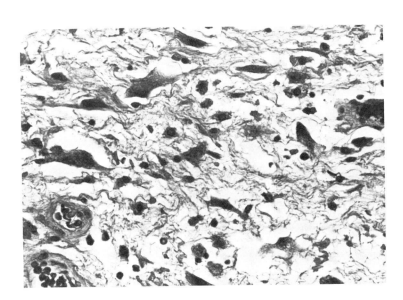

Figure 6–2. Atypical stromal cells in an antral choanal polyp from a 13-year-old boy. The cells are likely facultative fibroblasts and, although alarming in appearance, are non-neoplastic responses to injury.

and in the connective tissues. Extensive necrosis may obliterate other findings.

The fruiting heads of *Aspergillus* are considered pathognomonic. They are rarely seen in invasive disease, and most often are encountered when there is a noninvasive fungus ball in a sinus cavity.

NONHEALING GRANULOMAS

Even though attention is focused on the triumvirate of Wegener's granulomatosis, polymorphic reticulosis, and lymphoma in the diagnostic consideration of nonhealing granulomas of the sinonasal tract, it is to be remembered that worldwide these three disorders rank behind specific and nonspecific destructive inflammatory diseases as pathogenetic causes.[21]

MIDLINE (FACIAL) NONHEALING GRANULOMA

This term lacks specificity as either a clinical or surgical-pathologic designation. It is used only in a generic sense to indicate general location and aggressiveness. It is now clear that within this impressive category there are classifiable lesions, each with specific histopathologic features. Specific and nonspecific (sarcoidosis) granulomatous disease *must* always be ruled out by clinical and laboratory means. This done, three (and possibly four) clinicopathologic entities remain: Wegener's granulomatosis, polymorphic reticulosis, lymphoma, and a group currently classified as idiopathic midline granuloma (Table 6–1).[21]

WEGENER'S GRANULOMATOSIS

As originally defined, Wegener's granulomatosis required the presence of necrotizing granulomas, with vasculitis involving both arteries and veins in the upper and lower respiratory tract, coincident with a focal necrotizing glomerulitis. Early therapeutic experiences indicated that the disease brought death quickly, usually within a few months. Limited forms of the disease with a more benign course (without evidence of renal disease) were first recognized in 1966, and this recognition was later expanded so that now the disease is considered a clinical continuum or spectrum.[21–23]

Necrotizing granulomas with vasculitis form the common basis for diagnosis. A histopathologic diagnosis of Wegener's granulomatosis requires the demonstration of vasculitis.

Each of the major sites of involvement, i.e., upper respiratory tract, lungs, and kidneys, may be involved alone or in any combination, except that the focal necrotizing glomerulitis is nonspecific for diagnosis.[22] Disease may evolve from a single focus through the complete system complex or it may remain localized.

In most cases, signs or symptoms referable to upper or lower airway involvement attract the diagnostician's attention. Some patients have oral, ocular, otologic, or pharyngeal symptoms. Only a few individuals demonstrate pulmonary disease without evidence of upper airway involvement. Pansinusitis is quite common. In descending order of frequency, the maxillary, ethmoid, frontal, and sphenoid sinuses show involvement. In 31 of 52 patients studied by McDonald and colleagues,[23] there was sinonasal disease, either alone or in combination with disease at other sites, at some time during the course of the illness. Oculo-orbital involvement, either from a local vasculitis or from an extension from adjacent sinuses, is much more common in Wegener's granulomatosis than in polymorphic reticulosis. Secondary bacterial infection resulting from the damaged mucosal surfaces accompanies sinus, nasal, and oral disease. In the paranasal sinuses *Staphylococcus aureus* is most frequently responsible for the infections.[21, 24] Systemic involvement from Wegener's granulomatosis spares almost no organ system (Table 6–2).[21]

Even though the disorder exists in a clinical spectrum ranging from a mitigated or limited form to an overwhelmingly fulminant vasculitis with death by uremia, its tissue changes are distinctive. By light and electron microscopy, the apparent basic lesion is a necrotizing vasculitis.[21, 25, 26] Fine structure analysis indicates that intravascular lysis of leukocytes is an early event in the process of tissue injury.[25] This cytolysis is followed by platelet aggregation and adhesion, with fibrin deposition in vessels with an intact endothelium. Necrosis of endothelial cells also occurs early, and this leads to complete obstruction of vascular lumens and denudation down to the basement membrane of involved arteries and veins. Cytotoxic or steroid drug treatment halts the intravascular lysis and coagulation.[25]

The vascular compromise produced by the necrotizing vasculitis is responsible for the other histomorphologic expressions of the disease: mucosal ulcers, microabscess (often becoming confluent), coagulative necrosis within and extending to granulomas, giant cells, and a diffuse acute and chronic inflammation.

TABLE 6–1. Differential Features of Several Midfacial Necrotizing Disorders

	Wegener's Granulomatosis	Churg-Strauss Syndrome	Polymorphic Reticulosis	Idiopathic Nonhealing Granuloma
Upper airway	Diffuse, ulcerating, crusting lesions; predominantly sinuses and nose. Ocular manifestations common. Rarely erodes palate and facial soft tissues	Necrotizing, least prominent of group. Abnormal sinus radiographs and nasal polyps	Destructive, localized, or diffuse lesions with destruction of bone and extension through facial soft tissues	Destructive, localized, or diffuse lesions with characteristic extension through palate and facial soft tissue
Systemic	Small vessel vasculitis. Lungs. Kidney (necrotizing glomerulitis). May not have upper airway involvement. No asthma	Asthma is clinical hallmark. Peripheral eosinophilia. Lungs, skin, heart, GI tract, peripheral nerves. Renal disease is infrequent	May be localized to upper or lower airway or be systemic. May not have upper airway lesions	No systemic lesion. Disorder is localized to upper aerodigestive tract
Relation to lymphoma	None	None	May remain histologically atypical and disseminate or evolve to lymphoma with extranodal type spread	?
Basic lesion	Necrotizing vasculitis with granulomas, giant cells, and fibrinoid/coagulative necrosis. No atypical lymphoreticular infiltrate	Necrotizing extravascular granulomas and necrotizing vasculitis. Prominent tissue eosinophilia	Angiocentric, angiodestructive, atypical lymphoreticular infiltrate. Granulomas, giant cells, and primary vasculitis inconspicuous	Nonspecific acute and chronic inflammation. Granulomas, giant cells, and vasculitis are infrequent
Therapeutic response				
Steroids	+	+	0	Irradiation +, but disease is progressive
Cytotoxic drugs	+	?	0	
Irradiation:	0	–	+	

The vasculitis is the key and *must* be found and distinguished from the secondary vascular changes that accompany any inflammatory reaction. Giant cells and granulomas, by themselves, lack diagnostic specificity. They may be found also as reaction to nonspecific inflammation that may ensue from mucosal ulceration.

Small superficial biopsy specimens of sinus mucosa from patients with Wegener's granulomatosis are almost nondiagnosable. A deep biopsy is required to avoid granulation tissue and to allow search for the distinctive fibrinoid necrosis in involved vessels.

Finally, nasal and sinus necrosis with ulcers is common to nearly all the lesions or diseases capable of simulating Wegener's granulomatosis. From a quantitative and qualitative viewpoint, the destruction of mucous membrane and adjacent structures found in Wegener's granulomatosis is the least when compared with that found in polymorphic reticulosis, lymphoma, and idiopathic nonhealing granuloma.

TABLE 6–2. Organ System Involvement in Wegener's Granulomatosis

Organ/Tissue	Approximate Percentage of Patients
Paranasal sinuses	95
Nose and nasopharynx	90
Ears	38
Oculo-orbital area	40
Lungs	100
Kidney	80
Skin	50
Nervous system	25
Heart	30

CHURG-STRAUSS SYNDROME

A large number of vasculitides may affect the upper airway, but of the so-called respiratory vasculitides, the Churg-Strauss syndrome (allergic granulomatosis and angiitis) deserves special consideration in the differential diagnosis of Wegener's granulomatosis.[26] The diagnostic hallmark of the Churg-Strauss syndrome is clinical asthma. It is not seen in any of the other midfacial necrotizing disorders. Peripheral and tissue eosinophilia are often distinguishing features of the syndrome. Chest film findings are often abnormal (transient patchy infiltrates, multiple noncavity nodules). The systemic nature of the syndrome is evidenced by clinicopathologic involvement of skin, cardiovascular system, and gastrointestinal tract. Renal disease may be present but is less lethal than that of Wegener's granulomatosis. Necrotizing sinonasal lesions are not common but nearly two thirds of patients have nasal polyps with crusting and abnormal sinus radiographic findings.

Necrotizing extravascular granulomas with necrotizing vasculitis of small arteries and veins similar to that seen in Wegener's granulomatosis are the principal histopathologic findings. Some distinction can be made in that the Churg-Strauss granulomas have an allergic quality, i.e., more fibrinoid necrosis and epithelioid cells and eosinophilia.

POLYMORPHIC RETICULOSIS

Polymorphic reticulosis is not related to Wegener's granulomatosis but is similar to, if not congeneric with, lymphomatoid granulomatosis.[27] Mayo Clinic investigators present evidence that polymorphic reticulosis and lymphomatoid granulomatosis are the same disease.[23, 26] Indeed, both are characterized by necrotizing, angiocentric, and angiodestructive infiltrates composed of a pleomorphic population of cells consisting of small lymphocytes, plasma cells, and *atypical* lymphoreticular cells with mitoses. Angioinvasion and subendothelial infiltration by the atypical cells is frequently observed, and these events lead to a secondary vasculitis and occlusion of involved vessels.

In most cases of polymorphic reticulosis, the disease begins with signs and symptoms of intranasal obstruction or ulcerative lesions involving the palate or nasopharynx. Also common are nonspecific symptoms such as fever, fatigue, weight loss, and arthralgia.

The disease can involve the upper or lower respiratory tract alone or in combination but also can involve other anatomic sites, such as the skin, gastrointestinal tract, kidneys, liver, and central nervous system. The extra-airway lesions are infiltrates in the nature of a lymphomatous infiltrate and not like those of Wegener's granulomatosis. A focal, necrotizing glomerulitis is not found in polymorphic reticulosis.

Upper airway involvement in polymorphic reticulosis is locally ulcerative and aggressive in contrast to the diffuse, less destructive lesions found in patients with Wegener's granulomatosis. Histopathologically, granuloma formation is either absent or inconspicuous.

Of greater significance is the emergence of lymphoma in patients with polymorphic reticulosis/lymphomatoid granulomatosis.[26, 27] Such a sequela has never been observed in Wegener's granulomatosis and places polymorphic reticulosis in a category of lymphoproliferative disorders manifesting a spectrum of pathologic and clinical changes. Even without definite histocytologic criteria of lymphoma, however, polymorphic reticulosis is locally malignant and may disseminate like an extranodal lymphoma with satellites in bowel, skin, and other viscera, including the central nervous system, with a high mortality.[21, 26, 27]

IDIOPATHIC MIDLINE GRANULOMA

This is a term applied by Fauci and colleagues[24] to a disorder with destructive inflammatory lesions of the midline facial and upper airway tissues that cannot be classified into any of the above categories. It is not explainable as a neoplastic process but is a relentlessly progressive, localized inflammatory process that predominantly involves the nose, paranasal sinuses, and palate with erosion through contiguous structures, particularly the face. The disease remains localized without visceral lesions.

Most patients eventually manifest a pansinusitis, with destructive necrosis of the nasal septum or soft and hard palate or both. Aside from these local findings, most patients are free of systemic signs and symptoms, such as fever, malaise, and arthralgias, except when there is a superimposed infection. The superinfection responds to antibiotics, but there is persistence of the underlying process. Regional lymphadenopathy is not a feature.

Nonspecific acute and chronic inflammations are the predominant, if not sole, histopathologic findings. Some patients manifest granulomas and a small vessel vasculitis or atypical histiocyte-like cells. Because of the latter, idiopathic midline granuloma has been challenged as a bona fide entity; the challengers consider the biopsies to be unrepresentative and to be either misdiagnosed or inadequately sampled Wegener's granulomatosis, polymorphic reticulosis, lymphoma, or other masquerading malignancies.[28] This is denied by Fauci and associates[29] and also by us: we have seen four examples.

Idiopathic midline granuloma, as described earlier, is a uniformly fatal disorder, but local irradiation with relatively high dosage has been found to result in long-term, sometimes dramatic, clinical remissions in the majority of cases.[24]

The cause of idiopathic midline granuloma is unknown but may be related to an unidentified antigenic stimulus that provokes an abnormal and accelerated hypersensitivity reaction.[24]

SARCOIDOSIS

Any discussion of granulomatous disease in the paranasal sinuses and nasal cavity without inclusion of sarcoidosis would be remiss. The pathogenesis of sarcoidosis is as elusive as that of the aforementioned disorders. Purely in histopathologic terms, it is a disease characterized by the presence in affected organs or tissue of noncaseating epithelioid cell granulomas.[30] Deviation from this accepted classic pattern does occur, in the form of focal necrosis, usually of a fibrinoid or granular type, and a less than nodular pattern of the granuloma (Fig. 6–3). In nearly all biopsy specimens, exclusion of infective agents is required and can never be absolute. Diagnosis during life depends largely on clinical, radiologic, and immunologic findings.[30, 31]

Paranasal sinus involvement without concomitant nasal sarcoidosis is very uncommon, and solitary sinus sarcoidosis ranks lowest in incidence of involvement of the upper aerodigestive tract. Nearly all patients with sinonasal sarcoid have clinical evidence of systemic disease, and the clinical presentation may be that of any benign nasal process: stuffiness, discharge, crusting, or polyps. Involvement of facial bones has also been described, but spontaneous perforation of the septum is rare. Many patients have no symptoms referable to the lesions.[31]

Grossly, the nasal involvement varies from small, asymptomatic lesions to more extensive ones. The mucosa is granular and thickened, especially along the septum and inferior turbinates. Early in the involvement, there are nasal crusting, small ulcers, and a mucosal hypertrophy. Later, there are an atrophic rhinitis and fibrosis. Vasculitis and atypical lymphoreticular cells are absent.

MUCOSAL CYSTS AND MUCOCELES

Mucosal cysts and mucoceles of the paranasal sinuses are as much clinicoanatomic entities as they are histologically definable lesions. Some forms of mucosal cysts are equivalent to the oral/labial mucous retention cyst; others are histologically indistinguishable from mucoceles of the oral cavity in that they are mucus extravasation phenomena. Similarly, the paranasal sinus mucocele is basically a retention of mu-

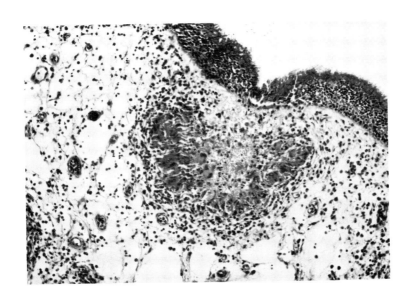

Figure 6–3. Sarcoidosis of maxillary sinus mucosa. An irregular, focally necrotic granuloma is beneath the epithelium.

coserous secretions within an initially epithe-lium-lined space. Fewer sinus mucoceles are extravasation lesions. Superinfection results in a pyocele of the involved sinus. The local man-ifestations of mucosal cysts of the sinuses and mucoceles, however, are dramatically different.

MUCOSAL CYSTS

Benign mucosal cysts of the maxillary antrum are well-documented findings in panoramic and periapical radiographs, where they are well-delineated radiodense shadows originating from the floor or a wall of the maxillary sinus.

The incidence of these lesions has been variously reported as from 1.9 to 9.6 per cent; we tend to the lower figure. The great majority of the cysts are asymptomatic and found inci-dental to x-ray examination of periantral tissues. Reports indicate they are most often discovered in subjects who are in their third decade and during time periods associated with allergic rhinitis and sinusitis.[32] Except for some evi-dence of an association with allergy, the cysts are usually unrelated to signs or symptoms of local or systemic antral or oral disease.[33]

Size is also variable, ranging from 50 to 1000 mm as measured on panoramic projections. Mucosal cysts usually demonstrate an attach-ment to the floor of the antrum, and the size is more a function of anatomic space and tissue expansion than of duration. The mucosal cyst of the antrum does not destroy bone.[32, 33]

Histologically, and likely pathogenetically, two types of mucosal cyst have been character-ized.[32] The first form, called secretory cyst, is a true cyst lined with epithelium and is a result of partial blockage of a draining mucosal duct. The second, a pseudocyst, is identical to a mucocele of the oral cavity and lips. This form has been termed nonsecretory cyst and is a consequence of escape of mucus into surround-ing fibrous connective tissue.

MUCOCELES

Paranasal sinus mucoceles are rare in chil-dren, and are found in adults with ages ranging from 13 to 80 years. Sites of involvement, in order of decreasing frequency, are the frontal, ethmoid, sphenoid, and maxillary sinuses. Ap-proximately 65 per cent of mucoceles are found in the frontal sinus and 30 per cent in the anterior ethmoid sinus.[34] Posterior ethmoid sinus mucoceles are uncommon.[35] Maxillary

sinus involvement occurs in 3 to 10 per cent of cases.[34]

Although the etiology and pathogenesis of a sinus mucocele are uncertain, the accepted theory points to an obstruction near or at a sinus outlet that causes retention of mucous secretion within the sinus cavity.[36] Osseous trauma, tumors, or a mucosal thickening (chronic inflammatory disease) in the areas of the sinus outlet are the major associated factors. In children, cystic fibrosis must be considered.[37]

Mucoceles often can be recognized by radio-logic appearances.[38] The involved sinus is opac-ified by entrapped secretions that have dis-placed all air. Accumulation of the secretions causes a gradual erosion of the sinus wall so that the mucoperiosteal margin decalcifies and fades, with disappearance of the normal scal-loped borders. With continuation of the proc-ess, the sinus appears more radiolucent, be-cause the bone loss cancels out replacement of air. At this time, the classic (frontal or ethmoid) mucocele appearance is usually seen: a smooth, expanded, oval or round area of bone erosion with an abnormal radiolucency.[38] The affected adjacent bone is generally osteolytic, but there is often a zone of sclerosing osteitis around the margins of the lesion. About 5 per cent of mucoceles manifest radiographically visible cal-cification of their walls. Computed tomography (CT) is helpful in evaluating the extent of the mucoceles.[39]

Unlike the mucous cyst, mucoceles are clin-ically symptomatic and dramatic lesions. Fron-toethmoid mucoceles most commonly present with proptosis and a mass in the upper medial quadrant of the orbit. Progressive enlargement compresses the orbital contents and may lead to visual impairment and even optic nerve atrophy secondary to stretching of the optic nerve.[36, 40]

The thinness of the lamina papyracea poses little resistance to an expanding mucocele and this accounts for the high incidence of orbital involvement. When the ethmoid sinus is in-volved, a mucocele often extends through the medial wall into the superior nasal cavity to erode the adjacent perpendicular plate or crib-riform plate.[35] An expanding frontoethmoid mu-cocele can expose the dura either by erosion of the ethmoid roof or dehiscence of the posterior wall of the frontal sinus.

Sphenoid sinus mucoceles can erode readily into the sella turcica and expand into the para-sellar, suprasellar, and orbital apex regions.

A chronicity of signs and symptoms usually precedes medical attention. The usual duration of symptoms of a sphenoid sinus mucocele prior to diagnosis is about 2 years. Patients with mucoceles of the sphenoid sinus manifest symptoms and signs secondary to pressure caused by the expanding mass. The structures involved are the dura, the internal carotid arteries, the cavernous sinus, the pituitary gland and the first through sixth cranial nerves, with the second and third most often compromised. Headache in these patients is attributed to a stretching of the dura over the sinus. The headache is usually retro-orbital and frontal. From 70 to 90 per cent of patients experience headache.[34, 38] Ophthalmoplegia occurs in more than 50 per cent of cases and is often variable in severity, but usually progressive. Blindness, if present, is usually gradual in onset, is usually unilateral, and is attributed to either direct pressure on the optic nerve or vascular obstruction with infarct of the nerve. A nasal mass is found in some patients, nasal stuffiness in 40 per cent of patients, anosmia in 10 to 15 per cent, a history of sinusitis in 20 per cent, and endocrine signs in 5 per cent.[34]

Patients with frontal sinus mucoceles also present most often with headache, localized in the region of the affected sinus. Less often, periorbital swelling, frontal sinus tenderness, and an external frontal mass cause patients to see their physician. Physical findings are periorbital swellings, proptosis, and diplopia.

The consequences of expansion of the frontal mucocele are readily seen in roentgenographic studies; erosion of the orbital roof, anterior frontal sinus table, and posterior wall of the sinus, along with evidence of osteomyelitis, is often present.[38, 41] Clouding of the sinus and a soft tissue mass in the sinus constitute the principal nonosseous findings.

Erosion of the floor of the frontal sinus, destruction of the anterior wall of the sphenoid, or dural exposure through the posterior ethmoid roof does not exclude the ethmoids as a site of origin of a mucocele. Ocular findings are prominent. Inferior and lateral displacement of the eye is present in nearly every case. The radiographic features include diffuse opacification of the ethmoids, lateralization of the medial wall of the orbit, and disappearance of the line of junction of this wall with the roof of the orbit. Medial displacement of the lateral wall of the nose is also common. Sites of extension of ethmoid mucoceles include the anterior and posterior group of ethmoid cells, the medial and superior walls of the orbit, and floor of the frontal sinus. Less often, extension into the antrum, erosion of the anterior wall of the sphenoid, and exposure of the dura are found.

The microscopic appearance of a sinus mucocele belies its destructive behavior. The mucosal lining varies from one with goblet and other mucous cell hyperplasia to flattened (pressure atrophy) cuboid epithelium. At times, considerable areas will manifest denudation and escape of mucus into the lamina propria. The sinus contents also vary from thick and mucoid to inspissated, tough gelatin-like material. Intracavitary hemorrhage discolors the contents and may add a high lipid content with secondary changes.

CHOLESTEROL GRANULOMA AND CHOLESTEATOMA

Both these terms, as applied to the paranasal sinuses, lack diagnostic precision.[42, 43] So-called cholesteatomas of the sinuses, particularly the frontal and ethmoid, are nearly always post-traumatic or congenital inclusions of epidermal tissues.[43] Cholesterol granulomas, like those found in the mastoid antrum and air cells and in the middle ear, can occur in closed cavities such as the maxillary sinus. Intramucosal hemorrhage is the most likely underlying basis for a maxillary sinus cholesterol granuloma (as it is in the mastoid air cells).[42] Microscopy shows the lesion to be a granulomatous reaction to liberated cholesterol.[42] The mucosa is thickened and also hemorrhagic.

PNEUMOCELE

The basis of a pneumocele is not completely known, but it is presumed to be a check-valve mechanism involving a physiologic block to rapid equilibration of sinus pressure. Pneumoceles (maxillary) are often associated with changes in intrasinus pressure, either from airplane decompression or incessant nose blowing.[44]

Clinical and radiographic findings are rather consistent. In addition to a triad of bone loss, hyperaeration, and expansion of the sinus, most patients also exhibit an expansion of the recesses of the sinus, profiling of dental roots, displacement of the orbital floor and middle meatus, and effacement of the ethmomaxillary angle.[44] Examination usually reveals dehiscence of the maxillary sinus, mostly along the inferolateral wall, bulging of the nasoantral wall into the nasal cavity, and enlargement or irregularity of the middle turbinate.

Pneumoceles of the frontal and sphenoid sinuses almost always follow trauma and, less commonly, infection.[45] Similar conditions apply to an escape of air from the middle ear or mastoid air system in the posterior part of the head.

EPITHELIAL TUMORS

Based on their phenotypic expression, epithelial tumors of the paranasal sinuses can arise from the modified respiratory mucosa, from metaplastic squamous epithelium, or from salivary-type tissues that are, in fact, functionally modified invaginations of the primordial ectoderm (Fig. 6–4). Numerically, however, squamous cell lesions far exceed those with an adenoid or glandular morphology.

Before discussion of definable epithelial neoplasms (squamous cell carcinoma, adenocarcinoma, and salivary-type tumors) of the sinuses, two borderline epithelial lesions require consideration: carcinoma in situ and papillomas.

CARCINOMA IN SITU

The regenerative ability of sinus mucosa is considerable. In persistent inflammatory states, however, this ability is exhausted, and an inferior squamous cell replacement occurs. Such foci of metaplasia often can be found in chronic sinusitis and in sinonasal polyps. Histologically *significant* squamous dysplasia or carcinoma in

situ in nasal polyps, however, is, of a low order of frequency. Busuttil, in a review of nasal polyps from 1710 patients, found that only 33 (1.8 per cent) manifested these changes.[46] The intraepithelial changes did not recur or progress to invasive carcinoma and local excision was curative. Whether the same changes in nonpolyp sinus mucosa have the same degree of banality is unknown. What is to be appreciated, though, is that similar to in situ carcinoma of the oral cavity and pharynx, intraepithelial squamous cell carcinoma of a sinus is unusual as an isolated lesion without adjacent invasive carcinoma.

SCHNEIDERIAN PAPILLOMAS

As indicated earlier, the mucosa of the nasal cavity and the paranasal sinuses differs from that of the remainder of the airway in that it is embryologically derived from ectoderm.[1] This uniqueness is carried over into the morphogenesis of papillomas of the sinonasal tract. We have elected to designate these lesions as schneiderian papillomas to signal their unique derivation, appearance, and biologic behavior as compared with other papillomas of the respiratory tract.[1, 47] The name honors one of the early investigators of the nasal and paranasal sinus mucosa and cannot be confused with any other anatomically located papillomas.[47]

Schneiderian papillomas account for up to 0.6 cases per 100,000 inhabitants per year in a

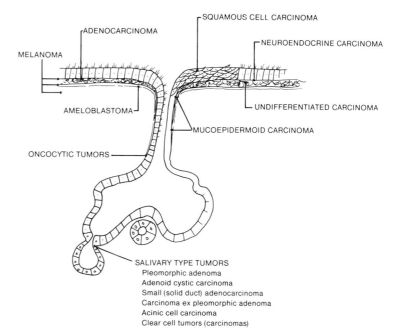

Figure 6–4. Schematic representation of the origin of epithelial or epithelial-like neoplasms of the paranasal sinuses. Melanomas and neuroendocrine carcinomas arise from neuroectodermal cells in the basal layer and ameloblastomas from odontogenic epithelium either in the mucosa or subepithelial stroma. Although nonsalivary carcinomas likely have their origin in stem cells, the tendency for squamous cell carcinomas to arise in metaplastic epithelium is illustrated. Salivary type tumors arise from reserve or stem cells in various portions of the duct system, which in turn originates from the ectodermally derived sinus mucosa.

SQUAMOUS CELL CARCINOMA
ADENOCARCINOMA
NEUROENDOCRINE CARCINOMA
MELANOMA
AMELOBLASTOMA
UNDIFFERENTIATED CARCINOMA
MUCOEPIDERMOID CARCINOMA
ONCOCYTIC TUMORS
SALIVARY TYPE TUMORS
  Pleomorphic adenoma
  Adenoid cystic carcinoma
  Small (solid duct) adenocarcinoma
  Carcinoma ex pleomorphic adenoma
  Acinic cell carcinoma
  Clear cell tumors (carcinomas)

well-defined representative geographic region.[47a] They arise from a proliferation of the reserve or replacement cells of the mucosa. Although capable of behaving like neoplasms, their neoplastic genesis is not confirmed. In its fullest expression, the proliferating cells assume two basic architectural patterns: inverting (Fig. 6–5) and fungiform or exophytic.[48] Mixtures also occur.

The two basic forms further segregate by a rather specific anatomic localization in the upper airway. Fungiform papillomas are usually restricted to the nasal septum or its environs. The lateral nasal wall and/or sinuses are the typical sites for inverted papillomas. Biologic behavior also correlates with site. Septal papillomas, although manifesting a nearly equal recurrence rate, tend to remain localized to the septum, and an association with carcinoma is very rare. By contrast, lateral wall papillomas often are not restricted to the site, often show sinus involvement, or are localized in a sinus. Of 212 lateral papillomas reviewed by Batsakis, 117 manifested both nasal and sinus disease, 62 were lateral nasal wall lesions only, and 32 were within the sinus without a nasal component.[47]

The predominant cell type in either lateral or septal papillomas is epidermoid (Fig. 6–6). Vestiges of the overlying respiratory-type epithelium may be found with a variable frequency. On occasion the entire papilloma (almost exclusively lateral wall and sinus) may be composed of modified columnar epithelium. If so constituted, the term *cylindric cell papilloma* is used.[1, 49]

The major clinical and therapeutic problem with any form of schneiderian papilloma is recurrence. These may be multiple and delayed. The rate of recurrence in major sinuses has ranged from 28 to 67 per cent, with lateral wall and sinus lesions having a higher rate than those of the septum.[1, 47, 49a]

Left untreated, the papillomas can be locally invasive and destructive. Erosion of bone and death by local extension are possible.

Ascribing a premalignant quality to schneiderian papillomas is generally unwarranted, but a patient with a lateral wall papilloma is definitely at risk for the development of an *associated* carcinoma (Fig. 6–7). Histologic documentation of the transformation of a papilloma to carcinoma has been reported only occasionally, and this event likely represents less than 2 per cent of cases.[47] The usual circumstance is that of a squamous cell carcinoma arising in the same anatomic region but without good evidence of origin from the papilloma. This is more common and approximates a frequency of 20

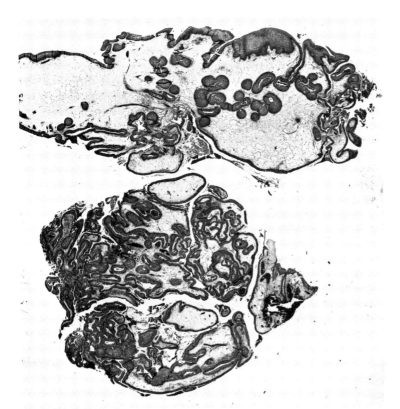

Figure 6–5. Lateral wall and inverting schneiderian papillomas.

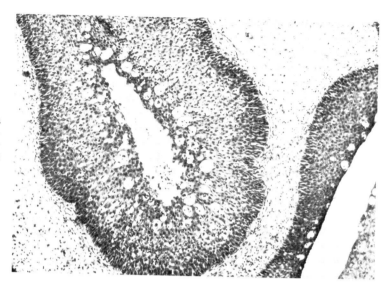

Figure 6–6. Higher power view of a typical lateral wall schneiderian papilloma. Note the nonkeratinizing epidermoid character of the lesion. The small microcysts are typical findings.

per cent.[47] An associated carcinoma with septal papillomas is so rare that it must be regarded as a medical curiosity. The cylindric cell papilloma also is rarely associated with carcinoma. The associated carcinomas are nearly always squamous cell lesions and of variable degrees of differentiation; their behavior is not unlike other squamous cell carcinomas of the sinuses. Rarely, carcinomas of other types may arise in association with papillary or undifferentiated features.[49b]

CARCINOMAS

In contrast to the neighboring nasopharynx, sinonasal cancer is not associated with strong genetic determinants or elevated antibody titers to Epstein-Barr virus. On the other hand, environmental agents peculiar to certain occupa-

tional settings often appear to play a role in sinonasal cancer.[49, 50] Table 6–3 shows only a partial listing, to which may be added chrome pigment manufacturing (chromates), dial painting (radium), isopropyl alcohol manufacturing (isopropyl oil), hydrocarbons, and chemical and petroleum manufacturing (nitrosamines, aromatic hydrocarbons, nickel catalysts).[49] Nonoccupational factors vary in their degree of correlation. The strongest is with intrasinus injections of thorium dioxide (Thorotrast). Snuff taking as a risk has geographic connotations, being higher in Africa than in Europe. Cigarette smoking as a risk needs further study. Tobacco may act synergistically, have a questionable direct effect, or have no effect at all.[49]

The evidence for industrial agents in the etiology of sinonasal cancer is most substantial for two occupations—nickel refining and wood-

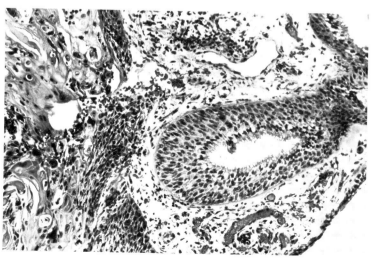

Figure 6–7. Moderately well differentiated squamous cell carcinoma arising adjacent to an inverting papilloma.

TABLE 6–3. Sinonasal Carcinoma and Relation to Occupation

Occupation	Site of Carcinoma	Histologic Type of Carcinoma
Nickel refiners	Nasal, ethmoids	Squamous and anaplastic
Furniture and other woodworkers	Ethmoids, nasal	Adenocarcinoma
Boot and shoe workers	Ethmoids, nasal	Adenocarcinoma, squamous
Textile and clothing manufacturers	—	Adenocarcinoma, melanoma

(From data presented by Roush GC: Epidemiology of cancer of the nose and paranasal sinuses: Current concept. Head Neck Surg 2:3, 1979.)

TABLE 6–4. Cancer of the Paranasal Sinuses and Nasal Cavity: Site Distribution According to Geographic Location

	Percentage in Nasal Cavity and Nose	Percentage in Paranasal Sinuses–Maxillary Sinus
Uganda	23	77 (64)
Japan (Osaka)	3	97 (97)
Norway	23	76 (71)
Sweden	33	61 (75)
Oxford, UK	12	86 (69)
England and Wales	40	53 (72)
United States	42	53 (76)
Hawaii	21	64 (89)

(From data presented by Muir CS, Nectoux J: Descriptive epidemiology of malignant neoplasms of nose, nasal cavities, middle ear and accessory sinuses. Clin Otolaryngol 5:195, 1980.)

working.[49–51] Nickel (carbonyl and subsulfide) exposures carry a significant risk.[50] The carcinomas are primarily squamous cell and are nasal rather than sinus in location (Fig. 6–8). The presumably airborne suspect carcinogen in the woodworking industry has not been defined. What is known is (1) wood dust slows mucociliary transport in nasal epithelium, (2) the carcinomas are predominantly adenocarcinomas, and (3) the site predilection is the ethmoid sinus/high nasal cavity region. The percentages of adenocarcinomas among furniture workers and boot and shoe manufacturers are given as 85 and 40 per cent, respectively.[49, 50] Suspected agents, common to both forms of endeavor, are aldehydes, aflatoxin, and chromium.[49]

The risk factors in the nickel industry and woodworking are independent of geography, but as Table 6–4 indicates there is considerable variation in site distribution of cancer in the sinonasal tract according to geographic location.[50] There is a striking localization of cancer in Japan and Oxford. In the former, the carcinomas are almost exclusively in the maxillary sinus. In the latter, the data reflect the extraor-

dinarily high incidence of adenocarcinomas related to woodworking.

Only a few studies on the incidence of cancer of the paranasal sinuses that are not biased by patient selection or geographic location exist. The study by Robin and colleagues[51] appears to be a singular exception. Table 6–5, derived from their report, compares carcinomas of the sinuses with those of the nasal cavity and vestibule. Tables 6–6 and 6–7, prepared from data presented by Muir and Nectoux[50] and Robin and colleagues,[51] present the types of cancer affecting the sinuses compared with the nose and nasal cavity. Table 6–8 indicates the good concordance between the reviews of sinonasal cancer by Lewis and Castro[52] and Robin and colleagues.[51] All these data reaffirm (1) the dominance of the antrum as a primary site, (2) the dominance of squamous cell carcinoma over other histologic types, (3) the rarity of primary cancer of the frontoethmoid sinus system, (4) the relative infrequency of salivary-type carcinomas and sarcomas and (5) the existence of a

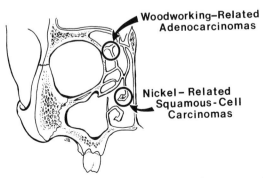

Figure 6–8. Predominant sites of origin of two types of industry-associated carcinomas of the sinonasal tract.

TABLE 6–5. Carcinomas of Paranasal Sinuses and Nasal Cavity: Distribution by Anatomic Site

Sinuses	Percentage	Nasal	Percentage
Maxillary antrum	60.3	Nasal cavity	19.5
Ethmoid sinus	14.9	Nasal vestibule	4.2
Frontosphenoid sinuses	1.1		
TOTAL	76.32	TOTAL	23.7

(Based on data presented by Robin PE, Powell DJ, Stansbie JM: Carcinoma of the nasal cavity and paranasal sinuses: Incidence and presentation of different histological types. Clin Otolaryngol 4:431, 1979.)

TABLE 6–6. Cancer of Paranasal Sinuses and Nasal Cavity:
Incidence by Histologic Type

	Percentage in Nose, Nasal Cavity, and Sinuses	Percentage in Nose and Nasal Cavity	Percentage in Antrum	Percentage in Other Sinuses
Squamous cell	57	60	57	41
Anaplastic/undifferentiated	10	9	10	15
Nonkeratinizing	2	3	1.5	3.5
Adenocarcinoma	9	9	6	20
Salivary carcinoma	2	1	2	3
Sarcoma	3	3	3	2.5
Lymphoma	2	2	2	2
Melanoma	1	3	0.5	1
Olfactory neuroblastoma	0.3	1	0.1	0

(From data presented by Muir CS, Nectoux J: Descriptive epidemiology or malignant neoplasms of nose, nasal cavities, middle ear and accessory sinuses. Clin Otolaryngol 5:195, 1980.)

small number of neoplasms that defy classification.

The lethality and poor prognosis of carcinomas of the sinuses are directly related to the early clinical silence or misleading signs and symptoms of these cancers, all of which allow considerable local extension before their discovery. It may indeed be said that carcinomas of the sinuses do not manifest *significant* evidence of their presence until they have broken out of the sinus of origin. More than 90 per cent of paranasal sinus carcinomas will manifest invasion through at least one wall of the involved sinus.[53] Only 4 of the 115 cases reported by Jackson and colleagues[53] were confined to the antrum.

Signs and symptoms of paranasal sinus carcinoma reflect this extension. For the maxillary

sinus carcinomas, these fall into several major categories: oral, nasal, ocular, and facial. The medial, anterior, and downward extensions of antral carcinomas produce the classic findings of this cancer: asymmetry of the face, a tumor bulge palpable or visible from the oral cavity, and a mass in the nasal cavity visible by anterior rhinoscopy. Each of these findings is present in 40 to 60 per cent of all patients, and one or more of them are found in nearly 90 per cent of patients.[54]

Just as the insidious growth by paranasal sinus carcinomas and the anatomic uniqueness of the sinuses defeat early diagnosis, so too do they hinder staging classifications.[55] Almost all staging schemes relate only to the maxillary sinus.[55, 56] Lederman's division of the region into supra-, meso-, and infrastructures includes tumors of the ethmoid sinuses and nasal cavity.[57]

TABLE 6–7. Cancer of Paranasal Sinuses and Nasal Cavity: Site and Histologic Type

Type of Cancer	Maxillary Antrum	Other Sinuses	Nasal Cavity and Vestibule
Squamous cell	225	32	62
Anaplastic/undifferentiated	27	13	22
Nonkeratinizing ("transitional")	18	16	14
Adenocarcinoma	10	21	8
Salivary carcinoma	15	4	6
Lymphoma	19	1	11
Melanoma	2	1	12
Sarcoma	29	6	9
TOTAL	345	94	144

(From data presented by Robin PE, Powell DJ, Stansbie JM: Carcinoma of the nasal cavity and paranasal sinuses: Incidence and presentation of different histological types. Clin Otolaryngol 4:431, 1979.)

TABLE 6–8. Cancer of the Paranasal Sinuses and Nasal Cavity: Histologic Distribution (%)

Type of Cancer	Percentage Lewis and Castro[52]	Robin et al[51]
Squamous cell	55	51
Anaplastic/undifferentiated	11	10
Nonkeratinizing ("transitional")	8	8
Adenocarcinoma	7	6
Salivary carcinoma	4	4
Lymphoma	5	5
Melanoma	2.5	2.5
Sarcoma	6	6
Miscellaneous or unclassified	2.5	6.5

(Modified from Robin PE, Powell DJ, Stansbie JM: Carcinoma of the nasal cavity and paranasal sinuses: Incidence and presentation of different histological types. Clin Otolaryngol 4:431, 1979; and Lewis JS, Castro EB: Cancer of the nasal cavity and paranasal sinuses. J Laryngol Otol 86:255, 1972.)

For the maxillary sinus, classifications take into consideration that malignancies situated in the posterosuperior part of the sinus carry a worse prognosis than those situated anteroinferiorly. The obvious reason for this is the difficulty in resecting the posterosuperior antral neoplasms because of proximity to the orbit, cribriform plate, and pterygoid region.

The majority of the squamous cell carcinomas of the sinuses are recognizable keratinizing carcinomas. They tend to be only moderately well differentiated (Fig. 6–9). Electronmicroscopic evaluation of nonkeratinizing forms and many of the undifferentiated carcinomas also indicates these carcinomas are of an epidermoid lineage. Histologic grading of these carcinomas, beyond that of keratinizing, non-keratinizing, and undifferentiated, has not been shown to have a prognostic impact, except that anaplastic sinus carcinomas have a more rapid clinical course.

Far more important than the degree of differentiation is the extent or stage of the carcinoma. Invasion of contiguous bone by neoplasms of the sinuses, regardless of histologic classification, is nearly always an ominous prognostic sign. For squamous cell carcinomas, the histomorphologic process of direct bone invasion involves three phases: (1) the periosteum is breached and the neoplastic cells infiltrate underlying bone; (2) in bone, the carcinomas evoke a striking increase in local osteoclasts, which erode bone trabeculae in front of the advancing neoplasm; and (3) the osteoclastic response subsides and the squamous cell carcinoma cells, alone, continue their spread into the bone.[58] A similar sequence has been described for squamous cell carcinomas invading metaplastic bone in the aging, focally ossified larynx.

Preliminary investigations of the mechanisms of the osteolytic process indicate that freshly excised squamous cell carcinomas of the head and neck contain an extractable prostaglandin (PG)–like material that activates osteoclasts.[58] This material is predominantly of the PGE type and seems to be elaborated in the immediate vicinity of the neoplasm, most likely from both carcinoma cells and host stromal cells. In vitro experiments confirm this but also point to differences between homogenous carcinoma cell lines and fresh tissue from a carcinoma.[58] This implies the presence also of nonprostaglandin osteoclast activators.

The introduction of chemotherapy and its increasing role in the management of sinonasal squamous cell carcinoma have required pathologists to become familiar with the effects of the drugs on the carcinomas. However, little solid *histomorphologic* information is available for changes induced by single agents. The best relates to bleomycin.

A major action of bleomycin is to stop or slow down cell progression at some phase before mitosis but subsequent to the initiation of DNA synthesis. Cells located in other phases of the cell cycle are relatively unaffected and RNA and protein synthesis are essentially not influenced. Bleomycin has an especially high specificity against epidermally derived cells, and squamous cell carcinoma cells are approximately 100 times more sensitive than normal cells, such as fibroblasts, or other neoplastic cells.

By light and electron microscopy, two principal effects of bleomycin are found: hyper-

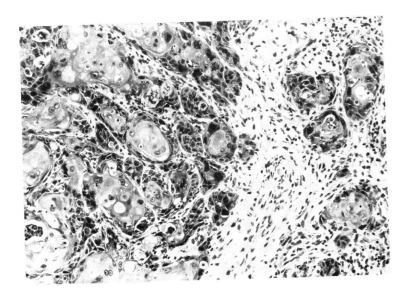

Figure 6–9. Keratinizing squamous cell carcinoma of the maxillary antrum.

maturation keratosis and hypertrophy of stroma.[59, 60] These occur in the carcinomas and in adjacent noncarcinomatous squamous mucosal surfaces. In the latter there is hyper-, ortho-, and parakeratosis in an otherwise regularly stratified epithelium. Scar tissue below the epithelium is prominent in all cases. The increase in collagenous fibrous tissue is likely a direct result of bleomycin accumulation in the area of the tumor.

The destruction of the neoplastic cells is not by a simple necrosis. It is a necrosis provoked via a keratinization of cells that are able to keratinize, hence the most favorable responses in keratinizing squamous cell carcinomas.[60] The keratin evokes a resorptive granulomatous reaction similar to that seen in foreign body granulomas. Multinucleated, non-neoplastic giant cells may be abundant. Following this phase, macrophages and other inflammatory cells remove the debris, and there is restitution of the tumor area with scar and a plasma cell–lymphoid reaction.

Electron microscopy confirms the maturation effect of bleomycin.[61] Remarkable cytoplasmic and nuclear alterations are observed in almost all neoplastic cells by 20 days after treatment. The development of tonofilaments is so extensive that their bundles come to occupy nearly all the cytoplasm except for some variously sized vacuoles. Nuclei also manifest fibrillar inclusions identical to those of bundles of the tonofilaments synthesized in the cytoplasm. A stepwise keratinization of the cellular tonofilaments follows. The addition of *cis*-platinum to the regimen is synergistic, and the process of differentiation is accentuated.[62]

The effectiveness of different forms of management of squamous cell carcinomas of the paranasal sinuses cannot readily be compared. This is in part because of a lack of a uniformly accepted classification and in part because of variations in sequence forms of surgical excision and radiation therapy. Taken in aggregate, however, paranasal sinus carcinomas have a poor prognosis. A 5-year survival of 35 per cent is unusual. One point is abundantly clear: failure to cure paranasal sinus cancer is almost always the result of failure to control disease at the primary site.[62a–c]

Clinically positive cervical lymph node metastases from squamous cell carcinomas of the sinuses are variously reported. From a review of 2642 patients in seven major series, Batsakis and colleagues[55] indicate that 25 per cent manifested clinical evidence of regional node involvement at some time during the course of illness. Thirteen per cent of patients demonstrated these on admission and a like percentage developed metastases later in the disease. Tong and colleagues[63] report nearly identical data based on a retrospective study of squamous cell carcinoma of the maxillary antrum. There is a twofold increase in lymph node metastases if the oral cavity is invaded. Distant metastases occur in approximately 10 to 18 per cent of patients.

On histologic, partial histogenic, and epidemiologic bases, the majority of nonepidermoid neoplasms of the paranasal sinuses can be divided into two basic groups: (1) glandular tumors having the histologic features of salivary gland tumors, e.g., pleomorphic adenomas and adenocystic carcinomas (Fig. 6–10), and (2) glandular tumors exhibiting the conventional and traditional histologic appearances of any visceral

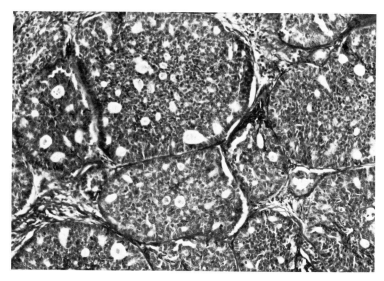

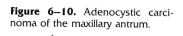

Figure 6–10. Adenocystic carcinoma of the maxillary antrum.

mucosal adenocarcinoma. The latter can be subclassified as indicated in Table 6–9. The majority of adenomatous neoplasms of the sinonasal tract arise from the mucosal lining of the sinonasal tract.[63a]

A glandular tumor in the sinonasal tract need not be biologically malignant, but malignant ones exceed benign tumors by 15 to 1. Specifically, pleomorphic and monomorphic adenomas are rare in the sinuses and unusual in the nasal cavity but have a predilection for the latter site. Adenomatous hyperplasia, sufficient to produce a clinical mass, is also infrequent.

Mucosal (nonsalivary) adenocarcinomas are the most numerous with an incidence of approximately 6 per cent of all nonepidermoid carcinomas of the sinonasal tract.[51] Adenocystic carcinomas occur at only a slightly lower rate and mucoepidermoid carcinomas at a rate only half that of the two dominant glandular carcinomas.

The comparatively lower incidence of salivary carcinomas and benign tumors is explainable, in large part, by the low density of salivary tissues found in the paranasal sinuses (Table 6–10). There are, nonetheless, site preferences within the sinuses. Adenocarcinomas are most numerous in the high nasal cavity and ethmoid sinus region, whereas adenocystic carcinomas have a moderate predilection for the maxillary antrum (medial wall and floor).

The muted character of sinus squamous cell carcinomas also applies to glandular carcinomas. Adenocystic carcinomas of the antrum, for example, smolder without clinical attention for 1 or more years in nearly 50 per cent of patients. Spiro and colleagues[64] have reported some degree of fixation or extension in nearly three fourths of their patients with primary adenocystic carcinomas in the paranasal sinuses, nasal cavity, and pharynx. In these sites, the carcinoma is rarely less than 2.0 cm when diagnosis is made, but gross in situ inspection is notoriously deceptive because of the insidious infiltrative nature of the majority of salivary type carcinomas. Perineural spread is usually evident along the maxillary and mandibular divisions of the trigeminal nerve, and the foramen ovale and foramen rotundum may be involved by extension to Gasser's ganglion.

The histologic appearances of any salivary-type tumor of the sinuses, benign or malignant, do not substantially differ from those of their respective counterparts in the major salivary glands. There are tendencies, however, for the pleomorphic adenomas to be more epithelial than stromal and the carcinomas to be of a higher histologic grade.

Lack of local control is the usual cause of death from salivary-type carcinomas. The incidence of metastases to lymph nodes from these carcinomas of the paranasal sinuses is not easy to discern from the literature. There is certainly a dependency on T stage, histologic type, local control, and site of origin. The latter refers primarily, but not exclusively, to the sparseness or richness of regional lymphatics. Table 6–11

TABLE 6–9. Histologic Subclassification of Adenocarcinomas of the Nasal Cavity and Paranasal Sinuses

Small duct ("solid duct") adenocarcinoma
Papillary adenocarcinoma
Mucopapillary adenocarcinoma
Mucoid (colloid) carcinoma
Poorly differentiated and undifferentiated (oat cell)
  adenocarcinoma
Neuroendocrine adenocarcinoma

TABLE 6–10. Goblet Cells and Mucoserous Glands of Nasal Cavity and Paranasal Sinuses

	Maxillary Antrum	Ethmoid	Frontal	Sphenoid	Nasal Cavity		
					Ant. Septum	Post. Septum	Post.-, Middle, and Inf. Turbinate
Mucosal thickness (mm)	0.3–0.8	0.3–0.8	0.2–0.7	0.2–0.7			
Median goblet cell density (cells/mm²)	9700	6500	5900	6200	4800	6200	10,000
Median mucoserous gland density (glands/mm²)	0.20	0.47	0.08	0.06		7–10	
Number of mucoserous glands		50–100	<50	<50		36000	

(Compiled from data presented by Mogensen C, Tos M: Quantitative histology of the maxillary sinus. Rhinology 15:129, 1977; Tos M, Mogenson C: Mucus production in the nasal sinuses. Acta Otolaryngol (Suppl) 360:131, 1979; and Tos M, Mogenson C, Novotny Z: Quantitative histologic features of the normal frontal sinus. Arch Otolaryngol 106:143, 1980.)

TABLE 6–11. Influence of Anatomic Site of
Salivary Carcinoma on Lymph Node Metastases

Site	Percentage of Cases with Lymph Node Metastases
Palate	7
Larynx and trachea	12
Sinonasal	8
Nasopharynx	40
Oropharynx	66
Tongue	55
Cheek and floor of mouth	40

(Modified from Rafla-Demetrious S: Mucous and Salivary Gland
Tumours. Springfield, Ill, Charles C Thomas, 1970.)

indicates the significantly higher frequency of
metastases from salivary carcinomas of oral and
naso-oropharyngeal sites.

The nonsalivary adenocarcinomas manifest
three basic growth patterns: papillary (Fig.
6–11), sessile, and alveolar mucoid.[55] Mucin
production is variable, and the level of differentiation ranges from only a modest deviation
from progenitor epithelium to poor differentiation. The papillary adenocarcinomas are usually
the best localized; sessile carcinomas involve a
broader surface and have a definitely greater
invasive quality. The alveolar mucoid carcinoma
is the least common and even more invasive.
In the three growth patterns, there is a resemblance to adenocarcinomas of the gastrointestinal tract. This resemblance is carried even
further in the occasional differentiated adenocarcinoma that on electron microscopic analysis
shows neuroendocrine granules and hormone
precursors.[66] Some undifferentiated carcinomas
may show similar features, but most lack evidence of a neuroendocrine origin and are not

oat cell carcinomas in the specific diagnostic
sense.[67]

Except for the papillary adenocarcinomas,
the local behavior and mode of death associated
with adenocarcinomas are like those for adenocystic carcinoma.

NEUROECTODERMAL TUMORS

The generic heading of neuroectodermal tumors includes a rather heterogenous group of
lesions. These range from benign encephaloceles to the highly malignant mucosal melanoma.

MELANOMA

Approximately 20 per cent of all melanomas
occur in the head and neck region, with about
6 per cent occurring in the mucous membranes.
Between 0.5 and 1.5 per cent of *all* melanomas
arise in the nasal cavity and paranasal sinuses,
where they constitute about 3.5 per cent of all
sinonasal tract neoplasms.[68, 69]

In the respiratory tract, melanomas arise
almost exclusively in the upper portions: nasal
cavity, paranasal sinuses, and less so in the
larynx. At these sites, the highest incidence
occurs in the fifth to the eighth decades. Men
are slightly more often affected.

Upper respiratory tract melanomas originate
from melanocytes normally present in the mucosa and submucosa of the nasal cavity, paranasal sinuses, and larynx.[70, 71] Pre-existing
melanosis, a finding often associated with mel-

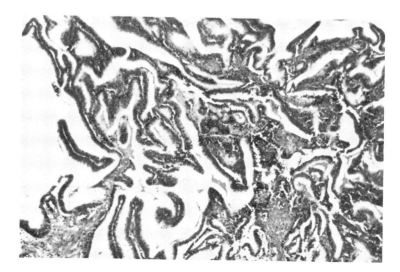

Figure 6–11. Papillary, focally mu-
cin-forming adenocarcinoma of the
ethmoid sinus.

anomas of the oral cavity, is not usually found in white patients with melanomas in the upper airway. African-Americans, however, often manifest ectopic pigmentation at sites corresponding exactly with the most common sites of intranasal melanomas.[72] Table 6–12 presents the site distribution of melanomas of the nasal cavity and paranasal sinuses. The dominance of nasal localization is evident. The maxillary antrum is more common than the other sinuses as an extranasal mucosal site. The dominance is accentuated when one assesses nasal and paranasal sites of involvement. Of 194 melanomas of the sinonasal tract, nasal localization was present in 124 cases, paranasal in 42, and involvement of both sites in 28 cases. Attention has been drawn to the concept or possibility that conjunctival melanoma may precede nasal cavity melanoma by months or years.[72a]

The histologic appearance of a sinonasal melanoma can be, and is, as variable as that of cutaneous melanomas. The cells may be spindled, round, or polygonal in shape (Fig. 6–12). A mixed cellular composition is common. Precursor lesions are rarely identified. In a number of lesions clear cell foci may be prominent or make up a major portion of the tumor. Nucleoli are prominent, and mitoses are frequent. In growth patterns, there may be a solid, whorled or storiform, alveolar, or organoid architecture.

Over two thirds of the sinus melanomas will manifest readily identifiable melanin. A small number will be apparently amelanotic. In these instances, fine structural study to identify premelanosomes or melanosomes may be necessary (Fig. 6–13).

A prognostic significance of various levels of invasion, as established for cutaneous mel-

TABLE 6–12. Location of Upper Airway Melanomas

Anatomic Site	Number of Melanomas
Nasal cavity (site not further specified)	62
Nasal septum	31
Maxillary sinus	26
Inferior turbinate	13
Ethmoid sinus	10
Laryngopharynx	7
Middle turbinate	6
Frontal sinus	2
Nasopharynx	1
TOTAL	158

nomas, does not apply for mucosal and especially sinus melanomas. This is due to an absence of histologic landmarks analogous to the papillary and reticular dermis. However, given sections of the primary lesion that are of satisfactory quality, microstage measurements can be made and correlated with prognosis. Depth of invasion is probably the single best correlate with prognosis, but mucosal melanomas seem to be even more capricious than cutaneous melanomas.[73] No patient is *ever* free of the liability of metastases and death.[74, 75] In many series, size, anatomic site of the primary lesion, and cytomorphology have not influenced the prognosis. Regional lymph node metastases, which are infrequent, also do not seem to have an impact on ultimate survival.

Differences in survival of patients with clinical stage I and stage II diseases are also not as striking as those seen in patients with cutaneous melanomas. Tumors with an invasion less than

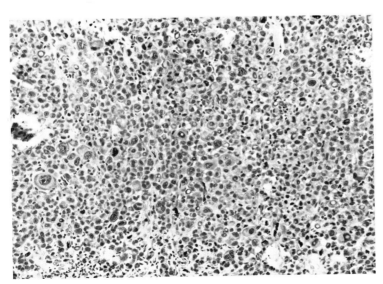

Figure 6–12. Melanoma of the lateral wall of the nasal cavity. This neoplasm also involved the adjacent sinuses. Note the lack of cohesiveness, cellular and nuclear pleomorphism, and prominent nuclei in the melanoma cells.

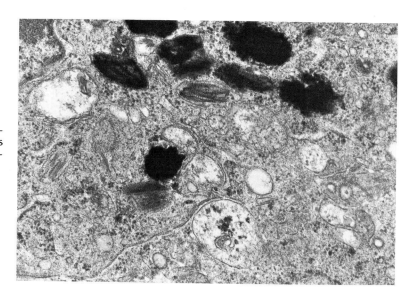

Figure 6–13. Electron-optic appearance of a melanoma. Cells contain melanosomes and premelanosomes. × 46,660.

0.5 mm have a better chance of 5-year survival. Other microscopic findings related to biologic aggressiveness are a lack of lymphoid reaction to the tumor and the presence of intralesional blood vessel and/or lymphatic invasion in nearly all cases.

The mean survival for patients with mucosal melanomas of the head and neck is shorter than that for cutaneous melanomas. Few patients have a prolonged course (more than 10 years). Local recurrences and *distant* metastases are the main causes of treatment failure.

Caution in excluding a metastasis to the mucosa is well advised. But judging from the literature, such an event is less common than a de novo primary lesion. Of the three major mucosal regions in the head and neck—sinonasal tract, oral cavity, and larynx—the last two are most often involved by a metastatic melanoma.

MELANOTIC NEUROECTODERMAL TUMOR OF INFANCY

A survey of the world literature indicates that the anterior maxilla is the most common site of origin for this peculiar tumor of neural crest origin.[76] Over 90 per cent of cases involve the head and neck, with nearly 70 per cent of the tumors in the maxilla. *Infancy* is an appropriate qualifying term in that 95 per cent of the patients have been under 1 year of age.[76a]

This tumor is often multifocal, which is partially accountable for a 10 to 15 per cent local recurrence rate. Until recently, the melanotic neuroectodermal tumor was universally considered as benign and of local significance only,

but 5 of 158 (3.2 per cent) tumors have been malignant.[76] Two of these malignant tumors originated in the maxilla.

Ultrastructural findings provide rather convincing evidence for a neuroectodermal origin for these lesions, i.e., few or no desmosomal attachments, specialized cell junctions, cytoplasmic filaments, and melanin formation.[76] Elevated urinary vanillylmandelic acid (VMA) levels in some patients add further support to neural crest derivation.

ENCEPHALOCELES

These benign, non-neoplastic ectopias of brain or a meninges may have either a traumatic or congenital basis. Early embryonic failure of mesodermal ingrowth between the neural tube and overlying ectoderm accounts for those presenting in infancy. The lesions are classified, by location, into three groups: occipital, sincipital, and basal. Sinus involvement can occur with the two latter types. In the sincipital variety, the defect is present between the frontoethmoid bones. Basal encephaloceles pass through the sphenoid or cribriform to present in the nasopharynx or nasal cavity, respectively. Rarely, a meningoencephalocele may be entirely confined to a sinus (frontal).[77]

MENINGIOMAS

A meningioma may involve the sinuses by extracranial extension of an intracranial tumor or apparently be primary in the sinus. As of 1990, 36 *primary* meningiomas of the nasal cavity and paranasal sinuses had been recorded in the world literature.[78-78e] In the paranasal sinuses, these meningiomas have most often presented in the frontal sinus, followed by the maxillary and ethmoid sinuses. Their cells of origin are the arachnoid cells in the sheaths of cranial nerves or ectopic within cranial periosteum.

Most of the meningiomas are either meningothelial or psammomatous subtypes (Fig. 6–14). All are variably invasive, but none have manifested either cytologic or other evidence of a biologic malignancy.

Tumors of Schwann cell origin, although of neuroectodermal origin, are discussed in the section dealing with Soft Tissue Tumors. The olfactory neuroblastomas are not discussed, even though invasion of the sinuses is quite often seen with this malignancy. We regard the olfactory neuroblastoma as being derived from olfactory epithelium and as such have *never* accepted a diagnosis of that neoplasm when the lesional tissue was *restricted* to a paranasal sinus without histologic or historic evidence of a previous or coexisting neuroblastoma high in the nasal cavity.

TUMORS OF BONE

The jaw and facial bones may be involved by virtually any osseous tumor, albeit at a much lower incidence than the axial and appendicular skeleton. The mandible is most often the site. Bones of the paranasal sinuses, with some exceptions, follow quite distantly with the maxilla leading. Some tumors, such as the myxoma and

giant cell reparative granuloma, are almost unique to the mandible and maxilla. In this section, we present the clinicopathologic features of myxoma, giant cell reparative granuloma, osteo- and chondrosarcomas, and osteoma.

MYXOMAS

These locally aggressive tumors may arise in bone, as well as somatic soft tissues. Those of bone are, for all purposes, tumors of the facial skeleton. The mandible, more often than the maxilla, is involved, and sites of predilection include the posterior and condylar regions of the jaw and the zygomatic process or alveolar bone of the maxilla. Maxillary tumors may fill the antrum.[79]

In either osseous or soft tissues, the gross and microscopic features of a myxoma are usually distinctive. Even though they may look circumscribed, these tumors are never delimited. On cut section, myxomas are gray-white or opalescent white. Their texture is rubbery, with a slimy mucoid surface.

Regardless of site, myxomas deviate little from a prototypical microscopic appearance. Parvicellularity and an abundant myxoid or mucoid intercellular matrix are the hallmarks (Fig. 6–15). There is an inconspicuous vascular pattern. The cells are usually stellate, with long, slender cytoplasmic processes, and their nuclei are small and bland. The only significant deviations are variable amounts of intralesional collagen and the finding, in some tumors, of odontogenic epithelium.

All myxomas are locally infiltrative lesions.

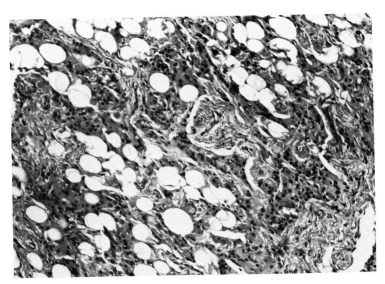

Figure 6–14. Extracranial meningioma of the frontal sinus with extension into regional soft tissue. Islands of meningothelial cells are separated by fibroadipose and connective tissue.

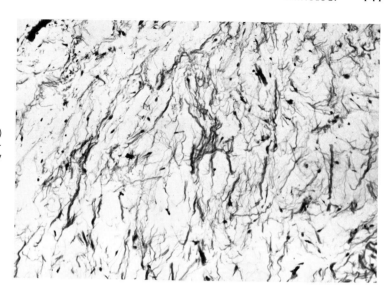

Figure 6–15. Central (intraosseous) myxoma of the maxilla. Slender fibroblastic cells are widely separated by a myxoid intercellular material.

There is no definable or accepted malignant variant.[80] Recurrences occur considerably less frequently for soft tissue myxomas than for gnathic myxomas. For the latter, up to a 25 per cent recurrence rate has been recorded.[79, 80] A recurrent myxoma usually makes its presence known clinically within 2 to 3 years but may be prompt or delayed.

GIANT CELL TUMORS

A true giant cell tumor of bone rarely, if ever, involves any of the sinuses. The majority are giant cell reparative granulomas (central or peripheral), and a lesser number represent misdiagnosis of other osseous lesions containing giant cells.

Giant cell granulomas chiefly affect adolescents and young adults. The maxilla leads all the sinuses as a site but follows the mandible, which is most frequently involved. The sphenoid bone is also cited, along with the temporal bones, as regions of affliction.[81, 82]

These radiolucent, usually well-demarcated lesions expand the involved cortical bone and may erode the bone. Fibrocyte-like cells with collagen production, multinucleated giant cells, hemorrhage, necrosis, and pigment deposition characterize the microscopic appearance. Osteoid and bone production can be found in about three quarters of the cases. Malignant features are absent. The great majority are essentially benign lesions, with only a 13 per cent local recurrence rate.

Differential diagnosis must always include the "brown tumor" of hyperparathyroidism.

OSTEOGENIC SARCOMA

This sarcoma arises in bone or soft tissues and is composed of malignant cells that produce an osteoid substance (Fig. 6–16). Osteoid, chondroid, or fibrous differentiation may predominate and thus yield osteoblastic, chondroblastic, and fibroblastic types of the sarcoma. They are classified also as endosteal or medullary, parosteal, periosteal, or extraosseous.[83]

Approximately 6.5 per cent of all osteogenic sarcomas are primary in the jaws. Excluding those sarcomas originating in a Paget's disease of bone matrix, the greatest number of cases occur during the third decade of life. Among children, osteogenic sarcoma is the most frequent primary bone malignancy of the maxilla. Of 412 osteogenic sarcomas of the craniofacial bones culled from the literature,[84, 84a, 84b] 146 occurred in the maxilla. The mandible, however, leads all sites. In the maxilla, the most frequent areas of involvement are along the alveolar ridge or within the antrum.

Paget's disease and pre- or postoperative irradiation for the treatment of other head and neck cancers are predisposing states. Painful swellings and signs and symptoms referable to encroachment into the nasal cavity and paranasal sinuses are the presenting complaints.

From a microscopic standpoint, osteogenic sarcomas of the bones of the sinuses do not differ significantly from those in the long bones. They may be predominantly osteoblastic and sclerosing or vascular and fibrosarcoma-like.

Local recurrences and distant metastases are the bane of the surgeon attempting to salvage patients with osteogenic sarcoma of the jaws.

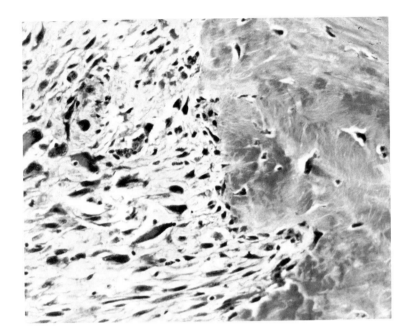

Figure 6–16. Osteogenic sarcoma of maxilla. Dense osteoid lies adjacent to neoplastic spindled cells.

Recurrences are high for maxillary lesions (80 per cent in the series of Caron et al[85]) and these appear within the first postoperative year. Distant metastases may be delayed but are usually manifest within 2 years. The average 5-year survival of patients with osteogenic sarcoma of the maxilla is 27 per cent.[83] When the sarcoma supervenes in Paget's disease, few patients are living after 5 years.[83]

CHONDROSARCOMA

All cartilaginous neoplasms of the jaws and facial skeleton are viewed with suspicion and a great deal of respect. This is necessitated by the notoriously difficult histopathologic distinction between a chondroma and a histologically low grade chondrosarcoma and by the rather consistent locally aggressive behavior of tumors of cartilage in these anatomic regions. Chondromas in the head and neck have been reported most often to occur in regions other than the maxilla and mandible, further indicating the suspect nature of cartilage tumors in these structures.

Chondrosarcomas of the jaws and maxillofacial skeleton are certainly uncommon. An estimate of their incidence would be 1.25 per cent of all chondrosarcomas in the body.[83] The maxilla is more frequently involved than the mandible by a ratio of 2:1, and there is a tendency for maxillary chondrosarcomas to occur more often in women. In the maxilla, the anterior area, the palate, and the vicinity of the lateral incisors and canine teeth are sites of predilection.[83]

Light microscopic features for the diagnosis include increased numbers of cells with plump nuclei, more than occasional binucleate cells, and multinucleated giant cartilage cells (Fig. 6–17). Cytologic grading based on cellularity, mitoses, and deviation from a cartilage phenotype is of prognostic significance.

Patients with sinonasal chondrosarcomas usually have a slow, progressive course, marred with multiple recurrences. Death results from uncontrolled local disease. Distant metastases are infrequent.

Five-year survival statistics tell only a partial story, because death may occur after that interval. Survivals of 62 per cent and 40 per cent at 5 years have been given.[86, 87] Prognosis improves almost in a direct relationship to the width of margin of normal tissue included by the surgical resection.

A distinctive type of chondrosarcoma, the *mesenchymal chondrosarcoma*, has a moderate predilection for the facial bones and adjacent soft tissues.[88] Histologic diagnosis of this lesion is established by the finding of a richly cellular neoplasm composed of undifferentiated mesenchymal cells, in which islands of relatively well-differentiated cartilage are found. The presence of this cartilage is essential and required for the diagnosis. The tumor requires complete surgical removal. Like chondrosarcoma, recurrences are numerous. Metastases, lymphatic and hematogenous, may appear after a long latent period.

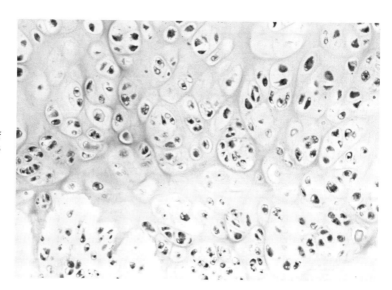

Figure 6–17. Chondrosarcoma of the maxilla. Neoplastic chondrocytes with atypical nuclei lie in clusters.

OSTEOMAS

A slowly growing lesion of bone, the osteoma is considered to be the commonest benign tumor of the nose and sinuses. The tumors are usually clinically silent and are detected only in radiographs of the sinuses. In that setting, an incidence of 1 per cent or less has been recorded.[89] The lesions are usually discovered in the third and fourth decades and there is a modest preference for men.

Statistics vary as to the frequency of particular sinus involvement. The figures given by Mikaelian and colleagues[90] are representative: frontal sinus, 39 per cent; ethmoid sinus, 24 per cent; maxillary sinus, nearly 5 per cent; and sphenoid sinus, under 1 per cent.

Whether neoplastic or not, the origin of osteomas is debatable. The tumors do tend to cluster about junctions of membranous and endochondral bone.

Osteomas of the sinuses are almost always single tumors and they usually exhibit a pedicle. Symptomatic tumors are those producing signs and symptoms of a space-occupying lesion obstruction of an ostium, or both. Osteomas arising from the posterior wall of the frontal sinus may attain huge sizes because of their relatively insensitive location. Those originating in the region of the frontonasal spine may grow upward into the frontal sinus, but also into the ethmoid air cells and nasal cavity. A few osteomas also arise in the superolateral angle of the orbit.

The association of craniofacial osteomas and Gardner's syndrome has been repeatedly confirmed. Less than 10 per cent of the afflicted patients, however, display the complete structural lesions of the syndrome (intestinal polyposis of small and large bowel, osteomas, soft tissue benign tumors, and sebaceous cysts of the skin). The syndrome is rarely diagnosed before the age of 30 years. In a survey of 280 patients with the syndrome, 40 (14 per cent) manifested bone abnormalities.[91] The multiple and solitary osteomas in this disease occur at the following sites, in descending order of frequency: frontal bone, mandible, maxilla, sphenoid, ethmoid, zygoma, and temporal bone. Osteomas usually precede the other syndromic manifestations.

Histologic descriptions of osteomas of the paranasal sinuses are variable but usually fall into compact (ivory), spongy, or mixed categories (Fig. 6–18). Compact osteomas are composed of dense, mature lamellar bone. No haversian system is formed, and marrow spaces are rare. Spongy or trabecular osteomas are predominantly cancellous or trabecular in architecture, and fatty marrow is found between the trabeculae.

The growth of osteomas is greatest at the time of maximal skeletal development and slows as skeletal growth reaches maturity.

Surgical intervention is indicated only in the presence of complications due to the osteoma.

SOFT TISSUE TUMORS

Table 6–13 lists the varieties of soft tissue sarcoma that may be found in the head and neck. Although they are classified by tissue type, nearly all likely originate from primordial or mesenchymal cells, which in their neoplastic

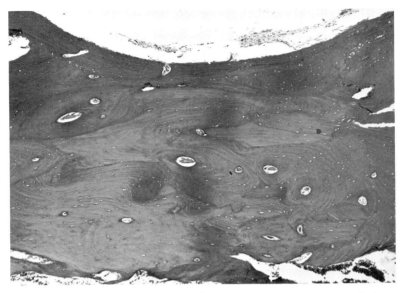

Figure 6–18. Compact type of osteoma composed of dense, mature lamellar bone.

expression contain light or electron microscopic evidence of a differentiation to adult tissue cells.

Except for specific entities, strikingly demonstrated by rhabdomyosarcoma, the head and neck, and especially the paranasal sinuses, are not regions of predilection for these sarcomas (Table 6–14).[92] In addition, nearly all the sarcomas arise de novo without passing through a phase of benign neoplasia. Rhabdomyoma, for example, is not a precursor of rhabdomyosarcoma. The neurogenic sarcoma, however, is often traceable to a maternal neurofibroma. Fibromatosis and chordoma are included in the listing, not because these lesions are classified as sarcomas but to acknowledge their sarcomatous behavior at the local site.

The rarity of either origin from or localization to the paranasal sinuses of most of the sarcomas in Table 6–13 precludes any worthy discussion of them except for rhabdomyosarcoma, fibrous and fibrohistiocytic tumors, neurogenous tumors, and one of the vasoformative lesions, hemangiopericytoma. Exclusion of the others is also purposeful, not only to underscore their unusual presence in the sinuses but also to caution the surgeon and pathologist against a too ready acceptance of diagnoses that may be in error. Angio- and leiomyosarcomas are illustrative examples. We are suspicious of the diagnosis of a primary angiosarcoma in the sinonasal tract. That sarcoma is principally a tumor of the skin and subcutaneous tissues of the scalp

TABLE 6–13. Sarcomas of Soft Tissue in the Head and Neck

Fibrous or Fibrohistiocytic
    Fibrosarcoma
    Fibrous histiocytoma
    (Fibromatosis)
	Neurogenous
	    Neurogenic sarcoma
	    (neurofibrosarcoma)

Adipose
    Liposarcoma
	Extraosseous Cartilage and Bone
	    Extraskeletal myxoid chondrosarcoma
	    Extraskeletal mesenchymal
	        chondrosarcoma
	    Extraosseous osteogenic sarcoma

Smooth Muscle Leiomyosarcoma	

Vasoformative
    Angiosarcoma, including
        lymphangiosarcoma
    Hemangiopericytoma
    Kaposi's sarcoma
	Notochord
	    Chordoma

	Tumors of Uncertain Derivation
	    Clear cell sarcoma
	    Epithelioid sarcoma
	    Alveolar soft-part sarcoma
	    Extraskeletal Ewing's sarcoma

Skeletal Muscle Rhabdomyosarcoma	
Synovial Synovial sarcoma	

TABLE 6–14. Anatomic Locations of 1619 Soft Tissue Sarcomas

Anatomic Site	Percentage of All Cases
Lower extremity	42
Trunk	30
Upper extremity	16
Head and neck	12

(From data presented by Rosenberg SA, Glatstein EJ: Perspectives on the role of surgery and radiation therapy in the treatment of soft tissue sarcomas of the extremities. Semin Oncol 8:190, 1981.)

and facial skin in elderly men. Richly vascularized sarcomas, melanomas, and even plasmacytomas histologically can masquerade as angiosarcomas. Leiomyomatous tumors, benign and malignant, are also primarily tumors of the skin and subcutaneous soft tissues. They arise from or near the walls of the blood vascular system.

Even though angiofibromas often extend into the paranasal sinuses, they are typically nasal or nasopharyngeal tumors and do not fall into the purview of this chapter.

RHABDOMYOSARCOMA

Little information is available on the sequence of specific structural features of skeletal muscle cells in their various stages of maturation. Figure 6–19 outlines these stages.[93] Transition from myoblast to a primary myotubule is seen in the seventh to ninth weeks of fetal life. Mononucleated, spindle-shaped cells with only a few myofibrils fuse end to end to form primary myotubules. On section (cross and longitudinal), the primary myotubules are characterized by glycogen granules, lipid droplets, and a few peripherally distributed myofibrils and scant sarcoplasm. Well-defined sarcoplasms with A, Z, I, and M bands in the myofibrils are few in number. There is only a rudimentary basal lamina. The next step in development, from the tenth week onward, involves a fusion of undifferentiated mononucleated cells with primary myotubules that lie side to side and a fusion of two myotubules, resulting in a more mature one. The apposed undifferentiated cells contain ribosomes, mitochondria, and a small amount of rough endoplasmic reticulum. Mature myotubes present as two or three cells in different stages of development in close contact with and enveloped by a common basal lamina. Typically, the largest cell is the primary myotubule. Attached to it are two smaller cells, one undifferentiated and often showing mitotic fig-

ures, and another containing only a few myofibrils. Between the eleventh and fifteenth weeks, the number of mature myotubules clearly predominate over those in earlier stages.[93]

From the sixteenth to twenty-second weeks, there are considerable structural and architectural changes in the muscle cells. Myofibrils become abundant in the myotubes; the latter grow smaller and the nuclei move from a central to a peripheral position. Undifferentiated cells persist, and they may manifest side-to-side fusion of two or more muscle cells, with formation of an immature muscle fiber.[93] Clusters of immature muscle fibers that appear to be in transition between the undifferentiated stage and the myoblast stage, with a few developing myofibrils, are seen even after the twenty-fifth week.[93]

The preceding discussion of normal myogenesis of skeletal muscle is offered to emphasize that rhabdomyosarcomas do not arise from developed skeletal muscle but rather for the most part recapitulate, in a neoplastic, aberrant manner, myogenesis from primitive mesenchymal cells. By definition, then, rhabdomyosarcoma is a malignant neoplasm whose *only identifiable* line of differentiation is that expressed by a rhabdomyoblast. This serves to separate it from certain other neoplasms that may also contain rhabdomyoblasts.

Accounting for over 50 per cent of all pedi-

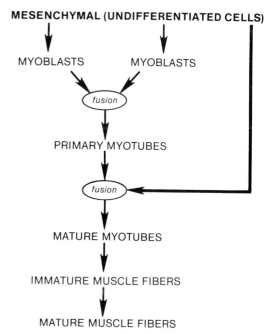

MESENCHYMAL (UNDIFFERENTIATED CELLS)

MYOBLASTS   MYOBLASTS

fusion

PRIMARY MYOTUBES

fusion

MATURE MYOTUBES

IMMATURE MUSCLE FIBERS

MATURE MUSCLE FIBERS

Figure 6–19. Progression of differentiation in normal myogenesis. Rhabdomyosarcomas may be considered as neoplastic caricatures of this process.

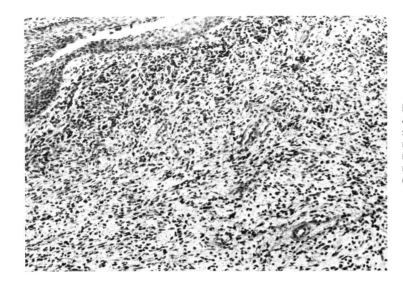

Figure 6–20. Rhabdomyosarcoma of antrum. Medial wall of the maxillary sinus has been destroyed and the neoplasm lies beneath metaplastic nasal mucosa. The condensation of neoplastic cells beneath the mucosa (cambium layer) is typical.

atric sarcomas, rhabdomyosarcomas are the most common malignant soft tissue neoplasms encountered in children, and in this age group, the head and neck are the sites of predilection.[94] The percentage distribution in 423 newly diagnosed rhabdomyosarcomas in children, as reported by Maurer and colleagues,[95] was orbit, 7 per cent; head and neck, 29 per cent; extremities, 23 per cent; genitourinary tract, 18 per cent; retroperitoneum and trunk, 14 per cent; and miscellaneous sites, 9 per cent.

Within the head and neck, the air cavities such as the middle ear, paranasal sinuses, and mastoid rank behind the orbit and eyelids, upper aerodigestive tracts, and soft tissues of the neck as sites of predilection. Dito and Batsakis indicated that 8.8 per cent of 170 cases arose in the sinuses and aural regions.[96]

Sinus rhabdomyosarcomas do not significantly differ grossly or microscopically from other rhabdomyosarcomas. They are aggressive, destructive lesions (Figs. 6–20 and 6–21).

The tumors have been classically divided into pleomorphic, alveolar, embryonal, and botryoid types. *Pleomorphic rhabdomyosarcomas* are the least common of all forms. They are usually found in the extremities, especially in the thighs, and are tumors of late middle age. Pleomorphic rhabdomyosarcoma is composed of spindle cells with marked pleomorphism, elongated strap or racquet cells with bright eosinophilic cytoplasm, and vacuolated "spider" cell forms. Cross-striations are present.

Alveolar rhabdomyosarcomas manifest collagenous septa that encircle or circumscribe cellular areas of neoplastic cells. These cells

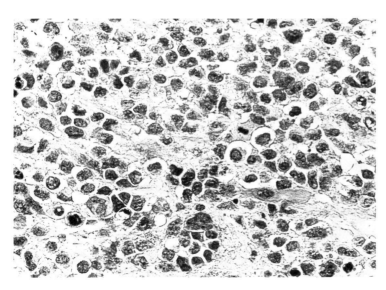

Figure 6–21. Embryonal rhabdomyosarcoma of the maxillary sinus. Only occasional cells have elongated eosinophilic cytoplasm with longitudinal striations.

tend either to adhere to the septa or to appear as free-floating cells within the spaces. The central cells may be multinucleated or strap cells. Classically a tumor of children or young adults, this variant can occur at any age. Attention has been directed to a clear cell variant of alveolar rhabdomyosarcoma in the sinonasal tract and its structural similarity to clear cell carcinoma by Chan, et al.[96a] The median age in Enzinger and Shiraki's[97] series was 15 years. At any site, the alveolar rhabdomyosarcoma is perhaps the most aggressive of all rhabdomyosarcomas. Metastases to lymph nodes are described in nearly three quarters of patients during the first postdiagnostic year, and distant spread to lungs, bones, and pancreas is common. Enzinger and Shiraki[97] report only 2 patients of 102 who survived 5 years. The median survival was only 8.7 months.

The most common form is *embryonal rhabdomyosarcoma*. It is primarily a neoplasm of infancy and early childhood (under 5 years of age). Embryonal rhabdomyosarcoma exhibits a striking predilection for the head and neck, less for the genitourinary area.[93] This variant is composed of rather small cells that either have stellate or slim, biopolar shapes. The cells are arranged in syncytial masses or anastomosing bands but do not exhibit an alveolar pattern. The cells may also be rounded and suggest a lymphocytic lymphoma. Nearly always, however, some cells will show a distinct eosinophilic cytoplasm with a fibrillary matrix. Not uncommonly, embryonal rhabdomyosarcomas show a peripheral zone where the cells layer out parallel to the surface, i.e., the cambium layer. Identification of cross-striations is not necessary for diagnosis. If found, however, the diagnosis is unassailable. Obvious rhabdomyoblasts and cross-striated cells may be evident only in metastatic foci.

Botryoid rhabdomyosarcoma is not a histologic variant. It is most often an embryonal rhabdomyosarcoma, distinctive only in its sites of origin beneath mucous membranes and protrusion into a space, e.g., sinus, nasal cavity, vagina.

Before the introduction of effective multimodal therapy, the prognosis for children with rhabdomyosarcoma was bleak. Standard surgical procedures, such as amputation of an extremity or radical resection for head and neck lesions, were predictably followed by rapid local recurrence, loss of local control, and metastases. The combination of a transferable staging system and knowledge that rhabdomyosarcomas are sensitive to the antineoplastic action of several drugs, particularly cyclophosphamide,

vincristine, actinomycin D, and doxorubicin, have altered the dismal outlook for many children with these sarcomas. To date, however, this more optimistic consideration has not been fulfilled to the same degree for rhabdomyosarcomas of the so-called parameningeal sites (nasopharynx, nasal cavity, paranasal sinuses, and middle ear–mastoid area).[98, 99] Fifty-seven of 141 cases (40 per cent) in the first Intergroup Rhabdomyosarcoma Study series had parameningeal site involvement.[97] Thirty-five per cent of these (20 of 57) showed evidence of a direct meningeal extension and 19 of the 20 patients were dead at the time of the Intergroup report. Median survival was only 9 months.

Patients with parameningeal rhabdomyosarcomas, including those arising in the paranasal sinuses, are clearly at risk, especially if they manifest abnormalities of the central nervous system, demonstrate enlargements of neural foramina, or have evidence of erosion of bone(s) at the skull's base. Definite meningeal involvement can be documented by the presence of neoplastic cells in the cerebrospinal fluid, by demonstration of an intracranial mass by computed tomography (CT) scan or arteriography, or by evidence of involvement of the spinal cord.

Berry and Jenkin's[99] data indicate that primary tumor radiation treatment parameters may be critical in determining the incidence of meningeal relapse in patients with parameningeal rhabdomyosarcomas. Their study, however, is flawed by small numbers of patients, varying degrees of selection, the inclusion of orbital tumors, and use of adjuvant chemotherapy in less than half of the patients. Nevertheless, using radiation as the primary modality, they obtained 5-year survivals of 43 and 12 per cent for primary rhabdomyosarcomas of the nasopharynx and middle ear–mastoid, respectively. The 3-year survival for patients with tumors of the paranasal sinuses was 40 per cent.

Because of the rapidity of death associated with parameningeal primary rhabdomyosarcomas, there is usually no evidence of distant spread in these patients. However, as well as a notorious rapid extension into contiguous structures, rhabdomyosarcomas (all sites) manifest a high incidence of distant metastases. An incidence of 20 per cent at the time of diagnosis is quite constant. Primary sites in the head and neck, even with the orbital tumors excluded, are the least likely (statistically) to manifest this morbid event.[94, 96] Metastasis to regional lymph nodes is also site dependent and does not correlate directly with size, extent, or histologic type. Regional lymph node metastases from head and neck primary sites (orbit not included) are said to be of a low order (3 to 5 per cent).[94]

FIBROSARCOMA

Little mention is made of fibroma in the current literature. This is appropriate because it is likely not a definable histologic or neoplastic entity. Most so-called fibromas are tissue reactions to local injury or other lesions in which variable degrees of collagenization and fibrosis are present. Before refinements in diagnosis and classification, fibrosarcoma was a popular diagnosis. It is much less so now, having been replaced by more precise histogenic and histologic diagnosis. By definition, a fibrosarcoma is a malignant soft tissue tumor that demonstrates variable production of collagen, does not manifest differentiation into other types of tissues, and has the ability to metastasize.

The head and neck, and especially the paranasal sinuses, are not areas of predilection for either adult or childhood fibrosarcomas.[100-102] Most occur in the extremities. Histologic appearances and diagnostic criteria, however, do not differ regardless of site of origin. The biologic behavior of the neoplasms, given the modifiers of the anatomic sites in the head and neck, are also similar.

Any sinus may be the apparent site of origin for fibrosarcomas, but these lesions tend to be either maxillary or ethmoid. The cases we have examined originated in the periosteum of the sinuses, i.e., a periosteal fibrosarcoma. A predisposing factor of importance is prior irradiation, as, for example, for fibrous dysplasia.[101, 102]

In general, fibrosarcoma of the nasal cavity and paranasal sinuses is a tumor of older people,

but there is a wide age range. Nasal obstruction with an intranasal neoplastic component is the most common clinical finding. Grossly, the tumors may be polypoid or diffuse. Bone destruction, either by expansion or by invasion, is often seen, especially when the tumors are attached to nasal or sinus walls. Fibrosarcomas invade by direct extension along fascial or cleavage places with ill-defined margins to form bulky, solid, pseudoencapsulated masses that eventually involve bone.

Marked pleomorphism is not a characteristic of fibrosarcomas even though they range from differentiated to poorly differentiated in their cellular composition.[103] The classic appearance is that of a spindle-celled neoplasm with cells arranged in interlacing fascicles to produce a herringbone pattern (Fig. 6–22). Collagen production varies. Mitoses are always found and at times may be frequent.

Histologic grading of fibrosarcoma is warranted because there is a correlation with recurrences and survival. Features utilized in the grading are degrees of cellularity and anaplasia, relative amounts of collagen and reticulin, frequency of mitoses, and degree of local infiltration. A well-differentiated fibrosarcoma (grade 1) manifests a rich reticulin framework, a low degree of cellularity, little or no anaplasia, and a low mitotic count. Increasing prominence of these permits classification into grades 2, 3, and 4. The influence of grade on survival is significant. For fibrosarcomas in aggregate, 80 per cent of patients with grade 1 tumors have a 10-year survival,[103] whereas no patient with a grade 4 sarcoma survives 10 years.

In adult fibrosarcomas, at all sites, local recurrences are high (55 to 75 per cent of

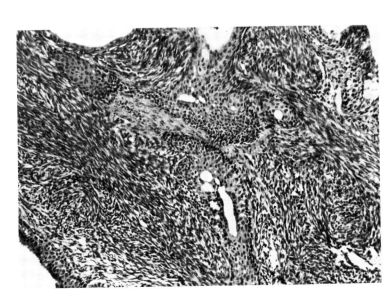

Figure 6–22. Fibrosarcoma of the maxillary and ethmoid sinus. Cellular neoplasm courses beneath the surface mucosa. The patient, a 57-year-old man, had six recurrences over a 20 year period.

patients). Five year survival statistics do not tell the full story of fibrosarcomas. Those of the paranasal sinuses tend to be of lower grades, and life, marred by the morbidity of recurrences, is usually not appreciably shortened.

Metastases appear to be related not only to histologic grade but also to effectiveness of local control. In one study, patients with uncontrolled local disease displayed a 59 per cent rate of metastases, compared with only 22 per cent in patients whose tumors were effectively managed locally.[104] Metastases may often be delayed (5 to 10 years or longer after the time of primary treatment). Survival obviously relates to local extent and control and metastases. In uncontrolled disease with metastases, the 10-year survival is reduced by half (65 versus 30 per cent).[105]

FIBROMATOSIS

This locally aggressive fibrous tissue lesion is also called well-differentiated fibrosarcoma by some pathologists. We use the latter only to indicate that the tumor is a locally and stubbornly aggressive tumor but not a metastasizing fibrous neoplasm. It is, in effect, an extra-abdominal desmoid.

Fibromatosis of the paranasal sinuses can occur in nearly any age group from childhood through adulthood. The maxillary antrum is the predominant sinus involved.[100]

The tumors appear as firm, tough, and white fibrous masses infiltrating adjacent tissues and encroaching on air passages. They may partially or completely fill the sinus cavity.

Microscopically, a fibromatosis is composed of relatively mature fibrous tissue with an abundant collagenous stroma. The spindle-shaped cells demonstrate little or no pleomorphism. Mitotic figures are infrequent. Invasion into adjacent tissues is always present. Some tumors may be so sparsely populated by cells that a scar is simulated. In these instances, only the clinical behavior of the lesion will indicate the true nature.

The fibromatoses of childhood deviate from the aforementioned in that they are more cellular and less well differentiated. These lesions may well qualify as fibrosarcomas because they manifest a progressive enlargement and mitoses are common. However, soft tissue tumors called fibrosarcomas occurring in the first 3 to 5 years of life appear to exhibit a biologic behavior less aggressive than those occurring in later life. The majority of lesions are either present at birth or are noticed within the first 3 months

of life. The head and neck and sinuses are not sites of predilection.[106]

Despite a noticeable mitotic activity and a lesser degree of differentiation, these fibrosarcomas behave like fibromatoses, albeit with occasional metastases. Even within the childhood and adolescent period, there are behavioral differences. Soule and Pritchard,[107] in their study of 110 patients under 15 years of age, found a local recurrence rate of 43 per cent and a rate of metastasis of 7.3 per cent for tumors occurring within the first 5 years of life. After the age of 10 years, both recurrences and metastases approach the rates seen in adults, a 50 per cent metastatic rate.

FIBROUS HISTIOCYTOMA

Tumors embraced by the term *fibrous histiocytoma* have a wide and variable histologic composition. The variance stems from the putative origin of these tumors, primitive mesenchymal progenitor cells. The maternal mesenchymal cells phenotypically differentiate into fibroblastic and histiocytic cells. Either of these cells may predominate, or they may be nearly equal in distribution. The spindled fibroblastic cells usually manifest, at least in focal areas, a cartwheel pattern (Fig. 6–23). The histiocytelike cells, which may be multinucleated, often show phagocytic activity and a foamy, lipid-containing cytoplasm.

Despite the recent observation that fibrous histiocytomas are among the most numerous of supporting tissue tumors, they are not common in the head and neck and are only occasionally reported as lesions of the paranasal sinuses. In 1977, Blitzer and colleagues[108] reviewed 32 cases of fibrous histiocytomas localized in various regions of the head and neck. Only six of them affected the paranasal sinuses, two originated from the ethmoids and four from the maxillary antrum. Since then, other sinus involvement has been documented.[109, 110]

The cell population of fibrous histiocytomas ranges from amitotic, cytologically benign lesions to ones with overt histologic malignancy in the forms of marked anaplasia and numerous mitoses. The malignant (capable of metastasis) potential of a fibrous histiocytoma is, however, more dependent on topographic features (size, superficial versus deep location) than on the more empiric histologic details. Kearney and colleagues[111] also consider that superficial tumors that subsequently have deep recurrences are more likely to manifest a higher degree of biologic aggressiveness.

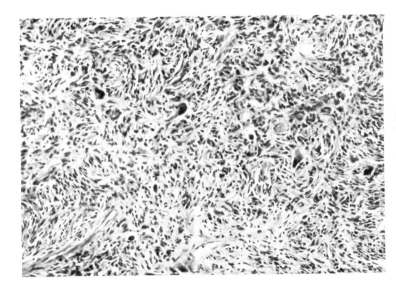

Figure 6–23. Fibrous histiocytoma of the paranasal sinuses. In this histologic form, fibroblastic, histiocytic, and giant cells can be seen. Note also the whorled areas.

Just as these tumors manifest a spectrum of histologic appearance, so too is there a spectrum of behavior. Most are locally aggressive with frequent recurrences. Blitzer and colleagues[108] recorded a 22 per cent incidence of metastasis from deep-seated head and neck fibrous histiocytomas. They indicated also that invasion of local structures was not a reliable criterion for malignant potential but noted that the more anaplastic and pleomorphic tumors followed a more malignant course.

The fibrous histiocytoma requires respect on the part of the clinician, especially if the tumor is deeply sited. Lymph node metastases from paranasal sites approximate 20 per cent, and this is equivalent to that seen in primary tumors of other regions.[110, 111] This lymphatic spread ranks the fibrous histiocytoma with rhabdomyosarcoma as being the soft tissue sarcoma most likely to spread to regional lymph nodes. Hematogenous dissemination is also found (2 of 21 cases).[110]

The number of cases from the sinuses is too small and follow-up too short to provide significant survival data. For tumors outside of the head and neck, 4-year survival of 65 per cent is given for superficial tumors and a 34 per cent survival for deep lesions.[111]

HEMANGIOPERICYTOMA

A surgical-pathologic diagnosis of hemangiopericytoma is never easy, and even when accurate, ascribing biologic malignancy on histologic grounds is often impossible. The problems in diagnosis are emphasized by Angervall and colleagues.[112] These investigators point out that in only 6 of 42 cases originally designated as hemangiopericytoma in the Swedish Cancer Registry was this diagnosis accepted.

Not only is the morphologic expression of these lesions quite variable, so too is biologic behavior. Age of patients and anatomic site appear to be considerable factors in modifying behavior. For example, hemangiopericytomas appearing in neonates are basically benign, regardless of their histologic appearance.[113]

The classic hemangiopericytoma exhibits a ramifying vascular bed, with considerable variation in the caliber of the endothelium-lined spaces (Fig. 6–24). The majority of the vessels are thin walled, regardless of their size. The tumor cells (pericytes) are arranged *about* these vascular spaces (perithelial) and are rather uniform, polyhedral cells. Reticulin fibers enmesh individual cells. Farther removed from the vasculature, the tumor cells have a more haphazard arrangement. Immunostaining has shown uniform, strongly positive results for vimentin; 10 per cent of cells stain for S-100 protein and focal, faint staining for actin has been noted.[113a]

Factors that correlate with malignant potential include mitoses, necrosis, tumor size, and, apparently, site of origin. Four or more division figures per 10 high power fields in a hemangiopericytoma are associated with a survival rate of 29 per cent, compared with a 77 per cent survival for patients having lesions with fewer mitoses.[113] Large areas of necrosis in a tumor are associated with poor prognosis. Tumors larger than 6.5 cm are also more biologically aggressive.

Only 15 to 25 per cent of all hemangiopericytomas occur in the head and neck, where they usually arise in extraoral and extrasinonasal soft tissues.[114] Judged on reported cases, the nasal cavity exceeds the paranasal sinuses as a

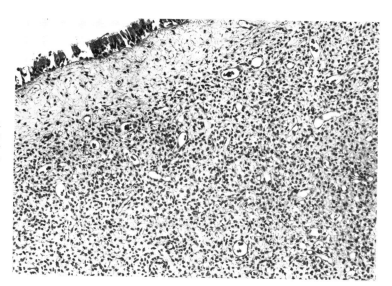

Figure 6–24. Hemangiopericytoma of the nasal cavity with extension into the maxillary antrum. The vascular character of the neoplasm is readily seen.

site by a 2:1 ratio. The sphenoethmoid and ethmoid regions lead the maxillary sinus by a 4:1 margin.

When hemangiopericytomas from all sites are considered, a recurrence rate of 25 to 50 per cent and a metastatic rate of 12 to 60 per cent are seen.[114] That the head and neck may be a site for less clinically malignant tumors is suggested by Batsakis and Rice.[114] Of 48 hemangiopericytomas of the sinuses or nasal cavity reported in the literature, 13 manifested local recurrences, 2 demonstrated metastases, and in 2 patients death was attributed to the neoplasm.

Reasons for these suggested differences are not readily apparent. The nasal cavity and paranasal sinuses are not usually favorable sites for supporting tissue neoplasms. It is possible that these regions favor the histogenesis of histologically low-grade hemangiopericytomas.[115] High-grade, anaplastic hemangiopericytomas are unusual to rare in the nasal cavity and sinuses. Longer follow-up periods may also negate a presumed better prognosis. Hemangiopericytomas of the head and neck may have long intervals of apparent local control before recurrences, and, with multiple recurrences, the disease can be life consuming.[114] The data of Eichhorn, et al. indicate that recurrence rates of sinonasal hemangiopericytomas approach the rates for that lesion at other sites, but that from the sinonasal site the rates of metastasis and mortality are lower.[113a]

SCHWANN CELL (NEUROGENOUS) TUMORS

Three supporting tissue tumors are considered in this category: neurofibroma, neurilem-moma, and neurogenous sarcoma (neurofibro-sarcoma). Of these three, the neurilemmoma is most often encountered in the paranasal sinuses and nasal cavity.

The histogenesis of these tumors is still being debated, although an origin from Schwann cells is favored by most. Schwann cell derivation has led to the use of the term *schwannoma* for the entire group. We have resisted this not only because complete proof is lacking for a Schwann cell origin, but also because the three tumors have distinctive clinical and light microscopic features.

Neurilemmomas are generally solitary, encapsulated tumors usually attached to, or surrounded by, a nerve. They are occasionally found in patients with von Recklinghausen's neurofibromatosis and rarely, if ever, undergo malignant transformation.

In contrast, neurofibromas are not encapsulated and are usually multiple. They are the prototype tumors of von Recklinghausen's disease and in a rather constant number of patients, one or more undergo malignant change.

With light microscopy, the differences between a neurilemmoma and a neurofibroma are usually readily evident. A capsule and a distinctive pattern—Antoni A tissue with palisading of nuclei about a central mass of cytoplasm (Verocay body) and a loose-textured stroma in which the fibers and cells form no distinctive pattern (Antoni B tissue)—are seen in neurilemmomas. Retrogressive changes are prominent and consist of necrosis, cystic degeneration, lipidization, and alterations of tumor vasculature. The secondary changes in neurilemmomas may be so prominent as to obscure the tumor's tissue type (Fig. 6–25).

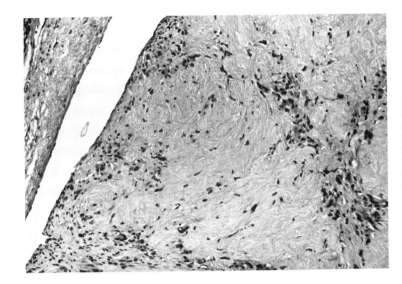

Figure 6–25. Neurilemmoma of the sinonasal tract. The lesion presented as a polypoid mass. Hyalinization of the tumor is prominent, and in advanced stages it, with other retrogressive changes, can obscure the cellular composition of these essentially benign tumors.

Neurofibromas are unencapsulated; they incorporate neurites rather than pushing them aside and manifest a spindle cell pattern of growth. They lack many of the retrogressive changes found in neurilemmomas, and the prominent vascular changes of the latter are less conspicuous.

Neurogenous sarcoma (neurofibrosarcoma) may or may not be associated with von Recklinghausen's disease. The association varies from 6 to 16 per cent.[103] The discrepancy is attributable, in the main, to two factors: (1) the tendency to select cases from patients with neurofibromatosis and (2) the great variation in clinical expression of von Recklinghausen's disease with an overlooking of minor manifestations. It still stands that the sarcoma arises in or from a neurofibroma rather than a neurilemmoma, and any age is susceptible. The predominant age period is in the early fifth decade.

Because the Schwann cell is presumed to be of neuroectodermal derivation, it is capable of several ectodermal or mesodermal phenotypic expressions. Most neurogenous sarcomas, however, may be indistinguishable from fibrosarcomas, except for a gross or clinical identification of origin from a nerve. Given the pluripotentiality of the Schwann cell, forms of neurogenous sarcoma may manifest rhabdomyomatous, osteogenic, liposarcomatous and other mesodermal differentiations, as well as epithelial glandlike formations and mucin-positive cells.[116, 117]

Mere nuclear pleomorphism or necrosis is certainly insufficient evidence for malignancy in a neurofibroma. Both these features are or can be prominent in benign neurogenous tumors. Increased cellularity and especially the mitotic index are the most reliable. Because mitoses in cells may not be uniformly distributed, a generous sampling of neurofibromas is necessary.[103]

Hillstrom, et al. indicate that only 4 per cent of nerve sheath tumors arising in the head and neck region are found in the paranasal sinuses, with only 40 such cases reported as of 1990.[117a] In our opinion, the literature's indication that primary nerve sheath tumors arising in the nasal cavity and paranasal sinuses are unusual entities is not entirely accurate. Many have been called fibromas, angiofibromas, or other lesions.

The majority of the lesions are neurilemmomas, not neurofibromas. Intranasal nerves, the ophthalmic and maxillary branches of the trigeminal nerves, and branches of the autonomic nervous system can give rise to the tumors. Because the olfactory nerves contain no Schwann cells, they can be excluded as a possible origin for these tumors.[118]

A combined nasoethmoid involvement is most common. This is followed, in order of frequency, by maxillary sinus, intranasal area, and sphenoid sinus.[118] Nearly all have been solitary tumors.

Early diagnosis and complete surgical excision is rarely followed by recurrence in the case of a neurilemmoma.

A relatively aggressive course characterizes neurogenous sarcomas and this is apparently accelerated if the sarcoma is associated with neurofibromatosis. In a Mayo Clinic series of 24 cases *not associated* with von Recklinghausen's disease, 9 patients died of their neoplasm and only 4 of 15 patients followed over a 5 year period were alive and well.[116] In 16 of 17 patients with neurogenous sarcoma and neurofibromatosis, death was attributable to the sarcoma.[117] Nine of these patients had extensive metastases.

LYMPHOMA AND EXTRAMEDULLARY PLASMACYTOMA

LYMPHOMA

The incidence of lymphomatous involvement of the paranasal sinuses is difficult to establish. Some indications are given by Sofferman and Cummings[119] and Fu and Perzin.[120] The former relate that 8 per cent of sinus malignancies are lymphomas; the latter give an incidence of 6.6 per cent of nonepithelial tumors involving the nasal cavity, paranasal, sinuses, and nasopharynx. In general, the first indication of lymphoma in the patients in both series was the paranasal sinus presentation.

The maxillary sinus is by far the predominant site of involvement. The clinical presentation is usually a diffuse swelling in the maxillary area in a patient in the fifth or sixth decade of life. Some patients also will have an intranasal component.

The lymphomas are non-Hodgkin's type and usually diffuse lymphocytic lymphomas (Fig. 6–26). Correlation between the degree and histologic type and response to treatment is usually not successful. Indeed, in our experience, it is unpredictable. Failure of local response to irradiation, however, is a poor prognostic indicator.

The great diversity among lymphomas within the paranasal sinus region in terms of clinical and pathologic presentation, immunologic parameters, and prognostic variation has been underscored. Some investigators note the problem with using the NCJ Working Formulation with this group, claiming close resemblance to the peripheral T-cell lymphomas described in Japan.[120a] Frierson and colleagues, on the other hand, found a predominance of B-cell immunophenotype in an American resident.[120b]

Survival for 1, 3, and 5 years after local control by irradiation is relatively favorable, but most patients succumb to either intercurrent disease or dissemination (to regional lymph nodes, viscera, or soft tissues).

EXTRAMEDULLARY PLASMACYTOMA

This is the term applied to plasma cell tumors that occur outside of bone. Of all extramedullary plasmacytomas, up to 80 per cent have been noted in the upper air passages and oral cavity. They represent nearly 4 per cent of all nonepithelial neoplasms of the nasal cavity and paranasal sinuses.[121] Arising in submucosal tissues at these sites, the plasmacytoma presents as a fleshy, yellow-gray to dark-red sessile, polypoid or pedunculated tumor (Fig. 6–27). Ulceration is not frequent, but underlying bone may be involved. Between 10 and 20 per cent of upper aerodigestive tract plasmacytomas will have multiple lesions elsewhere in the head and neck.[122]

The biologic behavior of an extramedullary plasmacytoma can be one of several patterns:

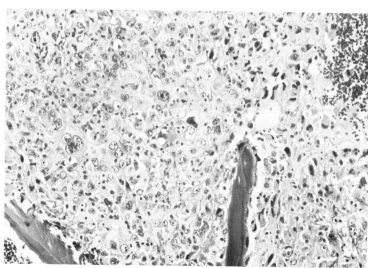

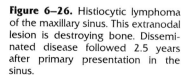

Figure 6–26. Histiocytic lymphoma of the maxillary sinus. This extranodal lesion is destroying bone. Disseminated disease followed 2.5 years after primary presentation in the sinus.

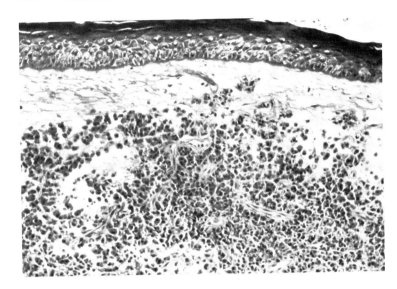

Figure 6–27. Extramedullary plasmacytoma beneath a squamous metaplastic epithelium.

(1) localized solitary disease, controlled by surgery, radiotherapy, or both, that does not recur or become disseminated; (2) locally recurrent disease, controlled by additional therapy; (3) aggressive, persistent, or recurrent disease killing the host via uncontrollable local extensions; (4) local disease with metastatic involvement of regional lymph nodes but without distant spread; and (5) local disease, recurrent or otherwise, followed by dissemination and the development of multiple plasma cell lesions or multiple myeloma or both.

Wiltshaw[122] indicates that 40 per cent of extramedullary plasmacytomas spread beyond their presenting site and its drainage lymph nodes. Of these, 81 per cent developed lesions in bone and 62 per cent had soft tissue and visceral deposits. There is an overall survival of more than 50 per cent at 10 years for extramedullary plasmacytoma patients.

Histologic appearance alone cannot be used as a reliable indicator of biologic activity. The typical extramedullary plasmacytoma consists of a monocellular proliferation of plasma cells set in a very sparse matrix (Fig. 6–28). Cellular and nuclear atypia may be minimal or prominent. Bi- and trinucleate cell forms may be present, and in some microscopic fields only a proximity to more definable plasma cells allows their definition. Local amyloid is found in about 15 per cent of cases.[121]

ODONTOGENIC TUMORS

Twenty per cent of ameloblastomas originate in the maxilla, where almost half the lesions are found in the molar region, one third in the area of the antrum, and the remainder at other sites,

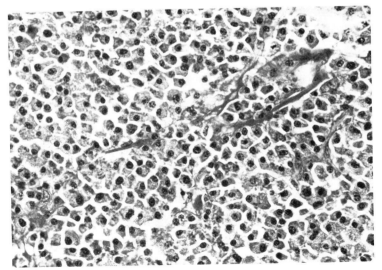

Figure 6–28. Extramedullary pleomorphism with typical features of a pure culture of plasma cells set in a moderately vascular but parvicellular stromal matrix.

including no more than 2 per cent in the anterior maxilla.[123]

The potential for disastrous consequences for a patient with an ameloblastoma of the maxilla is far greater than for patients with mandibular ameloblastomas. In the maxilla, the tumors typically occur in the cuspid and antral areas, where at least two factors predispose to local extension. The thick compact bone of the mandible is absent in the maxilla, and the intimacy with adjacent structures adds a clinical dimension not present for ameloblastomas of the mandible.

Although there is insufficient documentation using histologic criteria, there is certainly an indication that ameloblastomas of the maxilla are more aggressive than their counterparts in the mandible.[124, 125] Our experience and that of others has been that ameloblastomas of the maxilla tend to a greater cellularity and departure from conventional ameloblastomas.[126] Acanthomatous foci are also more often noted in the maxillary tumors.

More than histologic appearance, however, is the impact of recurrence following unsuccessful primary treatment. Results of curettage are such that that mode of therapy should be condemned. Sehdev and colleagues[124] report a 100 per cent recurrence rate and worse, a 63 per cent death rate or life with massive recurrences after curettement. In that context, it is worth quoting Shatkin: "The so-called 'conservative' treatment by curettage, at best, disfigures the patient and, at worst, kills him, whereas the so-called 'radical' treatment by adequate excision conserves the patient's appearance, function and life."[127] The only rational treatment is complete en bloc removal with a margin of uninvolved tissue.

The maxillary ameloblastoma, in most instances, does not radiographically present as an odontogenic tumor. Clinical presentation in the nasal cavity or even as a pterygomaxillary fossa tumor may lure the pathologist into a diagnosis of adenocarcinoma, adenocystic carcinoma, or even poorly differentiated carcinoma of the sinus (Fig. 6–29).

METASTASES TO THE PARANASAL SINUSES

The majority of hematogenous metastases to the paranasal sinuses are to bone, and these rank considerably behind metastatic disease to the mandible. In general, the apparent frequency of metastases to gnathic bones follows the incidence of the malignancy in the population, with breast and lung primary neoplasms being the most frequent.

Renal cell carcinoma, however, must be singled out when considering metastases to the sinonasal tract (Fig. 6–30). There is no question that the kidney leads, by a sizeable margin, all other reported infraclavicular sites as a source of metastases to the nasal cavity and paranasal sinuses.[128] Primary lesions in the lungs, breast, the rest of the urogenital tract, and the gastrointestinal tract follow distantly. Every paranasal sinus can be a site of involvement, but the antrum and nasal cavity are preferred loci.

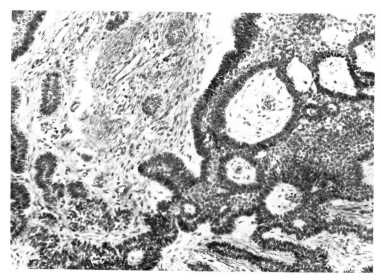

Figure 6–29. Ameloblastoma of the maxillary sinus manifesting anastomosing cords and trabeculae, peripheral cellular palisading, and microcytic areas. This lesion, misdiagnosed as adenocarcinoma, recurred four times and necessitated radical maxillectomy.

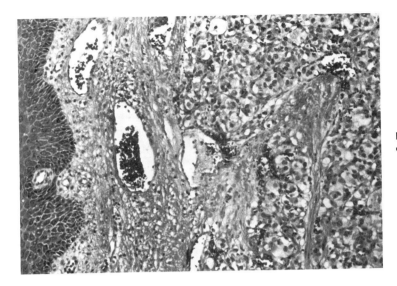

Figure 6–30. Metastatic renal cell carcinoma of the nasal cavity.

References

1. Batsakis JG: The pathology of head and neck tumors: Nasal cavity and paranasal sinuses, part 5. Head Neck Surg 2:410, 1980.
2. Donald PJ: The tenacity of the frontal sinus mucosa. Otolaryngol Head Neck Surg 87:557, 1979.
3. Mogensen C, Tos M: Quantitative histology of the maxillary sinus. Rhinology 15:129, 1977.
4. Tos M, Mogensen C: Mucus production in the nasal sinuses. Acta Otolaryngol (Suppl) 360:131, 1979.
5. Tos M, Mogensen C, Novotny Z: Quantitative histologic features of the normal frontal sinus. Arch Otolaryngol 106:143, 1980.
6. Toppozada HH, Talaat MA: The normal human maxillary sinus mucosa. An electron microscopic study. Acta Otolaryngol 89:204, 1980.
7. Haagensen CD, Feind CR, Herter FP, et al: The Lymphatics in Cancer. Philadelphia, WB Saunders, 1972.
8. Dixon FW, Hoerr NL: The lymphatic drainage of the paranasal sinuses. Laryngoscope 54:165, 1944.
9. van Nostrand AWP, Goodman WS: Pathologic aspects of mucosal lesions of the maxillary sinus. Otolaryngol Clin North Am 9:21, 1976.
10. Herson FS: Upper respiratory tract ciliary ultrastructural pathology. Ann Otol Rhinol Laryngol (Suppl 83) 90:part 2, 1981.
11. Littlefield, JW: Research on cystic fibrosis. N Engl J Med 304:44, 1981.
12. Leading article: Cystic-fibrosis variants—or variations. Lancet 2:1032, 1978.
13. Dann LG, Blau K: Exocrine-gland function and the basic biochemical defect in cystic fibrosis. Lancet 2:405, 1978.
14. Adams GL, Hilger P, Warwick WJ: Cystic fibrosis. Arch Otolaryngol 106:127, 1980.
15. Forman-Franco B, Abramson AL, Gorvoy JD, Stein T: Cystic fibrosis and hearing loss. Arch Otolaryngol 105:338, 1979.
16. Forest JB, Rossman CM, Newhouse MT, Ruffin R: Activation of nasal cilia in immotile cilia syndrome. Am Rev Respir Dis 120:511, 1979.
17. Heck WE, Hallberg OE, Williams HL: Antrochoanal polyps. Arch Otolaryngol 52:538, 1950.
18. Hardy G: The choanal polyp. Ann Otol 66:306, 1957.
19. Schramm VL, Effron MZ: Nasal polyps in children. Laryngoscope 90:1488, 1980.
20. Compagno J, Hyams VJ, Lepore ML: Nasal polyposis with stromal atypia. Review and follow-up study of 14 cases. Arch Pathol Lab Med 100:224, 1976.
21. Batsakis JG: Wegener's granulomatosis and midline (non-healing) "granuloma." Head Neck Surg 1:213, 1978.
22. DeRemee RA, McDonald TJ, Harrison EG Jr, Coles DT: Wegener's granulomatosis: Anatomic correlates, a proposed classification. Mayo Clin Proc 51: 777, 1976.
23. McDonald TJ, DeRemee RA, Weiland LH: Wegener's granulomatosis and polymorphic reticulosis—two diseases or one? Arch Otolaryngol 107:141, 1981.
24. Fauci AS, Johnson RE, Wolff SM: Radiation therapy of midline granuloma. Ann Intern Med 84:140, 1976.
25. Donald KJ, Edwards RL, McEvoy JDS: An ultrastructural study of the pathogenesis of tissue injury in limited Wegener's granulomatosis. Pathology 8:161, 1976.
26. DeRemee RA, Weiland LH, McDonald TJ: Respiratory vasculitis. Mayo Clin Proc 55:492, 1980.
27. Katzenstein A-LA, Carrington CRB, Liebow AA: Lymphomatoid granulomatosis. A clinicopathologic study of 152 cases. Cancer 43:360, 1979.
28. DeRemee RA, McDonald TJ: Midline granuloma. Ann Intern Med 85:128, 1976.
29. Fauci AS, Johnson RE, Wolff SM: In comment. Ann Intern Med 85:128, 1976.
30. Mitchell DN, Scadding JG, Heard BE, Hinson KFW: Sarcoidosis: Histopathological definition and clinical diagnosis. J Clin Pathol 30:395, 1977.
31. Miglets AW, Viall JH, Kataria YP: Sarcoidosis of the head and neck. Laryngoscope 87:2038, 1977.
32. Casamassimo PS, Lilly GE: Mucosal cysts of the maxillary sinus: A clinical and radiographic study. Oral Surg 50:282, 1980.
33. Kwapis BW, Whitten JB: Mucosal cysts of the maxillary sinus. J Oral Surg 29:561, 1971.
34. Natvig K, Larsen TE: Mucocele of the paranasal sinuses. A retrospective clinical and histological study. J Laryngol Otol 92:1075, 1978.
35. Canalis RF, Zajtchuk JT, Jenkins HA: Ethmoidal mucoceles. Arch Otolaryngol 104:286, 1978.
36. Bordley JE, Bosley WR: Mucoceles of the frontal sinus: Causes and treatment. Ann Otol 82:696, 1973.

37. Moller NE, Thomsen J: Mucocele of the paranasal sinuses in cystic fibrosis. J Laryngol 92:1025, 1978.

38. Zizmor J, Ganz AR: Mucoceles of paranasal sinuses. NY State J Med 72:1710, 1972.

39. Hesselink JR, Weber AL, New PFJ, et al: Evaluation of mucoceles of the paranasal sinuses with computed tomography. Radiology 133:397, 1979.

40. Blum ME, Larson A: Mucocele of the sphenoid sinus with sudden blindness. Laryngoscope 83:2042, 1973.

41. Siegel MJ, Shackelford GD, McAlister WH: Paranasal sinus mucoceles in children. Radiology 133:623, 1979.

42. Graham J, Michaels L: Cholesterol granuloma of the maxillary antrum. Clin Otolaryngol 3:155, 1978.

43. Campanella RS, Caldarelli DD, Friedberg SA: Cholesteatoma of the frontal and ethmoid areas. Ann Otol 88:518, 1979.

44. Meyers AD, Burtschi T: Pneumocele of the maxillary sinus. J Otolaryngol 9:361, 1980.

45. Jarvis JF: Pneumocele of the frontal and sphenoidal sinuses. J Laryngol Otol 88:785, 1974.

46. Busuttil A: Dysplastic epithelial changes in nasal polyps. Ann Otol 87:416, 1978.

47. Batsakis JG: Nasal (schneiderian) papillomas. Ann Otol Rhinol Laryngol 90:190, 1980.

47a. Buchwald C, Nielsen LH, Nielsen, PL, et al: Am J Otolaryngol 10:273–281, 1989.

48. Hyams VJ: Papillomas of the nasal cavity and paranasal sinuses: A clinicopathologic study of 315 cases. Ann Otol Rhinol Laryngol 80:192, 1971.

49. Roush GC: Epidemiology of cancer of the nose and paranasal sinuses: Current concept. Head Neck Surg 2:3, 1979.

49a. Phillips PP, Gustafson RO, Facer GW: The clinical behavior of inverting papilloma of the nose and paranasal sinuses: report of 112 cases and a review of the literature. Laryngoscope 100:463–469, 1990.

49b. Ward BE, Fechner RE, Mills SE: Carcinoma arising in oncocytic Schneiderian papilloma. Am J Surg Pathol 14:364–369, 1990.

50. Muir CS, Nectoux J: Descriptive epidemiology of malignant neoplasms of nose, nasal cavities, middle ear and accessory sinuses. Clin Otolaryngol 5:195, 1980.

51. Robin PE, Powell DJ, Stansbie JM: Carcinoma of the nasal cavity and paranasal sinuses: Incidence and presentation of different histological types. Clin Otolaryngol 4:431, 1979.

52. Lewis JS, Castro EB: Cancer of the nasal cavity and paranasal sinuses. J Laryngol Otol 86:255, 1972.

53. Jackson RT, Fitz-Hugh GS, Constable WC: Malignant neoplasms of the nasal cavities and paranasal sinuses. Laryngoscope 87:726, 1977.

54. Larsson LG, Martensson G: Carcinoma of paranasal sinuses and nasal cavities. Acta Radiol Ther 42:149, 1954.

55. Batsakis JG, Rice DH, Solomon AR: The pathology of head and neck tumors: Squamous and mucous-gland carcinomas of the nasal cavity, paranasal sinuses, and larynx, part 6. Head Neck Surg 2:497, 1980.

56. Harrison DFN: Critical look at the classification of maxillary sinus carcinomata. Ann Otol Rhinol Laryngol 87:3, 1979.

57. Lederman M: Tumours of the upper jaw: Natural history and treatment. J Laryngol Otol 84:369, 1970.

58. Tsaw SW, Burman JF, Easty DM, et al: Some mechanisms of local bone destruction by squamous carcinomas of the head and neck. Br J Cancer 43:392, 1981.

59. Bone RC, Byfield JE, Feren AP, Seagren SL: Bleomycin: Its utilization in the treatment of head and neck cancer. Laryngoscope 89:224, 1979.

60. Burkhardt A, Höltje W-J: The effects of intra-arterial bleomycin therapy on squamous cell carcinoma of the oral cavity. J Maxillofac Surg 3:217, 1975.

61. Yasuzumi G, Hyo Y, Hoshiya T, Yasuzumi F: Effects of bleomycin on human tongue carcinoma cells revealed by electron microscopy. Cancer Res 39:4645, 1979.

62. Shapshay SM, Hong WK, Incze JS, et al: Histopathologic findings after cis-platinum bleomycin therapy in advanced previously untreated head and neck carcinoma. Am J Surg 136:534, 1978.

62a. Spiro JD, Soo KC, Spiro RH: Squamous carcinoma of the nasal cavity and paranasal sinuses. Am J Surg 158:328–332, 1989.

62b. Sisson GA Sr, Toriumi DM, Atiyah RA: Paranasal sinus malignancy: A comprehensive update. Laryngoscope 99:143–150, 1989.

62c. Lavertu P, Roberts JK, Kraus DH, et al: Squamous cell carcinoma of the paranasal sinuses: The Cleveland Clinic experience. Laryngoscope 99:1130–1136, 1989.

63. Tong D, Blasko JC, Griffen TW: Cervical lymph node metastases in patients with squamous cell carcinoma of the maxillary antrum: The role of elective irradiation of the clinically negative neck. Int J Radiat Oncol Biol Phys 5:1977, 1979.

63a. Gnepp DR, Heffner DK: Mucosal origin of sinonasal tract adenomatous neoplasms. Mod Pathol 2:365–371, 1989.

64. Spiro RH, Huvos AG, Strong EW: Adenoid cystic carcinoma: Factors influencing survival. Am J Surg 138:579, 1979.

65. Rafla-Demetrious S: Mucous and Salivary Gland Tumours. Springfield, Ill, Charles C Thomas, 1970.

66. Schmid KO, Auböck L, Albegger K: Endocrine-amphicrine enteric carcinoma of the nasal mucosa. Virchows Arch (Pathol Anat) 383:329, 1979.

67. Koss LG, Spiro RH, Hajdu S: Small cell (oat cell) carcinoma of minor salivary gland origin. Cancer 30:737, 1972.

68. Snow GB, VanDerEsch EP, Van Slooten EA: Mucosal melanomas of the head and neck. Head Neck Surg 1:24, 1978.

69. Shah JP, Huvos AG, Strong EW: Mucosal melanomas of the head and neck. Am J Surg 134:531, 1977.

70. Goldman JL, Lawson W, Zak FG, Roffman JD: The presence of melanocytes in the human larynx. Laryngoscope 82:824, 1972.

71. Zak FG, Lawson W: The presence of melanocytes in the nasal cavity. Ann Otol Rhinol Laryngol 83:515, 1974.

72. Cove H: Melanosis, melanocytic hyperplasia, and primary malignant melanoma of the nasal cavity. Cancer 44:1424, 1979.

72a. Robertson DM, Hungerford JL, McCartney A: Malignant melanomas of the conjunctiva, nasal cavity and paranasal sinuses. Am J Ophthalmol 108:440–442, 1989.

73. Conley J, Hamaker RC: Melanoma of the head and neck. Laryngoscope 87:760, 1977.

74. Eneroth CM, Lundberg C: Mucosal malignant melanomas of the head and neck. Acta Otolaryngol 80:452, 1975.

75. Conley J, Pack GT: Melanoma of the mucous membranes of the head and neck. Arch Otolaryngol 99:315, 1974.

76. Cutler LS, Chaudhay AP, Topazian R: Melanotic neuroectodermal tumor of infancy: An ultrastructural study, literature reviews, and reevaluation. Cancer 48:257, 1981.

76a. Judd PL, Pedod D, Harrop K, Becker, J: Melanotic

neuroectodermal tumor of infancy. Oral Surg Oral Med Oral Path 69:723–726, 1990.

77. Shugar JMA, Som PM, Eisman W, Biller HF: Non-traumatic cerebrospinal fluid rhinorrhea. Laryngoscope 91:114, 1981.

78. Ho K-L: Primary meningioma of the nasal cavity and paranasal sinuses. Cancer 46:1442, 1980.

78a. Atherino CCT, Carcia R, Lopez LJ: Ectopic meningioma of the nose and paranasal sinuses (report of a case). J Laryngol Otol 99:1161–1166, 1985.

78b. Gronich MS, Pilch BZ, Goodman ML: Meningiomas presenting in the paranasal sinuses and temporal bone. Head Neck Surg 5:319–328, 1983.

78c. Leyva WH, Gnepp DR: Case 2. Arch Otolaryngol Head Neck Surg 113:206–209, 1987.

78d. Taxy JB: Meningiomas of the paranasal sinuses. A report of two cases. Am J Surg Pathol 14:82–86, 1990.

78e. Perzin KR, Pushparaj N: Non-epithelial tumors of the nasal cavity, paranasal sinuses and nasopharynx: A clinicopathologic study. XIII: meningiomas. Cancer 54:1860–1869, 1984.

79. Canalis RF, Smith CA, Konrad HR: Myxomas of the head and neck. Arch Otolaryngol 102:300, 1976.

80. Fu Y-S, Perzin KH: Nonepithelial tumors of the nasal cavity, paranasal sinuses and nasopharynx: A clinicopathologic study. VII. Myxomas. Cancer 39:195, 1977.

81. Waldron CA, Shafer WG: The central giant cell reparative granuloma of the jaws. An analysis of 38 cases. Am J Clin Pathol 45:437, 1968.

82. Andersen L, Fejerskov O, Philipsen HP: Oral giant cell granulomas. A clinical and histological study of 129 new cases. Acta Pathol Microbiol Scand (A) 81:606, 1973.

83. Batsakis JG, Solomon AR, Rice DH: The pathology of head and neck tumors: Neoplasms of cartilage, bone, and the notochord, part 7. Head Neck Surg 3:43, 1980.

84. Huvos AG: Bone Tumors. Diagnosis, Treatment and Prognosis. Philadelphia, WB Saunders Co, 1979, p 109.

84a. Batsakis, JG: Osteogenic and chondrogenic sarcoma of the jaws. Ann Otol Rhinol Laryngol 96:474, 1987.

84b. Maldonado, AR, Spratt, JS: Osteogenic sarcoma of the mandible and maxilla. Southern Med J 79:1453, 1986.

85. Caron AS, Hajdu SI, Strong EW: Osteogenic sarcoma of the facial and cranial bones. A review of forty-three cases. Am J Surg 122:719, 1971.

86. Fu Y-S, Perzin KH: Non-epithelial tumors of the nasal cavity, paranasal sinuses, and nasopharynx: A clinicopathologic study. III. Cartilaginous tumors (chondroma, chondrosarcoma). Cancer 34:453, 1974.

87. Kragh LV, Dahlin DC, Erich JB: Cartilaginous tumors of the jaws and facial regions. Am J Surg 99:852, 1960.

88. Bloch DM, Bragoli AJ, Collins DN, Batsakis JG: Mesenchymal chondrosarcomas of the head and neck. J Laryngol Otol 93:405, 1979.

89. Atallah N, Jay MM: Osteomas of the paranasal sinuses. J Laryngol Otol 95:291, 1981.

90. Mikaelian DO, Lewis WJ, Behringer WH: Primary osteoma of the sphenoid sinus. Laryngoscope 86:728, 1976.

91. Huvos AG: Bone Tumors. Diagnosis, Treatment and Prognosis. Philadelphia, WB Saunders Co, 1979, p 6.

92. Rosenberg SA, Glatstein EJ: Perspectives on the role of surgery and radiation therapy in the treatment of soft tissue sarcomas of the extremities. Semin Oncol 8:190, 1981.

93. Fidzianska A: Human ontogenesis. 1. Ultrastructural characteristics of developing human muscle. J Neuropathol Exp Neurol 39:476, 1980.

94. Batsakis JG, Regezi JA, Rice DH: The pathology of head and neck tumors: Fibroadipose tissues and skeletal muscle, part 8. Head Neck Surg 3:145, 1980.

95. Maurer HM, Moon T, Donaldson M, et al: The intergroup rhabdomyosarcoma study in a preliminary report. Cancer 40:2015, 1977.

96. Dito WR, Batsakis JG: Rhabdomyosarcoma of the head and neck. An appraisal of the biologic behavior in 170 cases. Arch Surg 84:582, 1962.

96a. Chan JK, Ng HK, Wan KY, et al: Clear cell rhabdomyosarcoma of the nasal cavity and paranasal sinuses. Histopathology 14:391–399, 1989.

97. Enzinger FM, Shiraki M: Alveolar rhabdomyosarcoma. Cancer 24:18, 1969.

98. Tefft M, Fernandez C, Donaldson M, et al: Incidence of meningeal involvement by rhabdomyosarcoma of the head and neck in children. Cancer 42:253, 1978.

99. Berry MP, Jenkin RDT: Parameningeal rhabdomyosarcoma in the young. Cancer 48:281, 1981.

100. Fu Y-S, Perzin KH: Nonepithelial tumors of the nasal cavity, paranasal sinuses, and nasopharynx. A clinicopathologic study. VI. Fibrous tissue tumors (fibroma, fibromatosis, fibrosarcoma). Cancer 37:291, 1976.

101. Cronin J: Fibrosarcoma of the paranasal sinuses. J Laryngol Otol 87:667, 1973.

102. Farr HW: Soft part sarcomas of the head and neck. Semin Oncol 8:185, 1981.

103. Enterline HT: Histopathology of sarcomas. Semin Oncol 8:133, 1981.

104. Van der Werf-Messing B, Van Unnik JAM: Fibrosarcoma of the soft tissues—a clinicopathologic study. Cancer 18:1113, 1965.

105. Pritchard DJ, Soule EH, Taylor WF, Ivins JC: Fibrosarcoma—a clinicopathologic and statistical study of 199 tumors of the soft tissues of extremities and trunk. Cancer 33:888, 1974.

106. Allen PW: The fibromatoses: A clinicopathologic classification based on 140 cases. Am J Surg Pathol 1:255, 305, 321, 1977.

107. Soule EH, Pritchard DJ: Fibrosarcoma in infants and children. Cancer 40:1711, 1977.

108. Blitzer A, Lawson W, Biller HF: Malignant fibrous histiocytoma of the head and neck. Laryngoscope 87:1479, 1977.

109. Schaefer SD, Denton RA, Blend BL, Carder HM: Malignant fibrous histiocytoma of the frontal sinus. Laryngoscope 90:2021, 1980.

110. Perzin KH, Fu Y-S: Non-epithelial tumors of the nasal cavity, paranasal sinuses and nasopharynx: A clinicopathologic study XI. Fibrous histiocytomas. Cancer 45:2616, 1980.

111. Kearney MM, Soule EH, Ivins JC: Malignant fibrous histiocytoma. A retrospective study of 167 cases. Cancer 45:167, 1980.

112. Angervall L, Kindbloom L-G, Nielsen J, et al: Hemangiopericytoma—a clinicopathologic, angiographic, and microangiographic study. Cancer 42:2412, 1978.

113. Enzinger FH, Smith BH: Hemangiopericytoma—an analysis of 106 cases. Hum Pathol 7:61, 1972.

113a. Eichhorn JH, Dickersin GR, Bhan AK, Goodman ML: Sinonasal hemanogiopericytoma. A reassessment with electron microscopy, immunohistochemistry, and long term follow up. Am J Surg Pathol 14:856–866, 1990.

114. Batsakis JG, Rice DH: The pathology of head and neck tumors: Vasoformative tumors, part 9B. Head Neck Surg 3:326, 1981.

115. Compagno J, Hyams VJ: Hemangiopericytoma-like intranasal tumors. A clinicopathologic study of 23 cases. Am J Clin Pathol 66:672, 1976.

116. D'Agostino AN, Soule EH, Miller RH: Primary malignant neoplasms of nerves (malignant neurilemmomas) in patients without manifestations of multiple neurofibromatosis (von Recklinghausen's disease). Cancer 16:1003, 1963.

117. D'Agostino AN, Soule EH, Miller RH: Sarcomas of peripheral nerves and somatic soft tissues associated with multiple neurofibromatosis (von Recklinghausen's disease). Cancer 16:1015, 1963.

117a. Hillstrom RP, Zarbo RJ, Jacobs JR: Nerve sheath tumors of the paranasal sinuses; electron microscopy and histopathologic diagnosis. Otolaryngol Head Neck Surg 102:257–263, 1990.

118. Batsakis JG: Tumors of the Head and Neck: Clinical and Pathological Considerations, 2nd ed. Baltimore, Williams & Wilkins, 1979, p 324.

119. Sofferman RA, Cummings CW: Malignant lymphoma of the paranasal sinuses. Arch Otolaryngol 101:287, 1975.

120. Fu Y-S, Perzin KH: Nonepithelial tumors of the nasal cavity, paranasal sinuses and nasopharynx. A clinicopathologic study. X. Malignant lymphomas. Cancer 43:611, 1979.

120a. Ratech H, Burke JS, Blayney DW, et al: A clinicopathologic study of malignant lymphomas of the nose, paranasal sinuses, and hard palate, including cases of lethal midline granuloma. Cancer 64:2525–2531, 1989.

120b. Frierson HF Jr, Innes DJ Jr, Milles SE, Wick MR: Immunophenotypic analysis of sinonasal non-Hodgkins lymphomas. Hum Pathol 20:636–642, 1989.

121. Batsakis JG, Fries GT, Goldman RT, Karlsberg RC: Upper respiratory tract plasmacytoma. Extramedullary myeloma. Arch Otolaryngol 79:613, 1964.

122. Wiltshaw E: The natural history of extramedullary plasmacytoma and its relation to solitary myeloma of bone and myelomatosis. Medicine 55:217, 1976.

123. Goodsell JF, Yamashita D-D, Moody R: Ameloblastoma of the anterior maxillae. J Surg Oncol 9:407, 1977.

124. Sehdev MK, Huvos AG, Strong EW, et al: Ameloblastoma of maxilla and mandible. Cancer 33:324, 1974.

125. Mehlisch DR, Dahlin DC, Masson JK: Ameloblastoma: A clinicopathologic report. J Oral Surg 30:9, 1972.

126. Regezi JA, Kerr DA, Courtney RM: Odontogenic tumors: Analysis of 706 cases. J Oral Surg 36:771, 1978.

127. Shatkin S, Hoffmeister FS: Ameloblastoma—a rational approach to therapy. Oral Surg 20:421, 1965.

128. Batsakis JG: The pathology of head and neck tumors: The occult primary and metastases to the head and neck, part 10. Head Neck Surg 3:409, 1981.

CHAPTER 7

INFECTIOUS DISEASES OF THE SINUSES

Harold C. Neu, MD, FACP

Sinusitis, a life-threatening infection in the preantimicrobial era, has become a much less serious illness in recent years. Nonetheless, antimicrobial agents, nasal decongestants, antihistamines, and other agents are widely used by patients and prescribed by general physicians and otolaryngologists for this disorder. Acute sinusitis usually is a complication of rhinovirus infection or other viral infection and occurs more frequently in individuals with allergic rhinitis and anatomic abnormalities of the nasal passages and much less frequently as a result of dental infection.[1] Since both children and adults average three colds per year, sinusitis is common. Fortunately, the serious complications of meningitis, brain abscess, and epidural and subdural abscess are rare. Sinus infection is most common in the fall, winter, and spring when upper respiratory viral illness is most common. In the summer, sinusitis may be associated with swimming. Whether sinusitis is more common in smokers is not established, but sinusitis is more frequent in adults than in children.

PATHOGENESIS

Paranasal sinuses normally are sterile because of the removal of material by the mucociliary apparatus. Studies have shown that a number of viruses are obtained from aspirates of sinuses.[5] Viruses can penetrate the mucous layer lining the sinuses and affect the normal ciliary function that protects the pseudostratified columnar epithelium. The motion of the cilia is altered by viruses such as adenovirus, influenza virus, coronavirus, and rhinoviruses. Bacteria enter from the oral and nasal cavities as the mucosal lining becomes swollen and inflamed with the polymorphonuclear leukocytes that enter the sinus cavity. Bacteria proliferate in the secretions, reaching levels of 10^5 to 10^8 CFU per ml of mucosal fluid.[3, 6]

In children, obstruction of the ostia is common when viral infection occurs, since the diameter is small—2.5 mm for the maxillary sinuses and approximately 1 to 2 mm for the ethmoids.[7, 8] Maxillary sinus infection in children or adults can originate from infection of the upper molar or bicuspid teeth, since the roots of these teeth are at the floor of the maxillary sinus.

Allergic reactions can cause mucosal edema and even polyp formation, which leads to infection. Septal deviation and foreign bodies also may lead to sinusitis. Indwelling nasal tubes and nasotracheal or larger feeding tubes can cause irritation and edema and result in sinusitis.[9, 10] This is particularly true in intensive care patients; nosocomial sinusitis is now a well-established entity.[10]

Repeated episodes of acute inflammation can progress to chronic sinusitis in which there is irreversible loss of ciliated epithelium with replacement by stratified squamous epithelium. The absence of cilia makes it impossible to maintain sterility of the sinus, so nasal and oral bacteria readily enter. Chronic sinusitis is somewhat analogous to chronic bronchitis in that acute infectious exacerbations caused by bacteria occur when environmental factors make the chronic condition worse.

In fungal sinusitis, it has been suggested that the underlying problem is narrowing of the ostia due to inflammation from other viral or bacterial infection, allergy, or anatomic deformity.[11] Fungi grow in the retained secretions within the sinus. Noninvasive fungal disease of the sinus is usually found in the maxillary or frontal sinuses; if it occurs posteriorly, it is confined to the sphenoid sinus or to one cell of the posterior ethmoid sinus.

MICROBIOLOGY

Most studies of the microbiology of sinusitis have involved adults[2, 5, 6] (Table 7–1). However, the bacterial flora of children with sinusitis has been carefully analyzed.[4] Many adults may harbor *Streptococcus pneumoniae* in the oropharynx during the winter months, but this is uncommon in children. *Streptococcus pneumoniae*, beta-hemolytic streptococcus, and *Haemophilus influenzae* are not usually present in the noses of normal, healthy children.[12] However, when children have respiratory illness, *S. pneumoniae* and *Haemophilus* spp. are recovered from 57 per cent and 25 per cent of children, respectively.[13]

Studies in which direct sinus puncture has been used to diagnose acute sinusitis in adults have shown that *S. pneumoniae* and *H. influenzae* account for half the infections.[2, 5] In a recent investigation of 238 patients with acute maxillary sinusitis, the most common pathogens were *H. influenzae* (50 per cent), *S. pneumoniae* (19 per cent), *S. pyogenes* (5 per cent), and *Moraxella branhamella catarrhalis* (2 per cent).[6]

In one of the pediatric studies, *Moraxella branhamella Catarrhalis* was recovered almost as frequently as *H. influenzae*.[4] Whether *H. influenzae* or *S. pneumoniae* is the most frequent organism isolated from acute sinusitis is unclear. Coagulase-negative staphylococci and *Staphylococcus aureus* were found in 8 per cent

and 1 per cent, respectively, and were in such low numbers that they were felt to be contaminants from the nasal secretions. It is now realized that older studies found staphylococci because specimens were obtained by irrigation rather than by direct aspiration.[14] *S. aureus* and coagulase-negative staphylococci (*S. epidermidis*) are commonly found in the normal flora of the nose of both adults and children.[15] Anaerobic species are not common in acute sinusitis, and in the aforementioned study only 2 per cent of sinuses were considered to have true anaerobic infection.

The frequency of isolation of *S. pneumoniae* has been between 20 and 40 per cent.[4–6] A trend for a higher percentage of *H. influenzae* in recent years could be related to better culture techniques or to an actual increase. *H. influenzae* is present in the nasal cavity of 5 per cent of subjects and in 20 per cent of epipharynx cultures of young healthy individuals; the same figures for *S. pneumoniae* are 0.5 per cent and 7 to 10 per cent, respectively. *S. pyogenes*, group A, is relatively infrequently cultured from acute cases of sinusitis. Indeed, the isolates found in the study of Jousimies-Somer and colleagues occurred during an outbreak of streptococcal pharyngitis in the military recruits they followed over 3 years.[6]

Anaerobes are cultured in up to 50 per cent of patients with chronic or dentogenic sinusitis.[16–20] The precise numbers of organisms are difficult to establish, since broth-enrichment methods have been used to culture the bacteria. Species found have included microaerophilic streptococci; anaerobic cocci; gram-positive, nonspore-forming rods; *Bacteroides* spp. such as *B. melaninogenicus*, *B. intermedius*, and *B. asaccharolyticus*; and fusobacteria.[6, 17–19] Anaerobic organisms are infrequent in acute sinusitis in children.[4, 20, 21] Indeed, the important consideration of the anaerobes is that they usually are coccal species and hence will be susceptible to the beta-lactams used to treat *H. influenzae* and *S. pneumoniae*.

The organisms found in nosocomial sinusitis have varied, but *Pseudomonas aeruginosa*, *Klebsiella pneumoniae*, *Enterobacter* spp., *Proteus* sp., *Serratia marcescens*, and so on have been recovered.[9, 10] In this situation the bacterial flora often will depend upon the antibiotics being used to treat other infections in patients. Unfortunately, in most of these studies, the sinuses have not been aspirated to determine the frequency at which anaerobic species are involved.

The number of different fungi that have been noted to cause sinusitis is large.[21–26] These in-

TABLE 7–1. Bacteriology of Acute Sinusitis

Organism	Adult (%)	Child (%)
Streptococcus pneumoniae	20–40	25–30
Haemophilus influenzae	20–50	15–20
Moraxella branhamella catarrhalis	2–10	15–20
Streptococcus pyogenes	2–4	2–5
Anaerobic cocci	<2	<2
Staphylococcus aureus	<1	<1

clude broad nonseptate hyphal organisms such as *Rhizopus* spp. and *Cunninghamella;* narrower septate hyphal organisms such as *Aspergillus* spp.; *Pseudoallescheria boydii; Penicillium* spp; *Fusarium* spp; *Cladosporium* spp.; *Curvularia* spp.; and organisms such as *Candida* spp., *Sporothrix,* and *Rhinosporidium seeberi.* Whether all these species are actually pathogenic is not clear, since many fungi can be cultured from mucosal surfaces of the nose and are probably inhaled commensals adherent to mucous secretions.

CLINICAL PRESENTATIONS

The clinical presentations of the different forms of sinusitis are varied. Most acute cases begin during a viral illness. Nasal discharge, nasal congestion causing alteration of voice, and cough are the usual symptoms in children. Wald has stressed that nasal discharge and daytime cough beyond 10 days suggest that sinusitis has complicated an upper respiratory viral illness that normally improves in 5 to 7 days.[27] In children under 10 years of age, persistent rhinorrhea is the most prominent symptom. Night cough is present in many upper respiratory infections, or it can be due to sinus drainage on the pharyngeal wall.

Facial pain is uncommon in children, whereas it is a frequent complaint of adults, who also note disorders of smell. Malodorous breath is common in small children. Fever is not present in half of adults and children in whom a diagnosis is established by radiographic findings and aspiration.

A less common presentation in children is periorbital swelling with erythema, which is more common in the mornings and actually may disappear during the day. Ethmoid sinusitis is associated with excessive tearing.

Symptoms of sinusitis are difficult to distinguish from viral respiratory infection. Chronic sinusitis is that which persists beyond 4 weeks. Nosocomial sinusitis is usually associated with leukocytosis and fever. Fungal sinusitis may present as symptoms of a foreign body, as chronic pain, or as an unexplained fever in an immunocompromised patient. Some noninvasive fungal sinusitis may not produce clinical symptoms.[21] Invasive fungal sinusitis may present with ocular symptoms, erosion of the palate, or cranial symptoms owing to frontal lobe involvement, with headache, altered sensorium, seizures, and localized neurologic findings.

DIAGNOSIS

Mucopurulent discharge is present in the nose or posterior pharynx of patients with sinusitis. Malodorous breath in the absence of bad dental hygiene or acute pharyngitis may be suggestive. Sinuses usually are tender to palpation or percussion. Lymph nodes are not enlarged. Transillumination of the maxillary and frontal sinuses may show opacity in acute infection. It is not of value in chronic disease. Periorbital swelling may be found in children.

Radiologic studies are essential, since they will show air-fluid levels or opacification in individuals over 1 year old.[28, 29] Mucosal swelling on a radiograph may be helpful in diagnosis if it is greater than 4 mm in children and 5 mm in adults. Acute exacerbations of chronic disease usually cannot be diagnosed radiologically.

Ultrasonography has been reported to be useful, since it can distinguish between mucosal thickening and retained secretions.[30] It may be of greater value in adults than in children.[30, 31]

Sinus aspiration is the most reliable way to establish the precise etiology of sinusitis. Maxillary sinuses can be aspirated in children over 2 years of age. Culture of nasal pus or rinsing of the sinus ostium does not yield correct information since the material is contaminated with the flora of the nose. Since the etiology of acute sinus disease is well established, there is little value in performing aspiration. Aspiration should be reserved for cases that fail to respond to therapy, when unusual infection is suspected, when intracranial extension is suspected because of a CT scan, or in the immunocompromised patient in whom fungus is suspected.

The maxillary sinus is punctured by the transnasal route with the needle below the inferior turbinate of the nose. A canine fossa puncture technique is also possible, especially in children. The frontal sinus is aspirated medially and just below the supraorbital rim of the eye. The aspiration site should be cleaned with iodine. Culture specimens should be collected via the needle or catheter. If secretions are not obtained by suction, 1 ml of normal saline can be instilled and aspirated. Material so obtained should be immediately plated in the laboratory, since fastidious bacteria will not grow if specimens are left for extended periods.

Material usually will be macroscopically purulent. Most material will have greater than 20 leukocytes per oil immersion field, and bacteria will be easily identified.[32] Occasionally, material is nonpurulent in appearance but will grow organisms. *S. pneumoniae* produces more purulence than does *H. influenzae.*[32] The macroscopic appearance of material should not be used to screen for culture, since negative smears may produce positive cultures containing 10^3 CFU per ml of fluid. The gram stain appearance of bacteria on smear usually correlates with culture results.

In fungal sinusitis, it is necessary to differentiate invasive from noninvasive disease. CT scanning has been extremely useful for this purpose.[22, 33, 34] Noninvasive disease involves a single soft tissue density, usually the maxillary sinus, although other sinuses have been involved. Involvement of several sinuses should suggest invasive spread. Magnetic resonance imaging may define extradural involvement caused by extension from the sinus, but owing to its bony detail computed tomography remains the test of choice. Nonetheless, surgical exploration is necessary. Surgical exploration may show that bone integrity is disrupted.

Noninvasive fungal sinusitis is not a serious condition. Diagnosis is based on finding a mass of mycelia in mucus within the sinus cavity. Therapy is surgical. Hyphae are not found on microscopic examination of the mucosa, submucosa, or bone. In contrast, in invasive fungal sinusitis the mucosa is hypertrophic, and hyphae are found in submucosa and bone specimens. It is important to use periodic acid–Schiff stains and methenamine silver stains, since some fungi may be missed on the routine hematoxylin-eosin stains.

TREATMENT

The goal of treatment is rapid sterilization of sinus secretions in order to prevent the serious complications of orbital and intracranial disease that occurred in the preantibiotic era and are rare today.[35] The selection of agent in most situations will be empiric, since the precise etiology will not be known.

In acute sinusitis, the agent selected must be one that inhibits *H. influenzae* and *S. pneumoniae*. Most of the commonly used antimicrobial agents diffuse into sinus tissue and secretions.[36–38] Penicillin V and erythromycin do not yield adequate concentrations to treat *H. influenzae*. Ampicillin yields adequate sinus levels, as do the other aminopenicillins, amoxicillin, and bacampicillin. However, the higher blood levels achieved with amoxicillin make it preferable to ampicillin. The orally administered cephalosporins that have adequate activity against the important pathogens are cefaclor, cefuroxime axetil, and cefixime. Cefaclor should be used at doses of 500 mg every 6 hours since it has proved less effective at lower doses. Cephalexin, cephradine, and cefadroxil are adequate for *S. pneumoniae* but inadequate for *H. influenzae* and *Branhamella* spp. Trimethoprim-sulfamethoxazole is adequate for most organisms encountered, particularly in adults,[5] but it may be ineffective in group A streptococcal infections. These, however, are infrequent. Erythromycin combined with sulfisoxazole (Pediazole) has been used for pediatric patients, since the erythromycin inhibits *S. pneumoniae* and the sulfisoxazole, *H. influenzae*.

The frequency of beta-lactamase–producing *H. influenzae* will influence therapy. Amoxicillin is not effective for these organisms. A combination of amoxicillin and clavulanate (Augmentin) has proved effective therapy of beta-lactamase–producing *H. influenzae* and *Branhamella*. Dosages of the drugs for children and adults are given in Table 7–2. Other agents that have been used are the tetracyclines minocycline and doxycycline, but the resistance of many *S. pneumoniae* to tetracyclines limits their use. Furthermore, tetracyclines cannot be used in children under 8 years of age. The duration of therapy for acute disease in most clinical studies has been 10 days. This is probably arbitrary, and there are no data to suggest that

TABLE 7–2. Treatment of Sinusitis

Agent	Adult	Child
Amoxicillin*	500 mg q12hr	40 mg/kg/day in 3 divided doses
Amoxicillin/clavulanate	500 mg q12hr	40/10 mg/kg/day in 3 divided doses
Trimethoprim-sulfamethoxazole	1 double strength tablet q12hr	8/40 mg/kg/day in 2 divided doses
Cefaclor	500 mg q6hr	40 mg/kg/day in 3 divided doses
Erythromycin/sulfisoxazole	—	50/150 mg/kg/day in 4 divided doses
Cefixime	200 mg q12hr OR 400 mg od	40 mg/kg/day in 2 doses
Cefuroxime axetil	500 mg q12hr	No suspensions
Ciprofloxacin	500 mg q12hr	Not to be used
Ofloxacin	500 mg q12hr	Not to be used
Temafloxacin	600 mg q12hr	Not to be used
Clarithromycin	500 mg q12hr	No suspensions

*If ampicillin is used, it should be at this dose every 6 hours or in divided doses.

7, 10, or 14 days is the optimal duration of therapy.

Recently, the quinolone antimicrobial agents ciprofloxacin and ofloxacin have become available. The use of these agents has been evaluated in sinusitis, and ciprofloxacin has proved comparable to penicillin in adults.[39] Although these two quinolones inhibit *H. influenzae* and *Branhamella* at concentrations of less than 0.12 μg/ml, the concentrations needed to inhibit *S. pneumoniae* often are 2 μg/ml. At doses of 500 mg of ciprofloxacin or 400 mg of ofloxacin every 12 hours, plasma concentrations are only slightly higher than the minimal inhibitory concentrations (MICs). Sinus tissue concentrations, however, are much higher and may explain the efficacy of the agents. Quinolones are not considered first-line therapy, and they are not to be used in children. Temafloxacin is more active than ciprofloxacin and ofloxacin against the gram-positive species causing sinusitis and has proved effective as therapy. None of these should be used in children.

Two new macrolides, clarithromycin and azithromycin, are active against *H. influenzae*, *Moraxella*, and *S. pneumoniae*. Both have proved effective in treatment of sinusitis and will be useful in the future.

Patients with acute sinusitis who require parenteral therapy because of toxicity or inability to take oral medications can be treated with broad-spectrum cephalosporins. Cefuroxime at 1.5 gm every 8 hours for adults or 100 to 200 mg/kg/day in three doses for children is reasonable. Other appropriate agents are cefotaxime, 1 gm every 8 hours, or ceftriaxone, 2 gm once daily. Patients who have had anaphylaxis to penicillins can be treated with trimethoprim-sulfamethoxazole, 15 mg/kg and 75 mg/kg per day in three divided doses. For the uncommon patient with staphylococcal sinusitis, oxacillin or nafcillin is an appropriate agent, and the penicillin-allergic patient can be treated with clindamycin, 600 mg every 8 hours. In the latter case, I would add aztreonam, 1 gm every 8 hours, to treat the associated *Haemophilus*.

Treatment of chronic sinusitis is a difficult problem. Surgical procedures discussed elsewhere in this text are used to facilitate sinus drainage. Antibiotics used to treat acute exacerbations of chronic disease should be the same as those used in acute illness. The role of anaerobic species in chronic disease favors agents such as amoxicillin/clavulanate, 500 mg every 8 hours, which inhibit anaerobic cocci, *Bacteroides*, and fusobacteria. There are reports of the use of imidazoles, such as tinidazole,[40] which is not available in the United States. However, the poor efficacy of metronidazole in anaerobic pleuropulmonary disease makes me question its use in chronic sinusitis; an agent like clindamycin is preferred.

Treatment of nosocomial sinusitis requires both the removal of nasotracheal or nasogastric tubes and use of an antimicrobial agent appropriate to the infection. Compounds that inhibit *Pseudomonas aeruginosa* often are necessary. Ticarcillin, ticarcillin/clavulanate, or piperacillin all are reasonable to use, as well as ceftazidine or imipenem. No studies have been conducted to establish an agent of choice in this infection.

Therapy of noninvasive fungal sinusitis is surgical, with removal of the mass and establishment of sinus drainage. There is no evidence that antifungal chemotherapy is needed.[22] Invasive fungal sinusitis has a difficult course, and the outcome often is related to control of the underlying host defects.[22, 23] Surgical removal of the infected tissue, with preservation of dura and orbital periostium, is necessary. Amphotericin B at a total dose of 2 gm for adults is recommended. *Pseudoallescheria boydii* should be treated with ketoconazole. Some investigators suggest that the frequency of relapse after amphotericin B makes it reasonable to administer drugs such as miconazole for up to 1 year. There are no studies with the newer antifungal agents itraconazole and fluconazole. In some patients, repeated surgery may be necessary as determined by follow-up CT studies that show the presence of new soft tissue material and further bony damage.

SUPPORTIVE THERAPY

Nasal decongestants and antihistamines are rarely needed for children.[27] Indeed, antihistamines should not be used in acute sinusitis since they impair drainage by thickening secretions. Phenylephrine (Neo-Synephrine) nose drops can be used as needed in adults. Control of nasal allergies will reduce the episodes of sinusitis in some individuals.

PREVENTIVE MEASURES

There are no ways to prevent sinusitis. The use of vasoconstrictors with colds has not been proved to reduce bacterial infection. Immunization against *H. influenzae* or *S. pneumoniae* has not been shown to affect the incidence of sinusitis. Use of aerosol amphotericin B will reduce nasal colonization with *Aspergillus* in neutropenic patients and may reduce the chance of development of both sinus and pulmonary infection. The correction of nasal abnormalities by surgery to produce adequate drainage will reduce sinus infections. Ultimately the most progress in this field will result from a reduction in viral illness, which impairs ciliary function and causes edema. Although nasally administered interferon can prevent rhinoviral infection, the interferon causes secondary swelling. Furthermore, at this time such therapy is not feasible from a financial standpoint.

References

1. Dingle JH, Badjer GF, Jordan WS Jr: Patterns of Illness: Illness in the Home. Cleveland, Western Reserve University, 1964, p 347.
2. Evans FO, Syndor JB, Moore WEC, et al: Sinusitis of the maxillary antrum. N Engl J Med 293:735–39, 1975.
3. Gwaltney JM, Syndor A Jr, Sande MA: Etiology and antimicrobial treatment of acute sinusitis. Ann Otol Rhinol Laryngol 90 (Suppl):68–71, 1981.
4. Wald ER, Milmo GJ, Bowen A, et al: Acute maxillary sinusitis in children. N Engl J Med 304:749–754, 1981.
5. Hamory BH, Sande MA, Syndor A, et al: Etiology and antimicrobial therapy of acute sinusitis. J Infect Dis 139:197–202, 1979.
6. Jousimies-Somer HR, Savolainen S, Ylikoski JS: Bacteriological findings of acute maxillary sinusitis in young adults. J Clin Microbiol 26:1919–1925, 1988.
7. Drettner B: Pathophysiology of paranasal sinuses with clinical implications. Clin Otolaryngol 5:272–284, 1980.
8. Rachelefsky GS, Katz RM, Siegel SC: Diseases of paranasal sinuses in children. Curr Prob Pediatr 12:1–57, 1982.
9. Caplan ES, Hoyt NJ: Nosocomial sinusitis. JAMA 247:639–641, 1982.
10. Kronberg FG, Goodwin WJ Jr: Sinusitis in intensive care unit patients. Laryngoscope 95:936–938, 1985.
11. Stammberger H: Endoscopic surgery for mycotic and chronic recurring sinusitis. Ann Otol Rhinol Laryngol 94 (Suppl 119):1–11, 1985.
12. Hays GC, Mullard JE: Can nasal bacterial flora be predicted from clinical findings? Pediatrics 49:596–599, 1972.
13. Box QT, Cleveland RT, Willard CY: Bacterial flora of the upper respiratory tract. A. Comprehensive evaluation by anterior nasal, oropharyngeal, and nasopharyngeal swabs. Am J Dis Child 102:293–301, 1981.
14. Lystad A, Berdal P, Lund-Iverson L: The bacterial flora of sinusitis with an in vitro study of the bacterial resistance to antibiotics. Acta Otolaryngol 188 (Suppl):390–400, 1964.
15. Bridger RC: Sinusitis: An improved regimen of investigation for the clinical laboratory. J Clin Pathol 33:276–281, 1980.
16. van Cauwenberge P, Verschragen G, van Renterghem L: Bacteriological findings in sinusitis (1963–1975). Scand J Infect Dis (Suppl)9:72, 1976.
17. Lundberg C, Carenfelt C, Engquist S, Nord CE: Anaerobic bacteria in maxillary sinusitis. Scand J Infect Dis (Suppl)19:74–76, 1979.
18. Mann W, Pelz K: Anaerobierinfection im Hals, Nasens, und Ohrenbereich. Laryngol Rhinol Otol 60:355–358, 1981.
19. van Cauwenberge P, Kluyskens P, van Renterghem L: The importance of the anaerobic bacteria in paranasal sinusitis. Rhinology 13:141–145, 1976.
20. Brook I: Bacteriologic features of chronic sinusitis in children. JAMA 246:967–969, 1981.
21. Wald ER, Reily JS, Casselbrant M, et al: Treatment of acute maxillary sinusitis in childhood: A comparative study of amoxicillin and cefaclor. J Pediatr 104:297–302, 1984.
22. Washburn RG, Kennedy DW, Begley MG, Henderson DK, Bennett JE: Chronic fungal sinusitis in apparently normal hosts. Medicine 67:231–247, 1988.
23. Blitzer A, Lawson W, Meyers BR, Biller HF: Patient survival factors in paranasal sinus mucormycosis. Laryngoscope 90:635–648, 1980.
24. Brennan RO, Crain BJ, Proctor AM, Durack DT: Cunninghamella, a newly recognized cause of rhinocerebral mucormycosis. Am J Clin Pathol 80:98–102, 1983.
25. Loveless MO, Winn RE, Campbell M, Jones SR: Mixed invasive infection with Alternaria species and Curvularia species. Am J Clin Pathol 76:491–493, 1981.
26. Bennett JL, Newman RK: Aspergillosis of the nose and paranasal sinuses. Laryngoscope 92:764–766, 1982.
27. Wald ER: Management of sinusitis in infants and children. J Infect Dis 7:449–452, 1988.
28. Shopfer CE, Rossi JO: Roentgen evaluation of the paranasal sinuses in children. Am J Roentgenol 118:176–186, 1972.
29. Kovatch AL, Wald ER, Ledesma-Medina J, et al: Maxillary sinus radiographs in children with non-respiratory complaints. Pediatrics 73:306–310, 1984.
30. Shapiro GG, Furukawa CT, Person WE, et al: Blinded comparison of maxillary sinus radiography and ultrasound for diagnosis of sinusitis. J Allergy Clin Immunol 77:59–64, 1986.
31. Berg O, Carenfelt C: Etiologic diagnosis in sinusitis: Ultrasonography as clinical complement. Laryngoscope 95:851–853, 1985.
32. Jousimies-Somer HR, Savolainen S, Ylikoski JS: Macroscopic purulence, leukocyte counts, and bacterial morphotypes in relation to culture findings for sinus secretions in acute maxillary sinusitis. J Clin Microbiol 26:1926–1933, 1988.
33. Kopp W, Fotter R, Steiner H, et al: Aspergillosis of the paranasal sinuses. Radiology 156:715–716, 1985.
34. Rolston KVI, Hepfer RL, Lawson DL: Infections caused by Drechslera sp.—case report and review of the literature. Rev Infect Dis 7:529, 1985.
35. Fairbanks DNF, Milmoe GJ: Complications and sequelae: An otolaryngologist's perspective. Pediatr Infect Dis 6:S75–S78, 1985.
36. Neu HC: Contemporary antibiotic therapy in otolaryngology. Otolaryngol Clin North Am 17:745–760, 1984.
37. Axelson A, Broson JE: The concentration of antibiotics in sinus secretions—ampicillin, cephradine, and erythromycin estolate. Acta Otol Rhinol Laryngol 83:323–328, 1974.
38. Ekedahl C, Holm SE, Bergholm AM: Penetration of antibiotics into the normal and diseased maxillary sinus mucosa. Scand J Infect Dis 14 (Suppl):279–283, 1978.
39. Falser N, Mittermayer H, Wenta H: Antibacterial treatment of otitis and sinusitis with ciprofloxacin and penicillin V—a comparison. Infection 16(Suppl 1):51–56, 1988.
40. Lundberg C, Markund G, Nord CE: Tinidazole in upper respiratory airway infection. J Antimicrob Chemother 10(Suppl A):177–184, 1982.

CHAPTER 8

EMBOLIZATION OF TUMORS AND VASCULAR MALFORMATIONS

Carol R. Archer, MD

Eric E. Awwad, MD

The lesions amenable to embolization are numerous, and it is not the purpose of this chapter to cover each in detail. Rather, the types of lesions amenable to embolization because they have proved to be responsive to the technique or to the facilitation of surgical removal will be introduced; some of the methods will be discussed, as well as a brief mention of some of the potential complications, especially cranial nerve palsies and occlusion of the internal carotid artery or its branches.

The recent advances in the techniques of controlled catheter embolization have contributed significantly to the management of head and neck tumors, as well as the control of epistaxis from a variety of causes, including idiopathic hemorrhage, neoplasm, vascular malformation, and trauma. The catheter techniques have been refined, and, although they may differ somewhat among angiographers, they are proving to be significantly safer and to provide a distinctly less hemorrhagic field at the time of surgery. Tumors, such as craniofacial hemangiomas, neurinomas, esthesioneuroblastomas, juvenile angiofibromas, branchial paragangliomas, and vascular lesions, both traumatic and spontaneous, are the commonest lesions to be embolized.

For embolization of lesions involving the paranasal sinuses to be successful, a thorough knowledge of their multiple vascular supplies is mandatory. This must be followed by superselective catheterization of these vessels so that all arterial feeders can be identified. What is not as widely appreciated is the extent of anastomoses between the external carotid and internal carotid arteries. These represent a potential source of serious complications, owing to the fact that emboli passing from the external carotid artery beyond the site of the lesion may cause permanent cranial nerve palsies and those passing into the internal carotid artery or its major branches may produce permanent neurologic deficits. Skin necrosis can result from aggressive embolization that includes its arterial supply, especially when small particles or fluids are utilized.

The limits of resolution of the angiographic technique do not allow visualization of vessels smaller than 100 microns; thus, although they cannot be seen directly, they may be responsible for a vascular stain that reliably delineates the extent of the lesion and occurs during the late arterial or venous phases. If direct arterial supply to the lesion is not delineated by angiography, embolization cannot be performed.

TECHNIQUE

The methods of embolization vary depending upon the type of the lesion and the choice and experience of the operator. Most interventional angiographers employ the femoral arterial route, although occasionally an intracarotid approach is used. An introducer sheath placed in the femoral artery allows exchanges and manipulations of the catheters without extensive trauma to the artery and also permits finer manipulation of the catheters.

Many different types of catheters are in use, but Lasjaunias and Berenstein divide them into two main categories: conventional catheters and balloon catheters. The latter can be subdivided into two main groups: those that are used primarily for control of blood flow or for tolerance testing and those used as the embolic agents themselves.[1] The former allows passage of both liquid and particulate embolic materials. Such technologic innovations as open-end guidewires[2] and Tracker catheters (Target Therapeutics, Los Angeles)[3] have vastly improved the successful catheterization of distal and small branches.

A large number of embolic agents differ in their specific characteristics. The choice of the specific agent depends on the goals of therapy as appraised by the angiographer. Biodegradable materials (Gelfoam) achieve temporary occlusion. Nonbiodegradable materials (polyvinyl alcohol foam [PVA], isobutyl-2 cyanoacrylate [IBCA], N-butyl cyanoacrylate [NBCA]) are used for a longer-lasting effect. Fluids (IBCA, NBCA) and small particles achieve better penetration into smaller vessels whereas large vessels can be occluded with larger strips of foam (Gelfoam, PVA) or detachable balloons. Cytotoxic agents (ethanol) cause a disruption of the adjacent tissues. Other embolic agents include Gianturco and "mini" coils, platinum wire, and silk threads. Often the various types of embolic material are used as mixtures or in conjunction with one another.

DANGEROUS ANASTOMOSES

The numerous anastomoses between the internal carotid and external carotid arteries have already been alluded to. Knowledge of these channels is of such importance that it was felt worthwhile to reproduce Table 8–1 from the text of Lasjaunias and Berenstein.[4]

Angiographic methods of protecting dangerous anastomoses prior to therapeutic embolization have been detailed by Lasjaunias and Berenstein[5] and are reproduced verbatim below with the kind permission of the authors:

(1) Mechanical blockage: This is frequently performed with large, usually absorbable, particulate matter.

(2) Reversal of flow: Occlusion by balloon or wedge-shaped catheter proximal to the anastomosis accomplishes this goal. The aim is to divert the flow of the embolic agent toward the lesion as opposed to the critical vessel, e.g., the vertebral artery. The reversal of flow will aid in pushing the embolic material toward the lesion. Careful monitoring under fluoroscopy will alert the operator to the fact that the flow is significantly slowing down, and at this point the procedure is discontinued.

(3) Protection of dangerous anastomoses by distal catheterization. Although it is not always possible to place a catheter distal to the dangerous anastomoses, the introduction of coaxial open-end guidewires and steerable microwires has improved this possibility.

(4) Occlusive balloon flow reversal: In hypervascular lesions lacking preferential flow, occlusive balloons may be placed proximal to the origin of the major feeding vessels, thereby forcing the collaterals to supply the critical territory. If the correct pressure of injection is used, all the contrast will enter the lesion, sparing the normal territory. The technique is then repeated with microparticles until the lesion is devascularized.

The potential for cranial nerve dysfunction prior to superselective embolization in the distribution of the external carotid artery can be tested with prior superselective infusion of cardiac lidocaine (Xylocaine), which is also useful for pain control and prevention of spasm.[6] Be aware that embolization of the ascending pharyngeal artery with small particulate or fluid agents may produce lower cranial nerve palsies.[5]

EXAMPLES

Endovascular embolization is a useful part of the treatment of tumors of the paranasal sinuses, vascular malformations, and uncontrolled epistaxis of various causes. In some instances it is the treatment of choice.

Its usefulness has been particularly well documented with juvenile angiofibroma. Preoperative embolization of juvenile angiofibromas permits complete surgical removal of the lesion, decreases the possibility of uncontrollable intraoperative hemorrhage, and probably reduces the incidence of tumor recurrence. Aggressive embolization also may be used in reducing portions of tumors that have invaded the base of the skull and are not approachable surgically.

TABLE 8–1. Dangerous Vessels of the Craniofacial and Upper Cervical Arteries

Region	Arterial Trunk (External Carotid)	Specific Dangerous Branch	Specific Course	Peripheral Nervous System Supply*
Orbit (ophthalmic artery branches)	Internal maxillary artery	Infraorbital artery (orbital branch)	Inferior orbital fissure	
		Sphenopalatine artery (ethmoidal anastomoses)	Ethmoidal canal	
		Middle meningeal artery (meningo-ophthalmic)	Superior orbital fissure	V_1th
		Middle meningeal artery (recurrent meningeal)		
		Anterior deep temporal artery (orbital branch)	Transmalar	
Parasellar region (internal carotid siphon)	Internal maxillary artery	Middle meningeal artery (cavernous ramus)	Foramen spinosum	GG, V_3th
		Accessory meningeal artery (cavernous ramus)	Foramen ovale or Vesalius	V_3th, V_mth, V_2th
	Ascending pharyngeal artery	Artery of the foramen rotundum	Foramen rotundum	V_2th
		Superior pharyngeal (carotid branch)	Foramen lacerum	Σ (ANS), GG
		Jugular artery (lateral clival branch)	Jugular foramen	VIth, IXth, Xth, XIth
		Hypoglossal artery (medial clival branch)	Hypoglossal foramen	XIIth
Temporal bone (intrapetrous internal carotid artery)	Internal maxillary artery	Anterior tympanic artery	Anterior tympanic canal	Chorda tympani
		Vidian artery	Vidian canal	Vidian nerve Foramen lacerum
	Ascending pharyngeal artery	Superior pharyngeal (mandibular anastomosis)		
		Inferior tympanic artery	Jacobson's canal	Jacobson's nerve
	Posterior auricular or occipital arteries	Stylomastoid branch	Facial canal	VIIth
Upper cervical spaces (vertebral artery)	Occipital artery	C1 anastomotic branch	First cervical space	C1
		C2 anastomotic branch	Second cervical space	C2
	Ascending pharyngeal artery	Hypoglossal artery (odontoid arterial arch system)	Third cervical space and hypoglossal foramen	XIIth, C3 (XIth, Xth, XIth)
		Musculospinal artery	Third and fourth cervical	C3 and C4, XIth
		Lateral spinal artery	Third and fourth cervical spaces anastomoses	C1-C2 nerve upper cervical spinal cord and medulla
	Ascending cervical artery	C3 anastomosis	Third cervical space	C3
		C4 anastomosis	Fourth cervical space	C4 (phrenic nerve)
	Posterior cervical artery	C2 anastomosis	Second cervical space	C2
		C3 anastomosis	Third cervical space	C3
		C4 anastomosis	Fourth cervical space	C4
	External carotid trunk	C4 collateral	Fourth cervical space	C4

*GG, gasserian ganglion (Vth); Σ (ANS), pericarotid autonomic parasympathetic nervous plexus.
(With kind permission from Lasjaunias P, Berenstein A: Surgical Neuroangiography. Vol 1. [Functional Anatomy of Craniofacial Arteries Ser.] New York, Springer-Verlag, 1986, p 242.)

Thin-section axial and coronal computed tomography (CT) and magnetic resonance imaging (MRI) define the extent of the lesion. CT is preferred to identify bone involvement, whereas MRI better differentiates between extension of the tumor into a sinus, as opposed to opacification secondary to osteal obstruction. Angiographic series to delineate the arterial supply to the tumor and particularly to identify dangerous external carotid artery–to–internal carotid artery anastomoses follow. The contralateral side should be studied if the tumor crosses the midline. There is a strong correlation between the angiographic blush of the tumor and its true extent; a tumor blush extending above the skull base indicates intracranial extension. Additionally, there is a good correlation between the obliteration of the blush and the adequacy of the embolization procedure, provided selective feeding vessels can be appropriately catheterized.

Embolization is usually performed using polyvinyl alcohol (PVA) or Gelfoam particles. Surgery is performed 3 to 5 days after embolization. Steroid administration during the interval between embolization and surgery is sometimes advocated. Shrinkage of the tumor is usually observed within 12 hours. Temporary occlusion with appropriately located large pieces of Gelfoam can be useful to protect dangerous anastomoses from small-particle embolic material and can be used proximal to the small embolic particles to promote thrombosis within the tumor and decrease the possibility of inadvertent retrograde particulate migration. Liquid embolic agents are dangerous because of the proximity of the arterial branches of the skull base to the cranial nerves and because of the external-to-internal carotid artery anastomoses. They can be useful, however, if aggressive therapy is necessary because of tumor invasion of the base of the skull.[7, 8, 9]

Other hypervascular tumors are also candidates for embolization as a part of the treatment regimen. Paragangliomas are hypervascular and invasive (Fig. 8–1) and are not sensitive to radiation therapy. They should benefit, therefore, from presurgical embolization, as should other vascular lesions such as esthesioneuroblastomas, hemangiomas, hemangiopericytomas, and hemangioendotheliomas.[10, 11]

Arteriovenous and capillary malformations (Fig. 8–2) can be treated by an endovascular approach. The ultimate goal is selective occlusion of the abnormal vessels, with preservation of the blood supply to normal tissues. From the angiographic display of each vascular territory, embolization is planned choosing the safest and most direct endovascular route. Dangerous collateral pathways must be avoided. The embolic agent chosen should be able to reach the vascular nidus; otherwise the vascular malformation will persist via alternate supply routes. Consequently, small microparticles or liquid agents are used. Recanalization following nonresorbable particulate embolization or the use of nonresorbable liquid agents has been noted, probably secondary to blood thrombus interspersed between the embolic agents. Subsequent recanalization then may occur through the pathways of the blood thrombus. Any angiographically visible anastomosis between the external carotid branches and the intracranial arterial system will need to be protected if microparticles smaller than 100 microns or liquid agents are used. As the embolization proceeds, feeding vessels, which may not have been angiographically evident initially, may enlarge and become visible. Post-treatment evaluation of the effectiveness of the procedure is performed by injection of the vessels that are known to be in hemodynamic balance with the occluded vessels. Incomplete obliteration of the vascular lesion need not mean failure, because a significant reduction in blood flow may render surgical resection not only possible but successful.[12]

Balloon embolization is the treatment of choice in carotid cavernous aneurysms. Most cases of pseudoaneurysms of the cavernous internal carotid artery caused by nonpenetrating injuries that present with epistaxis usually hemorrhage within 3 weeks of trauma; however, cases have been documented occurring 22, 30, and 40 years later. The etiology of the epistaxis is not appreciated in three fourths of these patients until 4 months after the initial episode. Surgical treatment of traumatic aneurysms carries an 18 to 24 per cent mortality, whereas a mortality of 41 to 50 per cent is noted with conservative care. These aneurysms are frequently accompanied by visual loss (usually noted immediately after the trauma), basilar skull fractures, and involvement of other cranial nerves. In one series, initial angiography failed to demonstrate the aneurysm in 6 per cent of the patients. Consequently, Chambers and colleagues emphasize the more frequent use of carotid angiography in patients with post-traumatic monocular blindness and delayed epistaxis.[13] Balloon embolization is also the treatment of choice in postsurgical damage to the carotid artery following trans-sphenoidal surgery (Fig. 8–3).[13–16]

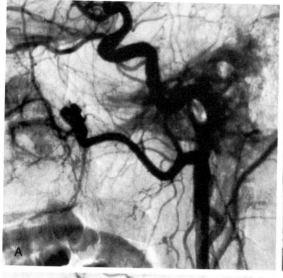

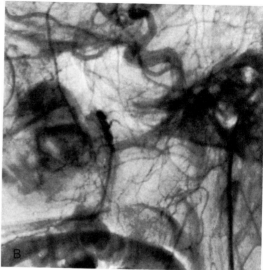

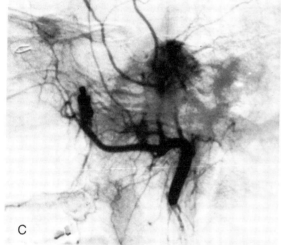

Figure 8–1. A 26-year-old woman with right nasal epistaxis. The arterial *(A)* and capillary *(B)* phases demonstrate the intense tumor stain of the malignant paraganglioma of the right maxillary sinus. Presurgical embolization was not performed. *C,* An arteriogram 1 year following total surgical removal of the tumor in the maxillary sinus demonstrates left parasellar metastasis.

Embolic treatment of cavernous internal carotid artery aneurysms (Fig. 8–4) includes balloon trapping of the aneurysm, with one balloon located between the aneurysm and the ophthalmic artery and another balloon located proximal to the aneurysm. A third balloon is placed within the internal carotid artery near the common carotid artery bifurcation to decrease the chance of thrombotic emboli from the internal carotid artery stump passing into the external circulation. This trapping procedure has the advantage over simple proximal occlusion either by balloon or surgical ligation in that it prevents retrograde filling of the aneurysm from the supraclinoid internal carotid artery. If the balloon can be inflated within the aneurysm, the aneurysm can be obliterated with sparing of the internal carotid artery. It is extremely important to allow sufficient time for a pseudoaneurysm to develop a thick wall to decrease the possibility of inadvertent aneurysm rupture. The risk of inducing hemorrhage is increased, however, and appropriate precautions should be considered, such as binasal Foley catheters inserted within the nasopharynx for control of the hemorrhage.[17, 18]

The advantages of balloon occlusion include the continuous neurologic assessment of an awake patient throughout the procedure, as well as arteriographic verification of the lack of aneurysmal filling and preservation of adequate cerebral perfusion. In cases in which marginal cross-circulation is present, a bypass from the superficial temporal artery to the middle cerebral artery can be performed prior to internal carotid artery occlusion.

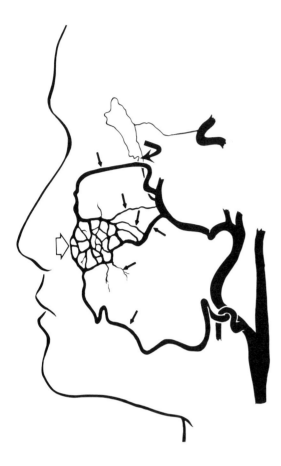

Figure 8–2. An arteriovenous malformation of the maxillary paranasal sinus. Note the multiple collateral channels within the nidus *(open arrow)*, as well as the multiple collateral vessels supplying the nidus *(small arrows)*. Proximal occlusion of the feeding vessels will lead only to enlargement of the collateral vessels. Many of these collaterals are not initially evident, since they are below the resolving capability of angiography. If there is not complete obliteration of the multiple channels within the nidus, the shunt will persist. Note the dangerous anastomosis with the cavernous internal carotid artery via the ethmoidal branches of the ophthalmic artery *(curved arrow)* through which small emboli could reach the intracranial circulation. This also could provide a source of collateral supply to the nidus, such as following proximal ligation of the facial and internal maxillary arteries.

Figure 8–3. Pseudoaneurysm of the internal carotid artery following surgical drainage of the sphenoid sinus. Note the clips about the ethmoidal arteries, as well as internal maxillary artery, following attempts to control the epistaxis after surgery without arteriographic evaluation to determine the true source of the hemorrhage. Extravasated contrast is noted within the nasal packing *(curved arrow)*.

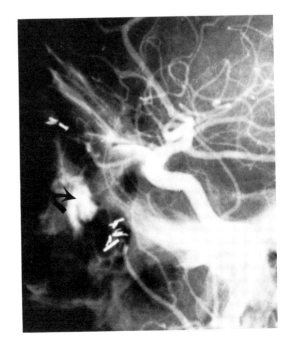

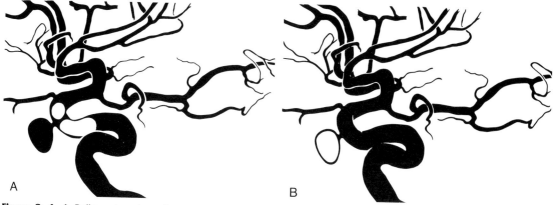

A

B

Figure 8–4. *A,* Balloon trapping of a cavernous internal carotid artery aneurysm, with sacrifice of the internal carotid artery. *B,* Balloon filling an aneurysm, with preservation of the internal carotid artery.

The balloon techniques also can be utilized in the treatment of carotid cavernous fistulas involving the internal carotid artery, although more conservative approaches should be considered first.[19] Transvenous approaches are useful if a transarterial approach is not technically feasible.[20, 21]

With most of the pseudoaneurysms of the external carotid artery (Fig. 8–5) it is not necessary to embolize the aneurysm cavity and risk

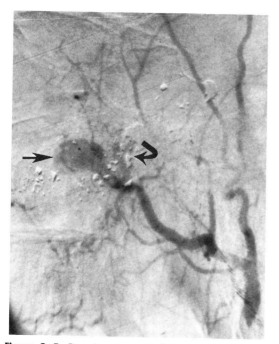

Figure 8–5. Pseudoaneurysm of the internal maxillary artery following a gunshot wound to the face, with a portion projecting into the maxillary sinus *(arrow)* and into the pterygomaxillary fissure *(curved arrow).* This can be readily treated by embolization of the internal maxillary artery proximal to the lesion.

rupturing the weak aneurysm wall. It is usually sufficient to occlude the feeding proximal vessel and allow clotting to occur from the reduced flow. This can be performed by means of balloons, coils, or alcohol plugs. The use of resorbable embolic materials, such as Gelfoam plugs, necessitates follow-up studies, owing to a propensity for recanalization of the feeding vessel.[22]

Embolization can also be useful in control of other causes of epistaxis that are not responsive to more conservative treatment, such as those secondary to neoplasm or vascular malformation. With spontaneous or hypertensive hemorrhage, it is rare to demonstrate the bleeding point angiographically because of the danger associated with removal of nasal packing. Knowledge of the presumed site of the hemorrhage is helpful, but its absence does not preclude vascular study. Angiographic mapping of the nasal region should be performed, including vessels that arise from the internal carotid, maxillary, facial, and ascending pharyngeal arteries. This should include the collateral supply if there has been previous ligation, such as of the ethmoid or maxillary arteries. The choice of embolic material will depend upon the primary lesion, the severity and site of the hemorrhage, and the presence of dangerous anastomoses.[9]

CONCLUSION

The main purpose of this chapter, as noted initially, is to introduce the rationale, methods, and possible complications of embolization of head and neck lesions in order to encourage the use of this technique in the treatment of vascular neoplasms and malformations. The reader is referred to the bibliography, which contains detailed and complete descriptions of the methods and potential complications of a much larger number of lesions affecting the head and neck region than were discussed in this chapter.

ACKNOWLEDGMENTS

The permission to use the material of Dr. P. Lasjaunias and Dr. A. Berenstein is greatly appreciated. We thank Jo Ann Shipp for her timely and thoughtful secretarial assistance.

References

1. Lasjaunias P, Berenstein A: Surgical Neuroangiography. Vol 2. (Endovascular Treatment of Craniofacial Lesions Ser.) New York, Springer-Verlag, 1987, p 5–18.
2. Jungreis CA, Berenstein A, Choi IS: Use of open-ended guidewire: Steerable microguide-wire assembly system in surgical neuroangiographic procedures. AJNR 8:237–241, 1986.
3. Kikuchi Y, Strother CM, Boyer M: New catheter for endovascular interventional procedures. Radiology 165:870–871, 1987.
4. Lasjaunias P, Berenstein A: Surgical Neuroangiography. Vol 1. (Functional Anatomy of Craniofacial Arteries Ser.) New York, Springer-Verlag, 1986, p 242.
5. Lasjaunias P, Berenstein A: Surgical Neuroangiography. Vol 2. (Endovascular Treatment of Craniofacial Lesions Ser.) New York, Springer-Verlag, 1987, p 48–54.
6. Horton JA, Kerber CW: Lidocaine injection into external carotid branches: Provocative test to preserve cranial nerve function in therapeutic embolization. AJNR 7:105–108, 1986.
7. Lasjaunias P, Berenstein A: Surgical Neuroangiography. Vol 2. (Endovascular Treatment of Craniofacial Lesions Ser.) New York, Springer-Verlag, 1987, p 119–121.
8. Bryan RN, Sessions RB, Horowitz BL: Radiographic management of juvenile angiofibromas. AJNR 2:157–166, 1981.
9. Davis KR: Embolization of epistaxis and juvenile nasopharyngeal angiofibromas. AJNR 7:953–962, 1986.
10. Lasjaunias P, Berenstein A: Surgical Neuroangiography. Vol 2. (Endovascular Treatment of Craniofacial Lesions Ser.) New York, Springer-Verlag, 1987, p 126.
11. Valavanis A: Preoperative embolization of head and neck: Indications, patient selection, goals and precautions. AJNR 7:943–952, 1986.
12. Lasjaunias P, Berenstein A: Surgical Neuroangiography. Vol 2. (Endovascular Treatment of Craniofacial Lesions Ser.) New York, Springer-Verlag, 1987, pp 24, 25, 37.
13. Chambers EF, Rosenbaum AE, Norman D, Newton TH: Traumatic aneurysms of cavernous internal carotid artery with secondary epistaxis. AJNR 2:405–409, 1981.
14. Debrun G, Fox A, Drake C, et al: Giant unclippable aneurysms: Treatment with detachable balloons. AJNR 2:167–173, 1981.
15. Debrun GM, Vinuela F, Fox AJ, Davis KR, Ahn HS: Indications for treatment and classification of 132 carotid-cavernous fistulas. Neurosurgery 22(2):285–289, 1988.
16. Simpson RK Jr, Harper RL, Bryan RN: Emergency balloon occlusion for massive epistaxis due to traumatic carotid-cavernous aneurysm. J Neurosurg 68:142–144, 1988.
17. Lasjaunias P, Berenstein A: Surgical Neuroangiography. Vol 2. (Endovascular Treatment of Craniofacial Lesions Ser.) New York, Springer-Verlag, 1987, pp 256–264.
18. Tantana S, Pilla TJ, Awwad EE, Smith KR Jr: Balloon embolization of a traumatic carotid-ophthalmic pseudoaneurysm with control of the epistaxis and preservation of the internal carotid artery. AJNR 8:923–924, 1987.
19. Higashida RT, Hieshima GB, Halbach VV, Bentson JR, Goto K: Closure of carotid cavernous sinus fistulae by external compression of the carotid artery and jugular vein. Acta Radiol (Diagn) (Stockh) [Suppl] 369:580–583, 1986.
20. Teng MMH, Guo WY, Huang CI, Wu CC, Chang T: Occlusion of arteriovenous malformations of the cavernous sinus via the superior ophthalmic vein. AJNR 9:539–546, 1988.
21. Halbach VV, Higashida RT, Hieshima GB, Hardin CW, Yang PJ: Transvenous embolization of direct carotid cavernous fistulas. AJNR 9:741–747, 1988.
22. Uflacker R: Transcatheter embolization of arterial aneurysms. Br J Radiol 59:314–324, 1981.

CHAPTER 9

GENERAL PRINCIPLES

Anthony F. Jahn, MD

A rational approach to paranasal sinus surgery requires thorough knowledge of sinus anatomy, physiology, and pathology. Surgical management is based not only on principles common to all forms of surgery, but also on those that are specific to the paranasal sinuses. The aim of this chapter is to place these specific principles in proper context.

Contemporary sinus surgery is the product of intrinsic and extrinsic influences. In part, it represents a natural historic evolution in the understanding of sinus diseases; in part, it reflects the impact of other disciplines, including pharmacology, radiology, and surgical technology. The synthesis of these forces represents contemporary principles of paranasal sinus surgery.

FUNCTION OF PARANASAL SINUSES

The first principle of surgery is restoration of normal function. It is generally accepted, however, that the paranasal sinuses serve no primary function in humans. This stance is the culmination of 2000 years of hypotheses concerning sinus function. Various authors have attributed the following functions to the sinuses: (1) production of mucus, (2) storage of mucus, (3) resonators for the voice, (4) lightening the skull, (5) humidification and warming of inhaled air, (6) accessory areas of olfaction, (7) conservation of heat from the nasal fossae, (8) definition of facial contours, and (9) "surge tanks" to dampen the pressure differential that develops during inspiration. Some (certainly not all) of these functions may take place to a minor

degree. They are, however, secondary properties of air-containing, mucosa-lined cavities. Human sinuses are phylogenic remnants.

To gain some idea of how sinuses arose, it is worthwhile to examine lower animals, which often possess sinus systems far more elaborate than those in humans. Although in humans we talk of the system of paranasal sinuses, in lower animals it becomes apparent that specific sinuses serve specific functions and ought not to be considered as a single system. Each set of sinuses represents an evagination of the nasal cavity for a specific purpose, and to seek a common function is misleading. Thus, Negus suggested that the ethmoid labyrinth originally evolved as an accessory olfactory surface in macrosmatic animals.[1] He believed that the maxillary sinus developed to accommodate the maxilloturbinal body (inferior turbinate). Reconsideration of sinus development in lower animals allows us to attribute reasonably the following functions to the sinuses:

Ethmoid Labyrinth. The ethmoid labyrinth probably developed as an accessory olfactory surface, with a secondary function of heating and humidifying inspired air. Humidification has olfactory implications also, as odors are held and concentrated in humid air, and water-soluble odors are delivered to the olfactory sensory epithelium.

Frontal Sinuses. The frontal sinuses represent an anterior tract of the ethmoid cells and have no olfactory function in any species. They probably developed as mechanical protection for the brain and as rigid support for horns and antlers (Fig. 9–1). The force of collision is borne by the rigid walls of the sinus that extend into the horns, and the energy is dissipated at the bone-air interfaces, protecting the brain from concussion. As Negus pointed out, if the function of frontal sinuses was merely to lighten the skull they would not be there at all, and the frontal bone would have remained a single plate.[1]

Maxillary Sinuses. The maxillary sinuses exemplify the body's economy. They absorb the force of mastication, which in herbivores is constant and considerable. This force is exerted on the upper alveolar arch, then transmitted through the walls of the antrum and dissipated over the rest of the skull. The hard palate bears little force from below and does not need support from above. The maxillary antrum, therefore, represents an appropriate set of bony struts (the walls of the antrum), which has evolved in response to forces exerted from below. Thus, ungulates and other herbivores generally have large antra, whereas carnivores, which tear rather than chew, have small ones. More than just removing unnecessary bone, the excavation of the antrum has the effect of increasing its rigidity. Stress is borne maximally at the surface, and a hollow box has more surfaces than a solid cube. This concept is not identical to lightening the skull, although that may be an incidental benefit in animals with large skulls (in humans, the weight difference is negligible).

A second important function of the maxillary sinus in animals might be to interfere with the bone conduction of chewing noises to the inner ear. Although some sound energy is clearly transmitted through the antral walls to the temporal bone, much is lost at the bone-air interfaces of the antral cavity. This increase in effective impedance (previously attributed to the mastoid process also, by Barany[2]) would have obvious survival value to grazing animals listening for predators.

Sphenoid Sinus. The function of the sphenoid sinus is not known in any species and does not readily lend itself to postulation. Because the acuity of olfaction, force of mastication, and likelihood of planned frontal collision are all greatly reduced in humans, the sinuses have become vestigial, with insignificant secondary functions.

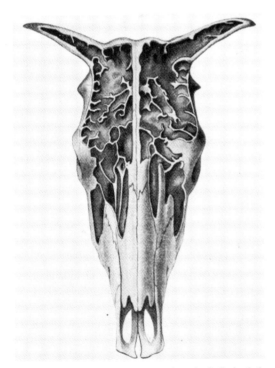

Figure 9–1. Frontal opened view of cow's skull, depicting extensive pneumatization of the skull and horns via the frontoethmoidal air cell tracts. (From Marx H: Die Nasenheilkunde. Jena, Fischer Verlag, 1949; modified from Paulli S: Über die Pneumacität des Schädels bei den Säugethieren. Gegenbaur's Morph Jahrbuch 28:147, 1900.)[16]

PRINCIPLES OF SINUS SURGERY—HISTORICAL DEVELOPMENT

Contemporary principles of sinus surgery have evolved over 2000 years and especially over the last century. A brief historical review of the surgery of the paranasal sinuses will help us understand the rationale of contemporary techniques.

The origins of sinus surgery must be sought in the technique of trephination as practiced by prehistoric peoples.[3] Pre- and postmortem trephination was common among tribes of the Old and especially the New World and had both ritual and practical significance. In some cases, releasing the evil spirits from the head undoubtedly had the therapeutic benefit of draining the pus of an intracranial abscess. The early priest-surgeon had some knowledge of the sinuses, as the skull depicted in Figure 9–2 shows. This Peruvian specimen, dating back to the Inca period around 1400 A.D., shows evidence of frontal sinus trephination with subsequent new bone formation around the edges of the defect. Surgery was apparently limited to the sinus and

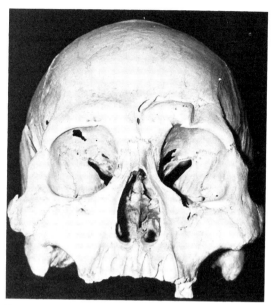

Figure 9–2. Pre-Columbian Inca skull demonstrating evidence of premortem trephination of the left frontal sinus and avulsion-curettage of the supra-orbital nerve. (Courtesy of Dr. Rinaldo Canalis, Archives of Otolaryngology, and the San Diego Museum for the History of Man.)

included curettage of the supraorbital foramen, suggesting that it may have been performed therapeutically for frontal sinus pain. Apart from a few tantalizing anthropologic artifacts, no records survive from prehistoric surgeons.

The ancient Greeks had no understanding of sinus structure or function. They appreciated the extrasinal manifestations of sinus disease but drew no inference as to the state of the sinuses.

The Greek perspective on nasal and sinus anatomy may have been inherited in part from the Egyptians, who extracted the brain piecemeal through the cribriform plate during mummification. Accordingly, Galen held that mucus was secreted by the pituitary gland in the brain and excreted into the nose via the cribriform plate. From there the mucus was collected in the sinuses and subsequently released into the nose. This theory remained unchallenged dogma until the sixteenth century. Only then did Fallopius conclusively demonstrate that the sinuses contained air rather than mucus.[4]

In 1660, Conrad Victor Schneider of Wittenberg began work on a five-volume tome on mucus, its origins and treatment. This massive work, which eventually totaled 1391 pages, put an end to the idea that nasal mucus originated in the pituitary gland. He showed that the olfactory processes were cranial nerves rather than mucous conduits (Fig. 9–3). From the

Greeks until the seventeenth century, nasal and sinus surgery consisted of recognizing and dealing with polyps and tumors as they presented in the nose.

The second phase of sinus surgery, discovery and treatment of sinuses as a primary site of infection, began in 1651. In that year Nathaniel Highmore described the maxillary antrum and related a case of suppurative maxillary sinusitis in a woman with carious teeth in the upper jaw.[5] Trephination of the antrum, either externally or through the socket of an extracted infected tooth, was apparently introduced in the 1650s by Zwingler and Meibomius.[6]

Antral trephination for suppuration remained the commonest sinus operation during the seventeenth and eighteenth centuries. Tumors of the sinuses were recognized in the nose, but their treatment lagged behind the treatment of suppurative sinusitis. The first surgical removal of a sinus tumor was by Plaignaud of Paris, related in his report of 1791.[7] This was a rapidly growing tumor of the antrum that was digitally removed through a canine fossa trephination and through the hard palate. The concept of total maxillectomy was first proposed in 1826

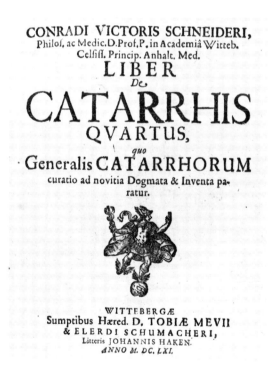

CONRADI VICTORIS SCHNEIDERI,
Philof. ac Medic.D.Prof.P. in Academiâ Witteb.
Celfiff. Princip. Anhalt. Med.

LIBER
De
CATARRHIS
QVARTUS,
quo
Generalis CATARRHORUM
curatio ad novitia Dogmata & Inventa paratur.

WITTEBERGÆ
Sumptibus Hæred. D. TOBIÆ MEVII
& ELERDI SCHUMACHERI,
Litteris JOHANNIS HAKEN.
ANNO M. DC. LXI.

Figure 9–3. Title page of Schneider's Liber de Catarrhis, printed in 1661. Apart from his contributions to the origins of mucus, Schneider's name has been linked with the schneiderian epithelium of the nose, and the schneiderian (inverting) papilloma.

by John Lazars of Edinburgh and successfully carried out by his contemporary, James Syme, 2 years later.[8] The main métier of the sinus surgeon of the eighteenth and nineteenth centuries, however, was drainage of sinus suppuration.[9] Antral suppuration was a recognized complication of dental disease; hence in chronic suppuration the antrum was opened through the alveolar ridge. If no infected tooth was present, a healthy one was extracted (usually the first or second molar) to create a permanent oroantral fistula. The patient kept the fistula open by daily irrigations or by the insertion of an obturator. When the anterior wall of the antrum was opened through the canine fossa, this also would be kept open and irrigated daily. The permanent external fistula method of antral lavage was not abandoned until 1893, when Caldwell proposed curettage of the infected mucosa followed by closure of the canine fossa incision and intranasal antrostomy—today's Caldwell-Luc operation.[10] Apart from surgical fistulization, lavage and poudrage of the sinuses through their natural ostia was frequently done for acute and chronic suppuration. The physician's confidence was based on a growing appreciation of the anatomy of the sinuses and their connections with the nasal cavity. In 1891, Frankel froze cadaver heads in a bucket of water and sectioned the resulting ice block with a carpenter's saw. This atlas of cross-sectional anatomy rivals modern histologic and radiologic depictions.[11]

The true foundations of modern sinus surgery were laid during these closing years of the ninteenth century. Every sinus was trephined, and frontal, ethmoid, and maxillary sinuses were curetted intranasally and also via external incisions. External operation of the frontal sinus was carried out both preserving the anterior table and sacrificing it. When the anterior table was sacrificed, the resultant deformity was corrected by injecting wax; Billroth's pupil Czerny was the first to propose the frontal sinus osteoplastic flap to prevent such defects.[14] Perhaps the greatest technologic advance in sinus surgery came through Roentgen's discovery of the x-ray. Prior to this, the content of sinuses could be visualized only by transillumination, and this method (diaphanoscopy) acquired a certain degree of sophistication if not infallibility. With the introduction of sinus x-rays, the frequency and extent of chronic sinus infections became apparent.

When Kuttner published the first radiologic atlas of paranasal sinuses in 1908, the illustrations depicted cases of gross involvement in frontal projections only. However primitive, these x-ray films were an enormous improvement over the vague shadows of the diaphanoscopist.[7] The x-ray films allowed an appreciation of the frequency of sinus disease, of the frequency of multiple sinus involvement, and of the appearance of postinflammatory changes.

The first major contribution of the twentieth century to operation on the sinuses was the concept of using the sinuses for access to deeper structures. The earliest example of this is the trans-sphenoidal approach to the pituitary, pioneered by the leading neurosurgeons of the early twentieth century. Phillip Golding-Wood[12] popularized the transantral approach to the pterygomaxillary space for his vidian neurectomy operation. Although this procedure is no longer in general use, the approach has remained in use for transantral ligation of the internal maxillary artery. Transethmoid approaches to the pituitary, as well as medial and inferior orbital decompression, are other examples of this aspect of sinus surgery.

Perhaps the most significant recent development in operations of the sinuses is the use of nasal telescopes to treat outlet obstruction in sinus disease. As is so often the case, the concept is not a new one: Messerklinger[13] was the first to draw attention to the fact that sinus disease is often the result of obstruction of the ostia in the middle meatus. Treatment of ostiomeatal obstruction is conceptually attractive, as it is analogous to relieving eustachian tube obstruction to treat middle ear disease. Part of the recent interest in functional endoscopic surgery of the sinuses is due to our ability now to treat the cause, not just the effect, of sinus disease, with modified arthroscopes and technologically advanced instrumentation (stronger light sources, lasers, and so on).

CURRENT PRINCIPLES

The indications for sinus operation are defined by our understanding of the disease process, its natural course, and how that course is altered by various treatment modalities. Operation may be indicated in acute or chronic disorders, and these indications may be absolute or relative (Table 9–1). The candidate for sinus operation has a problem that usually falls into one of three categories: infectious/inflammatory disorder of the sinus, neoplastic disease of the sinus, or a disorder of an area surgically approachable through an otherwise

TABLE 9–1. Indications for Paranasal Sinus Surgery

Absolute	Relative
Acute	Chronic infective sinusitis unresponsive to conservative treatment
Bacterial infection unresponsive to specific antimicrobial therapy	Chronic allergic rhinosinusitis with polyps, unresponsive to medical treatment
Impending or actual intracranial extension of sinus infection	Malignant tumors of sinuses (surgery for palliation or cure)
Mycotic infection in debilitated patient	Sinus fracture with cosmetic deformity (e.g., frontal sinus)
Infection with orbital or global involvement	Orbital floor fracture with herniation of orbital contents
Uncontrolled posterior epistaxis (transantral ligation of internal maxillary artery)	Orbital decompression for cosmesis of exophthalmos (Graves')
	Persistent oroantral fistula
Chronic	Vidian neurectomy
Persistent CSF leak following trauma	Transethmoid and/or trans-sphenoid pituitary surgery
Mycotic infection unresponsive to antimicrobial therapy	
Mucocele or pyocele with orbital encroachment	
Osteomyelitis of sinus wall	
Benign tumors (inverting papilloma)	
Orbital decompression for uncontrolled exophthalmos (Graves') with corneal damage	
Foreign body (tooth fragment) with persistent secondary infection	
Trans-sphenoid hypophysectomy for patient with visual field defects	

healthy sinus. While adhering to general surgical principles, the surgeon will vary the selection of techniques according to the specific condition. Although dealing in one particular modality of treatment, the surgeon must nevertheless approach the patient comprehensively, striving for accurate diagnosis, appropriate treatment, and competent management of subsequent complications or rehabilitative problems.

History. Chronic disease confined to the sinuses is often initially asymptomatic, whether inflammatory or neoplastic. As the history is taken, the surgeon elicits the time course for the development and progression of symptoms. Although the actual onset of the disease process (e.g., a maxillary sinus mass) usually precedes the first symptom by months or even years, the progression of the disease can be inferred from the rapidity with which symptoms change and new symptoms emerge. The nature of the symptoms helps pinpoint areas where the tumor or inflammatory process may have escaped the confines of the sinus. Because the patient may be overwhelmed by the dominant symptom, such as pain, he or she may neglect to volunteer information about less obvious but perhaps more significant symptoms, such as slight diplopia. The surgeon must therefore ask systematically about every possible symptom that may relate to the area under scrutiny. Such an anatomic approach applied to the maxillary

sinus would investigate the following: *sinus proper:* pain, pressure; *anterior wall:* cheek swelling, pain, skin changes; *medial wall:* nasal obstruction, nasal discharge, epistaxis, cacosmia, visible mass in nostril; *superior wall:* diplopia, proptosis, chemosis, pain or hypesthesia over cheek, decreased visual acuity; *lateral wall:* trismus, bulging mass; *inferior wall:* bulge in hard palate, ill-fitting dentures, loose teeth, hypesthesia or devitalization of teeth, bleeding from palatal erosion; *posterior wall:* midface pain or hypesthesia (V_2), loss of function of lower cranial nerves. Similar sequences can be generated for the frontal, ethmoid, and (to a lesser extent) sphenoid sinuses. Other salient historic features are occupational history, history of malignancy elsewhere, and decreased immune response (diabetes, alcoholism, immune suppression).

Physical Examination. The examination confirms historic findings and may elicit subtle signs that were not grossly symptomatic. The examination of sinuses and their contents is usually indirect, although in some cases proof puncture or diagnostic sinus lavage may yield useful information. Examination of the middle meatus using fiberoptic or rigid nasal endoscopes is useful, particularly in combination with the appropriate CT scans to demonstrate fully the ostiomeatal complex. Percussion or palpation over the sinuses may elicit tenderness in cases of acute sinus disease. Transillumination still may have a limited role in monitoring a resolving sinusitis in the office, for which repeated x-ray exposure is not justified.

Ancillary Studies. Radiologic assessment is of paramount importance. Routine sinus views have limited value and demonstrate only gross alterations in sinus aeration or possible bony erosion. These views, which involve a relatively low radiation exposure, have the additional advantage of demonstrating incidental asymptomatic disease in sinuses that may have been unsuspected. CT scanning at this time is the imaging modality of choice for evaluation of sinus disease. Special coned-down views of the middle meatus area are mandatory for endoscopic surgery. Since the anatomic variations in this region are virtually endless, the surgeon should review the films with the radiologist. Bacteriologic specimens can be obtained by swabbing the region of the ostia or by obtaining a sample of antral contents through proof puncture or antral lavage. If a mass is found protruding into the nose, this may be biopsied at the time of physical assessment.

Surgical Planning. The surgeon must tailor the operation to the disease and (equally important) to the patient. The type and extent of disease may dictate a certain procedure; however, the patient's physical condition, ability to withstand anesthesia, prolonged rehabilitation, and expectations or wishes must be considered. The procedure represents a synthesis of the disease's mandate, the surgeon's intent, and the patient's wishes.

To some patients with sinus cancer, the slightly greater chance of a surgical cure is not worth the physical and psychologic mutilation inflicted. Similarly, there are patients with chronic sinusitis who prefer to endure repeated antral lavage and medical treatment rather than a single curative surgical procedure. The health care system may permit more conservative, ongoing treatment in a civilized country, whereas in developing countries with haphazard follow-up and medical delivery, a more radical surgical philosophy may be more appropriate.[15]

In surgical planning, the surgeon must first consider the approach, including the incisions. The following priorities are weighed: visualization, instrumental access to remove the diseased area, flexibility to extend if necessary, and cosmesis. The standard surgical approaches already incorporate these considerations, but the surgeon's thinking should be fresh and appropriate to the problem.

When dealing with infectious/inflammatory disease, the surgeon's priorities are (1) complete and accurate removal of all diseased tissue, with maximal sparing of healthy tissue, (2) where feasible, opening the natural drainage pathways of the sinus (via endoscopic removal of ostiomeatal obstruction); if this is not possible, or the disease is judged to be too advanced, (3) creation of wide communication into the nose to permit gravitational drainage and ingrowth of healthy nasal mucosa (in acute infection, short-term drainage externally may be more expeditious); (4) if the effectiveness of (2) is in doubt, obliteration of the sinus to prevent ingrowth of mucosa and possible recurrence of disease; and (5) cosmetic considerations, after the first three priorities are satisfied (for example, the use of transnasal rather than external approaches, obliterating the frontal sinus via the osteoplastic flap rather than the Riedel operation, or placing external incisions above the hairline, in skin creases, and at the boundaries of regional esthetic units of the face).

When dealing with neoplasia of the sinuses, the surgeon should consider the following priorities: (1) complete removal of tumor, including areas of actual or suspected involvement beyond the confines of the sinus; (2) debulking the tumor to decrease tumor burden, in preparation for other treatment modalities, or to decompress areas of potential tumor extension; this often includes a planned fistula to permit visual monitoring afterward; and (3) the best possible reconstruction (surgical or prosthetic) to permit optimal functional and cosmetic rehabilitation.

In contemplating trans-sinal operation of the pterygomaxillary space or pituitary, the surgeon crosses a healthy sinus. The aims are (1) optimal visualization and instrumentation at the target area; (2) minimal trauma to the sinus and its lining; and (3) prevention of iatrogenic disorders of the sinus.

The many specific surgical procedures described in the following chapters all conform to these general principles. They impart meaning to the procedure contemplated and will give the surgeon conviction in treatment and a guideline for innovations.

FUTURE TRENDS

The future of paranasal sinus surgery is inseparably linked to advances in technology. Newer generations of CT scanners will permit ever more definitive assessment of sinus disease and lead to greater accuracy in planning, mapping, and prognosticating. Microsurgical techniques will continue to increase the importance of sinuses as a route of approach to hitherto inaccessible areas of the skull base. Advances in the fields of allergy and pathology will yield a more complete understanding of patients with inflammatory and neoplastic diseases and allow the surgeon to further refine the indications and techniques in the context of overall management of sinus disease.

References

1. Negus V: The Comparative Anatomy and Physiology of the Nose and Paranasal Sinuses. Edinburgh, E. & S. Livingstone Ltd, 1958.
2. Barany E: A contribution to the physiology of bone conduction. Acta Otolaryngol (Suppl) 26:1, 1938.
3. Canalis R, Hemenway WG, Cabieses F, et al: Prehistoric trephination of the frontal sinus. Ann Otol 90:186, 1981.
4. Marx H: Die Nasenheilkunde. Jena, Fischer Verlag, 1949.
5. Schmidt M: Die Krankheiten der Oberen Luftwege. 2nd ed. Berlin, Julius Springer Verlag, 1897.
6. Wright J: The Nose and Throat in Medical History. St. Louis, LS Matthews & Co, 1898.
7. Kuttner A: Die Entzundlichen Hebenhohlenerkrankungen der Nase in Röntgenbild. Berlin, Urban & Schwartzenberg, 1908.
8. Paparella M, Shumrick D: Otolaryngology. Vol 3: Head and Neck. Philadelphia, WB Saunders, 1973.
9. Mikulicz J: Zur operativen Behandlung des Empyems der Highmoreshöle. Arch Klin Chir 34:626, 1887.
10. Caldwell GW: Diseases of the accessory sinuses of the nose, and improved method of treatment of suppuration of the maxillary antrum. NY Med J 58:526, 1893.
11. Fränkel B: Gefrierdurchschnitte zur Anatomie der Nassenhöhle. Berlin, August Hirschwald Verlag, 1891.
12. Golding-Wood PH: Observations on petrosal and vidian neurectomy in chronic vasomotor rhinitis. J Laryngol Otol 25:232, 1961.
13. Messerklinger W: Endoscopy of the nose. Baltimore, Urban & Schwarzenberg, 1978.
14. Denker A, Brunings W: Lehrbuch der Krankheiten des Ohres und der Luftwege. 6th and 7th eds. Jena, Fischer Verlag, 1921.
15. Obiako MN: The rationale for radical surgery as the treatment of choice of chronic maxillary sinusitis in developing countries. Arch Otol 92:131, 1981.
16. Paulli S: Über die Pneumacität des Schädels bei den Säugethieren. Gegenbaur's Morph Jahrbuch 28:147, 1900.

CHAPTER 10

FRONTAL SINUS

William Lawson, MD, DDS

Operations of the frontal sinus are directed at the management of acute and chronic sinusitis and its complications (e.g., osteomyelitis, mucocele, pyocele, orbital and intracranial extension, intractability), the biopsy and removal of neoplasms, and the repair of fractures. The operations performed may be broadly divided into external and intranasal procedures. The various external procedures (Fig. 10–1) may be classified into those that (1) create a trephine type opening for drainage or excision of diseased tissue; (2) remove the anterior or orbital wall for access to the sinus; (3) create a hinged osteoperiosteal (osteoplastic) flap for instrumentation of the sinus without a cortical defect; (4) enlarge or reconstruct the nasofrontal duct; (5) obliterate the sinus cavity by (a) removing the anterior and/or inferior walls and collapsing the skin into it, (b) removing the posterior wall permitting cranialization of the sinus, (c) filling it with an autogenous or alloplastic graft material, or (d) inducing fibrosis or osteoneogenesis; and (6) combine these procedures. The intranasal procedures are directed at eliminating disease in the nose and contiguous paranasal sinuses and promoting drainage by removing obstructions to the nasofrontal duct and blockage within the nasal cavity.

HISTORY

Runge is said to have opened and obliterated the frontal sinus as early as 1750 (Table 10–1).[124] However, Ogston[110] is credited with publishing the first scientific paper on the external approach in 1884. He created a trephine hole through the anterior table and drained the sinus into the nose through the anterior ethmoid cells. Luc[85] described a similar procedure in 1896. In 1895, Kuhnt[78] reported removing the entire anterior wall through a brow incision and packing the skin to contact the posterior wall in an attempt to achieve obliteration. However, if the sinus were deep, obliteration would not be accomplished. In 1893, Jansen[67] created an osteoperiosteal flap of the anterior wall, which he collapsed against the posterior wall after removing the sinus contents, as well as its floor. Although this achieved obliteration of the sinus, it also resulted in a cosmetic deformity. Ritter[122] described in 1911 a purely orbital approach in which the inferior wall was removed along with the ethmoids, creating a large opening into the nose. In 1898, Riedel[120] reported removal of both the anterior and orbital walls of the sinus. This was effective in accomplishing sinus obliteration; however, it produced a marked cosmetic deformity. Killian[73] in 1903 described resection of the anterior and inferior sinus walls but with preservation of the supraorbital ridge and its periosteum, to minimize the cosmetic deformity. He also reconstructed the nasofrontal duct with a mucoperiosteal flap to maintain its patency. In 1895, Schonborn[131] and Brieger[20] reported a direct approach to the sinus by creating a hinged osteoperiosteal flap of its anterior wall.

The disfigurement produced by the removal of the anterior sinus wall, along with the failure to eradicate disease in a significant number of cases, led many workers to employ the transorbital approach. In 1908, Knapp[76] reported removal of the orbital wall in conjunction with an extensive external ethmoidectomy. The cosmetic acceptability of the procedure, along with removal of the frequently accompanying disease

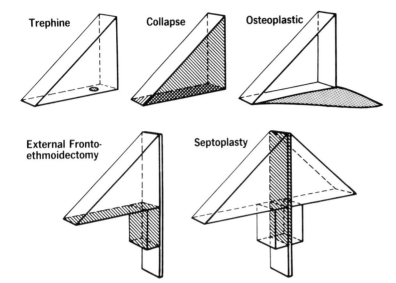

Trephine   **Collapse**   **Osteoplastic**

External Fronto-ethmoidectomy   **Septoplasty**

Figure 10–1. Diagrammatic representation of the various types of external frontal sinus procedures.

within the adjacent ethmoid sinuses, gained it many advocates, notably Lynch[88] and Howarth,[61] who widely popularized it. It soon became apparent that the keystone to the success of the external frontoethmoidectomy was the continued patency of the nasofrontal duct. Numerous modifications of the basic procedure attempted to ensure this (see later). In 1912, Lothrop[84] attempted to solve the problem by creating a common drainage cavity with the contralateral nasofrontal duct.

Continued problems with the transorbital approach led to resurgence of interest in the osteoplastic transfrontal approach. In addition to being esthetically satisfactory and giving wide operative exposure, this method achieved oblit-

eration of the sinus when properly performed. The various modifications of the procedure and methods of obliteration will be reviewed in this chapter.

Even though advances in surgery (e.g., operating microscope, power drill), anesthesia, and antibiotic therapy have improved the management of frontal sinus disease, the basic operative approaches (trephine, collapse, septoplasty, external frontoethmoidectomy, osteoplastic flap), which originated in the late nineteenth and early twentieth centuries, have persisted with only modifications to the present time. Comprehensive reviews of the early history of frontal sinus surgery were made by Lyman[87] and Williams and Holman.[153]

TABLE 10–1. Outline of the History of External Surgery on the Frontal Sinus

Trephine	Ogston (1884)	Trephine of anterior wall
	Luc (1896)	
Collapse	Kuhnt (1891)	Removal of anterior wall
	Riedel (1898)	Removal of anterior and inferior walls
	Killian (1903)	Removal of anterior and inferior walls with preservation of supraorbital ridge
Transorbital	Jansen (1902)	Removal of inferior wall, collapse of anterior wall
	Ritter (1911)	Removal of inferior wall, ethmoidectomy
	Knapp (1908)	
Osteoplastic flap	Schonborn (1894)	Osteoperiosteal flap of anterior wall
	Brieger (1895)	
Septoplasty	Lothrop (1912)	Removal of intersinus septum
Obliteration	Marx (1910), Tato et al (1954), Bergara and Itoiz (1955), Good and Montgomery (1956)	Adipose tissue
	MacBeth (1954)	Natural
	Adson and Hempstead (1937), Malecki (1959)	Cranialization

ANATOMY

The frontal sinuses are paired, irregularly pyramidal cavities situated within the squamous portion of the frontal bone above the orbits. They may pneumatize extensively, with extension laterally to the temporal area, superiorly toward the vertex of the skull and posteriorly to the sphenoid sinus. Each sinus may be compartmentalized by septa present within it. Such septa are recognized operatively by their generally convex configuration toward the midline, whereas the actual lateral wall of the sinus is concave in form.

The anterior table of the sinus is its thickest wall, with cancellous bone present between its cortical plates. The orbital plate of the frontal bone forms its inferior and generally thinnest wall. The posterior table also may be attenuated and lies in direct contact with the dura of the anterior cranial fossa.

A septum generally completely separates the right and left sinuses. Deviation of the interfrontal septum may cause narrowing of the nasofrontal duct. With the finding of deflection of the septum toward the operated side, the presence of an ethmoid cell behind the crista frontalis should be suspected. When the septum is displaced to the opposite side or absent, a median vertical shelf of bone may be present posteriorly, which can be mistaken for a septum. This bony ledge represents the anterior aspect of the olfactory groove (crista olfactorius) that may bulge into the frontal sinus. Mithoefer[99] and Williams and Holman[153] cautioned that injury to this thin plate of bone and the accompanying attenuated dura during surgery may lead to meningitis.

The nasofrontal duct begins as an ostium in the posteromedial aspect of the floor of the frontal sinus and extends for a variable distance before opening into the nasal cavity. The superior opening has a constant position, but the position of the inferior orifice is variable because of different methods of embryologic derivation of the sinus.

The ethmoid labyrinth is in intimate association with the frontal sinus because of a common embryologic development from the middle meatus. When the frontal sinus forms from an extension of the frontal recess, an ostium draining directly into the middle meatus is present. When the sinus develops from an infundibular ethmoid cell, a nasofrontal duct is created. The course and position of the latter are influenced by the growth and development of the anterior ethmoid air cells. A common anomaly is the upward displacement of an anterior ethmoid cell, producing obstruction of the ostium of the nasofrontal duct. With upward and forward growth of a posterior air cell, the middle turbinate may attach to the uncinate process and close off the upper end of the hiatus semilunaris. Enlarged subfrontal and infundibular cells may displace and obstruct the nasofrontal duct.

After 100 consecutive dissections of the frontal sinus, Kasper[70] found three patterns of origin. In 60 per cent of the cases, it arose from the frontal recess; in 38 per cent, from infundibular cells and the uncinate process; and in 3 per cent, from suprabullar cells. The clinical significance of these observations is that in over 62 per cent of the cases the ethmoidal infundibulum is a blind termination lateral to the frontal recess, not permitting the frontal sinus to be sounded from the nasal cavity. A supraorbital ethmoid air cell may occupy the entire orbital roof and may be the source of chronic infection to the frontal sinus.

Analysis of the causes of failure in the surgical management of frontal sinus disease[4, 150, 153] has revealed numerous factors: (1) closure of the nasofrontal duct, (2) presence of the sinus septa, which obstruct drainage, (3) narrow sinus extensions toward the vertex, which may form pockets of infection, (4) persistent islands of mucosa that may develop into cysts, (5) presence of supraorbital ethmoid cells, (6) reinfection from infected and obstructed ethmoid and sphenoid sinuses, (7) presence of resistant organisms, (8) occurrence of foci of osteomyelitis, and (9) presence of an infected interfrontal septum cell.

The same anatomic features that predispose an individual to frontal sinus disease limit the effectiveness of medical and surgical management. The presence of inflammatory disease in the nose and adjacent paranasal sinus, the occurrence of osteitis, and the microbiology of the infecting organisms all influence the outcome of therapy. Most complications of frontal sinus disease are associated with acute rather than chronic disease.[94] It soon becomes apparent that no single operation is adequate for the spectrum of pathology encountered. The principles of management and the indications, limitations, complications, and technical considerations of the various procedures will be individually considered.

INTRANASAL PROCEDURES

Measures to eliminate nasal obstruction and improve nasal drainage must be taken preliminary to direct surgery on the frontal sinus.[83] This includes the correction of anatomic abnormalities and the treatment of allergic, neoplastic, and osseous disorders. This may require septal surgery, partial resection of the middle and inferior turbinates, and the removal of polyps or tumors. Attention must also be directed to the treatment of chronic inflammatory disease within the maxillary, ethmoid, and sphenoid sinuses, as isolated involvement of the frontal sinus is uncommon. This may necessitate transoral or transnasal antrostomy, ethmoidectomy, and sphenoid sinusotomy. Mithoefer[99] expressed the view that the ethmoid sinus was the key to the frontal sinus and always performed a preliminary intranasal ethmoidectomy. The South American workers performed a transantral ethmoidectomy before undertaking a frontal osteoplastic flap.[14] Only when control of disease in the other paranasal sinus has been accomplished should a definitive procedure on the frontal sinus be undertaken, unless an orbital or intracranial complication is present.

The inconstancy and tortuosity of the nasofrontal duct does not readily permit its cannulation. Thus, most workers currently employ external trephination or attempt intranasal entry through the agger nasi cells[121] for drainage. Intranasal methods of trephination into the frontal sinus[54] are considered too dangerous and presently are of historic interest.

TREPHINE

The trephine procedure gains its greatest application in patients with acute frontal sinusitis and radiographic evidence of an air-fluid level. This includes the patient who continues to be symptomatic despite antibiotic therapy and the local application of vasoconstrictors to the nose or who has evidence of facial, orbital, or intracranial extension of the sinus infection. The trephine also may be used for drainage in patients with chronic sinusitis or frontal osteomyelitis with superimposed acute suppuration. It is indicated for exploration and biopsy of patients with chronic frontal sinus disease. Fractures of the anterior table of the frontal sinus may be reduced by instrumentation through the trephine opening, and the reduction may be maintained by the insertion and inflation of a balloon catheter in the sinus cavity if the fragments are unstable.

TECHNIQUE (Fig. 10–2)

After the induction of general anesthesia, a small, curvilinear incision (1 to 2 cm) is made underneath the medial aspect of the unshaved eyebrow. The subcutaneous tissues and orbicularis muscle are divided sharply, and the periosteum is incised and elevated to expose the sinus floor. The floor is penetrated with a large, round bur. The sinus is entered at this

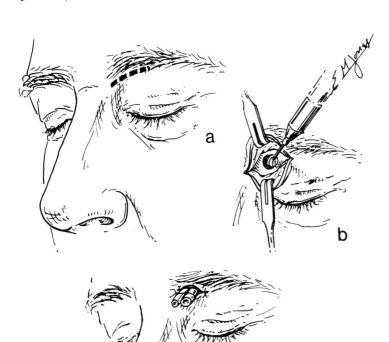

Figure 10–2. Frontal sinus trephine. *a,* Incision. *b,* Bur entry into the sinus. *c,* Double catheters anchored in position.

point, as it is the thinnest wall and contains no marrow spaces. In the preantibiotic era it was imperative not to enter the diploë, as the introduction of pus into it could produce osteomyelitis.[15] Loss of bone in this area does not produce a cosmetic deformity. Specimens are then taken for culture and sensitivity testing or for biopsy. Two small rubber catheters of different diameters are inserted into the opening and sutured to the adjacent skin. The incision is then closed with interrupted 4-0 nonabsorbable sutures.

The sinus is irrigated daily with saline through the larger catheter. Initially, the solution exits through the other catheter. However, as the mucosal edema subsides, the fluid will pass through the nasofrontal duct into the nose. The tubes are removed at this time. Failure to establish normal sinus drainage into the nasal cavity makes the patient a candidate for an external frontoethmoidectomy or osteoplastic flap procedure.

FRONTAL SEPTOPLASTY

Some authors[49, 117] have advocated the removal of the intersinus septum in patients with unilateral frontal sinusitis to provide drainage of the diseased sinus by the contralateral normally functioning one. In 1912, Lothrop[84] first reported removing the interfrontal septum along with the superior nasal septum to join the two nasofrontal ducts into a common opening. Newman and Travis[108] described removing the intersinus septum in cases of frontal sinus fracture with unilateral injury to the nasofrontal duct. Pope and Thompson[117] were successful with this method in treating 10 of 11 patients with chronic frontal sinusitis, who were followed for an average of 13.4 months. Goode and colleagues[49] extended its application to cases of bilateral chronic frontal sinusitis, by combining it with unilateral nasofrontal duct reconstruction. These workers also employed it in patients with nasofrontal duct injury following maxillectomy or ablative surgery for nasal tumors. They claimed satisfactory results with sinus septectomy in their series of 20 cases, but the majority of patients were followed less than 1 year.[49]

However, Williams and Holman[153] objected to a bilateral operation for unilateral disease because of the possibility of extending the infection to a previously uninvolved area. They observed delayed closure of the large common opening created by septectomy, similar to that seen with unilateral frontoethmoidectomy.

TECHNIQUE

The incision is made beneath the medial aspect of the unshaved eyebrow under local or general anesthesia. The skin and subcutaneous tissues are divided, and the periosteum is incised and elevated along the superciliary ridge. The sinus is entered medially through its floor with a round cutting bur. The opening is enlarged to 1.0 to 1.5 cm in diameter with a drill or rongeur until the intersinus septum is visualized. The septum is removed by bur or Kerrison rongeur, taking care not to injure the contralateral nasofrontal duct. A catheter tube drain is placed into the sinus and brought out through the incision, which is closed in layers. The catheter is removed when saline irrigation passes freely into the nose.

COLLAPSE PROCEDURE

Attempts were made to control chronic frontal sinus disease by obliterating the cavity by collapsing the overlying skin against the posterior wall. Initially, the anterior or orbital wall alone was removed;[67, 78] however, obliteration was successfully achieved only in patients with small sinuses. In 1898, Riedel[120] introduced a collapse procedure in which the anterior wall and floor of the sinus were removed, the mucosa stripped, and the soft tissues of the forehead apposed to the posterior wall. Although this procedure was more successful in eradicating disease, it was disfiguring and fell into disrepute. In an attempt to eliminate the cosmetic deformity, Killian[73] removed both the anterior and inferior walls but preserved the supraorbital ridge of bone. This procedure enjoyed brief popularity, but review of large series of cases by Lillie[82] and Anderson[6] revealed numerous complications and failure from residual pockets of infection. Subsequently, these ablative procedures were superseded by the nondeforming anterior osteoplastic flap with obliteration and the external frontoethmoidectomy with nasofrontal duct reconstruction, in the management of chronic inflammatory disease. However, the Riedel procedure continues to have application in patients with chronic osteomyelitis of the frontal bone who are refractory to antibiotic therapy and require resection of portions of nonviable bone.

TECHNIQUE

The operation may be performed through a direct brow or coronal approach similar to the

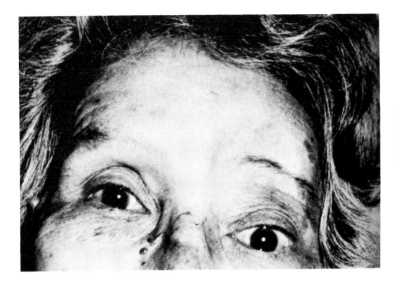

Figure 10–3. *A* 65-year-old woman developed proptosis and downward displacement of the left eye 20 years after a collapse (Riedel) procedure for osteomyelitis of the frontal sinus.

osteoplastic flap, depending on the extent of disease and esthetic considerations in a given case.

The flaps are elevated to expose the entire area of osseous involvement, and the osteomyelitic bone is removed with a rongeur until normal bleeding bone is encountered. This generally requires removal of the entire anterior table of the frontal sinus; occasionally the posterior table also must be resected.[103] The supraorbital ridges and the orbital wall of the sinus also must be removed even if uninvolved by disease, to achieve complete obliteration by permitting the soft tissues of the forehead to contact the entire posterior wall of the sinus. All bony ridges and septa must be drilled down and all mucosal remnants in all the recesses of the sinus must be removed, similar to the osteoplastic flap procedure. This requires drilling of the posterior table to remove microscopic tags of epithelium present in the pits produced by diploic veins. Supraorbital ethmoid cells also must be unroofed and their contents removed. Residual remnants of mucosa may result in mucocele formation despite seemingly complete collapse by the forehead and eyebrow skin against the posterior table or dura (Figs. 10–3 and 10–4). Specimens of the resected soft tissue and bone are sent for culture.

The operative field is copiously irrigated with saline. A Penrose drain is placed and the wound is closed in layers. Appropriate antibiotics are administered postoperatively for several weeks. After the patient is completely asymptomatic for 1 year, reconstruction of the defect by frontal cranioplasty may be undertaken.

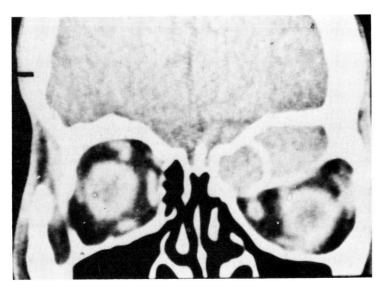

Figure 10–4. Computed tomography (CT) scan revealing the presence of two mucoceles that developed from retained mucosal remnants present beneath the forehead skin.

OSTEOMYELITIS

An acute or chronic pyogenic infection of the frontal sinus may extend to involve the surrounding bone.[21] The pathogenesis of the infection is by septic retrograde thrombophlebitis of diploic vessels leading into the medullary portion of the bone. It may then spread through the diploë to involve large portions of the cranium. Clinically, there is often a tender swelling over the involved sinus. An external pericranial abscess may form; it has a characteristic puffy or doughy appearance. In longstanding cases a fistula may develop.[21] Spread of the infection internally may result in such intracranial complications as meningitis and epidural, subdural, or brain abscess. In 25 cases of frontal sinus osteomyelitis reviewed by McNally and Stuart,[94] there was a fistula in 9, a subperiosteal abscess in 12, and an intracranial complication in 15.

Bacteriologically, the offending organisms are generally gram-positive cocci, especially *Staphylococcus aureus.* In the preantibiotic era, this complication of sinus disease carried a fearsome mortality, principally from intracranial extension.[152] Inner table involvement caused dural disease, with local abscess formation, meningoencephalitis, and thrombosis of the dural sinuses and the production of septic emboli and metastatic abscesses. Management during this period was by surgical drainage and extensive debridement of the involved bone, which was often microscopically involved far beyond the area of clinical disease.[103] This was performed through a coronal,[4, 72] eyebrow,[69, 138] or combined median forehead and eyebrow incision.[103]

Presently, osteomyelitis of the frontal sinus is treated by antibiotic therapy, with many cases responding to medical management alone. It may be necessary to perform a trephine if an air-fluid level is demonstrated radiographically within the sinus. In some cases a direct approach to the sinus may be necessary to debride the necrotic bone. Appropriate antibiotic administration should be maintained postoperatively for 6 weeks. After the infectious process is controlled, it may be necessary to perform an osteoplastic flap with sinus obliteration following removal of the diseased mucosa. When the osseous infection persists, it may be necessary to perform a collapse type of procedure after removal of all the necrotic tissue and nonviable bone (Figs. 10–5 through 10–7). The contour defect in the forehead can be reconstructed later by a cranioplastic procedure.

EXTERNAL FRONTOETHMOIDECTOMY

The transorbital approach to the frontal sinus through its inferior wall was first employed in Europe by Jansen[67] in 1902 and by Ritter[122] in 1911. In 1908, Knapp[76] described the procedure virtually in its present form in the American literature, although later workers[61, 88] have been credited with it. He made an incision along the medial and upper aspect of the orbit below the eyebrow (in distinction to the intrabrow incision

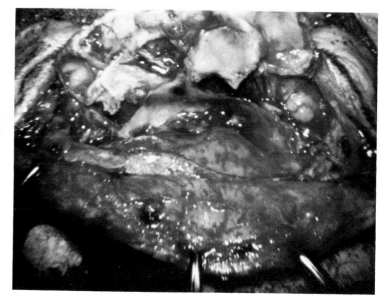

Figure 10–5. Patient with clinical and radiographic evidence of chronic frontal sinusitis. Surgical exploration through an eyebrow incision reveals extensive osteomyelitis of the anterior table.

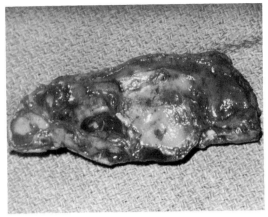

Figure 10–6. Removed portion of necrotic bone from patient in Figure 10–5.

of Killian); removed the floor of the frontal sinus, lamina papyracea, lacrimal bone and nasal process of the maxilla; and performed a complete ethmoidectomy. With an unusually high frontal sinus, an opening was also made in the anterior wall to facilitate removal of the mucosa. In 1921, Lynch[88] in the United States and Howarth[61] in England simultaneously reported their experience with the transorbital frontal sinusotomy and ethmoidectomy. In his 15 cases, Lynch[88] partially removed the sinus floor and curetted out all the mucosa and stressed drainage of the sphenoid sinus. Howarth,[61] in his review of more than 200 cases, resected the entire floor of the sinus, did not remove the mucosa, and stressed the importance of a preliminary intranasal ethmoidec-

tomy. Both workers temporarily placed a rubber tube drain into the nose.

The operative procedure has remained essentially unchanged since the early part of this century and continues to have many advocates. Most of the proposed modifications concerned maintenance of the patency of the nasofrontal duct and will be discussed later. Williams and Holman[153] suggested the use of a drill to remove all mucosal remnants from the sinus cavity and to detect and unroof an interfrontal septum cell, which if present, is a potential source of latent infection. They claimed excellent results in more than 50 cases so treated. Baron and colleagues[5] considered the external frontoethmoidectomy with flap reconstruction the procedure of choice for all frontal sinus pathology except the large osteoma.

INDICATIONS AND LIMITATIONS

The external frontoethmoidectomy gains its widest application in patients with frontal sinus disease who have small or extremely large sinuses. With a small sinus, it may be possible to remove all the diseased mucosal lining. With the large sinus, the successful recreation of the nasofrontal duct may obviate the need for the more extensive osteoplastic flap procedure. When the acute inflammatory disease has extended into the orbit, this approach provides both orbital drainage and decompression and permits the removal of disease in the ethmoid and frontal sinuses. It also offers a direct approach for the removal of the frontoethmoid mucocele and osteoma (Fig. 10–8). The access

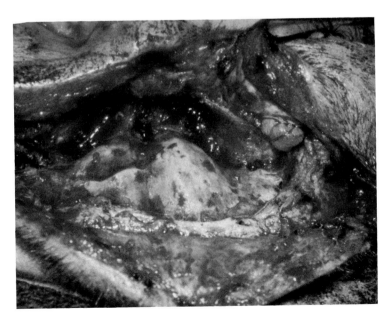

Figure 10–7. The anterior table and supraorbital ridges have been removed, and the posterior wall has been burred, preliminary to collapse of the forehead skin (same patient as in Figures 10–5 and 10–6).

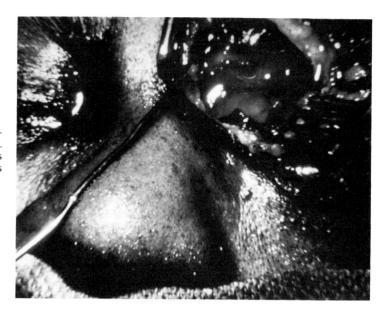

Figure 10–8. Frontoethmoidal mucocele causing proptosis of the left eye. Transorbital (Knapp) approach gives direct access to the lesion that has eroded the overlying bone.

gained to the superior nasal cavity through the external ethmoidectomy also finds application in the repair of cerebrospinal leaks, as well as sphenoid biopsy.

Another application of the external ethmoidectomy is to decompress mucoceles with intracranial extension, either as primary management or preliminary to performing an osteoplastic flap.[66] Following decompression, the sinus cavity contracts markedly, greatly facilitating performance of the osteoplastic flap operation with fat obliteration. This is especially well suited for patients with polypoid mucoceles, which tend to be bilateral and multisinus and have both orbital and intracranial extension. I have done this in two patients with excellent results, judged by regression of the mucocele cavities and resolution of the proptosis.

The advantages of the external frontoethmoidectomy are (1) it can be performed through a relatively small and cosmetically acceptable incision (Knapp incision); (2) it provides access to the ethmoid and sphenoid sinuses, as well as to the frontal sinus; and (3) it is not deforming, as the area of bone removal does not affect facial contour. The disadvantages of the procedure are (1) it is for unilateral disease; (2) it does not provide adequate exposure for the removal of all the mucosa in a large or septate sinus; (3) it does not produce sinus obliteration; (4) communication with the nose and other paranasal sinuses may result in infection by contiguous spread; and (5) the subsequent closure of the newly enlarged nasofrontal duct will cause recurrent infection or the formation of a mucocele.

There is considerable laboratory and clinical evidence of the limitations of the external frontoethmoidectomy operation. Several experiments have been performed in dogs to assess the effect of removal of the sinus mucosa and manipulation of the nasofrontal duct. Coates and Ersner[24] reported that complete removal of the mucosa of the frontal sinus was followed by only slight constriction of the cavity by a layer of fibrous tissue over which mucosa had regenerated. However, Hilding[58] found total removal of the lining mucosa to result in partial or complete obliteration of the cavity by dense fibrous tissue containing epithelium-lined, mucin-filled cystic spaces. Walsh[148] demonstrated that enlargement of the nasofrontal duct produced chronic infection of the sinus when the mucosa was intact. If it was radically removed, fibrous tissue containing bone, epithelium, and pus filled the sinus cavity. Mucosal removal without disturbance of the nasofrontal duct was followed by epithelial regeneration within the sinus. Neel and colleagues[106] also observed enlargement of the nasofrontal duct to result in partial obliteration of the frontal sinus, with hyperplastic mucosa containing large glands and cysts, fibrous tissue, new bone, and mucopus. Hilding and Banovetz[59] showed that removal of a strip of mucoperiosteum from the sinus resulted in the formation of bone-containing scar. With an annular loss of the mucosal lining, the scar produced was diaphragmatic, dividing the sinus into two cavities. Although epithelial regeneration occurred, it was poorly ciliated and resulted in mucous stasis.

Although the findings of these studies are

not in complete agreement, they permit certain conclusions. First, total removal of the mucosa often results in fibrous tissue proliferation; however, complete obliteration of the sinus cavity does not occur consistently. Second, there is a tendency toward the epithelialization of the sinus cavity following its denudation, from the mucosa of the nasofrontal duct or by retained microscopic tissue tags within the sinus itself. Consequently, if this method of open surgery is to be successfully performed, patency of the nasofrontal duct is essential. The finding by Walsh[148] that instrumentation of the duct led to chronic infection of the sinus has caused some workers[87] to advocate transorbital frontal sinusotomy without duct manipulation or enlargement. However, in many cases the chronic frontal sinus disease is the result of occlusion of the duct and requires its enlargement for drainage.

Clinically, the primary cause of failure of the external frontoethmoidectomy procedure has been repeatedly identified as closure of the nasofrontal duct by fibrous tissue or regenerated bone.[44, 56, 150] Harris[56] reported a 20 per cent failure rate after external frontoethmoidectomy. Goodale[44] on review of 182 cases from the Massachusetts Eye and Ear Infirmary, found a recurrence rate of 30.8 per cent following surgery for infection and 22.2 per cent for mucoceles. Williams and Holman[153] claimed that as many as one third of these procedures performed at the Mayo Clinic failed, given sufficient follow-up. Consequently, a variety of methods of stenting or resurfacing the newly enlarged nasofrontal duct have been devised in an attempt to maintain its patency.

Tubes constructed of various materials have been temporarily or permanently implanted. Rubber tubes were inserted by Howarth[61] and Lynch.[88] Tantalum foil tubes were implanted by Scharfe,[128] McNally and Stuart,[94] Harris,[56] and Goodale.[45] An acrylic obturator was inserted by Erich and New.[38] Portex tubes were employed by Wolfowitz and Solomon.[156] However, it soon became apparent that the improved biocompatibility of the stenting material and its prolonged use did not guarantee patency of the nasofrontal duct. McNally and Stuart[94] reported several cases in which duct closure occurred within a few weeks following tube removal, despite 6 months of implantation. This led several workers to place a permanent indwelling tube. Ingals[65] originally described the temporary intranasal insertion of a gold tube into the nasofrontal duct. The permanent placement of such a tube following external frontoethmoidectomy was later reported in 10 patients by Anthony[7] and in 2 by Lyman.[87] Barton[9] also described the successful permanent implantation of a Dacron tube in 34 patients.

Neel and colleagues[106] performed an experimental study of the comparative effectiveness of silicone tubing and sheeting in maintaining nasofrontal duct patency. Although Silastic tubes eliminated epithelialization and failed to prevent osteoblastic reaction, fibroplasia, and scar formation from occurring in dogs, the opposite was observed with rolled sheets of the rubber. Clinically, surgery failed in two of the three patients having silicone tubes placed for 6 to 8 weeks after external frontoethmoidectomy. However, in only 1 of 14 patients did use of rolled sheeting result in failure.

Attempts have been made to re-epithelialize the surgically enlarged duct by the placement of grafts and the rotation of flaps. Free mucous membrane grafts from the nose and lip were employed by Mithoefer[99] and skin grafts were placed by Negus[107] and Smith.[139] However, grafting has proved unsuccessful and has been replaced by flap techniques in which pedicled nasal mucosa is transposed into an enlarged sinus opening.

Sewall[135] and McNaught[95] demonstrated that the nasofrontal duct remained operative if one side was epithelialized. Sewall[135] devised a medially based mucoperiosteal flap to partially resurface the surgical neoduct. After the frontoethmoidectomy was completed, the lateral nasal wall was removed, creating a flap from the underlying mucosa, which was based on the septum and which could be turned upward into the frontal sinus. The flap was maintained in position with a Portex tube for 7 days. This procedure was popularized by Boyden,[18, 19] who reported complete success in 97 cases. McNaught[95] described a laterally based mucoperiosteal flap used in cases with large frontal sinuses and a narrow nasal vault, especially with bilateral involvement. The floor of the frontal sinus, interfrontal septum, and anterior bony nasal septum was removed (Lothrop procedure), creating a large common nasal and frontal cavity. This was lined with unilateral or bilateral flaps elevated from the nasal septum and based on the mucosa under the nasal process of the maxilla. Ogura and colleagues,[111] after performing a complete ethmoidectomy, opened the floor of the frontal sinus, removed portions of the nasal and lacrimal bones, the frontal process of the maxilla, the intersinus septum, and the perpendicular plate of the ethmoid and mobilized bilateral septal mucoperiosteal flaps into the frontal floor area. They claimed success in 19 of 20 patients eligible for follow-up. Dokianakis and colleagues[30] created a modification in which a mucoperiosteal flap taken from the upper portion of the middle turbinate was transferred to the intersinus septum. They claimed success in 22 of 24 patients. Porto and Duvall[118] reported a 14 per cent failure rate in 50 patients with chronic frontal sinusitis (including 22 mucoceles) undergoing external ethmoidectomy, with nasofrontal duct reconstruction using a mucoperiosteal flap, after an average follow-up of 8 years. Reports of the successful use of mucoperiosteal flaps for resurfacing the nasofrontal duct after external frontoethmoidectomy were also made by Williams and Holman[153] and Baron and colleagues.[8]

TECHNIQUE (Fig. 10–9)

The procedure is performed under general endotracheal anesthesia. After the face is prepared and draped, a tarsorrhaphy suture of 5-0 silk is placed to protect the cornea. A curvilinear incision is outlined with methylene blue just beneath the medial aspect of the unshaved eyebrow and is carried downward midway between the inner canthus and the dorsum of the nose along the nasal process of the maxilla to a point just below the inner canthus. The skin of the proposed incision, which measures 4 to 6 cm in length, is cross-hatched to facilitate skin approximation later. After the skin is divided, the underlying soft tissues are sectioned in layers. Branches of the angular blood vessels are ligated or electrocauterized for hemostasis. The periosteum is incised and elevated with a Freer elevator. Sutures of 3-0 silk may be placed to facilitate the retraction of the wound margins. The periosteum is readily elevated laterally until the lacrimal crest is reached, where added pressure on the instrument is required to detach the anterior and posterior portions of the medial canthal ligament. When this has been accomplished, the lacrimal sac is retracted laterally. The use of a narrow, malleable ribbon retractor or orbital retractor permits atraumatic retraction of the globe. Continued

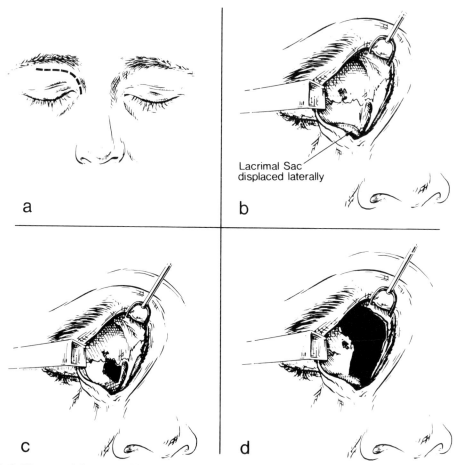

Figure 10–9. Diagram of the external (transorbital) frontoethmoidectomy. *a,* Incision. *b,* Exposure of the medial orbital wall. *c,* Entry into the ethmoid labyrinth through the lamina papyracea. *d,* Completed frontoethmoidectomy.

elevation of the periorbita along the medial aspect of the orbit exposes the lamina papyracea of the ethmoid. Periosteal elevation upward permits identification of the frontoethmoid suture. This is a key landmark, as the anterior and posterior ethmoid vessels run through it and superior to it is the anterior cranial fossa.

Knowledge of the anatomy of these vessels is indispensable in performing this operation (Fig. 10–10). In a classic study of 150 orbits, Kirchner and colleagues[75] found the anterior ethmoid foramen within the frontoethmoid suture line in 68 per cent of the specimens and 1 to 4 mm above it in the remaining 32 per cent. In 5 of 70 preserved orbits examined, the artery was absent. The distance from the maxillolacrimal suture line to the anterior ethmoid foramen was 14 to 18 mm in 64 per cent of the orbits; however, the distance ranged from 9 to 27 mm. The distance from the anterior ethmoid foramen to the posterior ethmoid foramen averaged 10 to 11 mm. The posterior ethmoid foramen was present in the frontoethmoid suture line in 87 per cent of the specimens and was immediately superior to it in the remainder. As with the anterior ethmoid foramen, it was never below the suture line. The posterior ethmoid artery was absent in 22 of 70 orbits studied. While the anterior ethmoid artery is larger than the posterior one, in four orbits the opposite was found. The distance from the posterior ethmoid foramen to the optic nerve was relatively constant, being 4 to 7 mm in 84 per cent of the skulls. However, the optic nerve entered the orbit at an acute angle to the medial orbital wall and actually lies 1 to 2 mm from the posterior ethmoid artery as it passes from the orbital soft tissues to its foramen. This places the optic nerve at considerable risk for injury with dissection, ligature passage, and electrocautery of

the posterior ethmoid artery. Caution also must be exercised in attempting to ligate or clip the anterior ethmoid artery when the frontoethmoid junction is very acute, as the risk for vessel rupture and retraction is great under these circumstances.

After the anterior ethmoid artery is identified, it is clipped or electrocauterized and divided. Care should be taken in cutting and retracting this vessel to prevent herniation of fat through the attenuated periorbita at this point. The periosteum is elevated backward to the smaller posterior ethmoid artery, which is identified but not ligated because of its proximity to the optic nerve. The periosteum covering the floor of the frontal sinus is now elevated.

The ethmoid labyrinth is entered through the lamina papyracea with a straight punch. The overlying cortical bone forming the medial aspect of the orbit is removed with angled punches (e.g., Kerrison rongeur). This is carried superiorly to the frontoethmoid suture line, posteriorly to the level of the posterior ethmoid artery, and anteriorly to the lacrimal fossa. The contents of the ethmoid labyrinth are removed, and it is converted into one large confluent cavity by removing the bony septa between cells. The nasal mucosa may be preserved if it is to be utilized for a flap to partially resurface the reconstructed nasofrontal duct. The bony dissection is continued upward anteriorly until the frontal sinus is entered medially. The floor of the sinus is opened with a right-angle type of punch forceps. The mucosa is completely stripped from the frontal sinus. It may be necessary to use a bur to enlarge the newly formed nasofrontal duct sufficiently. It is also generally necessary to resect the middle turbinate intranasally with an angled scissors. The attachment of the middle turbinate is another landmark, as the cribriform plate is situated medial to it. At this point it is possible to inspect the roof of the ethmoid labyrinth, cribriform plate, and face of the sphenoid sinus. The ostium of the sphenoid may be found medially in the plane of the posterior ethmoid artery. A Silastic tube, 1 cm in diameter, is placed into the newly reconstructed duct (Fig. 10–11) and anchored superiorly with a 4-0 nylon suture tied over a button in the eyebrow. The tube is left in position for 8 to 10 weeks and is removed intranasally. The wound is now reinspected, and meticulous hemostasis is obtained. It is preferable not to pack the nasal cavity to permit dependent drainage rather than risk increased intraorbital pressure. The periosteum is carefully approximated with 4-0 chromic cat-

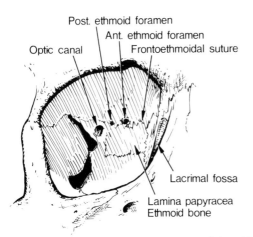

Figure 10–10. Anatomy of the medial aspect of the orbit.

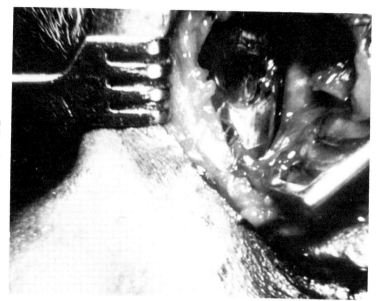

Figure 10–11. Following exenteration of the ethmoid labyrinth and removal of the floor of the frontal sinus, a Silastic tube is placed through the neoduct into the nasal cavity.

gut sutures. It must be securely reattached to anchor the medial canthal ligament. The skin is closed with interrupted sutures of 5-0 nylon. The incision is covered with an antibiotic ointment. It is best to leave the eye uncovered so that any intraorbital bleeding is immediately recognized and rapidly decompressed.

MODIFICATIONS

The basic operative procedure involves total or partial removal of the inferior wall of the frontal sinus in conjunction with a transorbital ethmoidectomy. The amount of bone removed from the medial wall of the orbit and the nasal pyramid depends on whether flap reconstruction of the lining of the nasofrontal duct is to be performed. Although the majority of workers enlarge the nasofrontal duct and employ some type of resurfacing or stenting, a small group avoids instrumenting it. Patterson[114] devised an orbital incision that extended from the inner canthus downward to the infraorbital rim. Through this opening he was able to remove the ethmoid labyrinth, unroof the nasofrontal duct, and expose the floor of the frontal sinus.

COMPLICATIONS

Complications of the external frontoethmoidectomy arise from subsequent closure to the nasofrontal duct and operative injury to regional structures. Loss of patency of the duct results in sinus obstruction with secondary mucocele formation.

Within the orbit, blood vessels, the lacrimal apparatus, and the trochlea are structures at risk. Incomplete ligation or electrocautery of the ethmoid blood vessels, or damage to the ciliary veins by traction on the globe, may result in bleeding within the periorbita, with formation of an orbital hematoma. Visual loss may be caused by retinal artery thrombosis from a retrobulbar hematoma or direct injury to the optic nerve from dissection or electrocautery too far posteriorly in the orbit. Injury to the lacrimal sac may produce scarring and stenosis, with epiphora or dacryocystitis occurring postoperatively. Damage to, or failure of, reattachment of the trochlea produces imbalance of the superior oblique muscle with diplopia developing. Failure to adequately reattach the medial canthal ligament may cause pseudohypertelorism. Care also must be taken to attach the ligament at the same level as the opposite side. Removal of bone above the frontoethmoid suture line posteriorly may result in injury to the dura of the anterior cranial fossa and cerebrospinal fluid leak.

OSTEOPLASTIC FLAP

The direct approach to the frontal sinus by creating a hinged osteoperiosteal flap of its anterior wall was first reported by Schonborn[131] in 1894 and Brieger[20] in 1895 in Europe. Subsequent modifications were introduced by Winkler,[155] Gussenbauer,[53] Czerny,[26] and Hoffman.[60] Winkler[155] and Beck[11] stressed the value of radiographs in performing the operation. In Latin America, an anterior osteoplastic approach to the frontal sinus accompanied by fat obliteration had been performed by Bergara[13] and Tato and colleagues[142] since the 1940s. At the time of his publication in 1955, Bergara[14] had operated on 104 patients.

In the United States, the procedure was first performed by Goodale and Montgomery[46] in 1958 and was popularized by thier subsequent publications.[47, 48] The collective experience with 100 cases treated at the Massachusetts Eye and Ear Infirmary was reported by Zonis and colleagues[157] and later with 250 cases by Hardy and Montgomery.[55]

Advantages of the osteoplastic flap technique include (1) direct visualization of both frontal sinuses; (2) access to the supraorbital ethmoids; (3) absence of a cosmetic deformity; (4) elimination of the need for the nasofrontal duct for drainage; and (5) obliteration of the sinus cavity. The disadvantages of the procedure relate to (1) its more extensive nature, with accompanying larger incisions and greater blood loss; (2) the need to remove all mucosal remnants within the sinus; and (3) complications, which include abnormal healing of the bone flap, scar camouflage, and nerve injuries.

The procedure may be performed directly through an incision in the eyebrow, or a forehead crease,[89] or indirectly by a coronal approach with the incision placed in or behind the hairline.[5, 42, 43, 113] Although a superiorly based bone flap has been designed,[123, 135] most workers employ one based inferiorly,[13, 142] after elevating the skin completely from the periosteum overlying the frontal sinus. A modification, originally devised by Kuster[79] and later reintroduced by Gibson and Walker[42] for the removal of a large osteoma, consisted of leaving the skin attached to the bone flap. This was popularized by MacBeth[89] and Bosley,[17] who later reported the results of 100 cases treated by this method. These latter workers do not implant the sinus but rely on natural obliteration.

Sinus obliteration has become an integral part of the frontal osteoplastic operation; however, the manner in which this is best achieved is controversial. Although there is considerable evidence supporting the efficacy of careful stripping of the sinus mucosa along with removal of the inner cortical layer and the implantation of autogenous material in accomplishing obliteration, as noted earlier, a small group of workers leaves the cavity empty in the expectation of auto-obliteration. A controversy also exists over the need to block the nasofrontal duct, to prevent regeneration of epithelium within the sinus. Although Montgomery[100] does not close

the duct in the belief that the revascularized implanted fat will prevent mucosal proliferation, the duct is plugged with fascia by Alford and colleagues[5] and Sessions and colleagues,[134] with muscle by Siirala,[137] and with bone by Grahne.[50] Consequently, it is essential to review the available laboratory and clinical data concerning the effectiveness of various materials and operative methods in accomplishing obliteration, in order to select the best therapeutic approach.

SINUS OBLITERATION

Frontal osteoplasty has been performed with and without the implantation of the sinus cavity. Osteoplasty without the placement of an embedded material relies on osteoneogenesis for obliteration. The materials implanted include a variety of autogenous and alloplastic substances. Alloplastic materials have been employed principally to eliminate the second procedure required to obtain an autograft.

Experimental Studies. Bergara and Itoiz[14] reported in 1955 that boiled homograft fat placed in the canine frontal sinus underwent fibrous transformation, whereas autograft fat persisted as adipose tissue. In 1963, Montgomery and Pierce[102] demonstrated in cats that implanted autogenous fat accomplished total obliteration of the sinus cavity and was resistant to infection and osteoneogenesis if the mucous membrane and the inner cortical bony lining were removed completely. Mucous membrane also failed to regenerate in the obliterated cavity. Montgomery and Ormon[101] considered adipose tissue to be an inhibitor of osteoneogenesis. Montgomery[100] stated that revascularization of the fat graft occurred within a few days by direct blood vessel anastomosis.

McNeil[96] confirmed this in the implanted feline frontal sinus. However, if the fat was traumatized or the cavity infected, it was transformed to fibrous tissue. He also experimentally implanted muscle, Gelfoam, and blood clot, all of which failed to achieve obliteration. Bovine cartilage was observed to be slowly transformed to bone.

Abramson et al[1, 2] showed that cancellous bone autografts and frozen allografts were transformed into organized bone and obliterated the canine sinus cavity. This was found to occur even in the presence of acute suppurative inflammatory disease, if the mucous membrane was completely removed.[37] Abramson et al[1] concluded that the absence of mucosal regeneration was the most important factor in achieving successful obliteration of the frontal sinus by grafting.

Sessions and colleagues[134] implanted fat, blood clot, synthetic collagen, and Silastic elastomer into the infected frontal sinuses of cats. They also demonstrated obliteration of the cavity if all the mucosa was removed.

Schenck[129] showed in dogs that the removal of the mucosa and the stripping of the periosteum of the canine frontal sinus resulted in incomplete obliteration if the nasofrontal duct was patent. Closure of the nasofrontal duct was found to promote osteoneogenesis. He concluded the osteoneogenesis could not be relied on to produce obliteration of the frontal sinus and demonstrated the formation of microcysts in experimental animals. He also showed that leaving a strip of mucosa in the sinus led to failure of obliteration of new bone formation in 100 per cent of the animals and caused mucocele formation.

Dickson and Hohman[29] implanted the denuded frontal sinus of cats with Gelfoam, blood clot, denatured fat, Teflon paste, paraffin, Silastic sponge, and Neocortef ointment. Partial obliteration was observed with Gelfoam, blood clot, and denatured fat. The implantation of Teflon paste, paraffin, and antibiotic ointment prevented sinus obliteration. Decreasing cavity obliteration by fibrous tissue and osteogenesis occurred with increasing time.

Janeke and colleagues[68] showed the ingrowth of osteoid tissue into proplast (a Teflon fluorocarbon polymer and vitreous carbon fiber combination) placed into the frontal sinus of cats. Schenck and colleagues[130] successfully implanted proplast in the denuded canine frontal sinus with and without a patent nasofrontal duct and noted bony obliteration in all animals within 1 year.

In summary, although various substances have been successfully used to obliterate the properly prepared sinus cavity, considerable experimental evidence supports the superior ability of implanted autogenous fat. The removal of all mucosal tissue is of paramount importance in all obliterative procedures. If the cavity is to be grafted, no special attention to the nasofrontal duct is necessary. However, if auto-obliteration by fibrous tissue or bone is to be relied upon, occlusion of the duct is vital. It was demonstrated early by Walsh[148] and Hilding[58] that the radical removal of the lining mucosa of the canine frontal sinus was followed by re-epithelialization of the sinus cavity and proliferation of fibrous tissue filled with epithelium-lined cysts, if the patency of the nasofrontal duct was preserved.

Donald[31] stressed the importance of drilling away the inner cortical layer of the sinus preliminary to obliteration. Simple curettage resulted in mucosal regrowth from epithelial remnants present in vascular pits in the bone through which diploic veins (veins of Breschet) passed. He observed total obliteration of the sinus in only 18 per cent of the cats implanted with fat after curettage alone.

In an experimental study of frontal sinus fractures in cats, Hybels and Newman[63] noted that fat implantation resulted in sinus obliteration, with incomplete survival of the fat but with fibrous tissue and new bone filling the remaining space as long as all the mucosa had been removed. The viable fat prevented mucosal ingrowth from the nasofrontal duct forming a blind pouch that drained into the nose. These workers also showed osteoneogenesis to achieve spontaneous obliteration in nongrafted sinuses. Osseous proliferation was most prominent in those sinuses in which the bone had been decorticated.

Clinical Studies. A variety of biologic and synthetic substances have been implanted in the human frontal sinus following osteoplasty. Tato and colleagues[142] filled the cavity with fibrin and gelatin sponge, coagulated blood, desiccated serum, and plasma, as well as fat. Naumann[105] also reported implanting plasma, fibrin, and Gelfoam in the frontal sinus. Siirala[137] reported successful obliteration of the frontal sinus in four patients with ossar, a protein-free bovine bone. Schwartzman and Silva[133] filled the sinus with preserved homograft bone. Grahne[50] reported successful osteoplasty in 11 patients in whom autogenous iliac bone was implanted. In his method, the anterior sinus wall was removed through a brow incision, the mucosal lining was microscopically excised, the nasofrontal duct was plugged with bone, the sinus was filled with cancellous bone, and the anterior wall was reconstructed with cortical plate.

Beeson[12] observed plaster of Paris implanted in the canine frontal sinus to accomplish obliteration by inducing osteoneogenesis. Coetzee[25] used this substance to fill the defects produced by large mucoceles in three patients.

With regard to synthetic alloplastic materials, Failla[39] reported good results in obliterating the traumatized frontal sinus with acrylic. Barton[10] reported successful obliteration with proplast in eight patients with chronic frontal sinusitis followed postoperatively for 1 to 5 years. However, the radiographic appearance of the obliterated cavity more closely resembled fibrous tissue than replacement with bone.

Autogenous adipose tissue is the substance most widely employed for frontal sinus obliteration. In 1910, Marx[91] reported implantation of the frontal sinus with fat to efface the defect produced by removal of the anterior table. Malecki[90] later employed this method in combination with tamponade of the nasofrontal duct by a periosteal-galeal flap. In the 1950s, Bergara[13] successfully employed abdominal fat and Tato and colleagues[142] achieved obliteration of the frontal sinus with autograft fat, homograft fat, and homograft fat mixed with the patient's blood through an anterior osteoplastic flap. Reoperation and biopsy of the previously implanted fat in two patients showed it to have remained viable.[142] The success of the South American workers prompted Goodale and Montgomery[46] to attempt frontal osteoplasty with autografting. They described their experience with seven osteoplastic flaps, of which five also had fat obliteration. Subsequent extensive clinical experience with autograft fat implantation has substantiated the findings in laboratory animals. Its effectiveness in obliterating the properly prepared sinus cavity has made it the standard material presently used.

Denneny[27] reported obliterating the frontal sinus in 11 patients with fat harvested from the abdomen or thigh by liposuction. He claimed no complications after 4 to 16 months of follow-up.

However, MacBeth[89] and Bosley[17] do not implant the sinus following the creation of an osteoplastic flap but rely on natural obliteration by osteoneogenesis. They indicate as advantages of this technique (1) the elimination of the need to implant an alloplastic or autogenous material; (2) the elimination of a second operation to secure a graft; and (3) a decreased incidence of ascending infection from the nose because of osseous occlusion of the nasofrontal duct. However, critics of this method cite the experimental studies that demonstrate the unreliability and incompleteness of auto-obliteration.

Another method of obliteration of the frontal sinus, called cranialization, involves removal of its posterior wall, permitting herniation of the brain and dura forward. This was originally performed in 1937 for osteomyelitis by Adson and Hempstead[4] through an intracranial approach. In 1959, Malecki[90] employed it for fractures of the posterior table after removing the sinus mucosa through a craniotomy. Donald and Bernstein[34] extended its use in 1978 to severe compound fractures of the anterior and posterior tables. The anterior table fragments are removed, cleansed, soaked in Betadine, and replaced as free grafts, following meticulous removal of the sinus mucosa, along with the posterior table, and occlusion of the nasofrontal ducts with temporalis muscle. They considered cranialization superior to fat obliteration in such traumatic cases because of the absence of the highly vascular bed necessary for the nourishment of adipose tissue. Donald[32] failed to observe difficulties with bone resorption or mucocele formation in 25 cases so treated.

INDICATIONS

Unlike the transorbital approach in which the frontal, ethmoid, and often the sphenoid sinuses are converted to a common draining cavity, in the osteoplastic approach the frontal sinus is treated as an independent entity. Consequently, ideal cases are ones in which the frontal sinus alone is involved, by chronic inflammation or by an osteoma (Figs. 10–12 and 10–13), a mucocele, or an ethmoid air cell occluding the nasofrontal duct. Cases with pansinus involvement by inflammatory disease also require intranasal, transantral, or external sphenoethmoidectomy. Failure to control infection in the adjacent sinuses may result in operative failure with the frontal sinus, with flap or graft necrosis. The osteoplastic flap with sinus obliteration also has a role in the management of fractures of the frontal sinus, especially those having extensive comminution of the anterior table or involvement of the posterior table or the nasofrontal duct.

In the series of 250 cases reported by Hardy and Montgomery,[55] an osteoplastic flap was performed for chronic infection in 190 (76 per cent), osteoma in 25 (10 per cent), trauma in 25 (10 per cent), and miscellaneous reasons (principally neoplastic) in the remaining 10 patients (4 per cent). Among the patients with chronic infection, 60 per cent had unilateral disease, and 61 per cent had mucoceles. In the group with osteomas, 76 per cent were unilateral, and in about 50 per cent secondary chronic sinusitis was present. In 23 patients, erosion of bone was present, 6 having dural exposure. Among the 100 consecutive osteoplastic flaps performed by the MacBeth technique and reported by Bosley,[17] surgery was performed in 6 patients for trauma, in 13 for osteoma, in 56 patients for unoperated frontal sinusitis, and in 25 patients for frontal sinusitis with previous surgery. However, at the time of surgery, frontal sinusitis was evident in 94 cases and localized osteomyelitis in 42 cases. Mucoceles were found

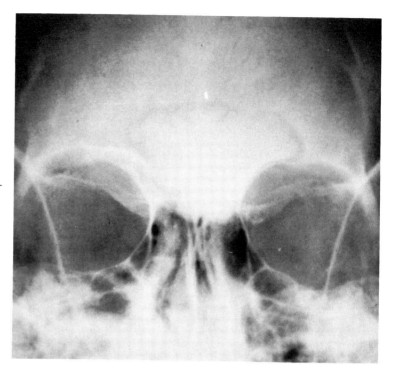

Figure 10–12. Large osteoma entirely filling both frontal sinuses.

in 13 of the 75 unoperated and in 4 of the 25 previously operated cases. In the 53 cases reported by Sessions et al,[134] 15 operations were for chronic sinusitis, 23 for trauma, 10 for mucoceles, and 5 for osteomas.

The use of the osteoplastic flap for traumatic injuries of the frontal sinus was reported by Valenzuela[145] and Failla.[39] Kirchner[74] extended its application to the removal of cholesteatomas

and dermoid cysts of the orbital roof with involvement of the frontal bone.

The osteoplastic flap has been frequently employed for revision frontal sinus surgery. Among the 250 cases of Hardy and Montgomery,[55] 42 per cent (104 patients) had prior frontal sinus surgery. This included the Lynch procedure in 46, trephination in 37, duct probing in 8, the Riedel procedure in 6, an osteoplastic

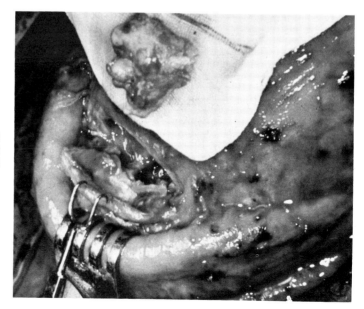

Figure 10–13. The osteoma was removed through a coronal approach. Attachment to the posterior table was severed by drill and osteotome.

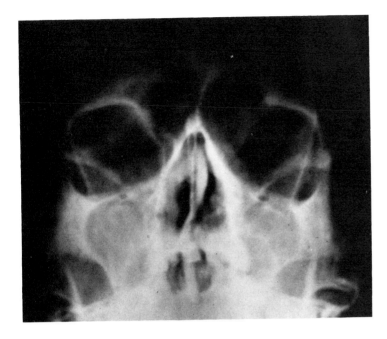

Figure 10–14. Plain radiograph of a patient with chronic bilateral frontal headache who developed lateral displacement of the left eye. Note the loss of scalloping of the borders of both frontal sinuses and destruction of the superomedial aspect of the left orbit.

flap in 5, and unspecified operations in 2 patients. Among the 25 cases of Bosley[17] undergoing revision surgery, 15 trephines, 6 Lynch procedures, and 4 osteoplastic flaps had been performed.

Even though the osteoplastic flap has gained wide application and success in treatment of mucoceles (Figs. 10–14 through 10–16), it is not an infallible modality. In a series of 56 frontal mucoceles reviewed by Bordley and Bosley,[16] there were 9 recurrences. This occurred in 4 of 22 osteoplastic flaps, 2 of 6 osteoplastic flaps with fat obliteration, 2 of 6 Lynch procedures, and 1 of 21 collapse procedures. Among 26 patients with mucoceles who had previous surgery, the mean interval to the treatment of the mucocele was 7.5 years, with a range of 1 to 42 years. Consequently, prolonged follow-up is mandatory in accurately assessing the efficacy of any procedure in curing frontal sinus disease.

The symptoms in operated cases reflect the presence of chronic sinusitis or its complications. Among the 250 patients of Hardy and Montgomery[55] who underwent frontal osteoplasty, there were frontal pain and headache in 61 per cent, forehead or periorbital swelling in 27 per cent, fistula in 5 per cent, and diplopia in 4 per cent. In 11 per cent of the patients, there was painless swelling or proptosis. In 12 per cent, the presenting symptoms were related to central nervous system or orbital complications (meningitis, brain abscess, orbital cellulitis, osteomyelitis). The great majority of the cases with extension of disease did not have an antecedent history of chronic sinusitis. Bilateral disease was present in 37 per cent of the cases. All 100 patients reviewed by Bosley[17] complained of headache; 13 had nasal discharge; in 27 periorbital swelling was present; and in 9 diplopia and proptosis occurred.

Another application of the osteoplastic flap is to cease the aeration and decrease the cosmetic deformity encountered with the abnormally enlarged frontal sinus. The excessively enlarged, aerated frontal sinus may be divided into three categories.[143] The hyper (pneumatized) sinus is one that has formed beyond the standard limits of development. In pneumosi-

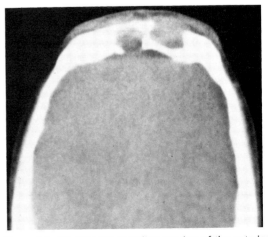

Figure 10–15. CT scan revealing erosion of the anterior table of the left frontal sinus and the posterior table of the right one.

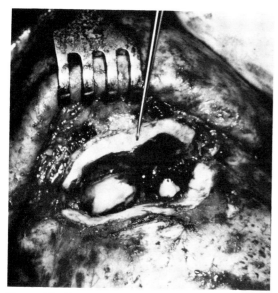

Figure 10–16. Surgical exploration through an osteoplastic flap, coronal approach, confirms the presence of bilateral frontal mucopyoceles.

nus dilatans, the entire sinus, or a portion, aerates beyond the confines of the frontal bone, producing cosmetic deformity or local symptoms. The pneumocele additionally causes thinning of the overlying bone. I have performed an osteoplastic flap with fat obliteration in the latter two conditions. The margins of the bone flap were drilled down to recess the anterior table into the sinus and reduce the frontal bossing.

SUCCESS RATE AND COMPLICATIONS

Bergara[14] reported operating on 104 patients (34 with fat obliteration), with only 2 failures.

Among the 53 cases of Sessions and colleagues,[134] there were two failures secondary to postoperative infection, which required removal of the graft. They noted asymptomatic retraction of the fat graft on radiographic study in some cases. Three patients developed embossment or prominence of the forehead because of calcification of the bone flap. These workers experimentally demonstrated bony thickening of the anterior and posterior tables of the feline frontal sinus following osteoplasty with implantation; however, the cause of the osteoneogenesis was unclear.

In the 100 cases reported by Bosley,[17] the procedure was considered successful in 93 patients, based on the accomplishment of complete frontal obliteration radiographically. In 15

patients there was continued headache, with radiologic evidence of incomplete frontal obliteration in 7 patients. In three of these cases, acute sinusitis developed. A second osteoplastic flap procedure was necessary in four patients for control of their disease. Eighty-one patients indicated complete satisfaction with the results of surgery.

Operative and postoperative complications developed in 18 per cent (47 of 250) of the cases of Hardy and Montgomery.[55] In the abdominal wall, a hematoma or seroma developed in 11 patients, and an abscess developed in 2 others. In the frontal wound, six patients developed a hematoma or seroma and eight formed an abscess. Six of these eight latter cases required revision surgery. Bone cuts were made outside the sinus in eight patients, the dura was increased in seven cases, and skin necrosis occurred in two others. One patient each had total anosmia, temporary ptosis, and temporary loss of frontalis muscle function. Among 208 patients with follow-up, 93 per cent remained asymptomatic. In 12 cases (6 per cent) there was persistent frontal pain unrelieved by medical therapy. Revision surgery in four of these patients failed to reveal any evidence of persistent disease. In three patients, there was persistent neuralgia resulting from the sectioning of the supraorbital nerve. Although all patients complained of abnormal frontal sensation, it disappeared within 12 months in 65 per cent but persisted in the remaining 35 per cent. From a cosmetic viewpoint, the scar was considered poor in 12 per cent and the forehead contour unsatisfactory in 6 per cent. Depression or elevation of the flap occurred most often with unilateral brow incisions. In 20 of 208 patients (9.5 per cent), revision surgery was performed 4 days to 14 years later (median, 2 years). Among six early revisions performed because of persistent purulent drainage through a fistula, five patients had fat necrosis and one had an unrecognized supraorbital pyocele. Among 14 delayed revisions, there were four patients with negative findings on explorations performed because of chronic pain, seven patients with chronic sinusitis, two with osteomyelitis, and one with infected fibrous dysplasia.

The criteria for success of the procedure are an asymptomatic patient and radiographic evidence of complete sinus obliteration (Figs. 10–17 through 10–19). The etiology of frontal pain or headache is difficult to assess in the patient lacking objective evidence of infection or any radiographic abnormality. This is especially true following a direct eyebrow approach to the sinus, in which the supraorbital nerves are

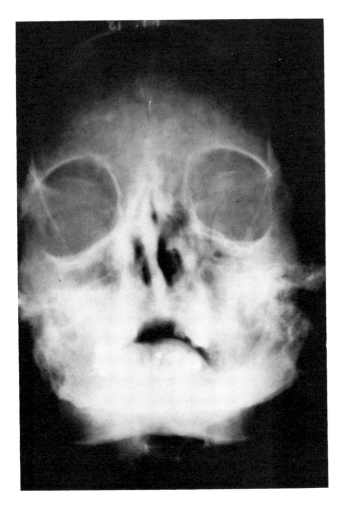

Figure 10–17. Plain radiograph of a frontal sinus following a bilateral osteoplastic flap with fat obliteration. The sinus is completely airless and appears isodense with the surrounding bone.

transected, postoperative anesthesia and paresthesia are usual, and neuralgias are not uncommon.

The incision for the direct brow approach must be carefully designed and repaired to minimize cosmetic deformity. Placement of the incision within the eyebrow may result in regional depilation by injury to the hair follicles, even with beveling of the incision. I have not encountered paresis of the eyebrow from injury

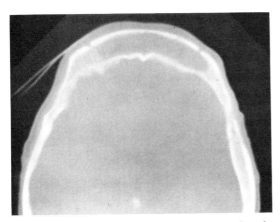

Figure 10–18. CT scan (narrow window) revealing fat and fibrous tissue completely filling an obliterated frontal sinus. Note that the bone cuts through the outer table.

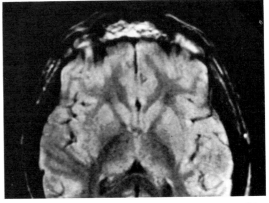

Figure 10–19. Magnetic resonance scan (balanced image—long TR, short TE), demonstrating high signal intensity of the fat obliterating both frontal sinuses. The interspersed black areas are strands of fibrous tissue.

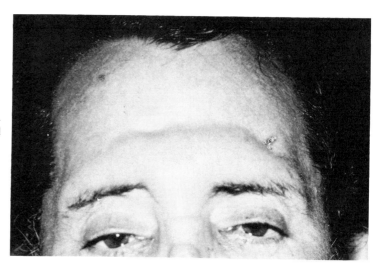

Figure 10–20. Embossment of an osteoplastic flap that developed several months after surgery.

to the frontal branch of the facial nerve; however, unilateral evaluation of the eyebrow occurred in one patient secondary to localized injury and fibrosis of the frontalis muscle.

Beveling of the bone flap has not resulted in penetration of the posterior table, even with a shallow sinus and with templates constructed from a standard Caldwell view. Embossment occurred in one case (Fig. 10–20) and was repaired by reduction of the hyperostotic anterior table by a drill and filling in of bony irregularities in the cranial contour with acrylic. Dividing the supraorbital rims with an oscillating saw and severing the intersinus septum with a curved chisel has eliminated fracture of the bone flap even without a bone cut at the nasion.

Whereas implanted adipose tissue has been found experimentally to survive clinically in an infected frontal sinus, chronic regional infection may impose too great a burden upon it. I performed a collapse (Riedel) procedure to remove residual osteomyelitic bone in several patients who had an osteoplastic flap with fat obliteration. In these cases the bone flap and fat graft had both necrosed (Figs. 10–21 and 10–22), and one patient also developed an epidural abscess. In several other patients, the failure of the procedure could be attributed to active suppurative disease in the ethmoid labyrinth, which resulted in septic necrosis of the fat graft. It is extremely important to assess the status of the other sinuses radiologically and to treat any disease there before undertaking definitive surgery on the frontal sinus.

TECHNIQUE

Preliminary to surgery a template is cut from a Caldwell view (anteroposterior) radiograph of

the frontal sinuses. It includes the supraorbital ridges and the root of the nose and facilitates accurate placement at the time of surgery. The intersinus septum and right and left sides are marked by scratching the film emulsion. The template is sterilized by placing it in an antiseptic solution (e.g., Betadine, glutaraldehyde).

In constructing the template, the type of Caldwell view radiograph taken is of utmost importance as it influences the degree of mag-

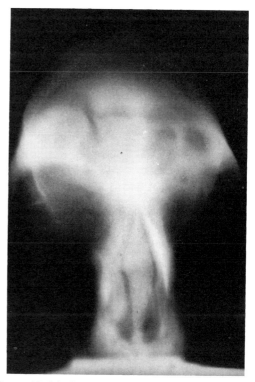

Figure 10–21. Coronal tomogram revealing fracture of the bone flap and areas of radiolucency where the fat graft has necrosed.

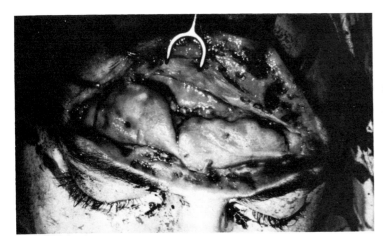

Figure 10–22. Failed osteoplastic flap procedure. The patient experienced fracture and migration of the anterior table, had necrosis of the fat graft, and developed osteomyelitis of the surrounding bone.

nification.[144] If it is made on the Franklin head unit, the magnification factor is 3.4 per cent, whereas with the standard PA Caldwell view made at a 40-inch film-target distance, it becomes 10.3 per cent. Should an AP view be taken at the same distance, the magnification factor climbs to 31 per cent. The type of projection is far more important than the film target distance. A radiograph taken on the Franklin head unit can be identified by the circular image. An important corollary is that the larger the sinus, the relatively greater the projection error. Hence, a sinus 6 cm in diameter will have a magnification error of 6 mm with the standard PA Caldwell view and under 2 mm with the Franklin head unit. This can be compensated for by beveling the bone cuts made through the anterior table to enter the sinus.

The patient's hair should be washed with hexachlorophene soap the day before surgery. The face, forehead, and scalp are prepared and draped after the induction of general endotracheal anesthesia. The abdomen is also prepared to obtain an adipose graft from the left subcostal area. The eyelids are closed with 5-0 silk tarsorrhaphy sutures. The operation is performed through an eyebrow or coronal incision (Fig. 10–23). The incision line may be infiltrated with 1 per cent lidocaine with epinephrine (1:100,000) to reduce bleeding.

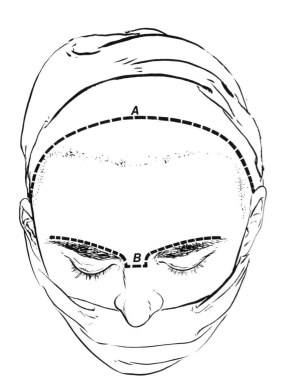

Figure 10–23. Outline of the coronal (A) and eyebrow (B) incisions for the osteoplastic flap procedure.

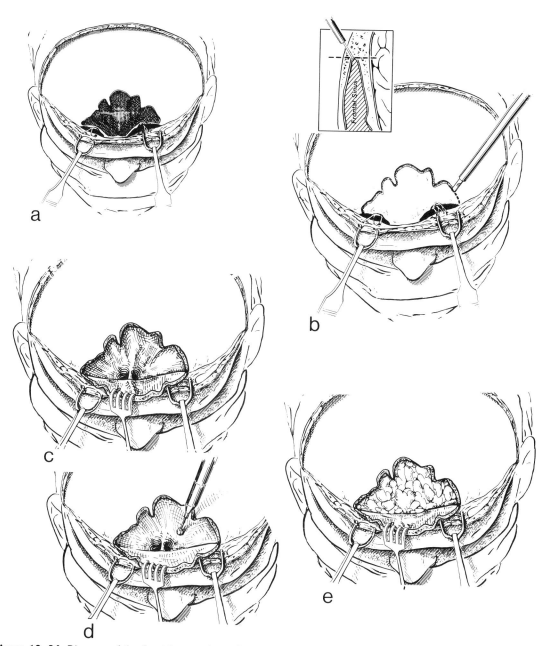

Figure 10–24. Diagram of the frontal osteoplastic flap, coronal approach. *a*, Scalp flap elevated, template positioned; note that the supraorbital nerves are intact. *b*, Bone cut made with an oscillating saw; inset shows beveling of bone by saw. *d*, Interior of sinus is burred clean. *e*, Fresh subcutaneous abdominal fat placed into the sinus cavity.

If a coronal incision is utilized (Fig. 10–24), it is placed approximately 5 cm behind the hairline. (The hair is previously shaved for a width to 2 cm along the projected line of incision.) After the drapes are sutured into position, an incision is made through the skin, subcutaneous tissue, and galea. This incision is curved laterally toward the superior margin of the anterior attachment of the pinna. The majority of bleeding occurs at the time of this initial incision and requires hemostasis by clamping and electrocautery of numerous individual vessels or by the placement of Raney clips along the wound margins. The dissection proceeds in the plane of loose areolar tissue above the pericranium with a curved Mayo scissors. Care must be taken not to injure the periosteum, which may be extremely thin in some areas over the frontal bone. Laterally, the undermining of the flap is more superficial, proceeding in the loose tissue overlying the temporalis fascia, avoiding injury to the branches of the superficial temporal blood vessels. The flap is elevated down to the superciliary ridges and root of the nose and is reflected over the face. Careful dissection is necessary in this region to prevent damage to the supraorbital neurovascular bundles.

The sterilized template is then carefully positioned along roofs of the orbits and nasal root and is transfixed in place by piercing it in two areas with a scalpel. The periosteum is incised along the periphery of the template and elevated for 1 to 2 mm. In the unilateral case, a series of perforations are made through the template along the etched line of the intersinus septum, which are later joined together with a scalpel. The bone is cut with an oscillating saw held at an angle of 45 degrees or less to the skull. Beveling the bone cut is extremely important to ensure stable repositioning of the flap and to prevent penetration of the posterior table. In some patients, the frontal sinus is extremely shallow superiorly, or a slight magnification error may have occurred in the fabrication of the template, making it imperative to cut the bone obliquely to avoid entering the anterior cranial fossa. The saw is also used to cut the dense bone along the supraorbital ridges to a depth of about 1 cm.

The bone flap is raised with a curved chisel, which is also used to section the intersinus septum. The bone flap, which is hinged along its attachment at the supraorbital ridges, is rotated outward and the sinus is inspected. Specimens for culture are taken, and the diseased mucous membrane is stripped from the sinus and all its recesses. Using a round bur, the inner table of the frontal sinus is drilled down, thinning the cortical plate and removing any septa within the sinus or on the bone flap. All crevices should be drilled, including posterior extensions of the sinus along the roof of the orbit, and any supraorbital ethmoid cells present are opened. This achieves removal of mucosal remnants and also exposes fine bleeding vessels, which serve to revascularize the fat graft. The sinus is then copiously irrigated with saline. At this point, the adipose graft is taken through a horizontal left subcostal incision. The fat should be fresh and handled gently. It is cut into fragments that are placed into all the recesses of the frontal sinuses and into the openings of the nasofrontal ducts. The bone flap is then returned to its original position, and the adjacent periosteum is approximated with 3-0 or 4-0 absorbable sutures. If the flap is unstable, a small bur hole is drilled and a 28-gauge stainless wire is placed to maintain it in proper position. The wound is again irrigated with saline, and a small Penrose drain is placed. The scalp flap is returned, and the incision is either closed with a continuous 2-0 or 3-0 nonabsorbable suture or with stainless steel staples. A light dressing is then placed over the forehead and anterior scalp.

In the approach through the eyebrow (Fig. 10–25), the face and forehead are prepared and draped in the usual fashion for frontal sinus surgery after the induction of general endotracheal anesthesia. Tarsorrhaphy sutures are placed bilaterally. The incision is outlined with methylene blue. For a *unilateral osteoplastic flap*, it extends along the entire length of the upper border of the unshaved eyebrow and arches downward to cross the root of the nose horizontally over the nasal process of the frontal bone to the opposite side. For a *bilateral osteoplastic flap*, the incision is carried superiorly and laterally along the upper border of the opposite eyebrow in gullwing fashion. The skin, subcutaneous tissues, and frontalis muscle are divided. The superior flap is retracted with double hoods, and the dissection is carried

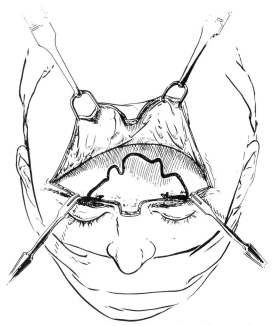

Figure 10–25. Elevation of the skin flap with an eyebrow (gullwing) incision for a bilateral osteoplastic flap. Note that this approach requires transection of the supraorbital nerves.

upward with a curved Mayo scissors in the areolar tissue between the frontalis muscle and pericranium. The inferior flap is elevated for a short distance to expose the supraorbital ridges. The flaps are elevated sufficiently to allow adequate space for placement of the template and the insertion of the oscillating saw. The incision of the periosteum, design of the bone cut, elevation of the anterior table, preparation of the sinus cavity, and obliteration with fresh abdominal fat are identical to those performed in the coronal approach. After the bone flap is returned and the periosteum approximated, the incision is closed in layers and an occlusive dressing is applied.

MODIFICATIONS

In the MacBeth technique,[17, 89] two crossed wires are placed in the midline of the patient's forehead between the eyes. A Caldwell view film is then taken, and a template is cut. The contours of the frontal sinuses are then traced on the skin, using the wire marker for proper orientation of the template. An incision is made coronally, or in a forehead crease. Needles are passed through the skin along the frontal sinus contour lines, the skin flap elevated, and the pericranium exposed to the needle points. The sinus is entered by perforating the anterior table with a bur at each needle point. These holes are joined, and the orbital rims and nasofrontal suture line are fractured. After the sinus is entered, the mucosa is stripped out, and all the bony surfaces are drilled down with a cutting bur. A transfrontal ethmoidectomy is then performed on each side. The osteoplastic flap is replaced, and the scalp incision is sutured. A further modification was introduced by Guggenheim,[52] who filled the sinus with a composite fat–fascia lata graft. The fascia was to serve as a hammock to prevent prolapse of the implant into the ethmoidectomy cavity.

In patients in whom mucoceles invade the dura and in whom there is considerable doubt that all the mucosa can be removed, Sessions and colleagues[134] obliterated the frontal sinus laterally with fat and placed a polyethylene tube through the enlarged nasofrontal duct in relation to the mucocele medially. Schaeffer and colleagues[126, 127] treated seven patients who had frontal sinus mucoceles with epidural extension: five by cranialization and marsupialization into the nasal cavity and two with resection of the dura and repair with a periosteal flap. This was accomplished through an osteoplastic flap in three patients and a frontal craniotomy in the remaining four.

In 1988, Kudryk and Mahasin[77] reported the use of a superiorly based osteoplastic flap in eight patients with unilateral disease. After an infrabrow incision is made, the floor of the frontal sinus is removed and the anterior table sectioned under direct vision and hinged upward. After this is performed, the sinus may be obliterated, the intersinus septum may be removed, or a mucoperiosteal flap may be rotated into a neoduct that is created. The proposed advantages of this method are that it eliminates the need for a template, lessens the possibility of a cerebrospinal fluid leak, and is performed through a cosmetically acceptable incision.

PRINCIPLES

If the osteoplastic flap is selected for the management of frontal sinus pathology, certain clinically established principles should be followed. The largest published experience with the osteoplastic frontal sinusotomy is that of Hardy and Montgomery.[55] They concluded that it is the procedure of choice for all chronic frontal sinus disease. The coronal incision was considered superior, not only for cosmetic reasons, but also because it provided wider exposure and eliminated postoperative supraorbital neuralgia. Nevertheless, 75 per cent of their cases were operated on through a brow incision. The increased blood loss accompanying the coronal incision must also be considered. Blood loss averaged 250 ml with a unilateral brow incision, 350 ml with a bilateral brow incision, and 650 ml with a coronal incision. They believed that all cases should have fat obliteration with fresh and atraumatically removed subcutaneous adipose tissue. This was done in 83 per cent of their cases.

Antibiotic therapy was instituted preoperatively, with the final agent selected from culture and sensitivity testing of specimens obtained during surgery. In 184 operative cultures, the frontal sinus showed no growth in 75; only *Staphylococcus albus* was noted in 38; and pathogens were isolated in 71 patients. Among this latter group were 61 gram-positive organisms (including 46 *Staphylococcus aureus*, 6 pneumococci, 5 α-streptococci and 4 β-streptococci), and 10 gram-negative organisms (4 *Escherichia coli*, 2 *Proteus*, 2 *Pseudomonas*, 1 *Klebsiella* and 1 *Bacteroides*). It was also deemed essential that all contiguous ethmoid cells and deep posterior extensions of the frontal sinus should be included in the common frontal cavity and obliterated with fat.

FRONTAL SINUS FRACTURES

Published experience with frontal sinus fractures has increased markedly in the last decade. Larger reported series include 46 cases by Hybels and Weimert,[64] 52 cases by Whited,[151] 54 cases by Larrabee and colleagues,[80] 78 cases by Luce,[86] 50 cases by Stanley and Becker,[141] 112 cases by Duvall and colleagues,[36] 41 cases by Shockley and colleagues,[136] 66 cases by Wilson and colleagues,[154] 72 cases by Wallis and Donald,[147] and 107 cases by Stanley.[140] This collective experience with over 600 cases gives greater insight into the therapeutic problems and complications posed by this form of injury, yet many controversies remain. The diagnostic value of modern imaging techniques and their impact on selection of treatment also will become readily apparent.

Fractures of the frontal sinus are often associated with other facial skeletal fractures as well as intracranial and thoracoabdominal injuries. Many patients also have fractures of the orbit, malar bone, and maxilla (Fig. 10–26). In the series of 72 cases of Wallis and Donald,[147] 76

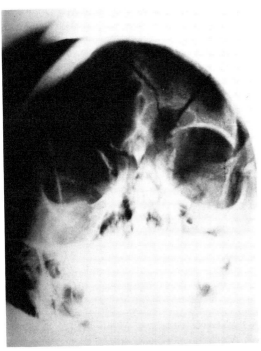

Figure 10–26. Extensive fracture of the skull involving the frontal sinus and nasoethmoidal complex.

per cent sustained loss of consciousness, 65 per cent other facial and skeletal fractures, and 33 per cent had a cerebrospinal fluid (CSF) leak. Among the 66 cases of Wilson and colleagues,[154] 50 per cent had fracture of the orbit, 35 per cent had fracture of the maxilla, and 30 per cent had a CSF leak. In the series of 78 cases of Luce,[86] 50 per cent had midfacial fractures, 41 per cent had nasoethmoidorbital fractures, 10 per cent lost an eye, half were compound, and one third had a CSF leak. The gravity of this injury is reflected in a significant accompanying mortality. Nine per cent of the 72 cases of Wallis and Donald[147] and 6.5 per cent of the 46 cases of Hybels and Weimert[64] died from their injuries.

The majority of frontal sinus fractures are the result of motor vehicle accidents, followed by assaults, sports, and home and industrial trauma. In all series of cases, the peak incidence was in the third and fourth decades of life, with a preponderance of men over women in a ratio of 4 to 10:1.[64, 80, 136, 147, 154]

The external appearance of the forehead does not correlate with the severity of the injury to the underlying bone and intracranial structures. Signs and symptoms of frontal sinus fracture include swelling, deformity, pain, paresthesia of the supraorbital nerves, CSF rhinorrhea or drainage through a laceration, headache, and eyelid edema.

Frontal sinus fractures are classified according to the anatomic nature and extent of injury, as these factors influence the type and incidence of complications and accordingly dictate therapeutic management. They are generally divided into fractures that involve the anterior wall, posterior wall, both walls, and nasofrontal duct. There are subgroups of fractures, which include nondisplaced and displaced fractures, linear and comminuted fractures, closed and open fractures, and those with or without a CSF leak. Adkins and colleagues[3] argued that all frontal sinus fractures should be considered compound because of the nasofrontal duct.

The relative incidence of the types of fracture varies widely in reported series, reflecting differences in patient sampling. Among the 72 cases of Wallis and Donald,[147] an isolated anterior wall fracture occurred in 18 per cent, an isolated posterior wall fracture in 3 per cent, anterior and posterior wall fractures in 36 per cent, nasofrontal duct injuries in 1.5 per cent, and fractures extending from the skin through the anterior cranial fossa in 40 per cent. In the series of 66 patients of Wilson and colleagues,[154] 21 per cent had an isolated anterior wall fracture, 5 per cent had an isolated posterior wall fracture, 29 per cent had combined wall fractures, 9 per cent suffered a nasofrontal duct fracture, and in 36 per cent the nasofrontal duct injury was combined with another fracture. Among the 41 cases of Shockley and colleagues,[136] 67 per cent had an isolated anterior table fracture, 28 per cent had combined anterior and posterior wall fractures, 5 per cent only had involvement of the posterior table, and 17 per cent had injury of the nasofrontal duct.

From a radiologic viewpoint, plain radiographs have limited diagnostic value with frontal sinus fractures unless a major injury has occurred, with marked fragmentation and dislocation of the anterior wall being present.[36, 64] Lesser injuries may go unnoticed, this being especially true with posterior table fractures. Stanley and Becker[141] detected fracture lines in 44 of their 50 cases with plain films. However, whereas only 9 patients were suspected of having a posterior wall fracture, it was found to be present in 28 patients on surgical exploration. In a study of 80 cases by Frenckner and Richter,[40] only 17 of 52 patients found to have anterior and posterior wall fractures on exploration were suspected of having this based on plain x-ray film examination.

By contrast, CT scanning readily and accurately detects these fractures, as well as injury to the adjacent brain, orbit, and facial skeleton.[109, 141] It can visualize disruption of the nasofrontal duct as well as the anterior and posterior walls. In a study by Harris and colleagues[57] of 12 patients with fractures of the base of the frontal sinus on CT scan, 10 were found to have nasofrontal duct injuries on surgical exploration, for a correlation rate of 85 per cent.

The presence of intracranial air (pneumocephalus) and an air-fluid level in the frontal sinus from layered CSF or blood in plain films or tomography are other indications of frontal fracture (Fig. 10–27). Shockley and colleagues[136] detected pneumocephalus in 17 per cent of their 41 cases. However, this is not a pathognomonic finding, as free air may enter the intracranial space from an opening anywhere in the skull base.

ANTERIOR TABLE FRACTURES

Nondisplaced anterior wall fractures are usually treated by observation.[81, 136, 140] Occasionally, a trephine is necessary if infection develops. This was performed in 3 of the 43 cases reported by Duvall and colleagues.[36] However, Adkins and colleagues[3] considered sinus clouding to be an indication for trephine. Peri and

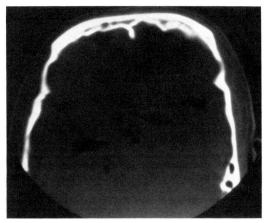

Figure 10–27. Isolated fracture of the posterior table of the frontal sinus with an accompanying pneumocephalus.

colleagues[115] advocated sinus drainage by the intranasal passage of catheters.

In a study of 52 anterior wall fractures by Whited,[151] 16 were open and displaced, 6 were closed and displaced, and 30 were nondisplaced. The open displaced fractures were reduced through the laceration, and the closed displaced were elevated through a trephine. The complication of suppurative sinusitis developed in only 3 of the 52 cases, of which 26 were open. By contrast, in an analysis of the suppurative complications of frontal sinus fractures in 51 patients, Larrabee and colleagues[80] noted that eight of the nine infections occurred with open fractures. Based on the further observation that 6 major suppurative complications developed in 15 nonoperated cases, they concluded that every case of frontal sinus fracture, even isolated anterior table fractures, should be explored.

It should be noted that this is a minority opinion. Clinical experience has shown that the majority of closed nondisplaced anterior table fractures heal uneventfully with conservative treatment. Antibiotics are generally administered because of the risk of bacterial contamination through the nasofrontal duct. With open nondisplaced anterior wall fractures, the laceration is carefully repaired and antibiotics given. In contradistinction, all displaced anterior wall fractures require repair to prevent cosmetic deformity. In the past, surgery was often more aggressive, with exploration of the sinus to determine whether a concomitant fracture of the posterior table or nasofrontal duct was present that would also require repair. The use of CT scanning provides this information noninvasively and accurately.

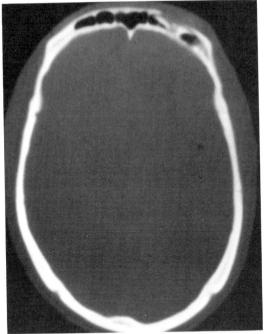

Figure 10–28. CT scan of depressed fracture of the anterior table of the frontal sinus.

Depressed fractures are treated by elevation and fixation (Fig. 10–28). Minimal fractures can be elevated through a bur hole made in the inferior-medial aspect of the sinus where the standard trephine is placed. A curved instru-

ment is inserted beneath the depressed segments, which are then outfractured. Should the fracture be unstable, a pediatric Foley or Fogarty catheter is threaded into the sinus and inflated beneath the fractured segments.[3, 116] Although most workers bring the balloon out through the trephine,[98, 112] some carry it through the nose.[23]

With comminuted fractures that are both displaced and unstable, the fragments are exposed, repositioned, and fixed with interosseous wiring, using 28-gauge stainless steel wire (Figs. 10–29 and 10–30). Despite direct wiring and balloon support, the outer sinus wall may tend to collapse, which has led workers to devise other methods of fixation. Ghorayeb[41] placed a wire sling beneath the anterior wall fragments for support, then placed and wired the bony segments together over the suspensory wires. Climo and colleagues[23] immobilized unstable depressed frontal bone fractures by fixation with Kirschner wires. McGrath and Smith[93] described passing a stainless steel wire transcutaneously through the periosteum or under a bony fragment and tying it over a perforated eye shield. Most recently, miniplate fixation of comminuted fractures has been employed.[51, 140] It should be noted that even performing an osteoplastic flap and filling the sinus with fat to cushion the unstable fragments do not guaran-

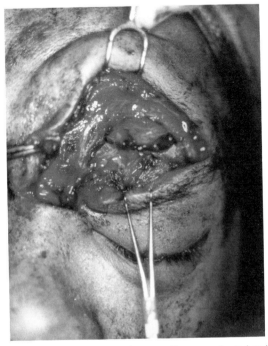

Figure 10–29. Operative view revealing comminuted and displaced bone fragments.

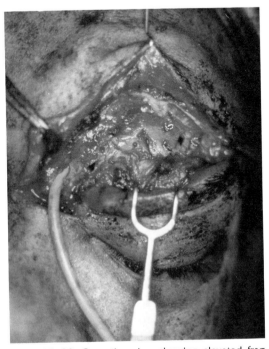

Figure 10–30. Operative view showing elevated fragments stabilized by interosseous wiring and the insertion of a pediatric Foley catheter passed through a trephine.

tee against forehead deformity and the need for a cranioplasty later. This complication and other attempts to reduce it will be further discussed.

The operative approach may be through a coronal or eyebrow incision, or through the laceration accompanying an open fracture. In the series of 72 cases of Wallis and Donald,[147] the operative approach was coronal in 48 per cent, through a laceration in 34 per cent, throught the eyebrow in 16 per cent, and transorbital in 2 per cent. The coronal approach has the advantage of scar camouflage and also provides access to other cranial, orbital, and midfacial fractures that may be present. The eyebrow approach provides direct access to the fracture. This is of benefit when the supraorbital ridge is extensively injured as it facilitates positioning and wiring of the fragments, with exploration of the orbit.

POSTERIOR WALL FRACTURES

An isolated posterior wall fracture in the absence of a corresponding fracture of the anterior wall is rare and is probably the result of the shearing forces in the skull from severe head trauma. Management will be considered in the following section on combined table fractures, which is the usual clinical occurrence.

ANTERIOR AND POSTERIOR WALL FRACTURES

The management of combined anterior and posterior wall fractures is controversial. Some investigators[36, 140, 154] believe that nondisplaced posterior wall fractures that were uncomplicated (e.g., no CSF leak, meningitis, or sinus infection) require no treatment, whereas others suggest operative intervention and sinus obliteration to prevent immediate or delayed intracranial complications. Displaced posterior wall fractures are universally considered an indication for surgical exploration, with workers differing only on what constitutes the operative procedure of choice.

Duvall and colleagues[36] recommended observation and antibiotics for a nondisplaced or a mildly displaced posterior wall fracture. Among nine such cases treated by this method, there were no complications. In two patients with this type of fracture, they performed a frontoethmoidectomy for drainage. Wilson and colleagues[154] reported that 5 of 19 patients with combined anterior and posterior wall fractures, in whom obliteration was not performed, did well.

In an experimental study in cats by Hybels and Newman,[63] both treated and untreated depressed posterior table fractures were observed to heal by the formation of new bone or fibrous tissue, sealing the subdural space from the sinus. No area of exposed brain or mucosal ingrowth was noted in the fracture site 6 months later. However, if the nasofrontal duct was impaired, mucoceles were observed to develop. In sinuses obliterated by fat grafts or allowed to obliterate spontaneously by osteoneogenesis, a layer of fibrous tissue generally developed between the sinus and the brain. This was enhanced by the placement of temporalis fascia over the fracture on the sinus side. However, in two instances the brain was attached to the fracture site despite fat obliteration and fascia grafting. The investigators speculated that this may have resulted from injury to the brain or arachnoid. Based on this study, Hybels[62] also recommended not exploring the nondisplaced or minimally displaced posterior wall fracture. However, a trephine was placed if the sinus remained cloudy on repeat x-ray examination.

Despite these experimental findings, many workers choose to explore and obliterate the frontal sinus with a nondisplaced posterior wall fracture to prevent delayed intracranial complications. I do not believe that this is a merely theoretic consideration after having seen several such cases, one with a fatal outcome, and accordingly I perform an osteoplastic flap with fat obliteration of all such fractures. Keay and colleagues[71] also reported two cases of meningitis developing 3 months and 14 years following untreated fractures, with one patient dying from the infection.

While it is considered mandatory to operate upon displaced frontal sinus fractures, the type of surgical procedure performed depends on the severity of the injury and the extent of damage to the contiguous structures, principally the dura, brain, and cranial vault.

A combined otolaryngologic-neurosurgical approach is indicated when severely displaced or penetrating fractures of the anterior and posterior walls of the frontal sinus are present in combination with an intracranial injury[97] (Fig. 10–31). This is performed through a unifrontal or bifrontal craniotomy. The frontal sinus is usually inspected by elevating the fractured segments of bone (Fig. 10–32). Denneny and Davidson[28] reported treating five such cases in which the calvarial bone flap was created at the upper border of the frontal sinus so that the sinus cavity could be inspected. A supplemental osteoplastic flap was created if indicated, and the sinus was obliterated with fat.

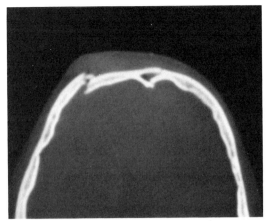

Figure 10–31. CT scan of displaced comminuted fracture of the anterior and posterior tables of the frontal sinus.

The landmark paper by Nadell and Kline[104] in 1974, on the management of the compound comminuted skull fracture, revolutionized thinking on the subject. In their series of 65 frontal fractures, 33 of which involved the frontal sinus, cribriform plate, or orbital rim, Nadell and Kline removed fragments of depressed bone, soaked them in povidone-iodine (Betadine), trimmed off sharp edges, and replaced them in a mosaic pattern to fill the defect. Before doing this, the mucosal lining of the sinus was removed, dural tears were repaired, the nasofrontal duct was packed with muscle, and the posterior sinus wall was removed. This provided space for the traumatized brain to expand and also preserved the bony contour of the forehead, with protection of the frontal lobes. This method of obliteration of the sinus cavity by permitting herniation of the brain anteriorly is termed cranialization. In none of their cases did meningitis or a brain abscess develop.

Advocates of cranialization, principally Donald,[32, 33] state that it is superior to fat obliteration, especially when there is an absence of frontal bone.[147] Fat grafts require a rich blood supply for revascularization and survival. In severe injuries with bone loss, the fat rests against relatively poorly vascularized subcutaneous tissue and dura rather than drilled-down sinus wall bone. The subsequent shrinkage of the remaining graft causes retraction away from the nasofrontal duct, with mucosal ingrowth and mucocele formation. In support of this concept, Donald and Ettin[35] showed experimentally in cats that when 50 to 100 per cent of the anterior and posterior frontal sinus walls were missing, epithelial regrowth occurred in 29 per cent and infection developed in 44 per cent of the animals following fat obliteration.

Donald and Bernstein[34] considered cranialization to be the method of choice for compound frontal sinus fractures with intracranial penetration. Donald,[33] in 1982, further outlined the operative procedure and reported his experience with 21 cases. He stressed the importance of drilling away the remaining bone to remove mucosal remnants so as to prevent mucocele formation. In a later review by Wallis and

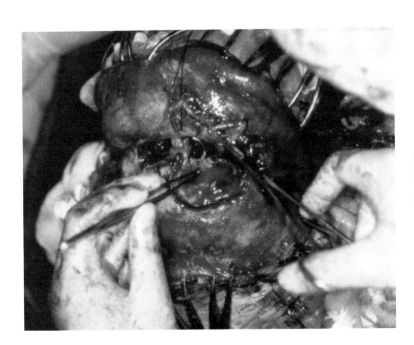

Figure 10–32. Operative view showing suturing of dural lacerations. Repair included a muscle graft to the nasofrontal duct and cranialization.

Donald[147] of 57 cases that involved the posterior table, they performed cranialization in 30 patients and an osteoplastic flap with fat obliteration in 24. The osteoplastic flap with fat obliteration was employed when there was (1) no intracranial penetration; (2) when there was no loss of large amounts of bone; and (3) for injuries of the posterior wall and nasofrontal duct.

The European workers Merville and Derome[97] and Peri and colleagues[115] reported a large experience with cranialization but gave no data regarding complications. Luce[86] reported no cosmetic or neurologic complications in eight patients undergoing cranialization. Levine and colleagues[81] mentioned employing cranialization in four patients with penetrating injuries but provided no other information. In the series of 112 cases of Duvall and colleagues[36] 20 patients had displaced fractures of the anterior and posterior walls, 13 of which underwent repair by an osteoplastic flap and fat obliteration and 7 by cranialization. In the obliteration group, one patient developed a mucopyocele 8 years later. In the cranialization group, five patients developed complications that included cosmetic deformity in two, CSF leak in three, and meningitis in one. The reasons for the marked disparity in the incidence of complications is unclear as all the patients had injuries of comparable severity.

However, Stanley[140] believed that the management of complex frontal sinus injuries with intracranial involvement should be directed to isolating the sinus from the cranial cavity so that potential complications have limited extension. Accordingly, he did not employ cranialization in any of his 157 cases but rather sealed communications between the nasal and cranial cavities with fascia lata grafts and placed free fat between the dura and the fascia. Bone grafts were also inserted between the frontal sinus and defects in the orbital roof and nose. In his operative method, Stanley[140] entered the frontal sinus through the anterior table fracture, removed anterior and posterior table fragments, repaired dural tears, and drilled out and obliterated the sinus with fat. Despite the loss of their periosteal attachments, the bone fragments that were replaced and wired together remained viable. A fascial graft (temporalis, rectus, fascia lata) was placed over the posterior table to bridge any gaps in the bone and across the sinus floor to support the fat and prevent ingrowth of epithelium from adjacent ethmoid air cells.

In the majority of cases of combined wall fractures without extensive bone loss, the os-

teoplastic flap with obliteration is the mainstay operative procedure. Weber and Cohn[149] showed the feasibility of performing this procedure even with fractures in children. However, differences exist with regard to the material used for sinus obliteration. Whereas otolaryngologists favor autogenous abdominal fat, neurosurgeons routinely employ skeletal muscle, and European workers[97, 115] implant iliac bone. In the study by Larrabee and colleagues,[80] abscess formation developed in one of ten patients in whom fat was implanted, in two of four patients in whom methyl methacrylate was implanted, in the one patient who had oxidized cellulose gauze placed; two patients in whom muscle and Gelfoam was inserted, respectively, remained infection-free. Stanley[140] calculated an incidence of complications of less than 1 per cent among 120 patients treated with fat obliteration.

Regarding the use of alloplastic sealing materials, successful fixation of frontal bone fractures with a cementing substance (methacrylate, tricalcium phosphate, and a ceramic filler) was reported in two patients by Vuillemin and colleagues.[146]

NASOFRONTAL DUCT FRACTURES

Fractures of this region are attended by obstruction of the sinus outflow, with the subsequent development of a mucocele. In this setting the osteoplastic flap with fat obliteration is generally considered the procedure of choice.[136, 140, 154] However, Adkins and colleagues[3] and Newman and Travis[108] recommended intersinus septectomy with a unilateral fracture, relying upon the contralateral healthy sinus and duct for drainage. Reconstruction of the nasofrontal duct with mucosal flaps also has been advocated.[81] However Stanley[140] cautions that stenting of the duct may worsen the injury and result in delayed complications. Similarly, septectomy does not guarantee against future sinusitis.

In a study of 50 frontal sinus fractures, 48 of which were surgically explored, Stanley and Becker[141] found that even displaced anterior table fractures did not produce injury to the nasofrontal duct unless there was a concomitant fracture of the nasoethmoidal complex or supraorbital rim. Of the 10 of 22 cases of anterior wall fractures in which duct injury was encountered, 5 patients had nasoethmoidal fractures, 4 had supraorbital rim fractures medial to the notch, and only 1 patient had an isolated displaced anterior table fracture. In contradistinction, combined fractures of the anterior and posterior walls almost always had a nasofrontal duct injury, and this occurred in 22 of 28 patients.

However, in the series of 52 anterior table fractures of Whited,[151] the nasofrontal duct was injured in 26 patients, with only 1 patient developing a complication.

The opinion of May and colleagues[92] to explore surgically all frontal sinus fractures, based on the finding of nasofrontal duct injury in 20 of their cases, with development of 4 late infections, is no longer tenable based on modern imaging techniques and a large collective clinical experience with these fractures.

SUPRAORBITAL RIM FRACTURES

Direct trauma to this upper facial buttress generally results in its fracture inward into the frontal sinus and downward into the orbit. In a study of 601 patients who had 1031 facial fractures, Schultz[132] found 36 (5 per cent) with fracture of the supraorbital and glabellar areas. As with other fractures of the frontal complex, plain radiographs have a low diagnostic yield, with the CT scan being the most reliable method of visualization of this type of injury.

Clinically, impairment of ocular mobility from injury to the superior rectus and superior oblique muscles is often present, as well as periorbital edema and ecchymosis, tenderness, and crepitation. The bony deformity is usually masked by local edema.

Management is by open reduction through a direct brow incision or existing laceration, with repositioning and wiring of the fractured segments.[98] Occasionally, a minor fracture can be elevated through a trephine alone. When lacerations are present, layered closure with repair of the muscles is important to prevent secondary deformity. Contiguous fractures of the remaining frontal sinus are repaired according to their location and severity, as outlined earlier.

COMPLICATIONS OF FRONTAL SINUS FRACTURES

Frontal sinus fractures carry the risk of early or late development of intrasinal, osseous, and intracranial complications. This includes chronic sinusitis, the formation of a mucocele or mucopyocele, osteomyelitis of the frontal bone, CSF leak, meningitis, intracranial abscess, and cavernous sinus thrombosis, as well as chronic headache syndrome, local pain, and pneumo-

cephalus. Stanley[140] stated that patients should be informed that they have a lifelong risk of delayed complications following frontal sinus fracture.

In their series of 72 cases, Wallis and Donald[147] reported meningitis occurring in 4 patients (6 per cent), infection in 7 patients (10 per cent), CSF leak in 7 patients (10 per cent) (three of which spontaneously stopped), deformity in 6 patients (8 per cent), pain in 4 patients (5 per cent), and diplopia in 1 case. They considered the incidence of complications acceptable considering the severity of injuries, of which 85 per cent were compound and 75 per cent traversing both sinus walls. It is of interest to note that while the average follow-up interval was only 22 months, four patients had already developed mucoceles.

Among the 66 cases of Wilson and colleagues,[154] only 21 patients had no complications. Twenty patients had chronic headache; 12, sinus infections; 10, chronic sinus drainage; 10, forehead depression; 7, wound infection; 4, diplopia; 4, seizure disorder; 3, meningitis; 1, ophthalmic pulsations; and 1, a brain abscess. No patient developed a mucocele, despite a mean follow-up of 38 months. Infections generally occurred within 3 weeks of injury; however, three patients developed a wound infection, meningitis, and brain abscess 5 to 12 weeks later. Their observation that patients treated by exploration alone had fewer complications than those undergoing obliteration appears to be related to the fact that the former group had injuries of lesser severity.

Chronic mucosal disease in the sinus may lead to the development of osteomyelitis within the surrounding injured bone. Keay and colleagues[71] reported this to occur 17 years after an untreated frontal sinus fracture. In this regard, entry into the sinus during a craniotomy also carries the risk of intracranial sepsis and osteomyelitis with the loss of the bone flap if the sinus is infected. Several of these cases were reported by Sataloff and colleagues.[125]

Mucocele or mucopyocele formation may arise both in untreated and treated patients. In the former, injury to the mucosa or bone about the nasofrontal duct can result in obstruction of sinus outflow, with secondary mucocele formation. In patients undergoing surgical exploration with obliteration, retained fragments of mucosa within the sinus may proliferate and undergo a cystic degeneration to form a mucocle.

Severely comminuted and displaced anterior table fractures, whether isolated or combined with a posterior table injury, often evince residual cosmetic deformity of the forehead following repair. Many workers prefer delayed reconstruction with acrylic,[119] operating in a noncontaminated and stable field. Other workers, including Luce,[86] Peri and colleagues,[115] Merville and colleagues,[97] perform primary grafting of the anterior wall defect with split calvarial and corticocancellous bone grafts. Stanley[140] and Gruss and Phillips[51] reported the successful use of bone plating and primary calvarial bone grafting in the repair of complex cranio-orbital fractures involving the frontal sinus. Still others collapse the frontal sinus and perform a primary[39] or secondary[22] acrylic cranioplasty.

References

1. Abramson AL, Eason RL: Experimental frontal sinus obliteration: Long-term results following removal of the mucous membrane lining. Laryngoscope 87:1066, 1977.
2. Abramson AL, Eason RL, Pryor WH, Messer EJ: Experimental results of autogenous cancellous bone chips transplanted into the canine frontal sinus cavity. Ann Otol (Suppl 17) 83:1, 1974.
3. Adkins WY, Cassone RD, Putney FJ: Solitary frontal sinus fracture. Laryngoscope 89:1099, 1979.
4. Adson AW, Hempstead BE: Osteomyelitis of the frontal bone resulting from extension of suppuration of frontal sinus. Surgical treatment. Arch Otolaryngol 25:363, 1937.
5. Alford BR, Gorman GN, Mersol VF: Osteoplastic surgery of the frontal sinus. Laryngoscope 75:1139, 1965.
6. Anderson CM: External operation on the frontal sinus. Causes of failure. Arch Otolaryngol 15:739, 1932.
7. Anthony DH: Use of Ingals' gold tube in frontal sinus operations. South Med J 33:949, 1940.
8. Baron SH, Dedo HH, Henry CR: The mucoperiosteal flap in frontal sinus surgery. (The Sewall-Boyden-McNaught operation.) Laryngoscope 83:1266, 1973.
9. Barton RT: Dacron prosthesis in frontal sinus surgery. Laryngoscope 82:1799, 1972.
10. Barton RT: The use of synthetic implant materials in osteoplastic frontal sinusotomy. Laryngoscope 90:47, 1980.
11. Beck JC: A new method of external frontal sinus operation without deformity. JAMA 51:451, 1908.
12. Beeson WH: Plaster of Paris as an alloplastic implant in the frontal sinus. Arch Otolaryngol 107:664, 1981.
13. Bergara AR: Osteoplastic operation on the large frontal sinus in chronic suppurative sinusitis: End results. Trans Am Acad Ophthalmol Otolaryngol 51:643, 1947.
14. Bergara AR, Itoiz AO: Present state of the surgical treatment of chronic frontal sinusitis. AMA Arch Otolaryngol 61:616, 1955.
15. Boies LR: Acute frontal sinusitis: The trephine operation for drainage in selected cases. Laryngoscope 52:458, 1942.
16. Bordley JE, Bosley WR: Mucoceles of the frontal sinus: Causes and treatment. Ann Otol 82:696, 1973.
17. Bosley WA: Osteoplastic obliteration of the frontal sinuses: A review of 100 patients. Laryngoscope 82:1463, 1972.
18. Boyden GL: Surgical treatment of chronic frontal sinusitis. Ann Otol 61:558, 1952.
19. Boyden GL: Chronic frontal sinusitis: End results of surgical treatment. Trans Am Acad Ophthalmol Otolaryngol 61:588, 1957.
20. Brieger: Über chronische Eiterungen des Nebenhohlen der Nase. Arch Ohren Nasen-Kehlkopfheilk 39:213, 1895.
21. Brunner H: Chronic osteomyelitis of the skull. Ann Otol 52:850, 1943.
22. Cipcic JA: Sinus fractures. Trans Am Acad Ophthalmol Otolaryngol 74:1055, 1970.
23. Climo MS, Block LI, Alexander JE: Extraosseous Kirschner wire fixation for an unstable depressed fracture of the frontal bone. Plast Reconstr Surg 52:200, 1973.
24. Coates GM, Ersner MS: Regeneration of the mucous membrane of the frontal sinus after its surgical removal (in the dog). Arch Otolaryngol 12:642, 1930.
25. Coetzee FS: Regeneration of bone in the presence of calcium sulphate. Arch Otolaryngol 106:405, 1980.
26. Czerny: Cited by Beck JC: A new method of external frontal sinus operation without deformity. JAMA 51:451, 1908.
27. Denneny JC: Frontal sinus obliteration using liposuction. Otolaryngol Head Neck Surg 95:15, 1986.
28. Denneny JC, Davidson WD: Combined otolaryngological and neurosurgical approach in treating sinus fractures. Laryngoscope 97:633, 1987.
29. Dickson R, Hohman A: The fate of exogenous materials placed in the middle ear and frontal sinus of cats. Laryngoscope 81:216, 1971.
30. Dokianakis GS, Helidonis E, Karamitsos D, Papzoglou G: Use of a new mucoperiosteal flap from the upper lateral nasal wall in frontal sinus surgery. Otolaryngol Head Neck Surg 89:912, 1981.
31. Donald PJ: The tenacity of the frontal sinus mucosa. Otolaryngol Head Neck Surg 87:557, 1979.
32. Donald PJ: Recent advances in paranasal sinus surgery. Head Neck Surg 4:140, 1981.
33. Donald PJ: Frontal sinus ablation by cranialization. Report of 21 cases. Arch Otolaryngol 108:142, 1982.
34. Donald PJ, Bernstein L: Compound frontal sinus injuries with intracranial penetration. Laryngoscope 88:225, 1978.
35. Donald PJ, Ettin M: The safety of frontal sinus fat obliteration when sinus walls are missing. Laryngoscope 96:190, 1986.
36. Duvall AJ, Porto DP, Lyons D, Boies LR: Frontal sinus fractures. Analysis of treatment results. Arch Otolaryngol 113:933, 1987.
37. Eason RL, Abramson AJ, Pryor WH: Experimental results of autogenous cancellous bone chips transplanted into the infected canine frontal sinus cavity. Trans Am Acad Ophthalmol Otolaryngol 82:148, 1976.
38. Erich JB, New GB: An acrylic obturator employed in the repair of an obstructed frontonasal duct. Trans Am Acad Ophthalmol Otolaryngol 51:628, 1947.
39. Failla A: Operative management of injuries involving the frontal sinuses. Laryngoscope 78:1833, 1968.
40. Frenckner P, Richter NG: Operative treatment of skull fractures through the frontal sinus. Acta Otolaryngol 51:63, 1960.
41. Ghorayeb BY: The use of a wire sling in anterior table fractures of the frontal sinus. Laryngoscope 97:1358, 1987.
42. Gibson T, Walker FM: Large osteoma of the frontal sinus: A method of removal to minimize scarring and prevent deformity. Br J Plast Surg 4:210, 1951.
43. Gibson T, Walker FM: The osteoplastic flap approach to the frontal sinuses. J Laryngol 68:92, 1954.
44. Goodale RL: Some cause for failure in frontal sinus surgery. Ann Otol 51:648, 1942.

45. Goodale RL: The use of tantalum in radical frontal sinus surgery. Ann Otol 54:757, 1945.

46. Goodale RL, Montgomery WW: Experience with the osteoplastic anterior wall approach to the frontal sinus. Arch Otolaryngol 68:271, 1958.

47. Goodale RL, Montgomery WW: Anterior osteoplastic frontal sinus operation: Five years' experience. Ann Otol 70:860, 1961.

48. Goodale RL, Montgomery WW: Technical advances in osteoplastic frontal sinusectomy. Arch Otolaryngol 79:522, 1964.

49. Goode RL, Strelzow V, Fee WE: Frontal sinus septectomy for chronic unilateral sinusitis. Otolaryngol Head Neck Surg 88:18, 1980.

50. Grahne B: Chronic frontal sinusitis treated by autogenous osteoplasty. Acta Otolaryngol 72:215, 1971.

51. Gruss JS, Phillips JH: Complex facial trauma: The evolving role of rigid fixation and immediate bone graft reconstruction. Clin Plast Surg 16:93, 1989.

52. Guggenheim P: Indications and methods for performance of osteoplastic-obliterative frontal sinusotomy with a description of a new method and some remarks upon the present state of the art of external frontal sinus surgery. Laryngoscope 91:927, 1981.

53. Gussenbauer: Cited by Beck JC: A new method of external frontal sinus operation without deformity. JAMA 51:451, 1908.

54. Halle M: External or internal operation for suppuration of the accessory nasal sinuses. Laryngoscope 17:115, 1907.

55. Hardy JM, Montgomery WW: Osteoplastic frontal sinusotomy. An analysis of 250 operations. Ann Otol 85:523, 1976.

56. Harris HE: The use of tantulum tubes in frontal sinus surgery. Cleve Clin Q 15:129, 1948.

57. Harris L, Marano GD, McCorkle D: Nasofrontal duct: CT in frontal sinus trauma. Radiology 165:195, 1987.

58. Hilding A: Experimental surgery of the nose and sinuses: III Results following partial and complete removal of the lining mucous membrane from the frontal sinus of the dog. Arch Otolaryngol 17:760, 1933.

59. Hilding AC, Banovetz J: Occluding scars in the sinuses: Relation to bone growth. Laryngoscope 73:1201, 1963.

60. Hoffman: Osteoplastic operation on the frontal sinuses for chronic suppuration. Ann Otol 13:598, 1904.

61. Howarth WG: Operations on the frontal sinus. J Laryngol 36:417, 1921.

62. Hybels RL: Posterior table fractures of the frontal sinus: II. Clinical aspects. Laryngoscope 87:1740, 1977.

63. Hybels RL, Newman MH: Posterior table fractures of the frontal sinus: I. An experimental study. Laryngoscope 87:171, 1977.

64. Hybels RL, Weimert TA: Evaluation of frontal sinus fractures. Arch Otolaryngol 105:275, 1979.

65. Ingals EF: New operation and instruments for draining the frontal sinus. Trans Am Laryngol Rhinol Otol Soc 2:183, 1905.

66. Jacobson AL, Lawson W, Biller HF: Bilateral pansinus mucocele with bilateral orbital and intracranial extension. Otolaryngol Head Neck Surg 90:507, 1982.

67. Jansen A: Neue Erfahrungen über chronische Nebenhohleneiterungen der Nase. Arch Ohrennasen-Kehlkopfheilk 56:110, 1902.

68. Janeke JB, Komora RM, Cohn AM: Proplast in cavity obliteration and soft tissue augmentation. Arch Otolaryngol 100:24, 1974.

69. Jones AC: Osteomyelitis of the frontal bone with report of 13 cases. Ann Otol 49:713, 1940.

70. Kasper KA: Nasofrontal connections: A study based on 100 consecutive dissections. Arch Otolaryngol 23:322, 1936.

71. Keay DG, Dale BA, Murray JA: Long-term complications of frontal sinus fractures. J R Coll Surg Edinb 33:95, 1988.

72. Kettel K: Osteomyelitis of the frontal bone. Surgical treatment: Which way of approach is the best? Arch Otolaryngol 31:622, 1940.

73. Killian G: Die Killianische Radicaloperation chronischer Stirnhohleneiterungen: II. Weiteres kasuistisches Material und Zusammenfassung. Arch Laryngol Rhinol 13:59, 1903.

74. Kirchner FR: Modified osteoplastic approach to the frontal bone, sinuses, and/or orbit. Laryngoscope 77:1706, 1967.

75. Kirchner JA, Yanagisawa E, Crelin ES: Surgical anatomy of the ethmoidal arteries. Arch Otolaryngol 74:382, 1961.

76. Knapp A: The surgical treatment of orbital complications in disease of the nasal accessory sinuses. JAMA 51:299, 1908.

77. Kudryk WH, Mahasin Z: Superiorly based osteoplastic flap for frontal sinus disease. J Otolaryngol 17:395, 1988.

78. Kuhnt H: Über die entzundliche Erkrankungen der Stirnhohlen und ihre Folgezstande. Eine Klinische Studie. Wiesbaden, JF Bergmann, 1895.

79. Kuster: Cited by Beck JC: A new method of external frontal sinus operation without deformity. JAMA 51:451, 1980.

80. Larrabee WF, Travis LW, Tabb HG: Frontal sinus fractures—their suppurative complications and surgical management. Laryngoscope 90:1810, 1980.

81. Levine SB, Rowe LD, Keane WM, Atkins JP: Evaluation and treatment of frontal sinus fractures. Otolaryngol Head Neck Surg 95:19, 1986.

82. Lillie HL: Postoperative complications of the radical external frontal sinus operations. Trans Am Laryngol Assoc 53:136, 1931.

83. Lillie HL, Anderson CM: The two-stage operation for suppurative frontal sinusitis with external manifestations. Arch Otolaryngol 5:152, 1927.

84. Lothrop HA: Frontal sinus suppuration. Ann Surg 59:937, 1912.

85. Luc H: Traitement des sinusites frontales suppurees chroniques par l'ouverture largest de la paroi anterieure du sinus et le drainage par la voie nasale (methode d'Ogston et Luc). Arch Int Laryngol 9:163, 1896.

86. Luce EA: Frontal sinus fractures: Guidelines to management. Plast Reconstr Surg 80:500, 1987.

87. Lyman EH: The place of the obliterative operation in frontal sinus surgery. Laryngoscope 60:407, 1950.

88. Lynch RC: The technique of a radical frontal sinus operation which has given me the best results. Laryngoscope 31:1, 1921.

89. MacBeth RG: The osteoplastic operation for chronic infection of the frontal sinus. J Laryngol 68:465, 1954.

90. Malecki J: New trends in frontal sinus surgery. Acta Otolaryngol 50:137, 1959.

91. Marx G: Fettransplantation nach Stirnhohlenoperation. Z Ohrenheilk 61:7, 1910.

92. May M, Ogura JH, Schramm V: Nasofrontal duct in frontal sinus fractures. Arch Otolaryngol 92:534, 1970.

93. McGrath MH, Smith CJ: A simple method to maintain reduction of unstable fractures of the frontal sinus. Plast Reconstr Surg 68:948, 1981.

94. McNally WJ, Stuart EA: A 30 year review of frontal sinusitis treated by external operation. Ann Otol 63:651, 1954.

95. McNaught RC: A refinement of the external frontoeth-

mosphenoid operation. A new nasofrontal pedicle flap. Arch Otolaryngol 23:544, 1936.

96. McNeil RA: Surgical obliteration of the maxillary sinus. Laryngoscope 77:202, 1967.

97. Merville LC, Derome P: Concomitant dislocations of the face and skull. J Maxillofac Surg 6:2, 1978.

98. Miller SH, Lung RJ, Davis TS, Graham WP, Kennedy TJ: Management of fractures of the supraorbital rim. J Trauma 18:507, 1978.

99. Mithoefer W: External operation on the frontal sinus: Critical review. Arch Otolaryngol 7:133, 1928.

100. Montgomery WW: Surgery of the upper respiratory system. 2nd ed. Philadelphia, Lea and Febiger, 1979.

101. Montgomery WW, Ormon PV: Inhibitory effect of adipose tissue on osteogenesis. Ann Otol 76:988, 1967.

102. Montgomery WW, Pierce DL: Anterior osteoplastic fat obliteration for frontal sinus: Clinical experience and animal studies. Trans Am Acad Ophthalmol Otolaryngol 67:46, 1963.

103. Mosher HP, Judd DK: An analysis of seven cases of osteomyelitis of the frontal bone complicating frontal sinusitis. Laryngoscope 43:153, 1933.

104. Nadell J, Kline DG: Primary reconstruction of depressed frontal skull fractures including those involving the sinus, orbit and cribriform plate. J Neurosurg 41:200, 1974.

105. Naumann HH: Gedanken zum gegenwartigen Stand der Stirnhohlen-Chirurgie. Z Laryngol 40:733, 1961.

106. Neel HB, Whicker JA, Lake CF: Thin rubber sheeting in frontal sinus surgery: Animal and clinical studies. Laryngoscope 86:524, 1976.

107. Negus VE: The surgical treatment of chronic frontal sinusitis. Br Med J 1:135, 1947.

108. Newman MH, Travis LW: Frontal sinus fractures. Laryngoscope 83:1281, 1973.

109. Noyek AM, Kassel EE: Computed tomography in frontal sinus fractures. Arch Otolaryngol 108:378, 1982.

110. Ogston A: Trephining the frontal sinuses for catarrhal diseases. Med Chron Manchester 1:235, 1884–1885.

111. Ogura JH, Watson RK, Jurema AA: Frontal sinus surgery. The use of a mucoperiosteal flap for reconstruction of a nasofrontal duct. Laryngoscope 70:1229, 1960.

112. Oppenheimer RP: Treatment of comminuted fractures of the anterior sinus wall. Trans Am Acad Ophthalmol Otolaryngol 80:507, 1975.

113. Pastore PN, Williams HL: Osteomyelitis of the frontal bone secondary to suppurative disease of the frontal sinus. Report of a case. Proc Staff Mayo Clin 13:7, 1938.

114. Patterson N: External operations on the frontal and ethmoidal sinuses. J Laryngol 54:235, 1939.

115. Peri G, Chabannes J, Menes R, Jourde J, Fain J: Fractures of the frontal sinus. J Maxillofac Surg 9:73, 1981.

116. Podoshin L, Altman MM: Balloon technique for treatment of frontal sinus fractures. J Laryngol 81:1157, 1967.

117. Pope TH, Thompson WR: Treatment of chronic unilateral frontal sinusitis by removal of the interfrontal septum. South Med J 69:755, 1976.

118. Porto DP, Duvall AJ: Long-term results with nasofrontal duct reconstruction. Laryngoscope 96:858, 1986.

119. Remsen K, Lawson W, Biller HF: Acrylic frontal cranioplasty. Head Neck Surg 9:31, 1986.

120. Riedel: In Schenke: Inaug Dissertation. Jena, 1898.

121. Ritter FN: The Paranasal Sinuses. Anatomy and Surgical Technique. St Louis, CV Mosby, 1973.

122. Ritter G: Erhaltung der vorderen Stirnhohlenwand bei der Radikaloperation. Verhandl Ver Deutsch Laryng 628, 1911.

123. Rongetti JR: Frontal sinus approach with minimal deformity. Arch Otolaryngol 72:380, 1960.

124. Runge: Cited by Stevenson RS, Guthrie D: A History of Otolaryngology. Baltimore, Williams & Wilkins, 1949.

125. Sataloff RT, Sariego J, Myers DL, Richter HJ: Surgical management of the frontal sinus. Neurosurgery 15:593, 1984.

126. Schaefer SD, Anderson RG, Carder HM: Epidural mucopyocele: Diagnosis and management. Otolaryngol Head Neck Surg 89:523, 1981.

127. Schaefer SD, Close LG, Mickey BE: The surgical management of epidural mucoceles. Laryngoscope 98:14, 1988.

128. Scharfe EE: The use of tantalum in otolaryngology. Arch Otolaryngol 58:133, 1953.

129. Schenck NL: Frontal sinus disease. III. Experimental and clinical factors in failure of the frontal osteoplastic operation. Laryngoscope 85:76, 1975.

130. Schenck NL, Tomlinson MJ, Ridgley CD: Experimental evaluation of a new implant material in frontal sinus obliteration. Arch Otolaryngol 102:521, 1976.

131. Schonborn: Cited by Wilkop A: Ein Beitrag zur Casuistik der Erkrankungen des Sinus Frontalis. Wurzburg, F Frome, 1894.

132. Schultz RC: Frontal sinus and supraorbital fractures from vehicle accidents. Clin Plast Surg 21:93, 1975.

133. Schwartzman J, Silva AD: A new homograft implant technic for ablation of the chronically infected frontoethmoid-sinal complex. Int Rhinol 8:101, 1970.

134. Sessions RB, Alford BR, Stratton C, et al: Current concepts of frontal sinus surgery: An appraisal of the osteoplastic flap—fat obliteration operation. Laryngoscope 82:918, 1972.

135. Sewall EC: The operative treatment of nasal sinus disease. Ann Otol 44:307, 1935.

136. Shockley WW, Stucker FJ, Gage-White L, Antony SO: Frontal sinus fractures: Some problems and some solutions. Laryngoscope 98:18, 1988.

137. Siirala U: Obliteration of the frontal sinus with ossar. Int Surg 47:425, 1967.

138. Skillern SR: Osteomyelitic invasion of the frontal bone following frontal sinus disease. Ann Otol 48:392, 1939.

139. Smith F: Chronic sinus disease—its present status. JAMA 100:402, 1933.

140. Stanley RB: Fractures of the frontal sinus. Clin Plast Surg 16:115, 1989.

141. Stanley RB, Becker TS: Injuries of the nasofrontal orifices in frontal sinus fractures. Laryngoscope 97:728, 1987.

142. Tato JM, Sibbald DW, Bergaglio OE: Surgical treatment of the frontal sinus by the external route. Laryngoscope 64:504, 1954.

143. Urken ML, Som PM, Lawson W, Edelstein D, Weber AL, Biller HF: Abnormally large frontal sinus. II. Nomenclature, pathology, symptoms. Laryngoscope 97:606, 1987.

144. Urken ML, Som PM, Lawson W, Edelstein D, McAvay G, Biller HF: The abnormally large frontal sinus. I. A practical method for its determination based upon an analysis of 100 normal patients. Laryngoscope 97:602, 1987.

145. Valenzuela L: Treatment of traumatic disease of the frontal sinus by adipose implant obliteration. Laryngoscope 77:1695, 1967.

146. Vuillemin T, Raveh J, Stich H, Cottier H: Fixation of bone fragments with BIOCEM. First observations on humans. Arch Otolaryngol 113:836, 1987.

147. Wallis A, Donald PJ: Frontal sinus fractures: A review of 72 cases. Laryngoscope 98:593, 1988.

148. Walsh TE: Experimental surgery of the frontal sinus: The role of the ostium and nasofrontal duct in post-operative healing. Laryngoscope 53:75, 1943.

149. Weber SC, Cohn AM: Fracture of the frontal sinus in children. Arch Otolaryngol 103:241, 1977.

150. Weile FL: The problem of secondary frontal sinus surgery. Ann Otol 55:372, 1946.

151. Whited RE: Anterior table frontal sinus fractures. Laryngoscope 89:1951, 1979.

152. Wilensky AO: Association of osteomyelitis of the skull and nasal accessory sinus disease. Arch Otolaryngol 15:805, 1932.

153. Williams HL, Holman CB: The causes and avoidance of failure in surgery, for chronic suppuration of the fronto-ethmosphenoid complex of sinuses: With a previous unreported anomaly which produces chronicity and recurrence, and the description of a surgical technique usually producing a cure of the disease. Laryngoscope 72:1179, 1962.

154. Wilson BC, Davidson B, Corey JP, Haydon RC: Comparison of complications following frontal sinus fractures managed with exploration with or without obliteration over 10 years. Laryngoscope 98:516, 1988.

155. Winkler: Beitrag zur osteoplastischen Freilegung des Sinus frontalis. Verhandl Deutsch Otol Gessellsch, 1904.

156. Wolfowitz BL, Solomon A: Mucoceles of the frontal and ethmoid sinuses. J Laryngol 86:79, 1972.

157. Zonis RD, Montgomery WW, Goodale RL: Frontal sinus disease: 100 cases treated by osteoplastic operation. Laryngoscope 76:1816, 1966.

CHAPTER 11

ETHMOID SINUS

William H. Friedman, MD, FACS

The ethmoid labyrinth has been called the keystone of the paranasal sinuses because of its central location and pivotal role in nasal and sinus function (Fig. 11–1). All the sinuses, the orbit, the nasal cavities, and the cranium share common borders with the ethmoid labyrinth. Its role in congenital, neoplastic, and inflammatory disease of the nose and paranasal sinuses cannot be readily separated from its contiguity with these structures. Unless pathologic changes in the ethmoids are confined to the most discrete of benign neoplasms, tiny congenital cysts, or isolated polyps, it is necessary to encroach on surrounding structures in performing surgery. This chapter will describe the ethmoidectomy operations, including intranasal, external, and transantral ethmoidectomy. In each of these procedures it is necessary to transgress a major bony sinus to completely exenterate the ethmoid labyrinth; in each, total or near total exenteration of the ethmoids is necessary if excellent results are to be obtained.

The role of ethmoidectomy in malignant disease is discussed elsewhere. However, because of its contiguity with other structures, the ethmoid labyrinth is seldom exenterated as an isolated procedure for the removal of malignant disease. Rather, it is more often a part of a more extensive operation such as partial, total, or radical maxillectomy. It may be performed in conjunction with orbital exenteration, osteoplastic frontal sinusotomy with obliteration of both the frontal and ethmoid sinuses, lateral rhinotomy, and craniofacial resection for tumors of the upper nasal vault, frontal cranial fossa, or both. Each of the ethmoidectomy procedures has specific advantages related to visualization and accessibility of adjacent structures.

HISTORY

Surgery of the ethmoid labyrinth dates to Hippocrates (460–370 B.C.),[1] who avulsed nasal polyps and probably adjacent ethmoid cells by using a sponge attached to traction strings. He utilized cautery with a hot iron and even employed a kind of polyp snare not too dissimilar from instruments in use today. Paulus and Aegina (625–690 A.D.) and Fallopius (1523–1562 A.D.) used similar techniques. Jansen[2] in 1884 probably performed the first transantral ethmoidectomy. This procedure was further popularized by Horgan[3] in 1926 and by Langenbrunner and Nigri[4] in 1976.

External ethmoidectomy was originally described by Ferris Smith in 1933[1] and has been continuously modified by many surgeons since that time. In 1912, Mosher[5] described the anatomy and intranasal surgery of the ethmoid labyrinth. Yankauer[6] demonstrated a complete exenteration of the ethmoids and removal of the anterior wall of the sphenoid in a stepwise procedure, which he termed sphenoethmoidectomy. Many workers have commented on and modified this procedure.[7–10] Van Alyea[11] in 1951 provided a detailed study of the bony lamellae of the ethmoid labyrinth, firmly grounding all ethmoid procedures in an appropriate anatomic framework.

The concept of ethmoid marsupialization, in effect the complete ethmoidectomy, was advanced by Friedman and colleagues[12] in 1986. The basis for ethmoid marsupialization arises from the surgical principle of incision and drainage of an abscess cavity. Because of the considerable mechanical disadvantage imposed upon

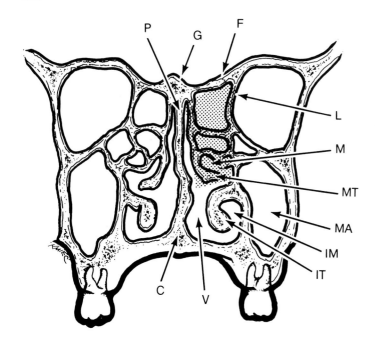

Figure 11–1. The ethmoid sinuses seen in coronal view. *P*, Perpendicular plate of the ethmoid; *G*, crista galli and adjacent cribriform plate; *F*, fovea ethmoidalis (roof of the ethmoids); *L*, lamina papyracea; *M, MT*, middle turbinate and medial anterior ethmoids; *MA*, maxillary antrum; *IM*, inferior meatus; *IT*, inferior turbinate; *V*, lower nasal vault; *C*, maxillary crest.

the ethmoid labyrinth by chronic disease, complete removal of the disease by isolated removal of a single ethmoid cell or the mucosal lining of an ethmoid cell, or polypectomy is not ordinarily considered sufficient or curative. Recently, the popularity of functional endoscopic sinus surgery[13] has led to controversy concerning both the method and extent of ethmoidectomy needed in controlling polypoid disease and chronic sinusitis. Endoscopic surgery is dealt with elsewhere in this textbook and will not be described in this chapter. However, endoscopic surgery of the paranasal sinuses is recognized as having both practical and historical importance in the continued development of surgery of the ethmoid labyrinth.

NASAL POLYPOSIS

The commonest indication for surgery of the ethmoid sinuses is nasal polyposis. Nasal polyps are typically saclike, prolapsed respiratory epithelium containing an edematous submucosa with a myxoid stroma. Chronic inflammatory cells and eosinophils may be present in large numbers. Polyps frequently arise in the middle meatus area and can also originate from the nasal septum, the upper and lower vaults, the lateral nasal wall, and the floor of the nose. Pathologic changes in polypoid nasal and sinus mucosa may include papillary, follicular, fibrous, cystic, and vascular alterations in prolapsed respiratory mucosa.[14] Symptoms induced

by polyps or hyperplastic rhinosinusitis include airway obstruction and recurring bouts of purulent pansinusitis and, in atopic individuals, may include the entire clinical spectrum of hyperirritable upper and lower respiratory epithelium with recurring bouts of asthma. Aspirin sensitivity, bronchitis, emphysema, recurring pneumonitis, and bronchiectasis are not uncommon in the patient with nasal polyps. Chronicity is a feature rather than a result of this disease and, in patients with polyps, attempts to subdivide chronic sinusitis according to etiology are fruitless. Williams[15] classified sinusitis as bacterial, allergic, or hyperplastic. However, these three entities may frequently be seen in the same patient. Davison[16] emphasized that early in his career he attempted to utilize the smallest amount of surgery needed to produce permanent relief of symptoms. Later, he became convinced that extensive disease required extensive surgery.

The term hyperplastic rhinosinusitis may be more appropriate than polyposis in chronic disease, as polypoid changes within the maxillary, sphenoid, and frontal sinuses occur simultaneously with overt polyp formation elsewhere.

Radiographically, hyperplastic rhinosinusitis ranges from isolated polyps to thickening of the mucosal linings and opacity of all the nasal sinuses. Fluid levels may be present in acute episodes of maxillary or frontal sinusitis or pansinusitis. Bony changes include progressive demineralization and loss of bony landmarks. So-called rarefying osteitis occurs in long-standing disease. This is associated with loss of frontal sinus architecture, particularly loss of the scalloped outlines of the superior frontal radiographic margins. Other demineralizing signs indicative of chronic disease include loss of ethmoid architecture, causing the ethmoid labyrinth to lose its lamellar, reticular quality and to be replaced by an amorphous, hazy, or radiodense cavity. The maxillary sinuses frequently have isolated polyps. However, the most common maxillary finding in hyperplastic rhinosinusitis is thickening of maxillary mucosa, sometimes to levels at which the mucosal walls nearly meet in the center of the maxillary sinus.

Nasal polypectomy[17] is of limited usefulness in control of nasal polyps because it does not permanently eliminate the probable causes of polyps: hyperreactive respiratory epithelium, chronic infection, and an altered immunologic state. Polypectomy does not remove underlying chronic osteitis and possible bacterial seeding from the mazelike ethmoid lamellae. These wafer-thin bony walls provide an expanded surface from which polyps can arise and may induce inflammatory changes because of osteitis and contiguous chronic infection. Finally, polypectomy is usually followed by recurrence of nasal polyps and is no more effective in controlling nasal polyps than intermittent dosages of corticosteroids. Because surgery for hyperplastic rhinosinusitis is never radical, the term *adequate* is more appropriate in describing total exenteration of these cells.[7] My experience indicates that adequate ethmoid surgery implies complete exenteration of the ethmoid labyrinth to control nasal polyposis and suggests that limited surgery produces limited benefits and more extensive surgery produces relatively greater benefits in the treatment of hyperplastic nasal and sinus disease.

Complete exenteration of the ethmoid labyrinth for hyperplastic rhinosinusitis is not necessarily curative. Friedman in 1975 reported an overall recurrence rate of 30.9 per cent following intranasal ethmoidectomy for patients with severe polyposis who had undergone previous polypectomy,[7] and in 1989 he reported a polyp recurrence rate of 18.1 per cent in asthmatics undergoing sphenoethmoidectomy for hyperplastic rhinosinusitis.[8] This should not discourage the surgeon, as ethmoidectomy provides an orderly and systematic removal of diseased ethmoid labyrinth, polyps, and inspissated infection and has proved useful in the management of polyps without demonstrable etiology and in the atopic and asthmatic patient with hyperplastic rhinosinusitis.

The specific ethmoidectomy approach utilized should be that with which the surgeon has the most familiarity and in which visualization of the ethmoids is best accomplished. Because of its ease of performance and relatively noninvasive and functional nature, endoscopic ethmoid surgery has become popular. This surgery has considerable disadvantages, including the limited field of view of the nasal endoscopes, the small size of the biting forceps, and the disadvantages that bleeding presents in maintaining clear optics. The intranasal, transantral, and external ethmoidectomies have specific indications and advantages. Many surgeons prefer the external ethmoidectomy because it allows visualization of orbital contents and provides an extra measure of safety in the avoidance of these structures. Its disadvantages include unilateral access, poor lower nasal visualization, and an external scar. Transantral ethmoidectomy is favored by some surgeons because of its simultaneous access to both the maxillary sinus and the ethmoid labyrinth. It too suffers the disadvantage of unilateral access and somewhat limited visualization, as the depths of the procedure are reached only by traversing the upper medial portion of the maxilla. Intranasal ethmoidectomy offers simultaneous access to both ethmoid labyrinths through natural orifices and does not require surgical entry until the ethmoids are reached. For polyposis or hyperplastic nasal and sinus disease, I prefer intranasal ethmoidectomy combined with transnasal maxillary antrotomy. For benign neoplasms, external ethmoidectomy is preferred because it offers anteroposterior visualization of the labyrinth and enables the surgeon to resect the labyrinth en bloc if necessary. For extensive, benign disease of the maxillary sinus involving the ethmoid labyrinth, the transantral ethmoidectomy provides additional exposure of the maxillary sinus, and disease in this structure is best visualized directly.

EXTERNAL ETHMOIDECTOMY

External ethmoidectomy is preferred for acute ethmoiditis resulting in orbital abscess or threatened orbital abscess, for biopsy of ethmoid neoplasms that are inaccessible intranasally, and for frontoethmoid disease requiring simultaneous access to the ethmoids and the frontal sinuses. In addition, the external ethmoidectomy can be combined with lateral rhinotomy for removal of locally invasive benign disease, such as the inverting papilloma, osteomas, and other mesenchymal tumors, and for closure of cerebrospinal fluid (CSF) leaks in the cribriform plate or fovea ethmoidalis regions. Because simultaneous access to the orbit and ethmoid contents is provided, the external ethmoidectomy is an excellent procedure for benign processes that involve both areas. This procedure alone or in conjunction with lateral rhinotomy is probably not adequate for the resection of most malignant neoplasms and must be combined with maxillectomy or orbital exenteration.

Technique

External ethmoidectomy is best performed under general anesthesia because orbital contents must be retracted. The incision[18] (Fig. 11–2) is curvilinear, extending from just below the eyebrow inferiorly along the lateral nasal wall halfway between the inner canthus and the dorsum of the nose. It can be extended laterally into the brow for frontal exposure to accomplish frontoethmoidectomy and can be carried inferiorly into the melonasal and nostril margin if lateral rhinotomy is required. Troublesome bleeding is usually encountered from the angular vessels lying above the periosteum at the nasofacial line. These should be ligated. If the incision is carried deep in the region of the brow, care must be exercised not to inadvertently incise deep to the supraorbital rim, as damage to the trochlea or superior oblique tendon can occur (Fig. 11–3). Periosteum overlying the frontal processes of the maxilla is

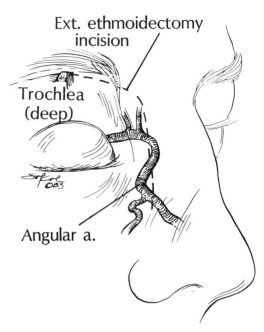

Figure 11–3. The relationship between the angular vessels and the external ethmoidectomy incision. The tendon of the superior oblique muscle lies deep to this dissection and is shown at its fulcrum in the trochlea just beneath the superior orbital rim.

incised. Once the periosteum is elevated, orbital contents are retracted (Fig. 11–4), taking care not to injure the lacrimal sac in the medial inferior portion of the operative field lying between the posterior and anterior lacrimal crest (Fig. 11–2). The usefulness of this approach is evident in dacryocystorhinostomy,

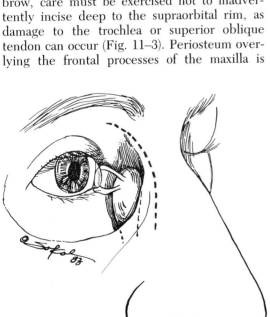

Figure 11–2. The external ethmoidectomy incision halfway between the medial canthus and the nasal dorsum. The lacrimal sac is shown deep to the anterior lacrimal crest. Ordinarily, dissection is aimed at avoiding this structure. In dacryocystorhinostomy, this approach is excellent.

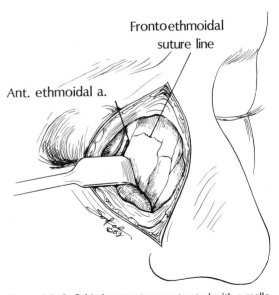

Figure 11–4. Orbital contents are retracted with a malleable or blunt retractor.

but it is not essential to manipulate or mobilize the lacrimal sac at the time of external ethmoidectomy. It may be necessary to incise the medial canthal ligament at its attachment to the anterior lacrimal crest. It is important to reattach this structure at the conclusion of the operation to avoid blunting or telecanthus.

With gentle retraction of orbital contents, blunt dissection is used to reveal the lamina papyracea forming most of the medial orbital boundary and the lateral wall of both the anterior and posterior ethmoid labyrinths. The anterior ethmoid artery is located in the frontoethmoid suture line (Fig. 11–5) approximately 2 cm posterior to the posterior lacrimal crest in adults. The posterior ethmoid artery is located approximately 1 cm posterior to this, and the optic foramen lies another 1 cm posterior to the posterior ethmoid artery. The anterior ethmoid artery is routinely ligated, or a vascular clip is applied. It is not necessary to ligate the posterior ethmoid artery, and its preservation may help in avoiding damage to the optic nerve.

When the operative field is fully visualized, the lamina papyracea is taken down with fine bone rongeurs, allowing visualization of the lateral ethmoid cells. These cells can be removed sequentially while keeping the limits of the dissection anterior to the posterior ethmoid artery. With the suction tip placed intranasally, the medial ethmoid cells can be removed and the nasal cavity entered. The middle turbinate is encountered and, if diseased, can be removed. If the middle turbinate is taken down, care must be taken to avoid transgression of the cribriform plate. The surgeon must be equally

careful in avoidance of the thicker fovea ethmoidalis[18] or ethmoid roof, as entry into the frontal cranial fossa can be accomplished inadvertently by this route, as well as by cribriform disruption. When all diseased soft tissue and bone are resected, the nose is packed with 0.5 inch petroleum jelly (Vaseline) gauze until the gauze is loosely visualized in the medial orbital fenestra. Orbital contents are released. A drain is not necessary. For skin closure, 4–0 chromic subcutaneous sutures are utilized with 5–0 silk or nylon suture for skin closure. Packing is removed in 2 days. Sutures are removed 3 to 5 days after surgery.

TRANSANTRAL ETHMOIDECTOMY

The transantral ethmoidectomy is most useful in orbital decompression. This procedure combines transantral ethmoidectomy with removal of the roof of the maxillary sinus, suspension of orbital contents on the infraorbital nerve, and multiple incisions of periorbita. Herniation of orbital fat into the space created by ethmoidectomy and removal of the floor of the orbit permits satisfactory decompression of orbital contents in patients with exophthalmos associated with Graves' disease. The procedure is quite effective in reducing exophthalmos by as much as 7 to 9 mm (measured by the exophthalmometer). The patient must be informed that eye muscle surgery may be required to restore conjugate gaze, because stretching of extraocular muscles by the disease process is not corrected by transantral ethmoidectomy.

In addition, many surgeons utilize transantral ethmoidectomy for chronic hyperplastic disease. I prefer to reserve this procedure primarily for patients requiring orbital decompression and for those with extensive benign maxillary disease that encroaches on the ethmoid sinuses.

TECHNIQUE

Transantral ethmoidectomy may be performed under either local or general anesthesia. For orbital decompression, general endotracheal anesthesia is preferred. This may be augmented with local infiltration of 1 per cent lidocaine (Xylocaine) with 1:100,000 epinephrine (the anesthesiologist must be informed that epinephrine is being used) introduced into the gingivobuccal sulcus, the lateral nasal walls, and

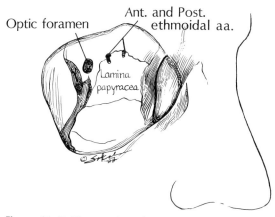

Figure 11–5. The anterior ethmoidal artery in the frontoethmoidal suture line. The posterior ethmoidal artery is also shown. There is a variable relationship between the posterior ethmoidal artery and the optic nerve. Dissection posterior to the posterior ethmoidal artery may result in injury to the optic nerve.

the middle and inferior turbinates. A Caldwell-Luc anterior maxillary antrotomy is performed through a sublabial incision. When the interior of the maxillary sinus is visualized and most of the anterior wall taken down, the upper medial wall of the maxillary sinus is approached halfway along the border between the medial and superior walls of the maxillary sinus (Fig. 11–6). At this point, the ethmoid labyrinth may bulge into the maxillary sinus; this is the region of the bulla ethmoidale. This structure presenting in the maxillary sinus may appropriately be called the bulla antrale. This bulla, or in its absence the anatomic area corresponding to it, is entered with a bone-cutting forceps such as a Myles punch. The surgeon has now entered the anterior ethmoid labyrinth through the maxilla. An orderly exenteration of cells posteriorly is safe because the orbital rim continues as the ethmoid contribution condenses in the medial orbital area just anterior to the lamina papyracea.

It is important that the surgeon not damage the orbital rim; an orbital rim fracture is not an acceptable complication of this procedure. The middle turbinate is used as the medial guide to the transantral ethmoidectomy, preventing access to the cribriform area. However, as in all ethmoidectomies, the roof of the ethmoid labyrinth, the fovea ethmoidalis, must be scrupulously maintained under direct vision. An inadvertent thrust of a surgical instrument cephalad can easily damage this structure, which is only slightly thicker than the cribriform plate.

Thorough exenteration of the ethmoid cells

is accomplished. Intranasal antrostomy is optional in this procedure because the entire middle meatus will have been removed. Many surgeons believe that dependent drainage postoperatively is better treated with an inferior meatal intranasal window. Packing is usually not required following transantral ethmoidectomy. However, if bleeding is not controlled at surgery, 0.5-inch gauze impregnated with an antibiotic solution may be used. This packing should be placed intranasally, first into the maxillary sinus, leading into the nose. Sharp bony ridges that may obstruct the removal of packing must be taken down. If packing is used, it should be removed on the third or fourth postoperative day.

INTRANASAL SPHENOETHMOIDECTOMY

The intranasal sphenoethmoidectomy, performed under local anesthesia, has proved invaluable in the treatment of hyperplastic nasal and sinus disease and is preferred for treating patients with recurrent nasal polyps, hyperplastic rhinosinusitis with asthma, and chronic purulent ethmoiditis.

TECHNIQUE

The patient is placed in a semisitting position. Preliminary intranasal anesthesia is achieved with 10 per cent cocaine on plain cotton gauze. A maximum of 2 ml of cocaine is used, most of which is squeezed from the cotton prior to insertion. Next, 2 ml of 2 per cent lidocaine (Xylocaine) with 1:50,000 epinephrine (Adrenalin) is introduced into the greater palatine foramen with a 1.5-inch needle traversing the pterygopalatine canal to the level of the pterygopalatine space. Anterior ethmoid infiltration is then accomplished by injecting 1 ml of the same mixture into the middle turbinate, into the lateral nasal wall, and laterally to a point near the infraorbital nerve. The septum is injected. A total of 5 ml per side is used.

A submucous resection of the nasal septum is performed if necessary. All polyps are removed with a mucosal biting forceps such as the Wilde forceps or snare. The middle turbinate attachment is then incised anteriorly and either snared or removed with a scissors (Fig. 11–7), leaving a 0.5-cm superior margin attached to the fovea ethmoidalis. A beaded probe

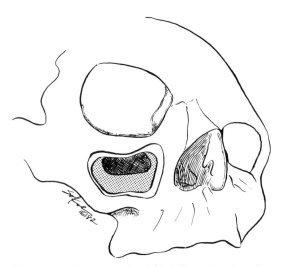

Figure 11–6. The transantral ethmoidectomy—entry into the ethmoids at a point halfway along the border between the roof and the medial wall of the maxillary antrum.

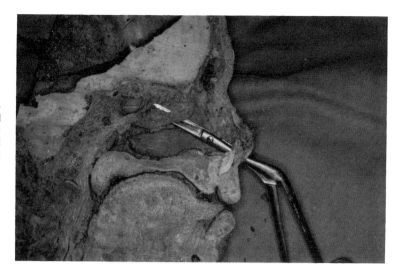

Figure 11–7. Either an angled scissors or a snare is ideal for removal of the middle turbinate. In this cadaver specimen, a 0.5-cm residual middle turbinate attachment to the fovea ethmoidalis is preserved.

with beads at 7 cm, 9 cm, and 11 cm is next inserted. At an angle of approximately 30 degrees measured from the floor of the nose, the sphenoid face is encountered at about 7 cm (Fig. 11–8) from the nostril margin. Bone-cutting forceps on a universal hand piece are used to remove posterior ethmoid cells anterior to the face of the sphenoid, so that visualization of the tip of the probe is accomplished. The probe tip is then placed into the sphenoid orifice, and, using the probe as a guide, a sphenoid punch is employed to remove the face of the sphenoid. The opening is enlarged with angled bone-cutting forceps (Fig. 11–9). Full visualization of the roof and lateral wall of the sphenoid enables the surgeon to remove posterior and anterior ethmoid cells in a three-dimensional block, always working from posterior to anterior. The lateral wall of the sphenoid may not be visible. However, the optic nerve, carotid canal, cribriform plate, lamina papyracea, fovea ethmoidalis, and cavernous sinus are not at risk as long as the forceps is never used outside the anterior extension of the planes of the roof and lateral sphenoid wall (Fig. 11–10). The medial boundary is the plane of the middle turbinate, the lateral boundary is the plane of the lateral sphenoid wall, and the superior boundary is the plane of the sphenoid sinus roof.

An attempt is made to exteriorize each ethmoid cell individually. The agger nasi, remnants of embryologic ethmoids, are resected anterior to the uncinate process and hiatus semilunaris (Fig. 11–11). The nasofrontal duct is not cannulated. Intranasal antrostomy is performed. The nose is not packed unless submucous resection of the septum was performed. Postoperatively, crusts are allowed to remain until

they can be removed with gentle suction. The patient is seen twice weekly until the nasal cavity is re-epithelialized. Bilateral sphenoethmoidectomy is usually performed at one sitting, requiring less than 60 minutes.

Meticulous postoperative care and control of underlying allergy, asthma, or infection are as important in controlling hyperplastic nasal disease as adequate resection of polyps and underlying ethmoid bone. This task is made simpler when exteriorization of the ethmoid, sphenoid, and maxillary sinuses has been accomplished.

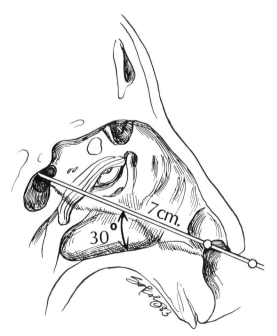

Figure 11–8. The sphenoid face encountered at 7 cm from the nostril margin at an approximate 30° angle from the nasal floor.

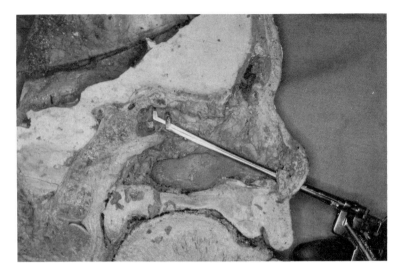

Figure 11–9. The sphenoid face removed (Cordes forceps).

COMPLICATIONS

The ethmoidectomy operations are all safe in proportion to the skill with which the surgeon visualizes important landmarks and observes anatomic planes in the dissection.

In the external ethmoidectomy, inaccurate placement of the incision can result in medial canthal scarring, and poor closure can result in hypertrophic scarring. Damage to the lacrimal apparatus or blunting of the medial canthus (telecanthus) is rare. Violation of the surgical planes may result in damage to third, fourth, fifth, or sixth nerves. Retrobulbar hematoma or surgical manipulation can result in optic nerve damage or blindness. Damage to the cribriform plate or fovea ethmoidalis with subsequent CSF leak may result from the careless placement of a probe or forceps.

In the transantral procedure, numbness of the gingivobuccal sulcus and alveolar ridge is

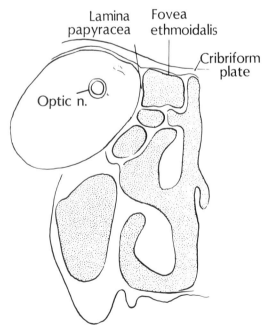

Figure 11–10. The position of optic nerve, cribriform plate, cavernous sinus, carotid canal, lamina papyracea, and fovea ethmoidalis during the sphenoethmoidectomy operation.

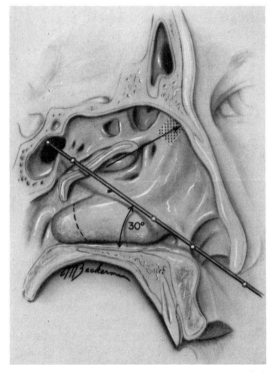

Figure 11–11. This diagram shows the location of the agger nasi cells *(stippled area)* lying anterior to the hiatus semilunaris on a direct line from the anterior tip of the disattached middle turbinate to the nasal dorsum. These cells are the only ethmoid cells in the external nose.

TABLE 11–1. Complications of Intranasal and Transnasal Sphenoethmoidectomies Performed Between 1969 and 1988 (N = 1300)

	Major	Minor
Intranasal Sphenoethmoidectomy (N = 1163)	4 CSF leaks 2 Frontal mucoceles 2 Cases atrophic rhinitis 3 Cases epistaxis (requiring IMA ligation) Total: 11/1163 (0.94%)	17 Asthma attacks 3 Cases orbital edema 4 Cases epistaxis Total: 24/163 (2.05%)
Transantral Sphenoethmoidectomy (N = 137)	1 CSF leak 1 Case epistaxis (requiring IMA ligation) Total: 2/137 (1.45%)	7 Cases postoperative pain/numbness 1 Case epistaxis Total: 8/137 (5.8%)

(From Friedman WH, Katsantonis GP: Intranasal and transnasal ethmoidectomy: A 20 year experience. Laryngoscope 100(4):343, 1990.)

common, as it is in Caldwell-Luc surgery performed without ethmoidectomy. Damage to orbital contents and orbital adnexa should not occur because the orbit should not be entered. However, damage to the cribriform plate and fovea ethmoidalis may occur as in external and intranasal ethmoidectomy. The danger of oroantral fistula or damage to tooth roots (particularly the second bicuspid tooth) is a possibility in this procedure as it is with the Caldwell-Luc procedure without ethmoidectomy.

The intranasal sphenoethmoidectomy has the same inherent dangers as external or transantral ethmoidectomies in that inappropriately or carelessly placed instruments may result in damage to orbital contents, extraocular muscle function, or vision. CSF leak can also occur and is usually the result of transgression of the cribriform plate or fovea ethmoidalis. If the leak does not exceed 1.5 cm it can usually be repaired via an external ethmoidectomy approach utilizing fascia lata for closure. The dreaded complications just listed are rare and except in unusual circumstances are not considered routine (Table 11–1). Acceptable complications following ethmoidectomy by any route include orbital cellulitis, sinusitis, and crusting that may last from 2 to 6 weeks. Prolonged crusting (atrophic rhinitis) is rare but can occur and may last up to 1 year. Antibiotics, gentle suctioning, and control of underlying medical problems are

usually sufficient to control these infrequent complications.

DISCUSSION

The role of ethmoidectomy is primarily the elimination of benign hyperplastic disease, removal of inspissated pus and debris, reduction of ethmoid surface area, and removal of osteitic bone, with provision of adequate drainage from all the paranasal sinuses. In addition, resection of the ethmoid labyrinth enables excellent postoperative evaluation of the posterior vault areas and, along with intranasal antrostomy, enables visualization and access to the maxillary sinuses. The intranasal sphenoethmoidectomy has provided excellent control of polyps (Table 11–2).[19] Recently, this procedure has been effective in the treatment of patients with the sinobronchial syndrome, particularly those with asthma, chronic sinusitis, and posterior nasal discharge. In these patients, prolonged reduction or elimination of steroid requirement is often achieved, along with reduction in the number of episodes of sinusitis, asthma, and related conditions (Table 11–3).[19] Many of these patients are sensitive to acetylsalicylic acid, and excellent results have been achieved even in this sometimes seriously ill group of patients. In the past, objections

TABLE 11–2. Recurrence Rate of Hyperplastic Disease (In Patients with Chronic Hyperplastic Rhinosinusitis) Between 1969 and 1988 (N = 1299)

	Intranasal Sphenoethmoidectomy	Transantral Sphenoethmoidectomy
Asthmatics	71/390 (18.2%)	8/42 (19.0%)
Nonasthmatics	110/772 (14.2%)	15/95 (15.8%)
Total:	181/1163 (15.5%)	23/137 (16.8%)

*Six operations performed in three patients for recurrent purulent pansinusitis are not included.
(From Friedman WH, Katsantonis GP: Intranasal and transnasal ethmoidectomy: A 20 year experience. Laryngoscope 100(4):343, 1990.)

TABLE 11–3. Effect of Intranasal Sphenoethmoidectomy on Steroid Requirement

	Asthmatic	Nonasthmatic
Elimination of steroid requirement (6 months to 4 years)	13/28	6/6
Marked prolonged reduction of steroid requirement	13/28	
Increased steroid requirement	0/28	0/20
Steroid requirement unchanged	2/28	

St. Louis University Medical Center, Sphenoethmoidectomy patients, 1977–1981. Note that in 20 nonasthmatic patients frequent steroid bursts were eliminated.

have been raised to the role of intranasal surgery in the asthmatic patient, as this surgery can precipitate asthma intraoperatively. The surgeon must be prepared to deal with acute asthma attacks on the operating table. This is usually readily accomplished with administration of intravenous aminophylline and hydrocortisone, and possibly subcutaneous epinephrine. In no case has irreversible status asthmaticus been precipitated.

There has been mild controversy over the sacrifice of the middle turbinate at the time of ethmoidectomy. I believe that this is acceptable, particularly in patients with massive nasal polyposis. This structure usually plays no aerodynamic role in the patient with hyperplastic rhinosinusitis, because it is bathed in massive secretions and redundant prolapsed mucous membrane. It is necessary to remove the middle turbinate to visualize the sphenoid sinus adequately. In one third to one half of the middle turbinates removed, pneumatization is evident, making the turbinate a fully developed ethmoid cell. Removal of the middle turbinate expands the ethmoidectomy procedure (Fig. 11–12) by volumetrically eliminating more of the ethmoid labyrinth. Leaving a pneumatized cell and possibly disease in the middle turbinate violates the precepts of ethmoid surgery, which requires complete exenteration of the ethmoid labyrinth.

References

1. Harrison DFN: Surgery in allergic sinusitis. Otolaryngol Clin North Am 4:83, 1971.
2. Jansen A: Zur Eriffung der Nebenhohlen der Nase bei chronischer Eiterung. Arch Laryngol Rhinol 1:135, 1894.
3. Horgan JB: Surgical approach to the ethmoidal cell system. J Laryngol Otol 41:510, 1926.
4. Langenbrunner DJ, Nigri P: Transantral ethmoidectomy: An overlooked procedure? Trans Am Acad Ophthalmol Otolaryngol 4:744, 1977.
5. Mosher HP: The surgical anatomy of the ethmoidal labyrinth. Ann Otol Rhinol Laryngol 38:869, 1929.
6. Yankauer S: Demonstration of intranasal surgery on wet specimens. Laryngoscope 40:642, 1930.
7. Friedman WH: Surgery for chronic hyperplastic rhinosinusitis. Laryngoscope 12:1999, 1975.
8. Friedman WH, Katsantonis GP: Intranasal and transantral ethmoidectomy; A 20 year experience. Laryngoscope 100(4):343, 1990.
9. Eichel BS: The intranasal ethmoidectomy procedure: Historical, technical and clinical considerations. Laryngoscope 82(10):682, 1972.
10. Freedman HM, Kern EB: Complications of intranasal ethmoidectomy: A review of 1,000 consecutive operations. Laryngoscope 89(3):421, 1979.
11. Van Alyea OE: Nasal Sinuses. 2nd ed. Baltimore, Williams & Wilkins, 1951.
12. Friedman WH, Katsantonis GP, Rosenblum BN, Cooper MH, Slavin R: Sphenoethmoidectomy: The case for ethmoid marsupialization. Laryngoscope 96(5):473, 1986.
13. Kennedy DS: Functional endoscopic sinus surgery. Arch Otolaryngol 111:643, 1985.
14. Ash JE, Raum M: An Atlas of Otolaryngic Pathology. Washington, DC, American Academy of Otology, American Registry of Pathology, and Armed Forces Institute of Pathology, 1949, p. 131.
15. Williams HL: The relationship of allergy to chronic sinusitis. Ann Allergy 24:521, 1936.
16. Davison FW: Hyperplastic sinusitis—a five-year study. Ann Otol Rhinol Laryngol 72:462, 1963.
17. Vancil M: External operation of the nasal sinuses. J Laryngol 60:449, 1945.
18. Ritter FN: Surgical anatomy of the nasal sinuses. Otolaryngol Clin North Am 4:3, 1971.
19. Friedman WH, Katsantonis GP, Slavin RG, et al: Sphenoethmoidectomy: Its role in the asthmatic patient. Otolaryngol Head Neck Surg 90:171, 1982.

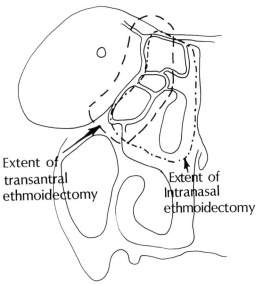

Figure 11–12. Extent of intranasal ethmoidectomy with exenteration of the entire ethmoid labyrinth, including the middle turbinate, compared with the extent of transantral ethmoidectomy. The medial limits of dissection are greater in the intranasal procedure, whereas the lateral limits are more easily visualized than in transantral ethmoidectomy.

Extent of transantral ethmoidectomy

Extent of intranasal ethmoidectomy

CHAPTER 12

TRANSORBITAL APPROACH TO THE ETHMOID SINUS—THE PATTERSON PROCEDURE

Donald F.N. Harrison, MD, PhD, FRCS

The advent of antibiotic therapy has led to the virtual exclusion of chronic ethmoiditis as a verified pathologic entity. However, recurrent nasal polypi, or the need to remove the ethmoid labyrinth for orbital decompression or access to the pituitary fossa, has maintained a need for radical ethmoidectomy. The present popularity for intranasal endoscopic surgery has arisen from the unsatisfactory results and morbidity associated with unskilled intranasal surgery upon the ethmoid. Despite considerable enthusiasm, which as yet has not been tested against the parameter of time, total removal of the ethmoid labyrinth is feasible only by an external approach. Even then it is limited by anatomic boundaries. Harrison, when examining variations in siting of anterior and posterior arteries with respect to the optic foramen in 94 specimens, found a range of 2 to 9 mm when measured from the posterior aspect of the lamina papyracea to the optic nerve.[1]

Poorly developed sphenoid sinuses allow posterior extension of the posterior ethmoid cells, with the latter then making up the medial wall of the optic canal (Fig. 12–1). Similar dangers exist in relation to the level of the 1-mm-thick cribriform plate, which on both computed tomography scan and coronal histologic sections is found to vary with respect to the medial orbital wall (Fig. 12–2). Despite these hazards, often unsuspected during intranasal operations, complications are minimized by the orbital periosteum, which not only protects the globe and periorbital tissues but acts as an effective barrier to penetration by neoplasms, infection, and surgical instruments!

The value of the Patterson transorbital approach to the ethmoid lies in the almost invisible scar and direct access to both ethmoid and medial orbital floor.[2] It is of interest that he prefaced his original description in 1939 by saying, "Where possible, operations upon the

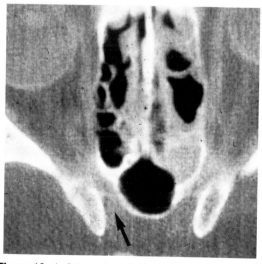

Figure 12–1. Submentovertical tomogram to show the intimate relationship between a posterior ethmoid cell and optic canal *(arrow)*.

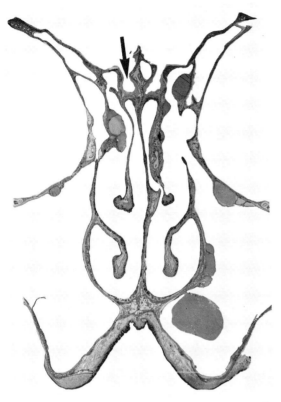

Figure 12–2. Coronal section of midface showing relationship of cribriform plate *(arrow)* to ethmoid labyrinth. Section cut at 5 μm.

nose should be avoided." Needless to say, this observation was not enthusiastically received, and initially this operation had a hostile reception, with accusations of technical difficulty and restricted access to the anterior ethmoid cells. The latter is certainly untrue for it is particularly ideal for these cells as well as for dacrocysto-rhinoscopy!

INDICATIONS

Although Lund considers that indications are similar to those for the more common Lynch-Howarth procedure, access to the frontal sinus is not good nor always possible without extending the incision.[3] This obviates the cosmetic advantage of the Patterson's operation. Removal of the ethmoid labyrinth, anterior wall of the sphenoid sinus, and orbital floor medial to the infraorbital nerve is all possible under direct vision. The risk of damage to the orbital contents, lacrimal sac, optic canal, or cribriform plate is minimal, and the virtually invisible scar makes this operation valuable, carrying little

morbidity. Problems associated with the Lynch-Howarth incision, such as edema, paresthesia, and damage to the medial palpebral ligament or webbing, are not seen, although it must be said that careful placement of the incision for this operation is said to minimize such problems.[4] Patterson himself said that there were only two places where incisions should be placed for ethmoid operation: the supraorbital ridge or the cheek, both areas of minimal scarring.

Despite access to the maxillary antrum via removal of part of the orbital floor, this is not an ideal approach for management of antral disease, although polypi and mucosa can be removed, but without direct visualization.

TECHNIQUE

Manipulation of the orbital contents makes this an operation unsuitable in most instances for local anesthesia. Operating time and visualization are considerably assisted by hypotensive anesthesia; infiltration of vasoconstrictors is not necessary.

The skin incision is placed within the nasojugal fold, a natural skin crease that begins about a quarter of an inch below the inner canthus. Since this depression is found even in young people, the final scar always should be virtually invisible (Fig. 12–3).

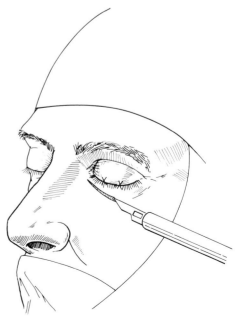

Figure 12–3. Skin incision placed in nasojugal fold.

Following preliminary tarsorraphy to protect the cornea from damage or pollution from blood or infection, the skin and subcutaneous tissue are incised down to the underlying orbicularis oculi muscle. It is important that the incision is confined to the skin crease, since extension superiorly may damage the medial tarsal ligament, while lateral extension past the infraorbital foramen provides no additional access.

Before separating the fibers of the orbicularis, palpation of the orbital margin minimizes accidental damage to the orbital septum, since the relationship of the nasojugal fold to the underlying orbital margin is variable.

Sharp separation of muscle fibers, with further dissection using a fine dissector, reveals the face of the maxilla just inferior to the orbital rim. Damage to the angular vein at the medial end of the incision may occur during this dissection and requires ligation. The divided muscle fibers can be held apart with a small self-retaining retractor, although this is cumbersome and a hand-held retractor takes up less space.

The periosteum on the face of the maxilla is now incised and careful elevation carried out as far as the medial tarsal ligament and laterally to the infraorbital foramen. The orbital rim varies considerably in both thickness and angulation. Separation must avoid damage to the periosteum at its attachment to the rim to avoid prolapse of fat. The orbital floor is now revealed and allows the introduction of a small, malleable copper retractor. Laterally, the tendon of the inferior oblique muscle is seen (except in 9 per cent of patients in whom the muscle is entirely intraperiosteal) and must be left undisturbed. Medially lies the lacrimal sac, and further dissection reveals the frontonasal process of the maxilla and the lacrimal crest.

As elevation of the orbital periosteum advances, the gap between the inferior oblique muscle and the lacrimal sac widens to reveal orbital floor and medial orbital wall as far as the posterior ethmoidal vessels (Fig. 12–4). Even under normotensive anesthesia there is no need to ligate either the anterior or posterior vessels, since removal of surrounding bone allows vascular contraction and hemostasis.

The lacrimal sac should now be carefully separated from its fossa, using a curved elevator. Previous intranasal surgery may have resulted in damage to both lacrimal bone or orbital plate of ethmoid, and care must be taken in these cases to avoid tearing the sac or periosteum. Once the sac has been freed, the frontal process of the maxilla adjoining the sac can be removed with drill or gouge, allowing entry to the nose and anterior ethmoid cells. Removal

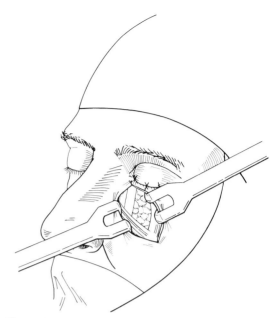

Figure 12–4. View obtained of lacrimal sac and inferior oblique muscle after elevation of orbital periosteum.

of the lamina papyracea is now possible under direct vision, but it should stop at the level of the posterior vessels or when the compact sphenoid bone surrounding the optic foramen is reached. Damage to this bone by grasping forceps can result in a "fissure fracture" extending back to the nerve, and further removal of the posterior ethmoid cells must be carried out intranasally and medial to this portion of the orbital wall. During these procedures the orbital contents are protected with the largest convenient malleable copper retractor, for damage to the periosteum may lead to prolapse of orbital fat. This is not necessarily dangerous, for it is done deliberately in orbital decompression, but it makes visualization difficult and should be avoided.

The access and direct visualization provided by this approach allows removal of all ethmoid cells, turbinates, and orbital floor medial to the infraorbital nerve (Fig. 12–5). Direct access to the frontal sinus is not usually possible, but removal of the anterior wall of the sphenoid sinus is facilitated and is an essential part of radical ethmoidectomy. Intranasal removal of polypi or remaining ethmoid cells can be performed without risk to the cribriform plate, since this area is under direct visualization.

Magnification has not been found necessary and may even confuse, hindering good orientation. Nasal packing is rarely needed, since bleeding is minimal.

Approximation of the fibers of the orbicularis

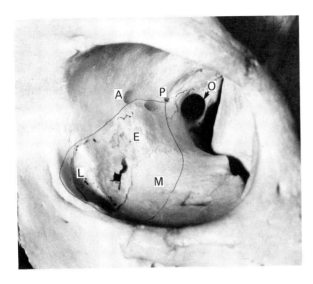

Figure 12–5. Area of bone removed outlined. *L*, Lacrimal bone; *E*, lamina papyracea; *M*, roof of maxillary antrum; *O*, optic canal; *A*, anterior ethmoidal foramen; *P*, posterior ethmoidal foramen.

oculi is carried out using 4-0 chromic catgut, and this tends to close skin edges. However, skin suturing is desirable, using 5-0 silk or nylon, and these sutures can be removed within 3 to 5 days. The end closest to the lash margins should be cut short to minimize irritation, and the cheek ends should be left long to facilitate removal.

COMPLICATIONS

Personal experience of 186 operations found only temporary epiphora from muscular edema in about 30 per cent of patients.[5] Repositioning of the inferior oblique muscle when it is sited entirely within the orbital periosteum may occur, producing diplopia on looking upward and outward. Temporary diplopia has been recorded by others as a result of trauma to this muscle during elevation of periosteum from the orbital margin.[6]

There is little doubt that this operation is technically more difficult than the Lynch-Howarth procedure: initial access is more restricted until adequate mobilization is obtained. Its value lies in excellent cosmesis and the direct visualization of the medial orbital wall, lacrimal sac, orbital floor, and sphenoid sinus that can be obtained with maximum safety.

References

1. Harrison DFN: Surgical approach to the medial orbital wall. Ann Otol Rhinol Laryngol 90:415, 1981.
2. Patterson N: External operations on the frontal and ethmoidal sinuses. J Laryngol 54:235, 1939.
3. Lund VJ: Surgical management of sinusitis. Ballantyne J, Groves J (eds): Scott-Brown's Otolaryngology. Vol 4. Stoneham, Mass, Butterworths, 1987, Chapter 11.
4. Rubin JS, Lund VJ, Salmon B: Frontoethmoidectomy in the treatment of mucocoeles. Arch Otolaryngol 112:434, 1986.
5. Harrison DFN: The ENT surgeon looks at the orbit. J Laryngol (Suppl 3), 1980.
6. Hargrove SWG: Discussion on the treatment of nasal polypi. Proc Soc Med 47:1015, 1954.

CHAPTER 13

ENDOSCOPIC NASAL AND SINUS SURGERY

James A. Stankiewicz, MD

Since 1985, when endoscopic sinus diagnosis and operation were introduced into the United States by Heinz Stammberger of Graz, Austria, and David Kennedy of Johns Hopkins, a revolution has occurred in the way otolaryngologists now approach nasal and sinus diagnosis and operation.[1-3] This has resulted in an intensified effort by otolaryngologists to better understand sinus anatomy, sinus physiology, and the pathophysiology of sinus disease.

The interest in the paranasal sinuses is now at an all-time high. Important innovations in radiology, instrumentation, and philosophy have greatly contributed to our ability to diagnose and treat sinus disease.

It is important to put endoscopic sinus diagnosis and operation into proper perspective. In the initial clinical evaluation of patients, endoscopic evaluation is the best way to diagnose sinus pathology. Whether one uses a flexible or rigid telescope, endoscopic rhinoscopy enhances and surpasses anterior rhinoscopy. Computed tomography (CT) of the sinuses as described by Zinrich and colleagues, and modifications of this technique, are now at the peak of excellence in radiologic diagnosis.[4]

The role of endoscopic sinus surgery in the treatment of sinus disease needs clarification. Unfortunately, when endoscopic sinus surgery was introduced, it was mistaken for and misunderstood as the replacement for traditional sinus surgery. This created much confusion and dismay among many traditional sinus surgeons who had been performing good sinus operations for years. Endoscopic ethmoidectomy, sphenoidotomy, and maxillary antrostomy actually are newly acquired techniques that add to the ar-mamentarium for surgical treatment of sinus disease. The surgeon, depending upon experience and skill, can elect to perform only traditional techniques, combination traditional and endoscopic techniques, or only endoscopic techniques (see Chapters 6, 7, 8, and 9). The endoscopic techniques are clearly beneficial in making a natural antrostomy in the middle meatus, for progressive functional ethmoid operation, and for clearing frontal recess pathology. Although intranasal ethmoidectomy and sphenoidotomy can be performed with use of the microscope, headlight, or telescopes, telescopes can add to traditional techniques by "fine tuning" areas where disease persistence is possible or by functionally removing localized pathology. Whether traditional or endoscopic procedures are used, safe surgery comes only with experience derived from reading the literature, attending lectures, dissecting cadavers, and participating in careful, graduated patient surgery.

HISTORY

Hirschman, in 1901, using a modified cystoscope, made the first attempts at nasal and sinus endoscopy.[2] Several other early-century reports utilizing endoscopes for diagnosis and minor maxillary sinus procedures were also recorded in the German literature. Maltz in 1925 described a sinoscope and described its use for nasal and sinus diagnosis and maxillary sinus endoscopy. In the 1960s, Messerklinger began his work with endoscopic sinus diagnosis and surgery, but his work was not published in the English literature until 1978.[5] He performed excellent studies of mucociliary clearance, identifying tissue contact points as areas of disruption where mucous retention could occur, leading to infection if not reversed. He defined the anterior and middle ethmoid sinus in the middle meatus as the area most influential for mucociliary problems, the ostiomeatal unit. In 1985, Stammberger, a protege of Messerklinger, gave the first course on endoscopic diagnosis and treatment in the United States. Kennedy, working with Stammberger and Zinrich, began giving several courses, and these men were mainly responsible for the rapid dissemination of endoscopic sinus diagnosis and surgery.

Another German school of endoscopic operation was that of Wigand and his protege Thumfart, whose endoscopic philosophy initially was more representative of traditional intranasal ethmoid surgery.[6] At present, however, Wigand has adopted the Messerklinger approach.

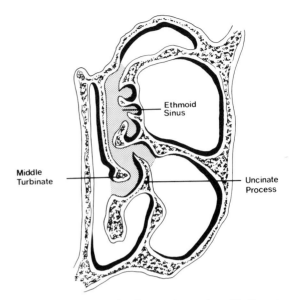

Figure 13–1. Figure of ostiomeatal complex with disease beginning in anterior ethmoid sinuses and secondarily blocking maxillary and frontal sinuses.

PHILOSOPHY

Endoscopic sinus surgery is based upon Messerklinger's studies of mucociliary clearance and the fact that most of the pathology occurs in the ethmoid sinus, especially anteriorly in the ostiomeatal unit. Most infections of the paranasal sinuses are rhinogenic.[1] The anterior ethmoid drains both the frontal sinus and maxillary sinus (Fig. 13–1). Given the right conditions, the narrow ostia and surrounding tissues may become obstructed; subsequent bacterial growth is then followed by mucosal hypertrophy. If allowed to persist, obstruction often will spread to the frontal recess, natural ostia, bulla ethmoidalis, posterior ethmoid, and sphenoid sinuses. Functional endoscopic sinus surgery (FESS), as termed by Kennedy, involves removal of disease proceeding anteriorly to posteriorly and limiting operation only to those areas involved[2, 3] (Fig. 13–2). This represents a major change from traditional intranasal ethmoidectomy, in which the custom is a total ethmoidectomy for even limited disease.

It is also important to understand that the concept of functional endoscopic sinus operation involves the accumulation of a data base involving history, physical examination—especially endoscopic rhinoscopy, and radiologic evaluation prior to any consideration of a surgical procedure. Surgical manipulation is performed only when a patient has failed medical therapy and evidence of disease is apparent on nasal endoscopy and corroborated with radiologic evaluation.

RADIOLOGY

Chapter 4 discusses radiology of the paranasal sinuses in depth. However, certain important facts require description or repetition. Computed tomography scan of the paranasal sinuses is the radiologic procedure of choice.[4, 7, 8] To evaluate a patient for sinus pathology properly, a coronal CT scan is performed to outline best the ostiomeatal complex, paranasal sinuses, septum, turbinate, roof of the nose, cribriform plate, and orbit. An axial scan will contribute information about the maxillary sinuses, extent of posterior ethmoid disease, and sphenoid involvement. The axial scan can be reconstructed from the coronal scan or done as part of the total scan. Bone windows are preferred, with window settings of 2000 to favor bone/soft tissue enhancement (Figs. 13–3 through 13–6). Many radiologists and otolaryngologists are developing screening coronal sinus CT scans, with special emphasis on the ostiomeatal unit.[9] The scans are not much more costly than screening sinus radiographs and provide much more information. Magnetic resonance imaging is not useful for sinus screening and has as its main benefit the delineation of tumor from sinusitis, which in certain cases may

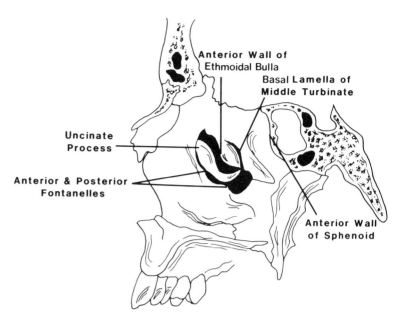

Figure 13–2. Progressive bony landmarks encountered as a surgeon moves from the anterior ethmoid to the sphenoid sinus.

be helpful. Good radiology is very important to the whole concept of endoscopic diagnosis, and it is important that it be performed well.

INSTRUMENTATION

Several endoscopes are available for performing endoscopic procedures, whether for diagnosis or treatment. Most surgeons prefer the 0°

and 30° rigid scopes by Karl Storz for diagnosis and operation. Many also like the 25° scope by Wolf. For clinic use, if but one scope had to be chosen, it would be the 25° or 30° by Richard Wolf and Karl Storz, respectively. I find the flexible laryngoscope also works nicely for diagnosis. The 70° scope is most valuable when viewing the frontal recess and the maxillary sinus through the ostia. Suction forceps are invaluable. Suction irrigation handles for the

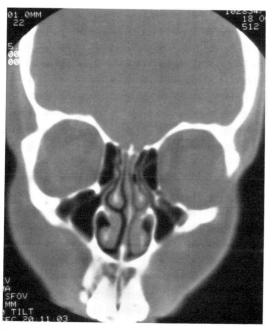

Figure 13–3. Coronal view with bone window at 2000.

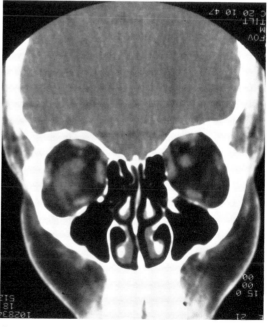

Figure 13–4. Coronal view with soft tissue window at 250.

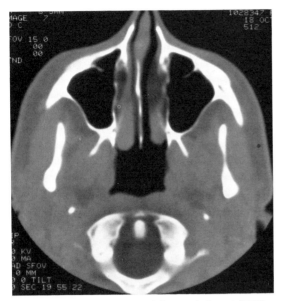

Figure 13–5. Axial view with bone window at 2000.

endoscopes work best if the middle turbinate is not present. Right-angle forceps are valuable for working in the maxillary sinus through the ostia and in the frontal recess. Curved suction tubes are helpful in clearing the superior ethmoids, cannulating the frontal sinus, and perforating the natural fontanelle area of the maxillary sinus.

INDICATIONS

Diagnostic endoscopic sinoscopy with or without biopsy can be performed for lesions isolated in the maxillary sinus. This can also be performed in conjunction with ethmoidectomy to help diagnose disease related to the maxillary sinus ostia, to assist removal of disease through the newly created natural ostia, and to help find the ostial area in difficult cases, allowing for creation of a safe and correct antrostomy.

The indications for endoscopic ethmoidectomy are the presence of acute or chronic disease, apparent on history, physical examination, and/or CT scan, that does not respond to an appropriate course of medical therapy. In some patients, a CT scan does not indicate obvious disease, but disease is apparent upon physical examination with diagnostic endoscopy. This may be most apparent in cases of recurrent acute sinusitis in which between episodes the sinuses are clear. The type of ethmoidectomy performed is related to the site of disease. Since the endoscopic ethmoidectomy

is a functional procedure, disease removal should be limited to the extent of disease. If disease is limited to the infundibulum and bulla ethmoidalis, only these need be removed. Disease involving the whole of the ethmoid is treated as in traditional ethmoidectomy with complete marsupialization of the ethmoid cells. Acute sinus disease with orbital involvement can be treated endoscopically but only by the most experienced surgeons.

Endoscopic sphenoidotomy is indicated for disease in the sphenoid sinus only or in conjunction with ethmoid disease.

Frontal sinus disease removal is limited to that disease that involves the frontal recess. Frontal mucoceles can be marsupialized, but careful follow-up is necessary because of the tendency for the nasofrontal opening to want to scar closed.

In my experience, several disease entities can be treated endoscopically. Mucoceles of the sphenoid, ethmoid, and maxillary sinuses can readily be treated endoscopically.[10, 11] Most disease processes in the maxillary sinuses are amenable to endoscopic operation, limiting the need for the Caldwell-Luc procedure. Nasal and choanal polyps and sinusitis are nicely treated endoscopically. Inverting papilloma and selected neoplasms can be treated endoscopically provided close follow-up is performed. Malignant nasal and sinus lesions can be debulked and biopsied via the endoscope. Fungal balls and early nasal and sinus fungal involvement in immunocompromised patients are re-

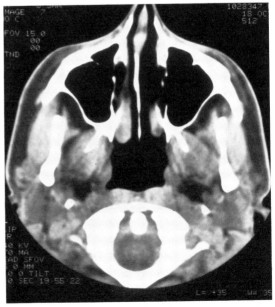

Figure 13–6. Axial view with soft tissue window at 250.

sponsive. Choanal atresia can be approached initially utilizing endoscopic surgical procedures. Ethmoid osteoma is amenable to endoscope removal if there is no intraorbital extension or involvement of the cribriform plate. Orbital decompression for Graves' disease can include endoscopic operation.[12]

TECHNIQUE

ANESTHESIA

Intranasal endoscopic sphenoethmoidectomy can be performed under general or local standby anesthesia. When the patient has general anesthesia, the surgeon loses the sensitivity of the orbit and base of skull as warning signals. However, if diligent, observant operation is performed, with attention paid to the anatomy, general anesthesia is safe. One of the main arguments for local anesthesia is the decrease in blood loss. I have found that unoperated patients with limited disease or those with first-time nasal polyposis with no blood pressure problems can be done equally well under both types of anesthesia. Patients with extensive disease or previous operations, and those who use steroids or aspirin, have more trouble with a general anesthetic. However, general anesthesia is better able to control blood pressure, and in older patients who are hypertensive a general anesthetic actually may work better than a local one.

Under general anesthesia, greater palatine foramen blocks are used (Fig. 13–7). The septum, turbinates, areas of nasal polyposis, and the uncinate process area all are injected after pledgets of 10 per cent cocaine have been placed in the nose for about 5 to 10 minutes. All patients are sprayed with Neo-Synephrine or Afrin nasal sprays while in preop holding to begin vasoconstriction. The same preparation time is necessary for a general as for a local anesthesia.

Under a local anesthesia, greater foramen blocks are used along with blocks of the infraorbital nerve, alveolar nerves, septum, turbinates, and infundibular area, with great care taken also to place blocks in the posterior septum and posterior middle turbinate. After removal of 10 per cent cocaine pledgets, a No. 8 Foley catheter is inserted into the nasopharynx and blown up with 8 ml of saline to prevent secretions from entering the oropharynx. The use of nitrous oxide concurrently with the administration of sedation prior to injection helps patients better tolerate the local anesthetic. Sodium bicarbonate added to lidocaine with epinephrine decreases the pain of injection. Superomedial orbital blocks with 2 ml of lidocaine, as described by Chung and colleagues, also can be used to decrease ethmoid nerve pain and artery bleeding.[13] However, ecchymosis and occasionally orbital hematoma can result from the injection, and the surgeon should be wary of this. One of my patients experienced temporary diplopia that in my opinion resulted from this procedure. If orbital blocks are used, the first few should be performed under the direction of an ophthalmologist or knowledgeable otolaryngologist until the technique is perfected.

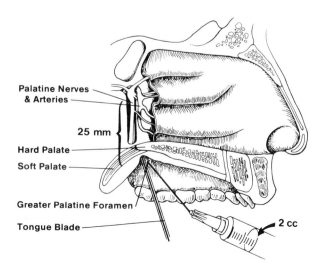

Figure 13–7. Injection of the greater palatine foramen for local anesthesia. (From Stankiewicz JA: Greater palatine foramen injection made easy. Laryngoscope 98: 580–581, 1988.)

DIAGNOSTIC RHINOSCOPY

Topical Afrin or Neo-Synephrine and topical lidocaine are sprayed into the nose in the clinic. After 5 to 10 minutes, the endoscope is introduced into the nasal cavity. The 4-mm rigid 'scope is used to examine the nose in a routine manner. The rigid 'scope is most easily placed in the middle meatus by rolling it over the inferior turbinate and up into the meatus. The anterior or frontal approach can be painful and may require outfracture of the middle turbinate. Because of a septal deviation or narrow nasal cavity, the 4-mm endoscope may not provide anything other than an anterior examination, which may still provide important information. An alternative is to use the 2.7-mm endoscope for examining these patients. Although the view is not as good as with the 4-mm endoscope, some additional information may be gained. The flexible laryngoscope also will provide an excellent examination, although the optics are not as good as with the rigid 'scope. The nasopharynx, sphenoid, middle meatus, and anterior nasal cavity usually can be seen well, and often the examination can be obtained even with a septal deviation. Abnormal anatomy, e.g., paradoxic turbinates and concha bullosa, and any evidence of pathology should be clearly noted.

MAXILLARY SINOSCOPY

This procedure is performed to evaluate the maxillary sinus directly. A trocar with a cannula is placed in the canine fossa, and the anterior wall of the sinus is perforated (Fig. 13–8). The cannula is left in place, and the sinus can then be irrigated or examined endoscopically. Endoscopic forceps can be used for biopsy or cyst removal. Major removal of disease cannot be performed via this route: either a Caldwell-Luc procedure or a large, intranasal antrostomy is necessary. The procedure may be coupled with antrostomy for extensive evaluation of the maxillary sinus. Sinoscopy is performed easily under local anesthesia. It is important to aim posteriorly in the canine fossa to avoid entrance into the nasal cavity. Tooth pain and numbness are temporary postoperative patient complaints.

FRONTAL SINUS OPERATION

Endoscopic operation of the frontal sinus is limited to removal of disease involving the

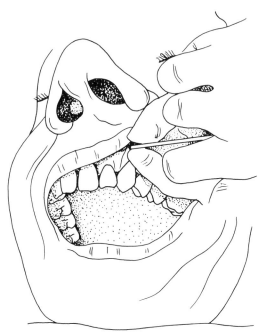

Figure 13–8. Technique for placement of sinoscopy trocar and cannula into maxillary sinus through the canine fossa, aiming laterally and posteriorly to avoid entrance into the nose. A twisting motion is used, and depth of entry is carefully controlled.

frontal recess and drainage of lesions that extend from the frontal sinus into the nose, such as a mucocele. The angled telescopes allow best visualization of the frontal recess. Angled forceps, large to small, allow entrance into the frontal recess and minimally into the frontal sinus. Frontal sinus lesions treated intranasally need close follow-up, because scarring and drainage obstruction can occur that require revision operation or external procedures.

LASER ENDOSCOPIC OPERATION

The laser has limited usefulness in sinus operations but is beneficial in patients who need turbinate operation or who have a bleeding diathesis and need an operation. The KTP laser is the most useful laser for this type of operation.[14] The CO_2, argon, and Nd:Yag lasers have not been used for intranasal sinus operation to any great extent. Levine reported on 128 patients treated with the KTP laser.[14] Sinus-related abnormalities, such as concha bullosa, polyps, choanal polyps, ostial obstruction, and synechia from previous operation, were treated successfully with the KTP laser.

PEDIATRIC ENDOSCOPIC OPERATION

Children with sinus disease that does not resolve with medical therapy can undergo intranasal sinus operation endoscopically. Sinus and nasal anatomy in children is the same as that in adults, but the structures are smaller. Radiologic evaluation with CT scan is most important. Only cooperative young children and older children will tolerate diagnostic endoscopy. The most difficult problem with operation is postoperative care, which can be impossible. One authority recommends an examination under anesthesia 2 to 3 weeks postoperatively to inspect the nasal sinus area.[15]

New endoscopic instruments geared toward children, along with standard instrumentation, have greatly improved surgical access. Ethmoidectomy, sphenoidotomy, and antrostomy are approached as for the adult. However, close observation is important because of the smaller anatomy. In making the antrostomy, the surgeon has to take care not to operate too anteriorly, because injury to the nasolacrimal duct can occur more easily in children. Also, since postoperative care is limited, synechia may be a problem; this can be avoided by using rolled Gelfilm or Merocel Otowicks. Merocel has to be removed, which may be a problem in some children.

Gross and colleagues reported on 57 children who underwent endoscopic sinus operation safely, with a 92 per cent improvement in symptoms.[15] Lusk and Muntz reported on 31 children who underwent endoscopic operation for sinusitis with a 74 per cent improvement on 6-month follow-up.[16] Pashley and colleagues report an 80 per cent success rate in 190 patients.[17] No major complications were noted. I have operated on 30 children with acute or chronic sinusitis with one nasolacrimal duct injury. In six cases of ethmoidectomy for acute sinusitis with periorbital cellulitis or abscess, all were successfully treated. Only experienced endoscopic surgeons should attempt these difficult cases. The child with surgical sinusitis can be treated successfully with endoscopic techniques.

ENDOSCOPIC ETHMOIDECTOMY

The Messerklinger technique as described by Stammberger and Kennedy is utilized in endoscopic ethmoidectomy.[1-3] This involves medial fracture of the middle turbinate, with

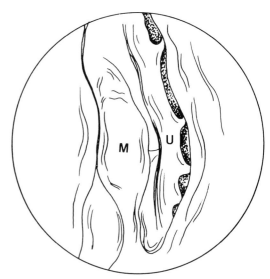

Figure 13–9. Infundibulotomy incision into the uncinate process. *M*, middle turbinate; *U*, uncinate process.

an incision made with a sickle knife into the uncinate process to create an infundibulotomy (Fig. 13–9). In a nose crowded with nasal polyps, a traditional or endoscopic polypectomy is performed prior to ethmoidectomy to open the nasal airway and allow for identification of landmarks. Once the uncinate process is removed, the bulla ethmoidalis is encountered and perforated (Fig. 13–10). The bulla is then opened and disease removed. A decision is made at this time to continue dissection either

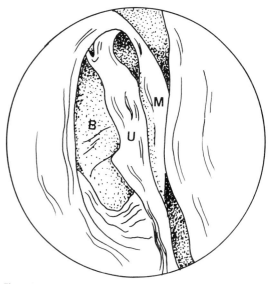

Figure 13–10. Anterior ethmoid exposure following infundibulotomy. *B*, bulla ethmoidalis; *U*, uncinate process; *M*, middle turbinate.

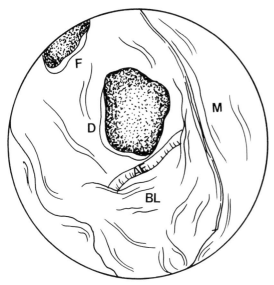

Figure 13–11. Basal lamella *(BL)* of middle turbinate *(M)*, showing relationship to anterior ethmoid artery *(AE)*, skull base, and dome of ethmoid *(D)*. F, Frontal recess.

posteriorly or superiorly. If the surgeon continues posteriorly, the basal or grand lamella of the middle turbinate is encountered; it usually measures about 6 cm from the nasal opening (Fig. 13–11).

The lamella is where the middle turbinate sweeps to the lateral wall of the orbit. The posterior ethmoid sinus is behind the lamella. Once the lamella is perforated, it is opened if disease is apparent. The posterior ethmoids are more expansive than the anterior ethmoids. At this point, if disease is obstructing or apparent in the sphenoid sinus, the sphenoid is entered, as will be described later. The frontal recess can be cleared of disease before going through the lamella or afterward. Diseased ethmoids obstructing the frontal recess are removed with upward-biting forceps. A small curved suction

tube can be upturned and used to palpate the fovea ethmoidalis to insure that diseased ethmoid cells are opened and the nasofrontal recess is open. The agger nasi cell area is palpated to determine whether disease is present. If so, the agger nasi cells are opened, taking care to observe for any evidence of periorbita. The sinus lateralis above the bulla ethmoidalis is perforated and cleared of disease, and dissection proceeds superiorly and posteriorly until the anterior ethmoid artery and base of skull (yellow) bone are encountered.

Most all of this operation is done under 0° or 25° telescopic guidance. I prefer the 0°. If the sphenoid is entered and sphenoidotomy is performed, the sphenoid can be used as a guide to the superior posterior ethmoids and base of skull. The 30° and 70° telescopes help give a better view of the fovea ethmoidalis, frontal recess, and superior ethmoid cell. Right-angle biting forceps can be used to facilitate disease removal in these areas.

Whether to remove or leave the middle turbinate is controversial and may vary from surgeon to surgeon. As a general rule, if the turbinate is uninvolved with disease it should be preserved. Some surgeons routinely remove part of the anteriorly middle turbinate to avoid synechiae.[18] Extensive disease with turbinate involvement requires partial removal of the turbinate. If the turbinate is removed, bleeding at the base of the sphenoid may occur, which requires control with cautery. The nasofrontal recess opens into the frontal sinus at 6 cm from the nasal aperture, and the posterior base of the skull is at 7 cm (Fig. 13–12).

ANTROSTOMY

It is important to define landmarks to make a good antrostomy. Remember that the natural

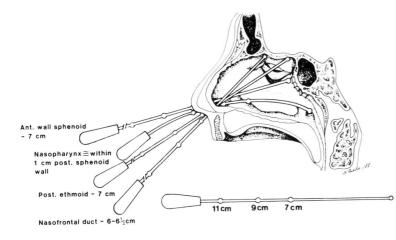

Ant. wall sphenoid
- 7 cm

Nasopharynx ≅ within
1 cm post. sphenoid
wall

Post. ethmoid - 7 cm

Nasofrontal duct - 6–6½cm

11cm   9cm   7cm

Figure 13–12. Beaded probe measurements to important anatomic sites. (From Stankiewicz JA: Complications of endoscopic sinus surgery. Otolaryngol Clin North Am 22:749–758, 1989.)

antrostomy is just inferior and slightly anterior to the bulla ethmoidalis in the infundibulum. A large area of soft tissue that covers a large dehiscence, which can vary, in the medial maxillary sinus wall is the fontanelles area. To avoid getting into the orbit, the entrance into the maxillary sinus is made in the fontanelle just above the inferior turbinate posterior to the anterior end of the middle turbinate. It sometimes can be extremely difficult to find the natural ostia, especially when disease is present or when there is long-standing sinusitis with a contracted maxillary sinus. Once the fontanelle is perforated with a small spoon or curved suction under 0° or 25° endoscopic guidance, it is enlarged with a backward-biting forceps under guidance with a 30° or 25° endoscope (Fig. 13–13).

The antrostomy should be carried far enough forward to include the natural ostia in the infundibulum. Otherwise, a recirculation of secretions may occur from the natural ostia into the new antrostomy, thus continuing the patient's problems.[19] A circumferential removal of tissue in creating the antrostomy increases the chance of postoperative antrostomy closure. Inferior and anterior removal of tissue is usually all that is necessary. Hard bone anteriorly indicates the nasolacrimal duct. As a general rule, the antrostomy should not be made more anterior than the anterior end of the middle turbinate.

Occasionally, the soft tissue wall of the maxillary sinus cannot be penetrated with the blunt spoon or suction tube. Under endoscopic guidance, a sickle knife can be used to perforate the soft tissue, and then the antrostomy opening can be created. Disease in the maxillary sinus can be removed with upward and right-angle biting forceps under 30° and 70° endoscopic guidance. Increased removal can be enhanced with the addition of canine fossa sinoscopy or a traditional nasoantral window. Not all tissue and mucous membrane requires removal, because for the most part the maxillary sinuses will heal once they are adequately opened. In patients with contracted maxillary sinuses and long-standing disease, a sinoscopy with irrigation may be helpful in locating the appropriate area for antrostomy. Recurrent or persistent extensive disease, especially in the asthmatic patient, may require a Caldwell-Luc procedure, revision of the antrostomy, or an inferior meatus antrostomy.

SPHENOIDOTOMY

The sphenoid sinus can be opened as a continuation of ethmoidectomy or as a single procedure.[13, 20] The sinus can be approached directly with the 0° or 25° telescope medial to the middle turbinate. The ostia is cannulated and dilated with a Frazier suction tube, and then the sphenoidotomy is opened widely with upward or straight forceps or sphenoid punch, as in the traditional universal instrumentation. For sphenoidotomy alone, I prefer partial removal of the inferior part of the middle turbinate, which gives a wide exposure to the base

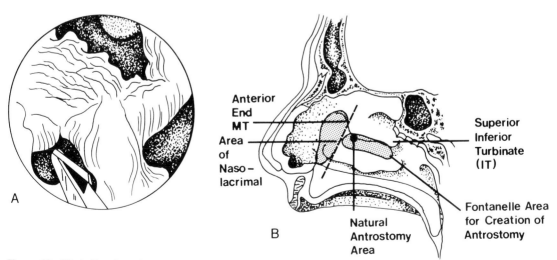

Figure 13–13. *A,* Creation of an antrostomy with backbiting forceps after perforation of the medial maxillary sinus wall through the fontanelles. *B,* Note areas to stay away from to avoid complication. Antrostomy is made with spoon or curved suction.

of the skull, posterior ethmoid, and sphenoid (Fig. 13–14). Postoperative evaluation is enhanced, since the sphenoid can be viewed directly. As part of ethmoidectomy, the sphenoid can be approached with the middle turbinate in place.

As one moves through the basal lamella into the posterior ethmoid, disease is removed in a wide swathe that usually includes the posterior part of the middle turbinate. At the level of the sphenoid anterior wall, 7 cm from the nares opening, a depression is usually apparent; this indicates the anterior sphenoid wall. This is then perforated. If the surgeon is operating too high, hard bone is encountered at the base of the skull, and perforation should be avoided. Also, toward the septum, the base of the skull and the cribriform plate may be low; if the surgeon is working too high, a CSF leak may result. The surgeon should not be higher than the lower part of the middle turbinate and, in general, should try to stay in an area between the superior inferior turbinate and the lower part of the middle turbinate.

Before perforating the anterior sphenoid wall, I prefer cannulating the sinus ostia with a beaded probe for the sake of safety. The posterior nasopharyngeal wall distance from the nares opening approximates that of the posterior wall of the sphenoid usually to within 1 cm. The sphenoid sinus is opened medially, inferiorly, and (very judiciously) laterally and superiorly (Fig. 13–15). Disease is removed as nec-

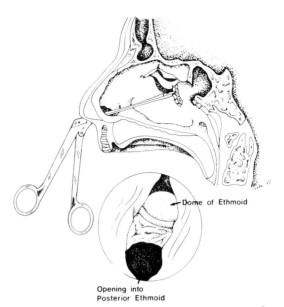

Figure 13–15. Opening into the sphenoid sinus after cannulating the ostia. (From Stankiewicz JA: The endoscopic approach to the sphenoid sinus. Laryngoscope 99:218–221, 1989.)

essary, avoiding manipulation to any great extent laterally and posterolaterally, in this way keeping away from the optic nerve and carotid artery, respectively.[21]

POSTOPERATIVE CARE

Endoscopic sinus operation requires that patients are seen frequently postoperatively to clean debris and clots, to break up adhesions and synechiae, and to monitor healing. If my patients have any bleeding, I usually use a small Merocel pack as a spacer and for hemostasis for 4 days. I see the patient weekly for intense cleaning of debris. I do not disturb any fixed clots; this precaution avoids hemorrhage. Irrigations are used to soften secretions and debris. Spacers such as Telfa or a small Otowick are used to prevent synechiae. Repeat endoscopic evaluation is performed at 2 weeks and repeated on follow-up visits. At 3 weeks it is not uncommon to note polypoid mucosa or infection in some patients. Steroids and antibiotics resolve this problem nicely for the most part. All patients are told that it will take 4 to 8 weeks for mucosal healing, but most patients have healed by 4 weeks. Recurrent or persistent disease may require revision operation if it is not controlled medically or with clinic debridement. Synechiae that can draw the middle turbinate

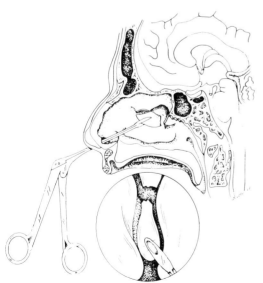

Figure 13–14. Partial removal of the middle turbinate in the approach to the sphenoid. (From Stankiewicz JA: The endoscopic approach to the sphenoid sinus. Laryngoscope 99:218–221, 1989.)

laterally, obstructing the ostiomeatal unit, and even a wide antrostomy require revision on occasion.

COMPLICATIONS

Complication rates of 2.7 to 3.7 per cent have been reported for traditional operation for intranasal ethmoidectomy.[22, 23] Anecdotally, several workers quote low complication rates for endoscopic intranasal ethmoidectomy, but only a few have written about this topic. Kennedy reports no complication in 16 patients in his earliest paper.[3] Stammberger reported 2500 endoscopic ethmoid operations with no serious complication.[1] However, complications were not specified. Schaefer and colleagues reported 14 minor complications in 100 consecutive patients, with synechiae being the most common complication.[24] One study reported a 9.3 per cent complication rate in 300 ethmoidectomies.[25] The most common complications were orbital hematoma, hemorrhage, and synechiae. In the second 150 ethmoidectomies reported in that study, the complication rate was 1.4 per cent, which is in line with traditional complication rates.

The same types of complications occur in traditional and endoscopic sinus operations; these have been discussed elsewhere.[20–27] Some points are relevant to endoscopic operation. The endoscopes are not telescopes, and the depth of field should be checked with either a headlight or a beaded probe. For right-handed surgeons, the telescopic view will take them superiorly into the lamina papyracea as they work posteriorly (Fig. 13–16). Simultaneous eye palpation while viewing the ethmoid and lamina papyracea can reveal dehiscence or absence of the lamina papyracea, periorbita, and orbital

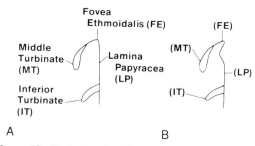

Figure 13–16. Anatomic differences on the left side of the nasal cavity concerning the papyracea. *A,* Through telescope, a right-handed surgeon views the apparent anatomy of the left side. *B,* The anatomy in reality, with the orbit pushing into the ethmoid superiorly and laterally. (From Stankiewicz JA: Blindness and intranasal endoscopic ethmoidectomy: Prevention and management. Otolaryngol Head Neck Surg 101:320, 1989.)

fat, which otherwise may not have been noted (Fig. 13–17). The eyes are always kept untaped and undraped. Because of the preservation of the middle turbinate in endoscopic surgery, synechia are all too common and sometimes require revision operation. Spacers are the best way to avoid this complication.

Traditional principles, such as palpating the inner canthus while suctioning to identify the lamina papyracea, watching the eye for movement when operating intranasally, noting the distances to sphenoid and nasopharynx, and never operating medial to the middle turbinate, are all very important and should be remembered.

DISCUSSION

Since the endoscopic technique has been used only since 1985, few papers discuss results of the endoscopic technique. In a 2-year follow-up of 100 patients, Rice reported that 83 per

Figure 13–17. Technique of simultaneous eye palpation and intranasal endoscopic examination. *A,* Endoscope in place examining the lamina papyracea of the lateral nasal wall. Note hole in lamina papyracea with mild fat exposure. *B,* Simultaneous eye palpation and endoscopic observation. If the hole in the lamina papyracea is apparent with periorbita or orbital fat exposed, early visualization of the defect is possible. (From Stankiewicz JA: Blindness and intranasal endoscopic ethmoidectomy: Prevention and management. Otolaryngol Head Neck Surg 101:320, 1989.)

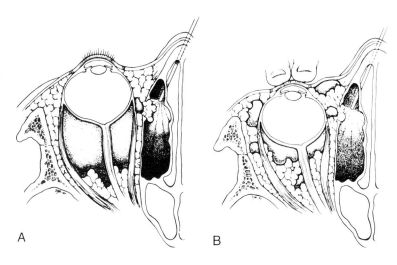

cent had a good result after a single procedure.[28] Toffel and colleagues reported on 170 patients, of whom 165 required bilateral surgery. In 41 patients followed for 1 year, 83 per cent had relief of headache, 78 per cent had relief of postnasal drainage, and 97 per cent, relief of nasal obstruction.[18] DeVries and Vleming reported on 300 patients who underwent endoscopic sinus operation, with a minimum of 6-months follow-up in 148 patients. Subjectively, 51 per cent reported good results and 27 per cent, moderate results. Objective examination in 148 patients showed a 51 per cent good result.[29] Schaefer and colleagues evaluated 100 consecutive patients followed for 5 months or more, who had an 83 per cent significant improvement.[24]

In over 500 of my patients undergoing endoscopic sinus operation, no patient has had a problem with asthma intraoperatively or postoperatively. With modern medications and surveillance, asthma poses a minimal risk to operation.

If the surgeon performs judicious endoscopic sinus operations, either alone or in combination with traditional operation, equivalent or better results than traditional operation should be possible owing to the functional nature of the procedure.[30] However, experience and skill need to be obtained, and careful, safe operating is most important. Surgeons need to know their limitations.

ACKNOWLEDGMENT

My thanks to Sue Whelton and Sandy Cello for their help in preparation of this manuscript.

References

1. Stammberger H: Endoscopic endonasal surgery: Concepts in treatment of recurring rhinosinusitis. Part I and Part II. Anatomic pathophysiologic considerations and surgical technique. Otolaryngol Head Neck Surg 99:143, 1986.
2. Kennedy D, Zinreich SJ, Rosenbaum A, Johns M: Functional endoscopic sinus surgery. Arch Otolaryngol 111:576, 1985.
3. Kennedy D: Functional endoscopic sinus surgery. Arch Otolaryngol 14:643, 1985.
4. Zinrich SJ, Kennedy D, Rosenbaum A, Gaylor B, Kumar A, Stammberger H: Paranasal sinuses: CT imaging requirements for endoscopic surgery. Radiology 163:769, 1987.
5. Messerklinger W: Endoscopy of the Nose. Baltimore, Urban and Schwarzenberg, 1978.
6. Wigand M: Transnasal ethmoidectomy under endoscopic control. Rhinology (Ger) 19:7, 1981.
7. Davidson T, Brahme F, Gallagher M: Radiologic evaluation for nasal dysfunction: CT vs. plain films. Head Neck 11:405, 1989.
8. Lusk R, Muntz H, McAlister W: Comparison of paranasal sinus radiograph and coronal scans in children.

Baltimore, ISIAN (International Symposium on Infection and Allergy of the Nose), Abstract 31, June 1989.
9. Chow J: Personal communication, 1990.
10. Stankiewicz J: Sphenoid sinus mucoceles. Arch Otolaryngol Head Neck Surg 115:735, 1989.
11. Kennedy D, Josephson J, Zinreich SJ, Mattox D, Goldsmith M: Endoscopic sinus surgery for mucoceles: A viable alternative. Laryngoscope 99:885, 1989.
12. Goodstein M, Kennedy D, Zinreich SJ, Miller N: A preliminary experience with endoscopic transnasal decompression of dysthyroid orbitopathy. Baltimore, ISIAN (International Symposium on Infection and Allergy of the Nose), Abstract 203, June 1989.
13. Chung S, Lee J, Hong S: Anterior ethmoid nerve block: Topographic anatomy in Koreans and clinical significance. Baltimore, ISIAN (International Symposium on Infection and Allergy of the Nose), Abstract 200, June 1989.
14. Levine H: Endoscopy and the KTP/532 laser for nasal sinus disease. Ann Otol Rhinol Laryngol 98:46, 1989.
15. Gross C, Gurucharri M, Lazar R, Long T: Functional endoscopic nasal sinus surgery (FESS) in the pediatric age group. Laryngoscope 99:46, 1989.
16. Lusk R, Muntz H: Pediatric endoscopic sinus surgery—a preliminary result. Baltimore, ISIAN (International Symposium on Infection and Allergy of the Nose), Abstract 194, June 1989.
17. Pashley N, Jaskunas J, Starbuck H: Functional endoscopic sinus surgery in infants and children. Baltimore, ISIAN (International Symposium on Infection and Allergy of the Nose), Abstract 195, June 1989.
18. Toffel D, Aroesty D, Weinmanner R, et al: Secure endoscopic sinus surgery as an adjunct to functional nasal surgery. Arch Otolaryngol Head Neck Surg 115:822, 1989.
19. Kennedy D, Zinreich SJ, Kuhn F, Shaalan H, Naclirio R, Loch E: Endoscopic middle meatal antrostomy: Theory, technique, patency. Laryngoscope (Suppl 43)97:1, 1989.
20. Stankiewicz J: The endoscopic approach to the sphenoid sinus. Laryngoscope 99:218, 1989.
21. Hassab M, Kennedy D: The internal carotid artery as it relates to endonasal sphenoethmoidectomy. Baltimore, ISIAN (International Symposium on Infection and Allergy of the Nose), Abstract 204, June 1989.
22. Freedman H, Kern E: Complications of intranasal ethmoidectomy; A review of 1000 consecutive operations. Laryngoscope 89:421, 1979.
23. Friedman W, Katsantonis G, Rosenblum B: Sphenoethmoidectomy: The case for ethmoid marsupialization. Laryngoscope 96:473, 1986.
24. Schaefer S, Manning S, Close L: Endoscopic paranasal sinus surgery; Indications and considerations. Laryngoscope 99:686, 1989.
25. Stankiewicz J: Complications in endoscopic intranasal ethmoidectomy: An update. Laryngoscope 99:686, 1989.
26. Stankiewicz J: Complications of intranasal endoscopic sinus surgery. Otolaryngol Clin North Am 22:749, 1989.
27. Stankiewicz J: Blindness and endoscopic intranasal ethmoidectomy: Prevention and management. Otolaryngol Head Neck Surg: 101:320, 1989.
28. Rice D: Endoscopic sinus surgery: Results at 2-year follow-up. Otolaryngol Head Neck Surg 101:476, 1989.
29. DeVries N, Vleming M: Experiences with endoscopic paranasal sinus surgery. Baltimore, ISIAN (International Symposium on Infection and Allergy of the Nose), Abstract 192, June 1989.
30. Ozawa M, Sano S, Horiuchi H, Haruna S, Honda Y: Endonasal sinus surgery. Baltimore, ISIAN (International Symposium on Infection and Allergy of the Nose), Abstract 58, June 1989.

CHAPTER 14

LASERS AND RHINOSINUSOLOGY

Howard L. Levine, MD
Bruce Sterman, MD

The concept of stimulated emission was proposed by Albert Einstein in 1917.[2] The application of this theory yielded the laser (light amplification by stimulated emission of radiation). A laser produces an intense, almost parallel, beam of electromagnetic energy of a specific wavelength. In 1964, Patel and colleagues from Bell Laboratories described the development of a high-powered, continuous wavelength carbon dioxide (CO_2) laser.[14] Over the following few years, the laser beam was modified for use as a surgical tool and controlled by mirrors and articulated arms.[15, 21] Following Jako's use of the CO_2 laser in human cadaver and dog larynges, the laser was added to the surgical armamentarium in otorhinolaryngology.[4]

LASER INSTRUMENTATION

Several lasers are adaptable for use in rhinosinusology. Fiberoptic delivery is possible with the neodymium: yttrium-aluminum-garnet (Nd:YAG), argon (Ar), and potassium titanyl phosphate (KTP/532) lasers, which allow fibers to be turned and bent to reach the recesses and spaces of the nose and sinuses. The carbon dioxide (CO_2) laser at present cannot be transmitted fiberoptically, only through the operating microscope or with rather cumbersome handpieces. Because of these limitations, it has minimal use in the nasal cavity.

Each laser can be characterized by its emission wavelength and tissue interaction, as well as the laser medium. The CO_2 laser is electri-

cally pumped with a medium of CO_2 gas. The emission is infrared energy (nonvisible) at 10,600 nm (10.6 μ). The major tissue absorber is water; therefore, the depth of penetration is only 0.01 to 0.23 mm. The Nd:YAG laser is optically pumped with a solid crystal medium of yttrium-aluminum-garnet with 1 to 3 per cent neodymium added. The laser energy is in the near-infrared spectrum (nonvisible), at 1060 nm (1.06 μ). The depth of tissue penetration is much greater, 2.5 to 4.2 mm, with less absorption by water and increased thermal coagulation. The CO_2 and Nd:YAG lasers require a beam of visible light to be coupled to them for aiming.

The electrically pumped Ar laser uses a gaseous argon medium. Its output is in the visible blue-green spectrum from 488 to 516 nm (0.488 to 0.516 μ). Thus, absorption is primarily from hemoglobin and melanin with little by water. Laser penetration is 0.03 mm in blood to 0.84 mm in tissue. The KTP/532 laser is optically pumped and solid state by passing a Nd:YAG beam into a potassium titanyl phosphate crystal. The emission is a visible emerald green color of 532 nm (0.532 μ). The greatest absorption is by hemoglobin and pigmented tissues, with a depth of penetration of from 0.3 to 2 mm.

The depth of thermal coagulation and damage is related to a laser's tissue penetration and scatter. The CO_2 laser is most effective as a cutting/vaporizing tool, although defocusing the beam will permit some coagulation. The Nd:YAG laser has the greatest degree of scatter and produces thermal damage for several millimeters of tissue. Thus, it functions best in coagulation. The visible light lasers, Ar and KTP/532, will produce all three functions (depending on the degree of focus) with intermediate thermal effect.

The flexibility of the KTP/532 laser has led to its predominance in endoscopic rhinologic surgery.[8] However, the Ar and Nd:YAG lasers could be used with similar surgical techniques. Nasal endoscopes (especially 0° and 30° ones with 4 or 2.7 mm shafts) provide a direct illuminated view of the nasal and paranasal sinus structures. The KTP/532 laser energy is delivered through 300, 400, or 600 μ flexible optical fibers via one of two approaches. The telescope and laser fiber may be inserted into separate channels of an endoscopic sheath (Fig. 14–1). This system keeps the telescope and laser as one unit, which limits the value of a fiberoptic delivery. It works for use in areas directly ahead of the endoscope's field of vision, but it does allow one hand to be free for suctioning or tissue manipulation.

The alternative system of instrumentation is the modified suction/laser handpiece with side-by-side suction and laser fiber channels (Fig. 14–2). By separating the endoscope and laser fiber, the surgeon may view structures with increased freedom in manipulating the handpiece. Straight, angulated, and curved suction/laser handpieces permit gentle tissue retraction and laser energy delivery to the various surfaces of the turbinates, septum, roof, floor, and side walls of the nose and sinuses.

An eye safety filter is attached to the nasal endoscope to protect the surgeon's operating eye from the laser (Fig. 14–3). The opposite

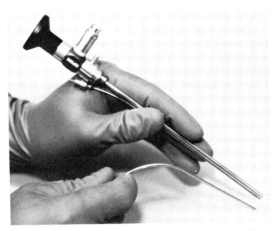

Figure 14–1. Endoscope and laser fibers inserted into separate channels of an endoscopic sheath.

eye may be protected with an eye safety monocle. There is a slight decrease in the amount of light transmitted to the surgeon while the safety filter is in place. All operating room personnel and the patient wear protective goggles of appropriate color.

PRINCIPLES OF SURGICAL TECHNIQUE WITH THE KTP/532 LASER

The power density of the laser energy determines whether tissue will be cut, vaporized, or coagulated. The power density may be decreased either by lowering the wattage or de-

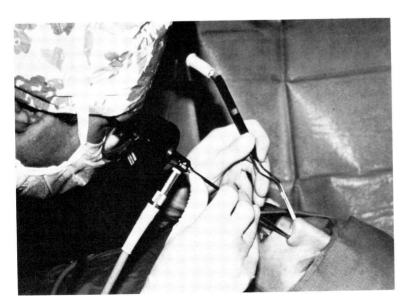

Figure 14–2. Suction/laser handpiece held separately from the endoscope.

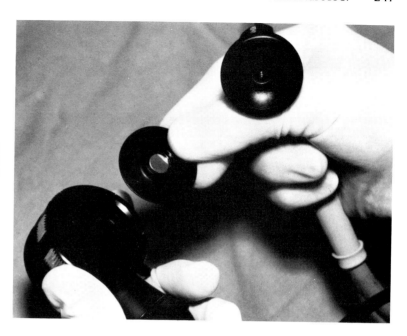

Figure 14–3. Eye safety filter that fits between the endoscope and the beam splitter to protect the operator's eye.

focusing the beam (i.e., enlarging the spot size). The KTP/532 laser is used at low power (4 to 6 W) with larger spot size (0.8 to 2 mm) when only coagulation is desired. When vaporizing tissue, an intermediate-power density is created with 5 to 8 W and laser beam of 0.6 to 1.0 mm. The fiber is placed in contact or near-contact to produce a small spot size (0.4 to 0.8 mm) at high voltage (9 to 12 W) to create high-power density for cutting. However, defocusing permits both vaporization and coagulation as needed without stopping to reduce the laser wattage.

The laser may be used in a coagulating mode to seal surface vessels prior to incising tissue. By alternating a defocused beam with one of higher-power density, the laser incision may be done in a relatively bloodless field. This technique is especially useful when removing neoplasms, angiomatous polyps, and conchae bullosae, or when trimming polypoid turbinates.

Vascular lesions, such as hereditary hemorrhagic telangiectasias, are lasered from peripherally to centrally with a low coagulating power density. The motion is circumferential from the edges of the lesion, approaching the central vessel or vascular stalk last.

LASER APPLICATION IN RHINOSINUSOLOGY

TURBINATE DYSFUNCTION

Patients with turbinate dysfunction secondary to allergic rhinitis, vasomotor rhinitis, or rhinitis medicamentosa have been treated by either laser photocoagulation or turbinectomy when these conditions are refractory to medical management. Lenz and colleagues used the argon laser in both in vitro and in vivo studies, believing that the blue-green wavelength would react best with the turbinate vascularity.[6, 7] In their patients with vasomotor rhinitis, a stripping technique was utilized, leaving intact mucosa between photocoagulated tissue. With sufficient laser treatments, patients became asymptomatic within 6 months. Lenz reported more than 2000 cases with vasomotor rhinitis treated by argon laser strip carbonization over an area 3 to 5 mm long, 2 mm wide, and 1 to 3 mm deep.[5] Results were presented for 411 of 700 patients followed during a 5-year period. A significantly improved or completely free nasal airway was obtained in 80 per cent. The results of laser treatment were improved by secondary surgery in an additional 6 per cent. Local anesthesia was used, and nasal packing was unnecessary. The end result was not achieved until 1.5 to 2 years following surgery.

Wang treated chronic hypertrophic rhinitis with the CO_2 laser.[20] He used a high-wattage, tightly focused mode to produce submucosal tunnels in the inferior turbinates. This was performed under local anesthesia on an outpatient basis in 437 cases. He reported an "effective rate" of 95 per cent after one to three treatments.

KTP/532 laser photocoagulation for turbinate dysfunction has been described by Levine.[9] A cross-hatching method of horizontal and vertical stripes with the laser left normal mucosal islands in place to speed re-epithelialization. An intermediate power of 6 to 8 watts and a very slightly defocused spot size were used. Crusting occurred for 2 to 4 weeks until the surface re-epithelialized. Twenty six of the 33 patients had decreased nasal secretions and improved airways upon follow-up of more than 1 year.

Fukutake and colleagues examined both the histopathologic changes and clinical results from CO_2 laser treatment of patients with allergic rhinitis.[3] The inferior turbinate was vaporized by a defocused beam of 20 to 30 watts for 1 minute. The nasal mucosa regenerated within 2 months following treatment. Fibrous proliferation and scar formation within the superficial layer of the submucosa were still evident at biopsy even 1 year after surgery. There was improvement in symptoms after 1 month in 38 per cent of the 140 patients. Of the 35 patients followed for 1 year, 48 per cent had excellent and 27 per cent had good results. It was hypothesized that the symptomatic improvement is related to submucosal scar formation limiting autonomically induced engorgement and secretion.

CO_2 laser partial inferior turbinectomies were reported by Mittleman[11] and Selkin.[16] Selkin used the laser in a continuous mode at 15 to 18 watts, with the beam focused to a minimum spot size to maximize tissue removed, or defocused for hemostasis. The turbinate was vaporized anteriorly and inferiorly as an adjunct to septorhinoplasty for airway obstruction. These patients had an overnight stay in the hospital, whereas Mittleman's procedures were done on an outpatient basis. There were no postoperative complications. All patients in both series had initial improvement in nasal airways, but 7 to 10 per cent had significant return of nasal obstruction within 6 months to 1 year. It was concluded that these cases had an inadequate reduction of the inferior turbinate.

VASCULAR LESIONS

Hereditary hemorrhagic telangiectasis (HHT) is an autosomal dominant syndrome. The lesions consist of subepidermal dilated blood vessels with thin walls, causing hemorrhage from minor trauma. The repeated episodes of epistaxis from nasal telangiectasias are refractory to conventional therapies and often necessitate transfusions. Even those patients who have had relatively good success with a septodermoplasty may find telangiectatic areas developing around its periphery.

All the previously described lasers have been utilized to treat HHT. Ben-Bassat and colleagues in 1978[1] and Simpson, Shapshay, and colleagues in 1982[19] reported the use of the CO_2 laser for HHT nasal lesions. In 1984, Shapshay and Oliver chose the Nd:YAG laser for its deeper coagulation effect.[18] Power was kept between 20 and 25 watts at 0.3- to 0.5-second exposures, with the fiber tip 1 to 2 cm from the surface. Bleeding episodes were controlled in five of the six patients over the 6- to 9-month follow-up.

Parkin and Dixon compared the Nd:YAG and argon lasers in HHT patients.[13] They concluded that the argon laser was easier to control and obtained better photocoagulation without tissue destruction. The argon laser was used at 2.5 watts for 5 seconds, repeated every 10 seconds. Although retreatment was necessary at 4- to 6-month intervals, seven of the eight patients reported better control of their disease than with any previous therapy.

Levine treated 11 HHT patients with the KTP/532 laser.[9] Power of 4 to 6 watts and a distance of 0.5 to 1 cm from the fiber tip to the surface produced photocoagulation. All patients had marked decreases in the severity and frequency of their epistaxis over the 6- to 18-month period. Three required repeated treatments but were quite willing to do so in view of the ease and success of the quick outpatient procedure done with local anesthesia.

A variety of other vascular lesions have been treted with laser therapy. Levine used the KTP/532 laser to remove five intranasal hemangiomas and an angiomatous polyp.[8] The laser also controlled recurrent epistaxis in a patient without HHT after conventional therapies had failed.

CHRONIC SINUS DISORDERS

Paranasal sinus surgery requires adequate visualization and illumination, whether provided by headlight or nasal endoscopes. Control of hemorrhage during sinus surgery is also important to improve visualization. The laser permits excision of nasal polyps while maintaining a dry field. Even though removal of polyps with the laser is time consuming and tedious, the laser does have a role in debulking massive polypoid disease. The laser beam can be defocused and focused to alternate coagulation and cutting. In this fashion, partial removal of massive polyps as closely as possible to their base is accomplished. The remainder of the procedure is performed with conventional techniques.

Levine reported using the KTP/532 laser in 12 patients with massive nasal polyposis and in 4 with large choanal polyps.[5] One case was done without correcting the prothrombin time of a patient on warfarin (Coumadin). His polyp was removed measuring 3 × 3 × 7 cm under local anesthesia with only a 5-ml blood loss.

Another application of the laser in surgery for chronic sinus disease is to remove scar tissue that was formed from previous procedures. Levine describes KTP/532 laser ostioplasty for obstruction of the natural maxillary sinus ostium secondary to scarring.[8] Presumably, the laser technique induces less recurrent scar tissue, which encourages sinus drainage and aeration. The same method removed intranasal scar secondary to dacryocystorhinostomy or trauma, thus relieving epiphora and nasal obstruction. When appropriate, flexible intranasal splints were inserted to prevent adhesions during early healing.

MISCELLANEOUS LESIONS

Lasers also have been utilized to remove nasal papillomas, lymphangiomas, rhinophymas, pyogenic granulomas, and small carcinomas.[8, 17, 19] Granulation tissue from sarcoid, from Wegener's granulomatosis, or secondary to chronic cocaine abuse has responded well to laser vaporization while the primary cause was treated.[8, 19]

COMPLICATIONS OF LASERS IN RHINOSINUSOLOGY

The most feared complications in laser surgery are fire and burns. Even when general anesthesia is utilized for nasal laser surgery, the oral endotracheal tube is not directly exposed to the laser field, which essentially eliminates the risk of its ignition. Fire and laser burn hazard during endoscopic laser use can be greatly reduced if the laser is put in standby mode whenever the fiber is removed from the nasal cavity. Laser beams applied through the operating microscope may inadvertently become misaligned and strike the surgical drapes or the patient's face. This risk can be decreased by surrounding the operative field with moisturized gauze.

Laser misfires or ricochets into the eyes of the patient or operating room personnel are extremely rare.[12] However, it is prudent to have appropriate eye protection in place prior to the activation of the laser unit.

Preoperative topical nasal vasoconstriction lessens the likelihood of hemorrhage. Although the laser is intended to reduce bleeding, it may still occur. Adherence to the principles of careful technique with laser coagulation as needed will decrease but not eliminate this risk. Care must be taken to reduce the laser power density reaching the tissue surface to a coagulating energy level to achieve this effect. Working from the periphery toward the central vessels is essential in vascular lesions.

When brisk hemorrhage occurs, the laser will coagulate and char the surface of the blood pool but not penetrate to its source. Suction and clearing of the char permit laser coagulation energy to have an impact on the bleeding point. If the vessel caliber is too large or the hemorrhage too rapid, traditional methods of hemostasis, such as electrocautery or packing, will be necessary.

The tissue effect of all lasers is the generation of heat. Therefore, excessive heat generation may overcome tissue cooling and result in tissue damage beyond that intended. Potential consequences include septal perforation, tissue slough, postoperative scarring, or damage to the structures adjacent to the paranasal sinuses.

Minton and Absten described three classic errors in technique that result in excessive tissue thermal damage.[10] The first is using more laser power than necessary, which yields overpenetration of tissue. To avoid this, begin with a lower power setting, then increase the energy to achieve optimal effect.

The second error is the exact opposite. By using too low a power, excessive laser time is required. This causes heat buildup, particularly when the laser is in the continuous mode. Using the laser in this mode for long periods allows insufficient time for dispersion of the heat generated. Appropriately higher power combined with intermittent laser use achieves the desired effect, with time between exposures for tissue cooling.

The third error is surface char from laser use. The laser interacts with the char to generate significant temperature increases that lead to tissue damage and scar formation. Clearing char from the area by suction and gentle manipulation prevents this complication.

The laser is a powerful surgical tool with a deceptively innocuous appearance. Safe and effective application of laser surgery requires constant vigilance.

HORIZONS IN LASERS IN RHINOSINUSOLOGY

The Nd:YAG laser with appropriate fibers may be used in removing nasal polyps by capitalizing on the high degree of scatter. Under this technique, the polyps would be desiccated, reducing hemorrhage and increasing visualization.

Adaptation of fiberoptic carriers for the CO_2 laser would greatly increase its applicability in nasal and sinus surgery.

SUMMARY

The laser has become an established surgical tool because of the inherent qualities of coagulation and reduction of hemorrhage while removing tissue. Fiberoptic delivery increases the flexibility of laser application. Careful selection of the appropriate laser and adherence to proper technique make the laser a valuable adjuvant in rhinosinusology.

References

1. Ben-Bassat M, Kaplan I, Levy R: Treatment of hereditary hemorrhagic telangiectasis of the nasal mucosa with the carbon dioxide laser. Br J Plast Surg 31:157, 1978.
2. Einstein A: Quantentheorie der Strahlung. Physiol Z 18:121, 1917.
3. Fukatake T, Yamashite T, Tomoda K, et al: Laser surgery for allergic rhinitis. Arch Otolaryngol 112:1280, 1986.
4. Jako GJ: Laser surgery of the vocal cords. Laryngoscope 82:2204, 1972.
5. Lenz H: Eight years' laser surgery of the inferior turbinates in vasomotor rhinopathy in the form of laser strip carbonization. HNO 33:422, 1985.
6. Lenz H, Eichler J, Knof J, et al: Endonasal Ar laser beam guide system and first clinical application in vasomotor rhinitis. Laryngol Rhinol Otol (Stuttg) 56:749, 1977.
7. Lenz H, Eichler J, Schafer G, et al: Parameters for argon laser surgery of lower human turbinates; In vitro experiment. Acta Otolaryngol (Stockh) 83:3, 360, 1977.
8. Levine HL: Endoscopy and the KTP/532 laser for nasal sinus disease. Ann Otol Rhinol Laryngol 98:46, 1989.
9. Levine HL: Lasers and endoscopic rhinologic surgery. Otolaryngol Clin North Am 22(4):739, 1989.
10. Minton JP, Absten GT: Surgical lasers: How they work. Am Coll Surg Bull 72(8):4, 1987.
11. Mittleman H: Carbon dioxide laser turbinectomies for chronic obstructive rhinitis. Lasers Surg Med 2:29, 1982.
12. Norton ML: Anesthesia problems in laser surgery. In Fried MP, Kelly JH, Strome M (eds): Complications of Laser Surgery of the Head and Neck. Chicago, Year Book Medical Publishers, 1986, p 55.
13. Parkin JL, Dixon JA: Laser photocoagulation in hereditary hemorrhagic telangiectasia. Otolaryngol Head Neck Surg 89:204, 1981.
14. Patel CKV, McFarlane RA, Faust WL: Selective excitation through vibrational energy transfer and optical laser action in N_2-CO_2. Physiol Rev 13:617, 1964.
15. Polanyi TG, Bredemeier HL, David TW: A CO_2 laser for surgical research. Med Biol Eng 8:541, 1970.
16. Selkin SG: Laser turbinectomy as an adjunct to rhinoseptoplasty. Arch Otolaryngol 111:446, 1985.
17. Selkin SG: Pitfalls in intranasal laser surgery and how to avoid them. Arch Otolaryngol Head Neck Surg 112(3):285, 1986.
18. Shapshay SM, Oliver P: Treatment of hereditary hemorrhagic telangiectasia by Nd:YAG laser photocoagulation. Laryngoscope 94:1554, 1984.
19. Simpson GT, Shapshay SM, Vaughn CW, et al: Rhinologic surgery with the carbon dioxide laser. Laryngoscope 92:412, 1982.
20. Wang Q: Laser in otolaryngology. Chin Med J (Engl) 92:857, 1979.
21. Yahr WZ, Strully J: Blood vessel anastomosis by laser and other biomedical applications. Assoc Adv Med Instr 1:1, 1966.

CHAPTER 15

SPHENOID SINUS

Andrew Blitzer, MD, DDS
Peter W. Carmel, MD, DMedSci
Kalmon D. Post, MD

In 1949, Van Alyea described the sphenoid sinus as the "most neglected sinus—neglected by disease at its deep location within the skull, and neglected by the physician because of its subtle presentation."[1] Knowledge of the anatomy of the sphenoid sinus and its pathophysiology will help remove it from obscurity and permit prompt diagnosis and treatment of its disorders, thereby reducing complications.

Developmentally, the sphenoid sinus is an outgrowth of the sphenoid bone in the posterosuperior part of the sphenoid recess. Pneumatization of the sphenoid varies in degree and can involve a portion, or the entire body, of the sphenoid and its processes. Thirteen important structures are adjacent to the sphenoid sinus: the dura, pituitary, optic nerve, cavernous sinus, internal carotid artery, abducens nerve, oculomotor nerve, trochlear nerve, ophthalmic nerve, maxillary nerve, sphenopalatine ganglion, sphenopalatine artery, and the nerve of the pterygoid canal. Some of these adjacent structures may indent the sphenoid sinus walls. Van Alyea reviewed numerous specimens and found that the carotid artery indented the wall in 65 per cent, the optic nerve in 40 per cent, the maxillary nerve in 40 per cent, and the vidian canal in 36 per cent. He did not observe any cases with actual dehiscence of the bony walls.[2–4]

The sphenoid sinus is situated in the nasal cavity, behind the posterior choana, and is not readily accessible to injury. The nasal air stream is directed below the ostia, so few bacteria or inhaled irritants are carried toward the sinus. The lining mucosa contains few glands, producing scant mucus compared with the maxillary sinus. Secondary infection uncommonly follows blockage of the sinus unless a virulent organism is involved.[3, 5]

When the sphenoid sinus is involved with a disease process, history and physical examination do little to establish the correct diagnosis. Once the sphenoid sinus has been incriminated, it is difficult to differentiate primary from secondary processes, as well as benign from malignant lesions.[6]

The most frequent symptom of sphenoid sinus disease is headache. The pain is most commonly localized in the retro-orbital area, followed by the frontal, vertex, and temporal regions. The character of the pain is best described as dull, deep seated, aching, and nagging. It often will awaken a patient from deep sleep and will not respond to salicylate therapy.[2, 5–7] The next most common complaints are ocular and include altered or decreased vision and diplopia. Visual symptoms frequently accompany space-occupying lesions, sixth nerve deficits being most common, followed by optic nerve deficits.[6, 7] Neuralgia of the trigeminal nerve or the sphenopalatine ganglion may also be related to sphenoid sinus involvement. Sluder,[2] in 1912, recognized this phenomenon and advocated cocainization or carbolization of the sphenopalatine ganglion.

A meticulous nasal examination may confirm the diagnosis of sphenoid sinus disease. Demonstration of the occlusion of the sinus by tumors or polyps, or the presence of suppuration in the superior nasal recess, will explain the patient's symptoms. Probing its ostium may elicit a release of purulent material from the sphenoid sinus.[5, 8]

Because physical examination is often quite difficult, early practitioners utilized blunt probes to "sound" the sinus, to detect purulence, to estimate the size of the sinus, and to palpate for any masses. However, radiography became a much more reliable method of analyzing the size and shape of the sinus and of determining any abnormalities. Plain and tomographic radiographs demonstrated the presence of intraluminal lesions and sclerosis and erosion of the bony walls.[5] With the advent of the computed tomography (CT) scanner, many previously undiagnosed lesions were easily visualized, as the scan is density specific. The adjunctive use of intravenous contrast material aided in the identification of vascular lesions, and the intrathecal insertion of metrizamide could demonstrate CSF leaks.[9]

The office examination has been greatly enhanced with the advent of fiberoptic telescopes. A 30-degree, wide-angle, 4-mm telescope can easily be passed in the nasal cavity past the middle turbinate to expose the face of the sphenoid sinus, the sphenoid ostium, and the sphenoethmoid recess.[10]

INFECTION

The most common disease of the sphenoid sinus is sinusitis. In 1892, MacDonald[11] could document only two cases. He stated that "great difficulty lies in our ignorance of the sphenoid in any individual case." This was written before radiographs were available, when the diagnosis was established on the basis of sounding. In the preantibiotic era, Teed[12] estimated that sphenoiditis was responsible for 15 to 33 per cent of all sinus infections, with many of the cases having intracranial extension and a high mortality. However, in a review of sinusitis treated at the Massachusetts Eye and Ear Infirmary from 1968 to 1980, Lew and associates collected 20 cases of isolated sphenoid sinusitis, which represented 2.7 per cent of all sinus infections.[13]

Factors that predispose to sphenoiditis include barotrauma, cocaine sniffing, radiotherapy, nasal occlusion by tumor, fractures, the use of steroids or immunosuppressive agents, and diabetes mellitus.[13]

The most common symptom of sphenoiditis is a dull aching headache,[14] which is unrelieved by aspirin and interferes with sleep in the early morning. The pain is often situated in more than one location and may involve the frontal, temporal, occipital, retro-orbital, and vertex areas. Associated with the pain is an inability to concentrate, lassitude, and anorexia. In acute infections there may also be fever, lethargy or coma, and nuchal rigidity.[13] The second most common symptom of infection is nasal discharge. There may be associated cacosmia, nasal crusting, and gross purulence.[13] Next most frequent is the occurrence of visual disturbances. These include central scotomas and paresis of the third, fourth, and sixth cranial nerves. There may be ptosis, proptosis and chemosis. Other related symptoms include pain or paresthesias of $V_{1, 2, 3}$ and vertigo.[7, 13, 16–18]

A complete blood count will generally show leukocytosis and increased neutrophils in many acute cases. However, a normal white blood cell count is often encountered in chronic disease.[13]

Radiographs taken during an acute infection often show no change, delaying the correct diagnosis. Occasionally, mucosal thickening or mild sclerosis is noted. In chronic cases, mucosal thickening is virtually always seen. There are often concomitant ethmoid sinus abnormalities, but the occurrence of air-fluid level or bony erosion is uncommon. Lew and associates[13] could not correlate the radiographic findings with the clinical severity of the disease. The CT scanner has now become a crucial part of the evaluation of sphenoid sinus disease and permits detection of subtle density changes.[7, 13, 15]

Cultures of the secretions found in acute infections often reveal *Staphylococcus aureus* and *Streptococcus pneumoniae*. In chronic cases, gram-positive and gram-negative organisms are both commonly isolated. Notable among the latter are *Escherichia coli* and *Proteus mirabilis*.[13]

Acute sphenoid sinusitis is often misdiagnosed as ophthalmic migraine, aseptic meningitis, or cavernous sinus thrombosis. In the chronic situation, the incorrect diagnoses have included atypical facial pain, migraine, trigeminal neuralgia, idiopathic oculomotor palsy, retro-orbital tumor, brain tumor, and carotid aneurysm.[13]

Fungal infections of the sphenoid sinus have also been reported, with the most common pathogen being *Aspergillus*. Aspergillosis has two clinical forms. In the noninvasive form, a fungus ball is found in the sinus, which clinically resembles a chronic bacterial infection (Figs. 15–1 and 15–2). The invasive form develops in debilitated patients, with the appearance of necrosis, hemorrhage, and systemic dissemination, and clinically mimics a malignant process. Mucormycosis has also been described in the sphenoid sinus and is generally lethal.[19–21]

The complications of sphenoid sinusitis in-

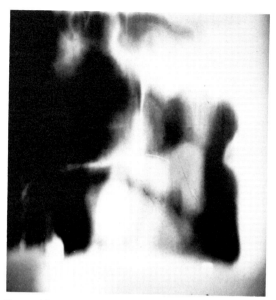

Figure 15–1. Lateral polytomogram showing a fungus ball in the sphenoid sinus.

clude cavernous sinus thrombosis, retrobulbar neuritis, meningitis, blindness, orbital apex syndrome, pituitary abscess with hypopituitarism, and carotid artery occlusion. Cavernous sinus thrombosis develops by spread of the infection to the valveless venous channels within the leaves of the dura, adjacent to the pituitary gland. The signs and symptoms of cavernous sinus thrombosis include proptosis, chemosis, lid edema, ophthalmoplegia, headache, meningismus, and spiking fevers. The orbital signs become bilateral by contralateral spread through the cavernous sinus. In 1961, Yarington[22] reviewed 878 cases of cavernous sinus thrombosis and found an 80 per cent mortality. With improved antibiotic therapy and prompt diagnosis, the mortality decreased to 13.6 per cent in a follow-up study in 1977.[7, 13, 16, 22]

Early diagnosis and aggressive treatment are the most important factors in reducing the morbidity and mortality of sphenoid sinus disease. A delay in treatment was associated with 80 to 100 per cent morbidity.[13, 23] The acute phase is managed with nasal decongestants and oral antibiotics. If severe retro-orbital, occipital, hemicranial, or vertex pain and fever or neurologic deficits are present, the patient should have a CT scan with contrast to rule out the possibility of cavernous sinus thrombosis. If this is detected, the patient is given a minimum of 2 weeks of parenteral antibiotic therapy. In the chronic situation, the patients are not critically ill, and there is a corresponding lower morbidity and mortality. These patients are initially

treated with antibiotics, followed by surgical drainage if necessary.[13]

The sphenoid sinus can first be "sounded" with a blunt metal probe passed through its ostium to determine the presence of pus. If pus is found, a long cotton carrier saturated with epinephrine and/or cocaine solution is placed over the ostium to decongest the surrounding mucosa and facilitate drainage. If drainage is not established, sinus cannulation and irrigation may be necessary.[24, 25] Cannulation may be difficult because of a deviated nasal septum, narrow olfactory groove, narrow sphenoethmoid recess, small or deeply placed ostium, hypertrophied middle turbinate, overhanging ethmoid air cells, or nasal polyps. These structural abnormalities may require surgical correction to improve visualization and allow proper instrumentation. The anterior wall of the sphenoid sinus is 7 cm from the anterior nasal spine, with the posterior wall 2 cm beyond. The ostia are 30 degrees from the floor of the nose and slightly lateral to the midline. An x-ray film taken with a probe in position will confirm its proper placement. If the ostium is too small for cannulation, it should be enlarged with a pouch (Fletcher or Hajek forceps). A direct puncture technique is too dangerous and can cause injury to surrounding vital structures, such as the cavernous sinus or carotid artery. Once the cannula is in place, the sinus is irrigated slowly with warm saline.[4, 8, 26–28]

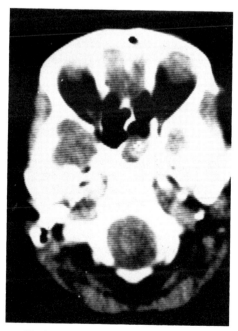

Figure 15–2. Axial computed tomography (CT) scan showing fungus ball in the sphenoid sinus.

A true pyocele of the sphenoid sinus often is accompanied by visual disturbances, which include exophthalmos, decreased vision, or ophthalmoplegia. The patient may also complain of episodic headache. The first case of sphenoid pyocele was described at autopsy by Lieutand in 1735.[29] The mortality and morbidity of the sphenoid pyocele is related to the development of intracranial complications, which include meningitis, pituitary necrosis, cerebral or extradural abscess, hydrocephalus, pontine infarction, cerebrospinal fluid (CSF) rhinorrhea, and osteomyelitis. Management includes antibiotic therapy and surgical drainage.[29–32]

MUCOCELE

The mucocele is the most common space-occupying lesion of the sphenoid sinus. It is uncommon, but not rare, with 70 to 80 cases reported in the literature. The first description of a sphenoid mucocele was by John Berg in 1889.[33, 34]

In the past, many mucoceles of the sphenoid were diagnosed at autopsy. However, a careful history and physical examination and appropriate radiologic studies should allow early diagnosis and treatment.[5] In a review by Blum and Larson,[35] it was found that 70 to 90 per cent of the patients with mucoceles had headache; 50 per cent had ocular symptoms; 20 per cent presented with a history of sinusitis; 10 to 20 per cent with anosmia; and 5 per cent with endocrine abnormalities. Other reported symptoms are nasal congestion, facial numbness, confusion, and CSF rhinorrhea. The accompanying headache is characteristically retro-orbital or frontal. The visual disturbances include ocular field defects, ophthalmoplegia, and proptosis. Continued compression of the optic nerve may lead to blindness.[7, 8, 34, 36] The physical findings include nasal septal deformities, mucopurulent discharge, bilateral or unilateral sixth nerve palsy, ptosis, facial paresthesia, and decreased vision or visual field defects.[35–37]

The pathogenesis of sphenoid mucoceles is uncertain; proposed causative factors include chronic infection or inflammation, traumatic or surgical injury, and congenital goblet cell cysts. As the mucocele enlarges, there is pressure resorption of the surrounding bone, exposing and stretching of the dura with pain, and involvement of contiguous vital structures.[34]

Dramatic presentations of mucoceles include sudden blindness and orbital apex syndrome, spontaneous pneumocephalus, and bilateral carotid artery occlusion.[35, 38]

Radiographs of the sphenoid bone are usually diagnostic; plain films in the lateral and submentovertex positions are useful only for screening purposes. The superior orbital fissure, optic foramen, walls of the orbit, floor of the sella turcica, walls of the sphenoid sinus, wings of the sphenoid, and the internal carotid artery canal should be evaluated for the presence of erosion. Tomographic findings include a mass in the sinus, an air-fluid level, clouding or mucosal thickening, bulging of the bony contours, and displacement or destruction of the intrasinus septum. The CT scanner provides accurate information concerning mass density, the integrity of the bony walls, and involvement of adjacent structures[7, 39–41] (Fig. 15–3).

The differential diagnosis of the mucocele includes craniopharyngioma, meningioma, glioma, chordoma, pituitary tumor, meningoencephalocele, and nasopharyngeal tumor.[34]

Treatment is sinusotomy, with removal or drainage of the mucocele. This may be accomplished by an intranasal, transorbital, transantral, or sublabial trans-septal approach. The external ethmoid approach is preferable if there are ocular symptoms because of better exposure of the orbit (Figs. 15–4 through 15–6).

Isolated sphenoid or sphenoethmoid pathology can also be approached via a Wigand endoscopic operation. Using a 25-degree and a 70-degree wide-angle fiberoptic illuminated telescope, the posterior half of the middle turbinate is obliquely transected using a turbinate

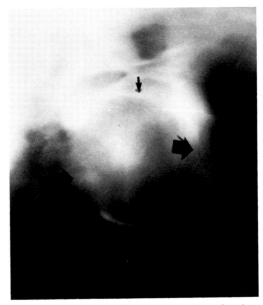

Figure 15–3. Tomographic coronal section showing a large mucocele of the sphenoid sinus. Note expansion and loss of bone.

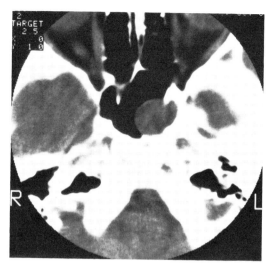

Figure 15–4. Axial CT scan of expanding lesion of the sphenoid.

scissors. The sphenoid ostium is then visualized and probed. An ostium punch is then used under direct vision to open the anterior face. The telescopes are used to inspect the interior of the sphenoid. Diseased tissue can be removed under direct vision to minimize potential risk to the optic nerve, cavernous sinus, or internal carotid artery. If there is concomitant ethmoid disease, the cells are dissected using a Weil-Blakesley forceps, from posterior to ante-

rior, along the fovea ethmoidalis as a superior border.[37, 42]

OTHER BENIGN LESIONS

Other benign conditions involving the sphenoid sinus include polyps, tumors, congenital lesions, and fibro-osseous disorders. Polyps can be isolated to the sphenoid sinus or occur in association with polyps of the posterior ethmoid cells. The patient with occlusive polyps of the sphenoid usually has a long history of postnasal discharge. On examination, purulent material is seen in the sphenoethmoid recess. Radiographs may be negative or show sinus clouding. Exploration may reveal polyps within the sinus or occluding its ostium.[7]

Most inverting papillomas of the sphenoid sinus represent extension of antral or ethmoid tumors; however, several cases of primary tumors of the sphenoid have been reported. The symptoms are usually subtle, consisting of vague headache or visual abnormalities (diplopia or decreased vision). Treatment for these lesions should be aggressive, as they are locally invasive and tend to recur. About 10 per cent show atypia, with 4 to 5 per cent undergoing malignant transformation. Because inverting papillomas tend to spread by metaplasia of the adjacent mucosa, excision of a wide margin of the normal tissue is indicated. This is difficult

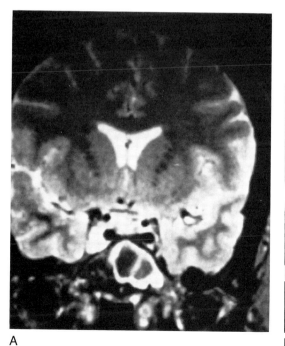

A

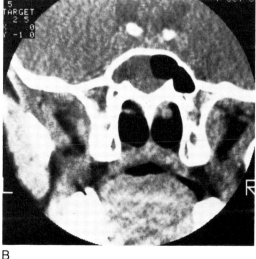

B

Figure 15–5. *A,* Coronal magnetic resonance image (MRI) showing a bi-lobed mucocele of the sphenoid sinus. *B,* Coronal CT scan of expanding lesion of the sphenoid.

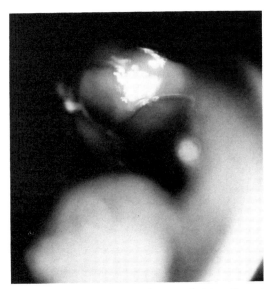

Figure 15–6. Intraoperative photograph taken through an operative microscope. A Hardy speculum is in place and, through a sphenoidotomy, the mucocele is visualized.

to achieve in the sphenoid sinus because of the vital adjacent structures and therefore may account for the 30 to 62 per cent recurrence rate. This lesion is not radiosensitive, and radiotherapy may result in osteoradionecrosis and radiation-induced malignant lesions. Long-term results with the CO_2 laser have not yet been reported.[45, 46]

An encephalocele may also occur as a space-occupying lesion of the sphenoid. It arises by herniation of brain through the congenital sphenopharyngeal dehiscence in the base of the skull. The possibility of such developmental lesions makes it imperative to have good radiologic studies of the skull base before attempting surgical extirpation of a sphenoid mass.[33, 48]

Fibro-osseous disorders may also involve the sphenoid. In fibrous dysplasia there is replacement of the normal bone with metaplastic woven bone. Although this process most commonly arises in membranous bone, several cases have been described in the sphenoid.[7, 49, 50]

Presenting symptoms include fronto-occipital headaches, diplopia, and sixth nerve palsies. Treatment consists of biopsy and curettage.[7]

Ossifying fibromas, which occur most commonly in the maxilla and mandible, have also been reported in the sphenoid. Radiographically, they are unilocular lesions with a cortical margin and lack evidence of periosteal reaction. Clinically, headaches and visual disturbances are the most common presenting complaints. Surgical excision is the treatment of choice.[33]

Other benign lesions reported in the sphenoid include neurilemommas,[51] giant cell tumors,[52] rhinoliths,[7] aneurysmal bone cysts,[53] chordomas,[54] hemangiomas,[56] and hemangiopericytomas.[57]

MALIGNANT LESIONS

Malignant neoplasms of the sphenoid sinus include both primary and metastatic lesions. Although squamous cell carcinoma can arise within the sinus, it generally represents an extension from a primary lesion in the nose or nasopharynx. Metastases from the breast, thyroid, lung, kidney, and prostate have also been reported.[55, 58, 59]

In a study of primary malignant tumors of the sphenoid sinus from the Mayo Clinic, there were two squamous cell carcinomas, two lymphoepitheliomas, one adenocarcinoma, and one undifferentiated carcinoma. Malignant melanoma, reticulum and osteoblastic sarcoma, transitional cell sarcoma, and basal cell carcinoma have also been reported.[7, 54]

Vague referred pain and visual complaints are the most common symptoms. In contrast to benign desease processes, there is usually a rapid progression of the symptoms. Nasal congestion, tinnitus, conductive hearing loss, and facial numbness may also occur.[7, 60, 61]

Radiographs are useful for diagnosis. In the series of Wyllie and associates,[7] five or six patients had radiographic evidence of a mass and/or bone destruction. Arteriography or CT scanning with contrast will demonstrate the presence of intracranial invasion, vessel displacement, or a tumor blush.[62] A sphenoidotomy provides tissue for biopsy and helps visualize the extent of the disease. Although en bloc resection often may be impossible, decompression of the tumor is often helpful. However, this surgery may be complicated by hemorrhage, infection, or CSF leak. The reported results of treatment vary from a 20 per cent survival in Watson's[7] series to 0 per cent survival after 33 months in Wyllie's[7] series.

INTRASELLAR LESIONS

Intrasellar lesions may erode through the sellar floor and present as sphenoid masses; consequently, the trans-sphenoid route has become a major approach for their removal. Most of these lesions are benign, slow-growing tumors, and their removal should be delayed until an adequate neurologic, endocrinologic, and radiologic evaluation has been completed.

PITUITARY ADENOMAS

Benign tumors of the pituitary constitute by far the largest group of sellar lesions requiring trans-sphenoid surgery. The availability of radioimmunoassay techniques and recent advances in computed scanning of the sella turcica have greatly facilitated early diagnosis of these tumors. The efficacy and safety of sellar microsurgery have contributed to an increasing preference for surgical intervention rather than other forms of therapy.[64]

These tumors may be quite well demarcated from the normal pituitary and are often described as being encapsulated. The "capsule" acquired by these microadenomas is derived from the connective tissue scaffolding of the compressed pituitary parenchyma. However, many diffuse tumors that blend into the normal gland are also encountered. With larger lesions, the remaining normal pituitary is often squeezed into a small portion of the sella, or it may be attenuated over the surface of the tumor. With continued growth, the tumor outstrips its blood supply, and areas of hemorrhage and infarction appear. The development of sudden massive hemorrhage and necrosis is termed pituitary apoplexy. However, recent work on this syndrome indicates that it is more probably caused by necrosis and edema than by hemorrhage, which may be a late occurrence in this syndrome.[65]

Classically, pituitary tumors have been classified on the basis of their cellular staining reaction and were termed chromophobic, acidophilic, or basophilic.[66, 67] More recently, application of the immunoperoxidase technique to pituitary tumors has allowed the identification of specific hormones within the pituitary cells. Pituitary tumors now may be classified as containing prolactin, growth hormone, ACTH, FSH, or TSH. In addition, certain well-differentiated "null" cells have also been delineated.[67, 68] With advances in endocrinologic testing and modern immunohistochemical and immunoelectromicroscopic techniques, the incidence of adenomas without evidence of hypersecretion or endocrine activity has decreased to about 25 per cent of pituitary adenomas.

The functionally active group of pituitary tumors comprise the largest percentage of pituitary adenomas. They represent about 75 per cent of all pituitary tumors. Preoperative endocrinologic testing, as well as clinical symptomatology resulting from the adenoma's hypersecretion of hormones, helps identify and classify these tumors. It is this functional classification, confirmed with immunohistochemical and immunoelectronmicroscopic techniques and not traditional light microscopic pathology, that separates these tumors.

Prolactinomas represent about 40 to 50 per cent of all patients with pituitary adenomas. Under light microscopy, prolactin cell tumors are chromophobic or acidophilic. Secretory granules are sparse and spherical and measure 150 to 350 nm, as seen on immunoelectronmicroscopy. Somatotropic adenomas, resulting in acromegaly, account for 15 to 25 per cent of pituitary adenomas. Under light microscopy, these tumors may be termed acidophilic or chromophobic. Using immunoelectronmicroscopy, two distinct cell types can be identified: densely and sparsely granulated adenomas.[69]

Cushing's disease or Nelson's syndrome, caused by corticotropin-secreting adenomas, represents only about 5 per cent of all pituitary adenomas. Under light microscopy, corticotrophs are basophilic. Immunoelectronmicroscopy shows these tumor cells to be similar to corticotropic, nontumorous pituitary cell types containing numerous spherical secretory granules that vary in density, measure 250 to 700 nm, and line up along the cell membrane.[69]

The rarest of pituitary adenomas are those that secrete solely thyrotropin or gonadotropin. Each type accounts for less than 1 per cent of pituitary adenomas. Finally, there are mixed endocrinologically active tumors. These represent about 10 to 15 per cent of all pituitary adenomas.[69]

Larger pituitary tumors invade the dura of the sellar floor and extend into the cavernous and circular sinuses. These invasive tumors are usually not termed malignant but often are difficult to eradicate. They have been compared with meningiomas of the orbit and nasal region, which are benign histologically but extremely invasive into regional structures (Fig. 15–7). More than 15 per cent of pituitary tumors are invasive, and their treatment requires radiation therapy after surgery.

CRANIOPHARYNGIOMAS

The craniopharyngioma is one of the commonest intracranial tumors of childhood but is not limited to the younger years, with more than half the patients in large reported series

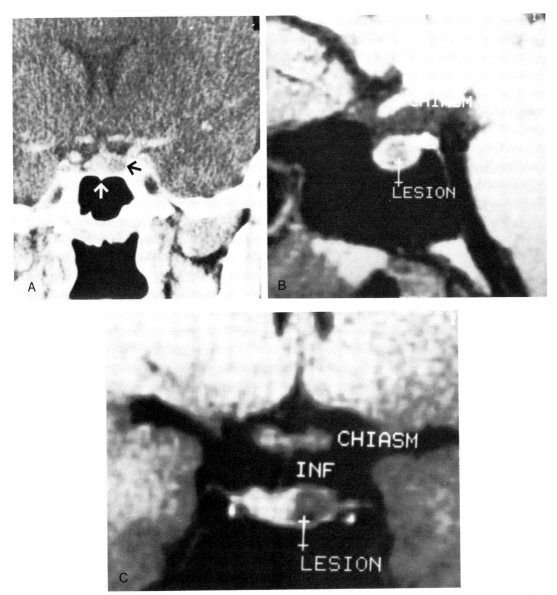

Figure 15–7. *A,* Coronal CT, with enhancement, demonstrating the pituitary gland with a microadenoma in the left side *(black arrow).* Note that the stalk is deviated slightly toward the right. The white arrow demonstrates the vertical septation in the sphenoid sinus. *B,* Sagittal MRI demonstrating the pituitary gland with a microadenoma. The optic chiasm is well visualized above. *C,* Coronal MRI demonstrating the same pituitary gland and microadenoma. The pituitary stalk *(inferior)* is seen shifted from left to right.

over 20 years of age.[70] There is no apparent sexual predilection. These tumors are slow growing and well encapsulated and become symptomatic by enlargement in the extra-axial cranial space. As they expand, they compress or displace the optic chiasm, sellar contents, pituitary stalk, and other basal brain structures. A minority of tumors have both suprasellar and intrasellar components. An even smaller number are located entirely within an expanded sella. Total primary surgical extirpation is the

goal of treatment.[71] Subtotally removed craniopharyngiomas tend to recur and require postoperative radiotherapy. For tumors located entirely within the sella or those with limited suprasellar extension, this may be accomplished via the trans-sphenoid approach. Craniopharyngiomas may be either cystic or solid. Cystic lesions are filled with a fluid that may range in color from dark brown to light tan or even clear and are rich in birefringent cholestrin crystals. Most of the tumors in childhood show calcified areas on radiography, and CT scanning also reveals that many of the adult lesions have granular calcifications. The capsule of the craniopharyngioma may be densely adherent to adjacent normal brain tissue and blood vessels. The gliotic adhesions that form between the tumor and the hypothalamus and chiasm are less likely to restrict tumor removal than the tough, mesenchymal fibrosis that occurs when these tumors adhere to major vessels at the base of the brain.

OTHER EPITHELIAL NEOPLASMS

This group of relatively rare lesions includes epidermoid and dermoid cysts that arise in the sellar and suprasellar regions. Although these are congenital lesions, their clinical appearance is usually delayed until the fifth or sixth decade. Epidermoid and dermoid cysts are extremely slow growing and will often conform to the subarachnoid spaces, spreading out as a flattened layer over an enormous expanse of the base of the brain. Epidermoid cysts are filled with a cheesy, desquamated epithelium. Dermoid cysts differ by the presence of additional structures, such as follicles, sebaceous glands, and exocrine glands.

MENINGIOMAS

Nearly 10 per cent of meningiomas occur in the region of the sella. They rarely arise within the sella itself, with most attached to the diaphragma sellae, to the tuberculum sellae, or to the inner third of the sphenoid ridge. A few unusual cases of meningiomas occurring entirely within the sella, or with a relatively small suprasellar extension, have been reported.

UNCOMMON TUMORS OF THE SELLAR REGION

Other types of tumor found within the sella include chordomas, germ cell tumors, and tumors of primary brain origin, such as the astrocytoma or ganglioglioma. Chordomas arise from vestiges of the obliterated notochord, which forms the primitive axial skeleton. The congenital tumor remains dormant for years, is extremely slow growing, and presents an expansile, erosive, intraosseous neoplasm. It extends beneath the brain as an encapsulated tumor, but total extirpation is difficult because of osseous invasion. Not uncommonly, nasopharyn-

geal extension results from downward growth through the sphenoid bone. It occurs far more frequently by direct extension than as a primary nasopharyngeal chordoma.

Intracranial germ cell tumors are quite rare; when they occur in the hypothalamic region, they are generally termed ectopic pinealomas. These tumors, fortunately, are radiosensitive and have a favorable prognosis.

RADIOGRAPHIC EVALUATION

Technologic advances have produced a wide range of diagnostic procedures for visualizing the sella, sphenoid sinus, and parasellar region. Currently, the methods most commonly used are computed tomography (CT) and magnetic resonance imaging (MRI).

CT scanning, with its various adjunctive techniques, has been the most important diagnostic method for lesions of the sella and parasellar region (Figs. 15–8 through 15–11). When CT scanning was introduced two decades ago, it could only detect pituitary tumors larger than 2 cm in diameter. Rapid technologic advances allow fourth generation scanners to delineate tumors only a few millimeters in diameter. Commonly, a series of axial tomograms is obtained prior to the administration of contrast material. The contrast material is then given

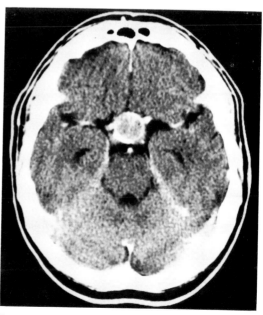

Figure 15–8. Axial CT, with enhancement, demonstrating a macroadenoma of the pituitary gland. It extends into the suprasellar cistern.

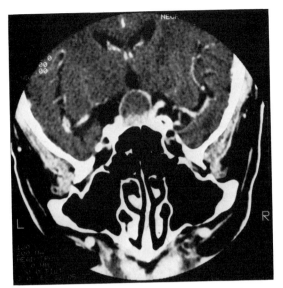

Figure 15–9. Coronal CT, with enhancement, demonstrating the same macroadenoma reaching and compressing the inferior portion of the third ventricle.

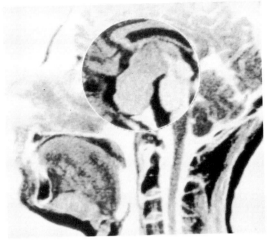

Figure 15–11. Sagittal MRI demonstrating a huge pituitary adenoma reaching the top of the third ventricle.

also visualized (Fig. 15–12). The sensitivity of CT in the evaluation of intrasellar and suprasellar tumors resulted in its replacing pneumo-

intravenously (approximately 40 gm of iodine), and a new series of films is obtained in both axial and coronal planes. This technique yields scans of high resolution, and small portal size decreases the artifacts caused by the surrounding bone. In this fashion, the intrasellar structures are visualized.[72] In most patients, the entire pituitary gland enhances following contrast injection, and parasellar structures, including the cavernous sinus, internal carotid artery and branches, pituitary stalk, optic nerves and chiasm, and the suprasellar cistern system, are

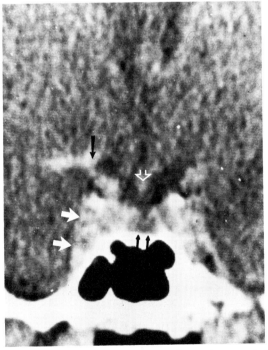

Figure 15–12. Coronal contrast-enhanced computed scan of a young woman with a prolactin-secreting pituitary adenoma. The cavernous sinus normally enhances *(white arrows)*; the dark circular structures within the sinus are the third, fourth, and sixth cranial nerves. The carotid artery and its bifurcation into the anterior and middle cerebral arteries are seen on right *(black arrow)*. Enhancement normally demonstrates the median eminence and upper pituitary stalk *(open arrow)*. The pituitary gland enhances as well, and prolactin-secreting adenomas often appear as darker lucent areas *(double arrows)*.

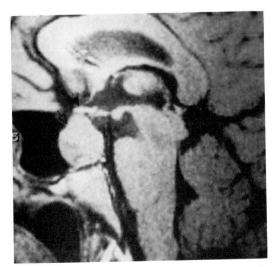

Figure 15–10. Sagittal MRI demonstrating a macroadenoma of the pituitary gland *(open arrow)* reaching the optic chiasm *(closed arrow)*.

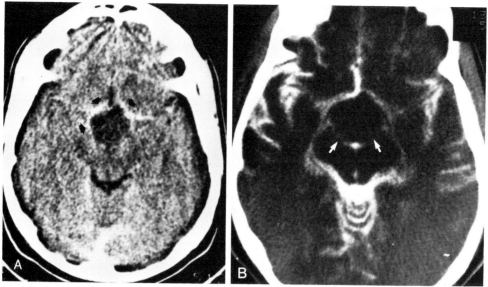

Figure 15–13. *A,* Contrast-enhanced axial computed scan of a patient with a cystic craniopharyngioma. The tumor does not enhance but is outlined by the displaced arteries of the circle of Willis *(arrows). B,* Axial computed scan following intrathecal metrizamide injection. The tumor mass is clearly defined in front of the brain stem. The tumor has spread to the cerebral peduncles *(arrows),* although a CSF plane can be seen between the posterior wall of the tumor and the peduncles.

encephalography as a diagnostic modality (Fig. 15–13).

Progress in CT scanning has continued steadily. Thin slices in both the axial and coronal view, both with and without contrast, offer excellent visualization of the sellar region. With this technique, tumors greater than 3 to 5 mm often can be visualized. Additionally, nuances of the bony architecture can also be particularly well seen when appropriate bone windows are obtained. Large tumors are easily visualized with their effect on the parasellar structures, including the cavernous sinus, internal carotid artery and its branches, pituitary stalk, and the optic nerves and chiasm. Microadenomas also can often be seen or inferred from a fullness of the gland unilaterally, with a shift of the pituitary stalk to the contralateral side.

CT scan, however, cannot always rule out aneurysm, and therefore angiography often has been necessary in the past to exclude that possibility. Currently, however, the MRI scan can be used to visualize the sella and parasellar structures as well as the vascular structures. As opposed to CT scanning, the imaging of vascular structures is quite excellent with the MRI scan, often more than adequate to eliminate the possibility of aneurysm.

MRI scan is done in the axial, coronal, and sagittal planes. Both small tumors as well as large tumors in the surrounding structures can be extremely well visualized. Where available, this has supplanted the use of CT scan for evaluating microadenomas. MRI scanning, however, is still expensive and not always available, and therefore CT scanning is quite useful.

Carotid angiography may yield additional information about the nature and configuration of the intrasellar pathology. Aneurysms can mimic sellar and parasellar tumors, causing similar erosive patterns. If MRI scanning is not available or not conclusive, then angiography must be performed to eliminate this possibility. Additionally, angiography may demonstrate a tumor blush characteristic of a certain type of tumor, such as meningioma.[73]

ENDOCRINE EVALUATION

Every patient who is suspected of having an intrasellar lesion should undergo a careful endocrine evaluation. In many instances, the signs of pituitary hyperfunction may be overt, such as acromegaly or Cushing's or Nelson's syndrome. However, the endocrinopathy may be more subtle, especially with the occurrence of hypofunctional pituitary disorders. Patients with low thyroid levels may have little clinical symptomatology but are at high risk during elective intrasellar operations. Preoperative endocrine tests should be done in the basal state and often must be supplemented by appropriate provocative tests.[67, 74] Almost all these patients will need complete re-evaluation in the post-operative period as well. Restoration of endocrine function is an integral part of the therapeutic management of patients with intrasellar lesions. An outline of the routine evaluation is shown in Table 15–1.

SURGERY

Many of the surgical approaches to the sphenoid were developed for trans-sphenoidal surgery of sellar lesions.[75, 76] The development of trans-sphenoid surgery in the early years of this century was prompted by several coincident factors: neurologic examination permitted localization of chiasmatic lesions; roentgenographic plates could demonstrate sellar enlargement; and pathologic studies had established the incidence of several types of slow-growing, benign lesions in the sellar region. However, surgeons remained reluctant to attempt to reach the center of the cranial base, which required major elevation of the brain; Krause, who credited himself with the first transfrontal approach to a pituitary tumor in 1905,[77] described the difficulties: "The cerebral pressure proved to be enormous; my assistant made forcible traction with the spatula with both hands, using his entire strength, yet managed to gain only a finger's breadth of additional space." The patient died 13 hours postoperatively. Although Krause was not the first to use this approach (Horsley had used it successfully in 1889),[78] his

description makes clear that surgeons were anxious to find a method that would not require brain retraction, preferably an extracranial approach. In 1906, Giordano[79] approached the sphenoid via an osteoplastic flap of the anterior wall of the frontal sinus and nose. The ethmoid cells were removed, as was the anterior wall of the sphenoid (a transfrontal transethmoid approach).

The transnasal route was used first by Schloffer[80] in 1907. In his approach, a lateral rhinotomy was performed, and the turbinates, septum, ethmoids, and anterior wall of the sphenoid were removed. Schloffer published a roentgenograph showing the eroded sella and the path of the approach illustrated by a probe (Fig. 15–14). A subsequent autopsy of this patient revealed that the size of the lesion had been underestimated, with the residual tumor being considerably larger than the portion removed[81] (Fig. 15–15). This problem would be encountered often in the history of transnasal surgery, but Schloffer's operation, done in daylight without the aid of artificial illumination or reflectors, was a remarkable accomplishment.

Later in 1907, von Eiselberg,[82] stimulated by Schloffer's report, used a modified transnasal approach. His second case was of great interest, as it involved Frolich's famous patient with the syndrome known as adrenogenital dystrophy. Von Eiselberg's operation utilized a transverse incision along the brow, as well as an incision

TABLE 15–1. Endocrine Evaluation in Sellar Lesions

Endocrine Axis	Basal Tests	Provocative Tests
Adrenal	Serum cortisol Urinary 17-ketosteroids Urinary 17-OH corticosteroids	Dexamethasone suppression (high/low) Metyrapone test
Thyroid	Serum T_4 (total) Serum T_4 (free) TSH	
Growth	Serum GH	GTT Glucose suppression
Gonadal	Serum LH Serum FSH Serum testosterone Serum estradiol	
Prolactin	Serum prolactin	

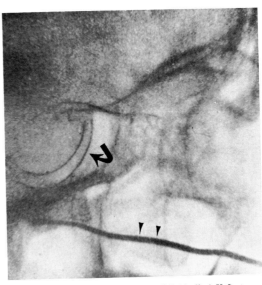

Figure 15–14. Roentgenogram of Schloffer's[80] first case (1907). This radiograph was retouched prior to publication to emphasize the erosion and "double-floor" of the sella (curved arrow). Note that a flexible metal probe was inserted to demonstrate the path of the operative approach (double arrowheads).

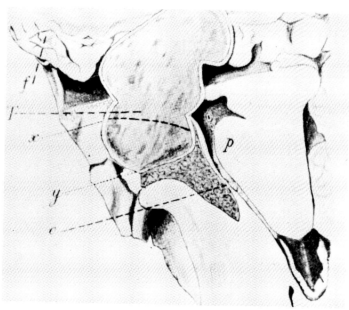

Figure 15–15. Sagittal view of autopsy on Schloffer's[81] case. The patient had a CSF leak for almost 2 weeks postoperatively, which stopped spontaneously. His vision and headaches worsened 2 months after operation, and he died 10 days later. The tumor *(T)* was much larger than Schloffer had thought at operation. Less than 20 per cent of the tumor was removed, as indicated by the dotted line. The massive tumor had obstructed the foramina of Monro, causing hydrocephalus.

along the edge of the nose (Fig. 15–16). The combination of a frontal sinusotomy with a lateral displacement of the entire nose provided direct midline access. The turbinates and septum were resected and the sphenoid and sella were entered (Fig. 15–17). A cystic tumor was encountered, which contained dark fluid on aspiration. Biopsy of the cyst wall diagnosed a "precancerous" pituitary tumor, a pathologic diagnosis no longer used. Some contemporary writers have regarded the lesion in this famous

case as a craniopharyngioma,[83] whereas others have interpreted it as a cystic pituitary adenoma with old hemorrhage.[84] Whatever the pathology, the operation was certainly disfiguring.

Improvements in technique followed rapidly in the next several years. In 1908, Stumme[85] proposed the use of a Bellocq tamponade in the

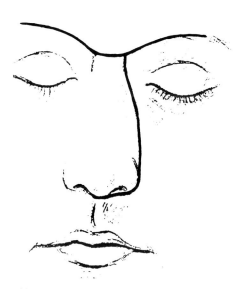

Figure 15–16. Illustration of the skin incision in the von Eiselberg[82] operation. The initial incision was along the left side of the nose and across its base. A crossbow incision was then made along the brow, and the entire nose was turned to the right.

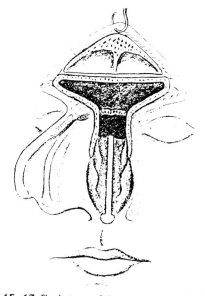

Figure 15–17. Final stage of dissection in von Eiselberg's approach. The nose had been turned to the right and the septum, turbinates, and ethmoid and sphenoid sinuses largely removed. Note that the frontal sinus also has been opened and partially resected, apparently to improve the light reaching down to the sella. The patients who survived had persistent foul odors from their noses due to atrophic rhinitis and were cosmetically disfigured.

epipharynx to prevent aspiration. In 1909, Kanaval[86] introduced an incision along the base of the nose to expose the nasal septum. The septum was resected, pulling the nose upward, and a portion of the middle turbinates was removed. The following year Halstead[87] used Kanaval's resection but placed the incision in a more cosmetically acceptable location, beneath the upper lip. Kanaval's report apparently also stimulated Kocher,[88] in Berne, Switzerland, who described a submucosal resection of the septum to reach the sphenoid (Fig. 15–18).

In 1910, utilizing the best features of the procedures of Stumme, Kanaval, Halstead and Kocher, Cushing[6] performed a submucosal nasal septal resection using an epipharyngeal tamponade, via a sublabial incision. The same year in Vienna, Hirsch[90] introduced an endonasal operation, performed either in two or three stages, that reached the sphenoid via a single nostril, resecting a portion of the septum en route (Fig. 15–19). He removed the intrasinus septum, and the sella was opened using chisels and rongeurs. Septal flaps were employed for repair of a CSF leak should it occur.[90]

Thus, in the brief span from 1907 to 1910, the basic operative steps of the trans-sphenoid approach had been established. However, the problems of meningitis and CSF leak made this procedure increasingly unpopular with surgeons. In the 1920s, Cushing's return to the transfrontal route strongly influenced the neurosurgical field. Hirsch,[91] fleeing Europe in the late 1930s, continued the transeptal approach in Boston for another quarter of a century. He reported 277 operated cases with a 5.4 per cent mortality and a 65 per cent success rate.

Advances in technology and the introduction of antibiotics fostered the return to extracranial pathways to the pituitary. In the 1960s, Guiot,[92] in Paris, introduced the image intensifier, providing accurate visualization of the placement of instruments in the intracranial cavity. Hardy and Wigser[93] brought this technique back to Montreal, adding microsurgical technique, and reported the unique safety and efficacy of the trans-sphenoid operation. This microsurgical technique has gained wide acceptance and is the operation being performed in large numbers throughout the world today.

Although the trans-septal route is generally favored, other approaches to the sphenoid may be useful. The transethmoid approach was first used by Chiari[94] in 1912 and later redescribed by Nager[95] in 1940 and by Bateman[96] and Kirchner and Van Guilder[97] in the 1970s. In 1963, Montgomery[98] combined a transethmoidosphenoid hypophysectomy with a septal mu-

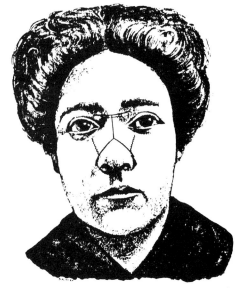

Figure 15–18. Illustration of Kocher's[88] transnasal, submucosal approach. The solid lines indicate skin incisions, which created two lateral flaps. The bone was then cut along the nasal and lacrimal bones *(wavy lines)*. The mucosa was lifted from the septum, which was then resected. Kocher introduced the submucosal septal removal and discarded the opening of the frontal sinus.

cosal flap closure. Angell-James[99] described a transethmoidosphenoid approach to the pituitary combined with an intranasal technique. This method allowed microscopic viewing via the ethmoid opening and instrumentation via the nose, without obscuring direct vision. It also provided a much shorter operating distance and a more direct approach to the sphenoid sinus; however, it left an external scar and approached the sphenoid off the midline, placing the lateral structures at greater risk to injury.

Denker[100] described a transantroethmoidosphenoid approach to the pituitary in 1921. This method was repopularized in 1961 by Hamberger.[101] It is a very useful approach if antral disease also needs surgical treatment and allows wide exposure without an external scar. However, it places the surgeon far from the midline, putting the lateral structures at risk, and is a difficult approach for use with the operating microscope.

The transpalatal approach was first employed for correction of choanal atresia by Brunk[102] in 1909. Preysing[103] in 1913 and Tiefenthal[104] in 1920 later described this approach for trans-sphenoid surgery and it was repopularized by Trible and Morse[105] in 1965. It has the advantages of being midline, not leaving an external scar, and providing a wide operative field. It has disadvantages: it interferes with a functional

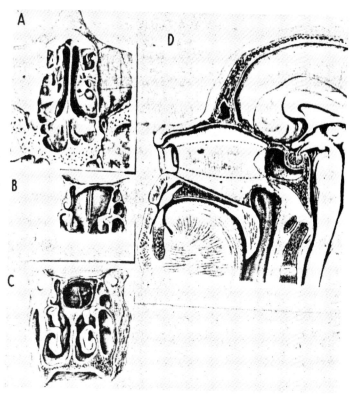

Figure 15–19. Hirsch's[90] trans-septal approach to the sella. Mucosal flaps were elevated *(A)*, the septum resected and the sphenoid entered *(B)*, and then the sella exposed *(C)*. This long tunnel (indicated by the dotted lines in *D*) was held open by a speculum. Initially Hirsch performed each step as a separate stage, but by 1911 he had combined them into a single procedure.

element (the soft palate), cannot be used in patients with trismus or macroglossia, and provides a difficult angle for the use of an operating microscope.

The transnasal approach to the sphenoid was popularized by Mosher[106] in 1912, as part of his work on the intranasal ethmoidectomy. It is an inadequate approach for pituitary surgery because it provides poor visualization.

A transnasal osteoplastic trans-sphenoid approach was described by MacBeth[107] in 1962. This approach is midline but creates an external scar. Tucker and Hahn[108] described an alar approach to trans-septal, trans-sphenoid pituitary surgery, but this also has the disadvantage of an external scar.

TECHNIQUE

The technique of trans-sphenoid surgery is deceptively simple; its increasing prominence in medicolegal situations underscores a high incidence of complications. Many of these complications appear to result from insufficient attention to such details as the proper positioning of the patient, identification of midline structures, and adequate intraoperative radiographic monitoring.

The patient is placed under general anesthesia in the supine position with the endotracheal tube at the left corner of the mouth. The head is slightly elevated and turned, so that the vertex points to the left. The head is also tilted to the left so that a right-handed surgeon can stand beside the operating table and operate in the sagittal plane without leaning on the patient's torso. The head is not ordinarily fixed in a locking device such as the Mayfield pin headholder; support with a foam rubber headrest is adequate. When the patient's head is positioned in front of a C-arm image intensifier, with the head perpendicular to the beam of the x-ray, the body is angled away from the surgeon. In many cases of significant suprasellar tumor extension, an intrathecal catheter is introduced in the lumbar region, with the tubing accessible to the anesthesiologist. During the initial positioning of the patient in front of the image intensifier, a small amount of air is injected into the intrathecal space and is observed to come over the top of the tumor (Fig. 15–20). This maneuver is repeated during the tumor removal portion of the procedure, as visualization of the upper surface of the tumor adds materially to the safe removal and completeness of suprasellar extensions of the lesion. The patient's thigh is then prepared and draped for the possible

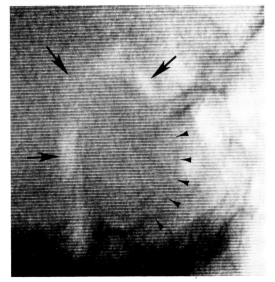

Figure 15–20. Lateral fluoroscopic view of a pituitary tumor as seen on an image intensifier during operation. Air has been injected via a lumbar intrathecal catheter and outlines the intracranial portion of a large pituitary tumor *(arrows)*. The thinned anterior and inferior surface of the sella *(arrowheads)* is outlined by air of the sphenoid sinus.

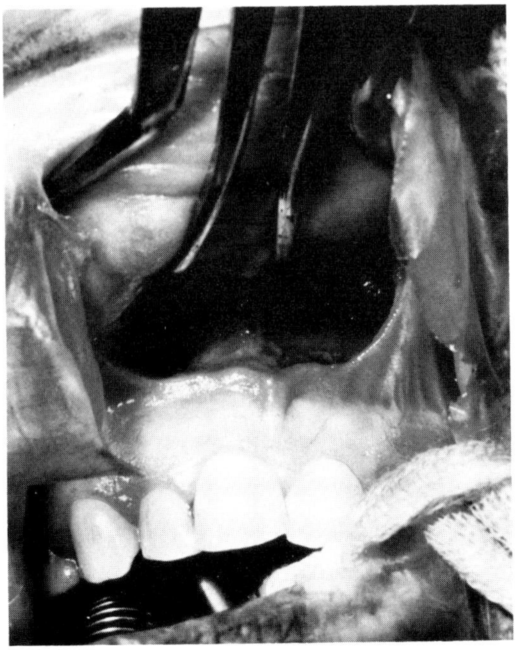

Figure 15–21. A sublabial incision performed with a retractor in place. The nasal spine is exposed.

removal of autograft muscle or fat, if required during the surgery.

The nasal mucosa can first be decongested with cotton pledgets saturated with 0.25 per cent Neosynephrine. This agent has been found to be the safest, as some patients with abnormal thyroid metabolism secondary to pituitary disease may be exquisitely sensitive to pressor agents or cocaine. The face, interstices of the nose, and sublabial area are next cleaned with betadine. The sublabial area is injected with 0.5 per cent lidocaine with 1:200,000 epinephrine (if the patient does not have thyroid abnormalities) from canine tooth to canine tooth and also intranasally along the nasal septum.

The field is next draped, with a hole in the sterile drape allowing access to the nose and sublabial area. A curvilinear incision is made several millimeters above the junction of the free and attached gingiva of the anterior maxillary teeth. This provides a cuff of gingiva for easy closure. The incision is carried through the periosteum to bone. An elevator is then used to sweep the mucoperiosteal flap superiorly, exposing the nasal spine, nasal floor, and piriform aperture bilaterally (Fig. 15–21). Bleeding is meticulously controlled by electrocoagulation, to allow for maximal visualization. An elevator is then used to raise mucoperiosteal flaps from the floor of the nose bilaterally. The

caudal end of the septum is exposed, and the right mucoperichondrial flap is elevated back to the bony septum. The fibers of the mucoperiosteum and mucoperichondrium that insert onto the maxillary crest are severed to allow elevation of the entire covering mucosa, giving wide exposure of the nasal septum (Figs. 15–22 and 15–23).

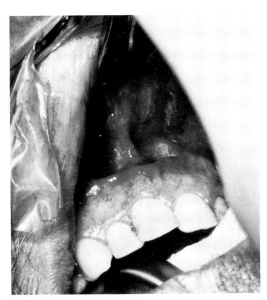

Figure 15–22. The caudal end of the septum exposed.

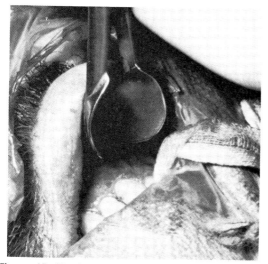

Figure 15–23. A speculum is in place, exposing the cartilaginous and bony septum.

If cartilage is desired for reconstruction of the sellar floor, a vertical incision is made through the septum 1 cm from its caudal edge. A left mucoperichondrial flap is then elevated posterior to the caudal strut, back to the bony septum. A Ballenger swivel knife is inserted to remove a portion of the cartilage, leaving an L-shaped strut for support of the external nose. The anterior septum is then displaced to the left, after separation of its attachments to the nasal spine. If a graft is not desired for repair, the entire cartilaginous septum is deflected toward the left side after being detached posteriorly from the perpendicular plate of the ethmoid and vomer.

In patients undergoing revision pituitary surgery, or those who have had a previous submucous resection, a transnasal approach may be preferable to a sublabial one. An alar incision will increase the access space for this procedure.

A long nasal speculum is then placed along the bony septum, and dissection of both mucosal flaps continues until the rostrum of the sphenoid is encountered. The bony septum is then removed with a rongeur, and the sphenoid and sinus ostia are exposed. A self-retaining speculum is positioned in the midline, and its location is confirmed by image intensification fluoroscopy (Figs. 15–24 and 15–25). Rongeurs are then used to remove the anterior wall of the sphenoid, giving wide access to the sella. The intrasinus septa are removed, leaving remnants for localization of the midline. The lining mucosa is carefully stripped from the posterior wall, and good hemostasis is achieved. The operating microscope is then brought into po-

sition (Fig. 15–26) either before or after the sphenoid is opened.

Note that when the tips of the speculum are opened to straddle the nasal septum, pressure from the superior turbinates and posterior ethmoid cells tends to displace them inferiorly. It is important that the speculum be repositioned within the sphenoid to allow adequate exposure of the anterior face of the sella. However, care should be taken not to place the speculum within the sphenoid, because a fracture to the base of the skull may ensue when opening the speculum. In addition, the midline landmark must be carefully demonstrated, usually marked by a crest of bone running from the rostrum of the sphenoid to the floor of the nose. Occasionally this landmark is not in the midline and its location should be verified by preoperative study of coronal sections of the CT scan.

The operating microscope is draped and an objective lens with a 300-mm focal length is placed. This provides an adequate working distance for the introduction and manipulation of instruments through the nasal speculum. In patients with significant suprasellar extension, additional air is injected through the intrathecal

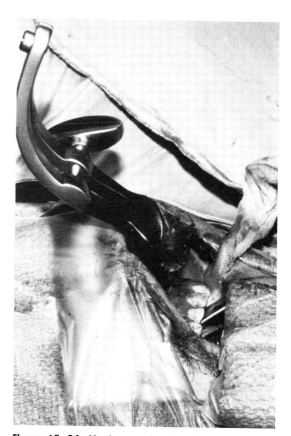

Figure 15–24. Hardy speculum in place, giving wide exposure of the sphenoid.

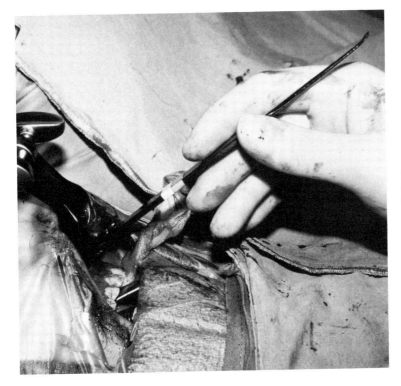

Figure 15–25. A Cottle elevator is used to remove the intrasinus septum and mucosa.

catheter at this time (Fig. 15–27). The amount of air introduced is small and may be given in 5-ml aliquots; 10 to 15 ml of air is usually sufficient. The image intensifier visualizes the inferior and superior limits of the anterior wall of the sella on lateral view.

The remaining sphenoid mucosa is generally removed to expose the bony sella. The floor of the sella is usually thin enough to be lifted off with a forceps or a small nerve hook. When the bone is thicker, it can be drilled away with a small diamond bur or removed with an osteo-tome and a small bone punch. Wide lateral bony exposure of the sella is advisable, with openings under 1 cm in transverse diameter suboptimal for adequate exploration. Bone is carefully removed superiorly to avoid damage to the circular sinus connecting the cavernous sinuses. In this region, dural adhesions to the tuberculum sella may rupture, producing sinus bleeding or a CSF leak.

When the sellar dura is exposed, a fine needle is inserted to aspirate the tumor trans-durally. This eliminates the possibility of either

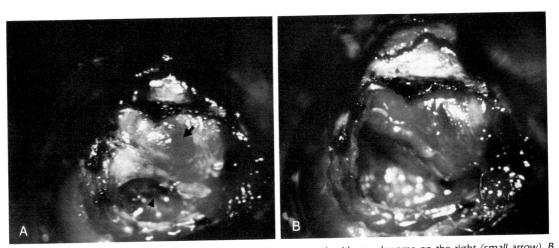

Figure 15–26. *A,* Operative view of the pituitary gland *(large arrow),* with an adenoma on the right *(small arrow). B,* The adenoma has been removed; a clean interface is seen.

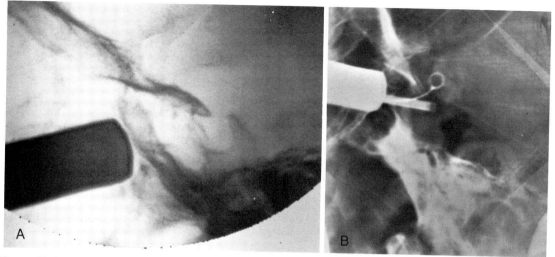

Figure 15–27. A, Intraoperative lateral fluoroscopic view of the speculum in place, directed toward the sella. B, Intraoperative lateral fluoroscopic view of the sellar region during trans-sphenoidal surgery. Air instilled through a spinal catheter can be seen outlining the superior and posterior portion of the tumor (arrow).

an intrasellar aneurysm or false localization with exposure of a cavernous sinus. The dura is then cauterized and opened with an X-incision or the excision of a rectangular window. Either an angled number 11 blade or a micro Beaver blade can be used to make this opening. The dural leaves are then cauterized, causing further dural retraction and preventing separation of the two dural layers. Preventing dural separation is extremely important, as dissection along this plane can lead to inadvertent entry into the cavernous sinus.

Most pituitary tumors are apparent on inspection of the anterior surface of the gland. Even if the tumor is within the substance of the anterior lobe, discoloration, softening, or bulging of the overlying pituitary parenchyma will reveal its presence. The tumor is entered; if it is cystic or soft, it is suctioned out, but it is usually soft and is curetted out. The plane around a typical microadenoma is usually defined. In most instances, this plane is easily found and the tumor shells out. It is usual for an experienced surgeon to differentiate adenoma from normal gland visually.

If there is significant suprasellar extension, the tumor is slowly excavated from the sella. Using the image intensifier, injected subarachnoid air above the sella will outline the dome of the tumor. The tumor is generally covered by thickened arachnoid and thinned remnants of the diaphragma sellae. As the tumor beneath it is removed, the dome of the tumor slowly descends (Fig. 15–28). Difficulty is encountered when the diaphragma sellae becomes redundant and collapses within the sella, with remnants of

the tumor obscured by the infolding of the diaphragm, and the arachnoid may be torn.

Removal of tumor laterally is often difficult, as the tumor may displace or invade the cavernous sinus. Care must be taken not to enter the cavernous sinus or damage the intracavern-

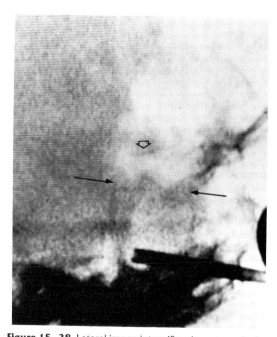

Figure 15–28. Lateral image intensifier view at conclusion of tumor removal, same case as Figure 15–20, with less magnification. The diaphragma sellae has returned to normal level (arrows), as outlined by intrathecal air above this level. Tumor has also been largely removed from within the sella itself. The outline of the pituitary stalk, descending to penetrate the diaphragma sellae, is outlined by air (open arrow).

ous nerves and vessels. Radiation therapy is usually needed for those tumors in which the dura is invaded, as an aggressive attack on the walls of the cavernous sinus is not warranted. Prolactinomas may be an exception.

If suprasellar extension of tumor either compresses the visual apparatus or obstructs the third ventricle, it is mandatory to decompress the tumor adequately. If the tumor is dense and fibrous and is not easily removed by suction or by curettage, it is necessary to bite away the adenoma with pituitary rongeurs of various shapes and sizes only within the sella. The suprasellar component would require a craniotomy for safe removal. Great care must be taken not to grasp the capsule or surrounding arachnoid because of the danger of tearing the arachnoid or damaging the surrounding neural and vascular structures.

It is often difficult to identify the normal pituitary gland in the course of removal of a larger tumor. With the microadenoma, a major portion of both the anterior and the posterior gland can be preserved. The diaphragma sellae and arachnoid are left intact to prevent a CSF leak. In patients in whom a CSF leak is seen during tumor removal, autograft fat or muscle and fascia lata are taken from the thigh to pack the sella to seal the leakage. This is also occasionally done when a very large sella might permit the prolapse of adjacent structures. If the leak is significant, a spinal drain is often left in for 2 to 4 days postoperatively to allow for sealing of the tear.

Following the removal of most functioning microadenomas, absolute alcohol is instilled into the tumor bed and aspirated after several minutes. Although there is limited tissue penetration by the absolute alcohol, it will fix the remaining functional tumor at the circumference of the tumor bed. It is imperative that meticulous hemostasis be achieved prior to closure; alcohol is very helpful with this. The floor of the sella is then closed with a piece of bone taken from the vomer during the exposure.

After closure of the sella, the speculum is removed and the nasal flaps and residual displaced septum are returned to the midline. Packing the nose with Merocel sponge around catheters allows the passage of air through the nose. The lip incision is closed with a 4-0 absorbable suture. A tip dressing is placed, and the general anesthetic is terminated.

A major advantage of the trans-sphenoid route is the benign postoperative course. Most patients are allowed fluids the afternoon following surgery and are out of bed and taking a soft diet the next day. The nasal packing is removed over a 2-day period. Postoperative evaluation includes a full endocrine profile and a CT or MRI scan of the pituitary to evaluate for residual tumor.

Although primarily we use the sublabial trans-septal, trans-sphenoid approach for pituitary surgery and exploration of lesions of the sphenoid, other approaches to the sphenoid may be best in some situations:

The transethmoid approach to the sphenoid is begun with a modified Lynch-type incision. The orbital periosteum is reflected, and the ethmoid and posterior ethmoid cells are removed back to the anterior face of the sphenoid using a rongeur. (See Chapter 11.) The sphenoid ostia are identified, and the anterior face is taken down as in the sublabial approach.[97]

The transantroethmoid approach is performed via a Caldwell-Luc approach (see Chapter 16). The medial wall of the antrum is removed to enter the ethmoid. The anterior and posterior ethmoid cells are opened and the septa removed, exposing the anterior face of the sphenoid (as in the transethmoid approach).[100]

The transpalatal approach is performed through a midline or U-shaped palatal flap. The mucosa is elevated, exposing the hard palate. The posterior edge of the hard palate is separated from its attachment to the soft palate. The greater palatine vessels are identified, and the posterior portion of the hard palate back to the edge of the foramina is carefully removed. This permits the neurovascular bundles to fall free posteriorly and allows additional retrodisplacement of the soft palate for wide exposure of the nasopharynx. A vertical incision is made over the posterior border of the septum along the vomer, and mucosal flaps are elevated from the face of the sphenoid. The vomer, the perpendicular plate of the ethmoid, and the sphenoid crest are removed to give exposure of the sphenoid. The anterior wall of the sphenoid is then opened, as in the previously described techniques.[105]

The trans-sphenoid approach has also been described for decompression of the optic nerve.[109] Donald[110] reported utilizing the transethmoid, trans-sphenoid approach for decompressing fractures that involve the planum sphenoidale portion of the anterior fossa floor, which encroach upon the optic nerve at the orbital apex. This surgery should be done as an emergency, as the blindness that follows trauma has a poor prognosis if not treated promptly.

RESULTS

Visual Defects. The most dramatic improvements following trans-sphenoid surgery often are seen in patients with visual defects. In the years prior to immunologic assay for functioning adenomas, the majority of patients who underwent pituitary surgery had a significant visual loss. However, the increased incidence of functioning microadenomas reported in most contemporary series has reduced the relative frequency. Long-standing visual deficits that have resulted in marked pallor of the optic disc due to atrophy will show a modest visual recovery. A larger number of patients will experience improvement postoperatively in cases with recent visual loss that lack optic atrophy. More than 70 per cent of the patients with visual deficits improve following trans-sphenoid decompression of the chiasm and visual apparatus.[111] Although some patients experience dramatic relief, in most the return of vision is gradual. Patients who have tumors with significant suprasellar extension generally undergo radiation therapy, with visual improvement occurring both during and after treatment.

A visual field loss following treatment used to be the major indicator of recurrence of a pituitary tumor. Because these tumors are often slow growing, a considerable following period is necessary adequately to evaluate this finding.[77] Several old series have indicated that the recurrence of visual symptoms following surgery and radiation therapy is 5 to 10 per cent.[112] Those tumors that compromise vision are the largest and most aggressive, consequently they carry a greater recurrence rate than the microadenomas. The patients are followed with serial scans, eye examinations, and endocrine testing, to diagnose a recurrence before it affects vision again.[112]

Acromegaly. Trans-sphenoid surgery for functioning microadenomas has provided dramatic improvement in the management of these endocrine disorders. Acromegaly is perhaps the most clear-cut of the hypersecreting pituitary endocrinopathies. The disease is always the result of a benign pituitary adenoma, and its effects are so debilitating and life-threatening that control of the tumor is virtually mandated.[113]

First described in 1886 by Marie, acromegaly is characterized by a hypersecretion of growth hormone (GH), enlargement of hands and feet, prognathism, thickened skin, galactorrhea, cardiac disease, abnormal carbohydrate metabolism, macroglossia, peripheral nerve entrapment, and arthralgias.[114, 115]

Because acromegaly causes a decreased life expectancy as well as significant disfigurement, early recognition and definitive therapy are important. The cardiovascular and cerebrovascular diseases caused by the associated arterial hypertension and diabetes, as well as the respiratory disease secondary to thoracic cage deformity, account for an increased morbidity and mortality.[16] When compared with the general population, there is a fivefold change for men and a twofold change for women in mortality rates.

Significant reduction of growth hormone levels in most acromegalies will cause some improvement of their acral overgrowth, fatigability, and weakness but not of most of the bony changes.

Surgery is considered the definitive treatment for growth hormone-secreting tumors. It offers the best chance for cure, with rates of cure varying from 44 to 99 per cent.[64, 117–119] Laws has shown a success rate of 87.5 per cent with microadenomas (less than 10 mm), versus only 68 per cent when the tumor has filled the sella or extended into the suprasellar cistern. In Wilson's series,[120] when trans-sphenoidal surgery was the first therapeutic intervention, there was a 94 per cent (96 of 102 patients) rate of remission, as judged by return of GH levels to normal. Sixteen of these ninety-six patients also had postoperative radiation therapy. The remaining 6 of 102 patients had partial remission, with GH levels falling to less than 50 per cent of preoperative values. The rate of response appeared related not only to the initial treatment modality but also to the grade and stage of the tumor. These studies suggest that, for patients who have not had previous therapy, trans-sphenoidal surgery should be the initial therapeutic modality.

The incidence of hypopituitarism is lower in the patient for whom trans-sphenoidal surgery was the first treatment modality (5 per cent), versus those who received postoperative irradiation (71 per cent) or pre-operative irradiation (66 per cent).[120] Surgical rates of success vary from 20 to 70 per cent and should be evaluated on an individual institutional basis. Long-term rates of recurrence are low if GH is normalized (less than 5 ng per ml) and dynamic testing is normal.[121]

Every effort should be made to treat acromegalics at the earliest possible phase of the disease, when selective removal of small microadenomas can be most readily accomplished.[64, 68, 113]

Cushing's Disease. Cushing's disease is characterized by pituitary ACTH-dependent hyperplasia of the adrenal cortices with hypercortisolism. Most patients have pituitary adenomas producing excess adrenocorticotropin. Hypothalamic pituitary adrenal function appears to be entirely normal once the effects of prolonged high amounts of ACTH and cortisol have worn off in all patients tested following selective adenoma resection.

Most of the clinical features of Cushing's disease are secondary to excessive secretion of glucocorticoids. Clinically, such patients present with central obesity, hypertension, hirsutism, easy bruisability, myopathies, diabetes mellitus, osteoporosis, and mental changes. It is considered an aggressive disease with a possible mortality of 50 per cent if left untreated for 5 years.

It is important that the origin of the Cushing's syndrome be delineated. Included in such a differentiation are (1) pituitary ACTH-dependent hyperplasia of the adrenals (Cushing's disease), (2) adrenal adenomas, or (3) ectopic ACTH secretion.

Surgical removal of the pituitary adenoma, when complete, can provide a cure. Surgical results clearly depend upon the experience of the surgical team, with success as high as 95 per cent, although this is not a uniform rate of success.[64, 122–124]

Mampalam[124] has described 216 cases of Cushing's disease treated with trans-sphenoidal microsurgical removal, resulting in an overall rate of cure of 76 per cent. In 166 patients with tumor confined to the sella, 86 per cent had the hypercortisolism corrected, with 15 requiring total hypophysectomy. With extrasellar extension, the rate is lower: 53 per cent. Hardy[123] reported an initial cure of 88 per cent in 59 patients with noninvasive tumors, whereas only one of four patients with an invasive tumor was cured. In our series, 87 per cent of patients have been cured surgically, with two requiring total hypophysectomy.

Such tumors are usually true microadenomas, and identification of tumor intraoperatively can be quite difficult. In fact, in 10 to 20 per cent of operated cases of Cushing's disease, negative explorations were reported. Such negative exploration may represent a small group in which the Cushing's disease is secondary to hypothalamic dysfunction. Usually, however, the negative exploration is because the microadenoma is not found or appreciated. Preoperative sampling of venous blood via retrograde catheterization of the inferior petrosal sinus may suggest the side of the tumor. ACTH level gradients between the peripheral blood and the sinus blood confirm the pituitary source, and a side-to-side gradient will allow the surgeon to perform a hemihypophysectomy rather than a complete hypophysectomy, to increase the success rate for curing the disease.[64, 125, 126]

Nelson's Syndrome. Patients in whom ACTH-secreting tumors become apparent following adrenalectomy for Cushing's disease are a particularly difficult group to handle therapeutically. In these patients, there is great difficulty in achieving normal ACTH levels following surgery; this is achieved only in approximately one fourth of the cases.[127] Most of the remaining patients have amelioration of the hyperpigmentation and other clinical signs of the syndrome, but the postoperative ACTH levels remain abnormal and they must undergo further treatment. The disappointing results seen in Nelson's syndrome, especially when contrasted with those in Cushing's disease, suggest that the former has a more aggressive tumor type.

Prolactin-Secreting Adenomas. Prolactin-secreting pituitary adenomas (prolactinomas) are the most common type of pituitary adenoma, comprising between 40 and 70 per cent in most series.[114] The clinical manifestations of prolactinomas are based on hyperprolactinemia and mass effect with large tumors. Hyperprolactinemia often produces menstrual dysfunction, including oligomenorrhea, primary or secondary amenorrhea, and galactorrhea. Menstrual cycle changes and galactorrhea in women appear more sensitive to mild hyperprolactinemia than do libido and potency changes in men. Prolactinomas in men are most often seen when they are very large, rarely in the microadenoma class. In women, the distribution is two thirds microadenomas with one third macroadenomas. Estrogen deficiency related to hyperprolactinemia may cause significant demineralization of bone.

The incidence of visual symptoms is much greater in men, consistent with the larger size of the tumors at the time of surgery. Numerous explanations have been proposed for this, including (1) psychologic barriers preclude admitting sexual impotence; (2) impotence is often interpreted as a psychologic phenomenon; (3) physicians are not as aware of the clinical entities in men as they are of those in women; and (4) hyperprolactinemia may have less influence on male physiology than it does on the female menstrual cycle.

Prolactin levels below 150 ng per ml may be secondary to stalk compression from other lesions. In men whose basal PRL values exceed 100 ng per ml, a prolactinoma is usually the cause of hyperprolactinemia. In women, hyperprolactinemia with basal values greater than 200 ng per ml almost invariably indicates a prolactinoma. There is controversy over the indications for surgical management of these tumors, with only slight evidence that hyperprolactinemia alone is a disease entity. Certainly its general systemic effects are minimal.

Many of the hypersecreting prolactinomas are the very largest tumors seen in the pituitary region. The indications for surgery in this group are identical with those of nonfunctioning adenomas and include mass effect, visual loss and headache.[68] At our institution, macroadenomas are pretreated with bromocriptine in the hope that shrinking the tumor will increase surgical success. Bromocriptine is not considered a primary modality of therapy for the macroadenoma. We currently use 7.5 mg per day and repeat the prolactin levels. If prolactin is significantly decreased or normalized, medication is continued and a CT scan is done after 4 weeks. If tumor shrinkage is demonstrated, the medication is continued for 3 months, at which time elective trans-sphenoidal resection is performed. If prolactin is not significantly altered or there is no shrinkage, surgical intervention is not delayed. In addition, if there is serious visual loss, bromocriptine may be initiated; if there is no rapid improvement in neurologic function we switch to surgical intervention. The cure rate from surgery for these large tumors is low, and other modalities such as continued bromocriptine or radiation therapy are often necessary.

The indications for surgery for hypersecreting microadenomas are related largely to amenorrhea or galactorrhea syndromes, when fertility is desired. Intractable copious spontaneous galactorrhea may be so embarrassing to the patient that it warrants operative intervention.

The results in the women studied show a 71 per cent cure rate for all, whereas an 85 per cent cure rate can be demonstrated for all the microadenoma subgroup. When the group is restricted to those with preoperative prolactin levels of less than 200 ng per ml, the overall cure rate is increased to 85 per cent, while that for the microadenoma group is increased to 89 per cent. The interval between surgery and return of menses is from 10 days to 3 months; the average time is about 1 month. The cessation of galactorrhea is more difficult to determine. Normal menses and fertility may be restored even when postoperative prolactin values remain slightly or moderately elevated. However, bromocriptine remains an excellent alternative. The success rate of normalizing prolactin and restoring menses is high. If preg-

nancy is achieved with bromocriptine therapy, the risk of significant tumor enlargement during pregnancy is low.[127] The controversy continues over the use of bromocriptine and the operative indications for this tumor.

COMPLICATIONS OF TRANS-SPHENOIDAL SURGERY

Complications are related to the nasal and neurologic portions of the procedure. The nasal complications are largely cosmetic and include saddle noses and tip deformities.[68] Fenestration of the septum, hemorrhage, infection, and CSF leak have all been reported.

The most serious problems following transsphenoid surgery are those related to damage of surrounding vascular structures. The carotid artery may be traumatized and undergo severe postoperative spasm, or it may be lacerated at the time of surgery. The cavernous sinus and its contents also serve as a source of complications. Venous hemorrhage may occur from it or from the circular sinuses. If the head is significantly elevated when the sinus is opened, air embolism may occur. The nerves that run within the cavernous sinus, including the third, fourth, fifth, and sixth cranial nerves, have all been reported to develop palsies following surgery. Intracranial complications include trauma to the optic chiasm, either directly or from pressure by a muscle plug. Late complications involving the visual apparatus can be caused by prolapse of the optic chiasm into the decompressed sella. Direct trauma to the hypothalamus, resulting in hyperthermia, memory loss, or altered mentation, also have been reported. CSF leak is not uncommon and occasionally can lead to meningitis; therefore, it must be treated vigorously when first observed.

Those cases in which an unexplained postoperative complication occurs require immediate intervention. CT scanning often will reveal the cause, especially hemorrhage. In patients with a CSF leak, occasionally antibiotic coverage alone has been effective, but they usually require a further operative procedure for repair.

References

1. Van Alyea OE: In discussion of operation for the sphenoid sinus by Arthur W. Proetz. Trans Am Acad Ophthalmol Otolaryngol 53:38, 1949.
2. Sluder G: Some anatomical and clinical relations of the sphenoid sinus to the cavernous sinus and the third, fourth, fifth, sixth and vidian nerves. Trans Am Laryngol Assoc 34:46, 1912.
3. Protez AW: The sphenoid sinus. Br Med J 2:243, 1948.

4. Van Alyea OE: Sphenoid sinus: Anatomic study, with consideration of the clinical significance of the structural characteristics of the sphenoid sinus. Arch Otol 34:225, 1941.
5. Maxwell JH, Hill BJ: The diagnosis of chronic inflammatory lesions at the sphenoid sinus. Ann Otol 68:411, 1959.
6. Levine E: The sphenoid sinus—The neglected nasal sinus. Arch Otol 104:585, 1978.
7. Wyllie JW, Kern EB, Djalilian M: Isolated sphenoid lesions. Laryngoscope 83:1252, 1973.
8. Hajek M: Pathology and Treatment of the Inflammatory Diseases of the Nasal Accessory Sinuses. St. Louis, CV Mosby Company, 1926.
9. MacRae D, Lampe H: Use of computer assisted tomography in the diagnosis of lesions in and around the sphenoid sinus. J Otolaryngol 9:412, 1980.
10. Gustafson RO, Kern EB: Office endoscopy—when, why, what, and how. Otolaryngol Clin North Am ·22:683, 1989.
11. MacDonald G: A Treatise on Diseases of the Nose and Its Accessory Cavities. London, McMillan and Co, 1892.
12. Teed RW: Meningitis from the sphenoid sinus. Arch Otol 28:589, 1938.
13. Lew D, Southwich FS, Montgomery WW, et al: Sphenoid sinusitis: A review of 30 cases. N Engl J Med 309:1149, 1983.
14. Pearlman SJ, Lawson W, Biller HF, Friedman WH, Potter GD: Isolated sphenoid sinus disease. Laryngoscope 99:716, 1989.
15. Baldwin RL, Bragg L: Sphenoid sinusitis: The importance of CT scanning. Alabama Med 57:35, 1988.
16. Ridpath RF: The sphenoid sinus. Laryngoscope 44:657, 1934.
17. Urquhart AC, Fung G, McIntosh WA: Isolated sphenoiditis: A diagnostic problem. J Laryngol Otol 103:526, 1989.
18. Mizoguchi K, Jojimam H, Tanaka M, Hotta M, Yano H, Toyomasu T, Shoji H, Kaji M, Kondo M: Sphenoid sinusitis associated with meningitis, visual disturbances and total ophthalmoplegia. Kurume Med J 35:211, 1988.
19. Miglets AW, Saunders WH, Ayers L: Aspergillosis of the sphenoid sinus. Arch Otol 104:47, 1978.
20. Blitzer A, Lawson W: Mycotic infections of the nose and paranasal sinus. In English GM (ed): Otolaryngology. Vol 2. Philadelphia, Harper & Row, 1982.
21. Larranaga J, Fandino J, Gomez-Bueno J, Rodriguez D, Gonzales-Carrero J, Botana C: Aspergillosis of the sphenoid sinus simulating a pituitary tumor. Neuroradiology 31:362, 1989.
22. Sofferman RA: Cavernous sinus thrombophlebitis secondary to sphenoid sinusitis. Laryngoscope 93:797, 1983.
23. Kibblewhite DJ, Cleland J, Mintz DR: Acute sphenoid sinusitis: Management strategies. J Otolaryngol 17:159, 1988.
24. Coakley CG: A Manual of Diseases of the Nose and Throat. New York, Lea Bros & Co, 1905.
25. Zalin H: On the complications of sphenoiditis. J Laryngol Otol 78:727, 1964.
26. Tremble GE: Irrigation of the sphenoid sinus: A simple and safe method. Ann Otol Rhinol Laryngol 79:840, 1970.
27. Montgomery W: Surgical treatment of sinus infections. In Ballenger JJ (ed): Diseases of the Nose, Throat, and Ear. Philadelphia, Lea and Febiger, 1977.
28. Skillern RH: The Accessory Sinuses of the Nose. Philadelphia, JB Lippincott, 1923.
29. Krueger TP, McFarland J, Ommaya AK: Pyocele of the sphenoid sinus. J Neurosurg 22:616, 1965.
30. Nelson DA, Kara-Eneff SC: Neurological syndromes produced by sphenoid sinus abscess. Neurology 17:981, 1967.
31. Teed RW: Meningitis from the sphenoid sinus. Arch Otol 28:589, 1938.
32. Macdonald RL, Findlay JM, Tator CH: Sphenoethmoidal sinusitis complicated by cavernous sinus thrombosis and pontocerebellar infarction. Can J Neurol Sci 15:310, 1988.
33. Gatti WN, Cronin JJ: Ossifying fibroma of the sphenoid sinus. Eye Ear Nose Throat Mon 54:60, 1975.
34. Weaver RG, Gates GA: Mucoceles of the sphenoid sinus. Otolaryngol Head Neck Surg 87:168, 1979.
35. Blum ME, Larson A: Mucocele of the sphenoid sinus with sudden blindness. Laryngoscope 83:2042, 1973.
36. Maisel RH, El Deeb M, Bone RC: Sphenoid sinus mucoceles. Laryngoscope 83:930, 1973.
37. Stankiewicz JA: Sphenoid sinus mucocele. Arch Otolaryngol Head Neck Surg 115:735, 1989.
38. Lundgren A, Olin T: Mucopyocele of sphenoid sinus or posterior ethmoidal cells with special reference to apex orbital syndrome. Acta Otolaryngol 53:61, 1961.
39. Simon M, Tingwald F: Syndrome associated with mucocele of the sphenoid sinus: Report of 2 cases and their radiographic findings. Radiology 64:538, 1955.
40. Meisels EL: Mukozele der Keilbenhohle. Fortschr Rontgenstr 34:905, 1926.
41. Jino GS, Goepfert H, Close L: CT of paranasal sinus neoplasm. Laryngoscope 88:1485, 1978.
42. Schaefer SD: Endoscopic total sphenoethmoidectomy. Otolaryngol Clin North Am 22:727, 1989.
43. Rice DH, Schaefer SD: Endoscopic Paranasal Sinus Surgery. New York, Raven Press, 1988.
44. Wigand ME: Endoscopic Surgery of the Paranasal Sinuses and Anterior Skull Base. New York, Thieme Medical Publishing, 1990.
45. McElveen JT, Fee WE: Inverting papilloma of the sphenoid sinus. Otolaryngol Head Neck Surg 89:710, 1981.
46. Edison BD: Primary inverting papilloma of the sphenoid sinus. Trans Am Acad Ophthalmol Otolaryngol 80:434, 1975.
47. DeBartolo HM, Vrabec D: Sphenoid encephalocele. Arch Otolaryngol 103:172, 1977.
48. Danoff D, Serbu J, French LA: Encephalocele extending into the sphenoid sinus. J Neurosurg 22:684, 1965.
49. Malcomson KG: Ossifying fibroma of the sphenoid. J Laryngol Otol 81:87, 1967.
50. Townsend GL, DeSanto LW: Malignant change in sphenoid sinus fibrous dysplasia. Arch Otol 92:267, 1970.
51. Calcaterra TC, Rich R, Ward PW: Neurilemmoma of the sphenoid sinus. Arch Otolaryngol 100:383, 1974.
52. Emley WE: Giant cell tumor of the sphenoid bone. Arch Otol 94:369, 1971.
53. Delorit GJ, Summers GW: Aneurysmal bone cyst of the sphenoid sinus. Trans Am Acad Ophthalmol Otolaryngol 80:438, 1975.
54. Alexander FW: Primary tumors at the sphenoid sinus. Laryngoscope 73:537, 1963.
55. Gibson W: Sphenoid sinus revisited. Laryngoscope 94:185, 1984.
56. Hayden RE, Luna M, Goepfert H: Hemangiomas of the sphenoid sinus. Otolaryngol Head Neck Surg 88:136, 1980.
57. Kimmelman CP: Hemangiopericytoma of the sphenoid sinus. Otolaryngol Head Neck Surg 89:713, 1981.

58. Bateman GH: Destruction of the pituitary in cases of carcinomatosis secondary to mammary carcinoma. J Laryngol 73:631, 1959.

59. Barrs DM, McDonald TJ, Whisnant JP: Metastatic tumors to the sphenoid sinus. Laryngoscope 89:1239, 1979.

60. Van Wart CA, Dado HH, McCoy EG: Carcinoma of the sphenoid sinus. Ann Otol 82:318, 1973.

61. Nichols RD, Fujita S, Muzaffar K, Olson NR: Destructive lesions of the sphenoid sinus. Trans Am Acad Ophthalmol Otolaryngol 78:359, 1974.

62. McCarthy DP, Gold L: Tumor stain in primary sphenoid sinus carcinoma. Arch Otol 101:512, 1975.

63. Sisson GA, Becker SP: Cancer of the nasal cavity and paranasal sinus. In Suen JA, Myers EN (eds): Cancer of the Head and Neck. New York, Churchill Livingston, 1981.

64. Post KD, Muraszko K: Management of pituitary tumors. Neurol Clin 4:801, 1986.

65. Onesti ST, Wisniewski T, Post KD: Clinical versus subclinical pituitary apoplexy: Presentation, surgical management, and outcome in 21 patients. Neurosurgery 26:980, 1990.

66. Cushing H: The Pituitary Body and Its Disorders: Clinical States Produced by Disorders of the Hypophysis Cerebri. Philadelphia, JB Lippincott, 1912.

67. Landolt AM, Wilson CB: Tumors of the sella and para area in adults. In Youmans JR (ed): Neurological Surgery. 2nd ed. Philadelphia, WB Saunders Co, 1980.

68. Laws ER Jr, Randall RV, Kern EB, Abboud CF: Management of pituitary adenomas and related lesions and emphasis on transsphenoidal microsurgery. New York, Appleton-Century-Crofts, 1982.

69. Kovacs K, Horvath E: Morphology of adenohypophyseal cells and pituitary adenomas. In Imura H (ed): The Pituitary Gland. New York, Raven Press, 1985, pp 25–55.

70. Sung DI, Chang CH, Harisiadis L, Carmel PW: Treatment results of craniopharyngiomas. Cancer 47:847, 1981.

71. Carmel PW, Antunes JL, Chang CH: Craniopharyngiomas in children. Neurosurgery 11:382, 1982.

72. Naidich TP, Pinto RS, Kushner BA, et al: Evaluation of sellar and parasellar masses by computed tomography. Radiology 120:91, 1976.

73. Powell DF, Baker HL Jr, Laws ER Jr: The primary angiographic findings in pituitary adenomas. Radiology 110:589, 1974.

74. Wilson CB, Dempsey LC: Transsphenoidal microsurgical removal of 250 pituitary adenomas. J Neurosurg 48:13, 1978.

75. Lee KJ: The sublabial transseptal transsphenoidal approach to the hypophysis. Laryngoscope 88 (Suppl 10):1, 1978.

76. Montgomery NW: Surgery of the sphenoid sinus. In Montgomery WW (ed): Surgery of the Upper Respiratory Systems. Vol 1. Philadelphia, Lea & Febiger, 1971.

77. Krause F: Hirnchiragie (Freilegung der Hypophyse). Deutsch Klin 8:1004, 1905.

78. Horsley V: On the technique of operations on the central nervous system. Br Med J 2:411, 1905.

79. Halstead AE: Remarks on the operative treatment of tumors of the hypophysis. SGO 10:494, 1910.

80. Schloffer H: Erfolgreiche operatione eines hyophysentumors auf nasalem Wege. Wien Klin Wochenschr 20:621, 1907.

81. Schloffer H: Weiterer Bericht über den Fall von operiertem Hypophysentumor (Plotzlicher Exitus letalis 2½ Monate nach der Operation). Wien Klin Wochenschr 20:1075, 1907.

82. von Eiselberg AF: My experience about operation upon the hypophysis. Trans Am Surg Assoc 28:55, 1910.

83. Plum F, Van Uitert R: Nonendocrine diseases and disorders of the hypothalamus. In Reichlin S (ed): The Hypothalamus. New York, Raven Press, 1978.

84. Reichlin S: Overview of the anatomical and physiologic basis of anterior-pituitary regulation. In Martin JB, Reichlin S, Brown FA (eds): Clinical Neuroendocrinology. Philadelphia, FA Davis, 1977.

85. Stumme E: Akromegalie und hypophyse. Arch Klin Chir 87:437, 1908.

86. Kanaval AB: The removal of tumors of the pituitary body by an infranasal route. JAMA 53:1704, 1909.

87. Halstead AE: Remarks on the operative treatment of tumors of the hypophysis: With the report of two cases operated on by an oronasal method. Trans Am Surg Assoc 28:73, 1910.

88. Kocher T: Ein Fall von Hypophysis-Tumor mit operativer Heilung. Dtsch Z Chir 100:13, 1909.

89. Cushing H: The Weir Mitchell Lecture: Surgical experience with pituitary disorders. JAMA 63:1515, 1914.

90. Hirsch O: Eine neuen Methode der endonasalen Operation von Hypophysen-tumoren. Wien Med Wochenschr 59:636, 1909.

91. Hirsch O: Symptoms and treatment of pituitary tumors. Arch Otolaryngol 55:268, 1952.

92. Guiot G: Transsphenoidal approach in surgical treatment of pituitary adenomas; General principles, and indications in nonfunctioning adenomas. Excerpta Medica International Congress Series 303:159, 1973.

93. Hardy J, Wigser SM: Transsphenoidal surgery of pituitary fossa tumors with televised radiofluoroscopic control. J Neurosurg 23:612, 1965.

94. Chiari O': Uber eine Modification der Schloffer's chen Operation von Tumoren der Hypophyse. Wien Klin Wochenschr 25:5, 1912.

95. Nager FR: Paranasal approach to intrasellar tumors. J Laryngol 55:361, 1940.

96. Bateman GH: Transsphenoidal hypophysectomy. Otolaryngol Clin North Am 4:205, 1971.

97. Kirchner JA, Van Guilder JC: Transethmoidal hypophysectomy. Trans Am Acad Ophthalmol Otolaryngol 80:391, 1975.

98. Montgomery WS: CSF rhinorrhea. Otolaryngol Clin North Am 6:757, 1973.

99. Angell-James J: Transethmoidal hypophysectomy. Arch Otol 86:32, 1967.

100. Denker A: Drei Fülle operiert nach transmaxillarer Method. Int Zentralbl Laryngol 37:225, 1921.

101. Hamberger CA: Transantrosphenoidal hypophysectomy. Arch Otol 74:2, 1961.

102. Brunk A: A new case of unilateral osseous choanal occlusion; An operation through the palate. Ztischr Ohret 59:221, 1909.

103. Preysing D: Beitrage zur Operation der Hypophyse. Verhandl Deutsch Laryng 20:51, 1913.

104. Tiefenthal A: Technik der Hypophysenoperation. Munch Med Wochenschr 67:794, 1920.

105. Trible WM, Morse AE: Transpalatal hypophysectomy. Laryngoscope 75:1116, 1965.

106. Mosher HP: The applied anatomy and intranasal surgery of the ethmoid labyrinth. Trans Am Laryngol Soc 34:25, 1912.

107. MacBeth RG: An approach to the pituitary via a nasal osteoplastic flap. J Laryngol 75:70, 1962.

108. Tucker HM, Hahn JF: Transnasal, transseptal sphe-

noidal approach to hypophysectomy. Laryngoscope 92:55, 1982.

109. Fukado Y: Results in 350 cases of surgical decompression of the optic nerve. Trans Asia Pac Acad Ophthalmol 4:96, 1972.

110. Donald PJ: Recent advances in paranasal sinus surgery. Head Neck Surg 4:146, 1981.

111. Laws ER Jr, Trautmann JC, Hollenhorst RW Jr: Transsphenoidal decompression of the optic nerve and chiasm: Visual results in 62 patients. J Neurosurg 46:717, 1977.

112. Svien HJ, Love JG, Kennedy WC, et al: Status of vision following surgical treatment for pituitary chromophobe adenoma. J Neurosurg 22:47, 1965.

113. U HS, Wilson CB, Tyrell JB: Transsphenoidal microhypophysectomy in acromegaly. J Neurosurg 47:840, 1977.

114. Barrow DL, Tindall GT: Acromegaly. Contemp Neurosurg 7:1, 1985.

115. Lie JT, Grossman SJ: Pathology of the heart in acromegaly: Anatomic findings in 27 autopsied patients. Am Heart J 100:41, 1980.

116. Wright AD, Hill DM, Lowy C, et al: Mortality in acromegaly. Q J Med 9:1, 1970.

117. Laws ER, Piepgras DG, Randall RV, et al: Neurosurgical management of acromegaly: Results in 82 patients treated between 1972–1977. J Neurosurg 50:454, 1979.

118. Hardy J, Somma M: Acromegaly: Surgical treatment by transsphenoidal microsurgical removal of the pituitary adenoma. *In* Tindall GT, Collins WF (eds): Clinical Management of Pituitary Disorders. New York, Raven Press, 1979, pp 209–217.

119. Baskin DS, Boggan JE, Wilson CB: Transsphenoidal microsurgical removal of growth hormone–secreting pituitary adenomas: A review of 137 cases. J Neurosurg 56:634, 1982.

120. Wilson CB: Transsphenoidal surgery for pituitary adenomas. Anesthesiol Rev 7:49, 1985.

121. Serri O, Somma M, Comotois R, et al: Acromegaly: Biochemical assessment of cure after long-term followup of transsphenoidal selective adenomectomy. J Clin Endocrinol Metab 61:1185, 1985.

122. Boggan JE, Tyrell JB, Wilson CB: Transsphenoidal microsurgical management of Cushing's disease: Report of 100 cases. J Neurosurg 59:195, 1983.

123. Hardy J: Cushing's disease: 50 years later. Can J Neurosci 9:375, 1980.

124. Mampalam TJ, Tyrrell JB, Wilson CB: Transsphenoidal microsurgery for Cushing disease—a report of 216 cases. Ann Intern Med 109:487, 1988.

125. Oldfield EH, Chrousos GP, Schulte HM, et al: Preoperative lateralization of ACTH-secreting microadenomas by bilateral and simultaneous inferior petrosal sinus sampling. N Engl J Med 312:100, 1985.

126. Abboud CF, Laws ER: Clinical endocrinological approach to hypothalamo-pituitary disease. J Neurosurg 51:271, 1979.

127. Molitch ME: Pregnancy and the hyperprolactinemic woman. N Engl J Med 312:1364, 1985.

CHAPTER 16

SURGERY FOR INFECTION AND BENIGN DISEASE OF THE MAXILLARY SINUS

Andrew Blitzer, MD, DDS

In the normal state, the maxillary antrum is an air-containing cavity lined with ciliated respiratory epithelium. In 1876, Bowditch of Harvard demonstrated the sweeping action of the ciliated membrane. In 1885, St. Clair Thompson and Hewlett showed that the sinuses were relatively bacteria free because of the propulsive action of these cilia. The cilia beat and move the mucous blanket in a spiral fashion toward the ostium and normally can clear the sinus in approximately 10 minutes.[1] Many factors influence the flow of the mucous blanket, including the intra-antral and intranasal pressure.[2] In 1937, McMurray demonstrated that if both maxillary antra were filled with Lipiodol and one nostril was blocked, 5 hours were needed to clear the antrum on the normal side, with complete failure of emptying observed on the blocked side. He concluded that the negative pressure generated in the nose on inspiration was necessary for the evacuation of material in the sinus. This factor is probably responsible for the chronic sinus disease observed in patients with anatomic or allergic nasal obstruction.[3]

The mucociliary blanket is produced by the goblet cells in the sinus mucosa and is composed of approximately 96 per cent water, 1 to 2 per cent inorganic salts and 2 to 3 per cent mucin. The secretions may vary from thin and watery to viscous and elastic. These variations are due to small changes in the mucous content. The blanket is composed of two layers: a viscous, mucinous outer layer and a serous inner layer,

which is in contact with the ciliary apparatus. The stickiness and electrostatic charge of the viscous layer filters microparticles by inducing adhesion to the surface. The mucous blanket also contains lysozyme, which inactivates most organisms in contact with the surface.[1]

This system functions well unless the mucous blanket or the cilia are altered or damaged. Excessive drying or dehydration, upper respiratory tract infections, chemical irritation, scarring, or trauma can damage the mucociliary apparatus severely. Edema and obstruction secondary to foreign bodies, packing, nasotracheal tubes, vasomotor or allergic rhinitis, rhinitis medicamentosa, or polyps can slow or paralyze the mucociliary blanket and therefore predispose the sinus to infection. Once the apparatus has failed, an overgrowth of bacteria occurs. The infectious organisms most commonly isolated in the nonimmunocompromised host are pneumococcus, staphylococcus, and *Haemophilus influenzae*. These bacteria produce vasodilation, edema, increased mucous production, and polymorphonuclear cell infiltration within the mucosa. Clinically, a dull aching to severely throbbing pain is felt in the cheek, teeth, and eyes. There is usually an accompanying profuse nasal discharge with a foul smell or taste. Occasionally, there will be otalgia or otitis media. The pain is intensified by increasing the venous pressure by bending or the Valsalva maneuver. In chronic infections, monocytic infiltration, fibrosis, squamous metaplasia of the antral mucosa, and an increased number of goblet cells are observed histologically. There also may be an osteoblastic response in the surrounding bone.[3]

Maxillary sinusitis often can be diagnosed by history and physical examination. In the preradiographic era, clinical evaluation was of paramount importance. The nose was carefully inspected to detect purulence near or emanating from the ostium. If purulent secretions were not observed, sounding was performed. A silver probe was passed into the meatus to determine whether pus would be released on its removal. The depth of the sinus, thickness of the sinus walls, or presence of intra-antral masses could be ascertained by the experienced examiner. The patient was also examined for hypertrophy of the midline meatus, swelling and sensitivity of the cheek, dilation of the bony walls, and change of shape or swelling of the alveolar process.[4]

Several methods were devised to determine the presence of purulent secretions within the antrum. The Politzer apparatus and glass tube and the rubber ball apparatus of Sondermann elicited pus at the sinus ostium by causing a negative pressure in the nasal cavity when the soft palate was elevated by swallowing.[4]

Glas introduced a tuning fork test for the detection of maxillary sinus obstruction. A tuning fork held at the root of the nose was supposed to lateralize to the diseased side in the patient with unilateral involvement; however, the test was generally found to be unreliable. Another unusual test, advocated by Kahone, was based on galvanic palpation. He proposed that the skin overlying an inflamed part would show increased redness and sensitivity to galvanic stimulation when compared with the noninflamed side. This was also found to be unreliable.[4]

With the advent of the incandescent light bulb, transillumination of the maxillary sinus was possible. The light was placed within the mouth or was directed through the cheek to detect sinus opacification. This method demonstrated the presence of opacification but could not differentiate fluid from solid areas. It is still applicable.[5]

With radiography, the diagnosis and evaluation of antral disease became much less speculative. The sophistication of present radiographic techniques, computed tomography, and magnetic resonance imaging provides precise diagnostic information (see Chapter 2).

Today, the patient's history, physical examination (including rhinoscopy and possible sinoscopy), radiographs, CT and MRI scans, smears and cultures of secretions, and biopsies when necessary allow for rapid and accurate diagnosis. Treatment planning should consider the host status, anatomic and functional factors, and the nature and virulence of the offending organisms.[6]

TREATMENT

In most cases, conservative therapy is the treatment of choice. This consists of antibiotic therapy for 10 to 14 days, accompanied by local and systemic decongestant agents. If medical therapy fails, or if a specimen for culture is needed, antral irrigation should be performed. In the immunocompromised host, patients with anatomic obstruction, or those infected by a virulent organism, surgery may be necessary at an earlier time.[7]

ANTRAL IRRIGATION

Failure of a sinus infection to clear with conservative methods implies damage to the mucociliary blanket or obstruction of the ostium, which produces puddling of undrained mucopus within the antrum. In these refractory cases, irrigation of the sinus will remove retained products of the infection, such as necrotic tissue, nonviable and viable organisms and their toxins, and cellular debris.[8] In 1885, Hartmann performed the first antral irrigation via the membranous portion of the middle meatus. Oil was injected to displace the secretions from the sinus floor.[9]

After sinus irrigation, a regeneration of functional cilia generally occurs within 2 weeks, to sweep the cavity clean of any residual debris. With chronic sinus disease, irrigation should be performed early, because of the presence of scarring and avascular areas.[8]

TECHNIQUE

Anesthesia is obtained by the application of topical 4 per cent cocaine solution on cotton pledgets, followed by mucosal infiltration with a local anesthetic solution. A curved cannula (sharp or blunt) is inserted upward, midway in the middle meatus. The cannula tip is rotated laterally and then pulled forward to engage the natural ostium. Once in the ostium, the catheter tip should point downward, anteriorly and laterally; however, it is not always possible to cannulate the natural ostium.[4, 8–12] In a study of 114 skulls, Myerson found 14 in which there was a high obstructing wall of the uncinate process and 15 in which the probe could not find the ostium. He predicted that cannulation could be successfully accomplished in about 80 per cent of patients.[13, 14] Van Alyea also stated that about 20 per cent of subjects could not be cannulated because of anatomic variations but that cannulation could be performed in the remaining 80 per cent with minimal trauma. Prolonged probing would lead to local trauma, offsetting the benefits of irrigation.[9] However, Mosher contended that it was difficult if not impossible to cannulate the natural ostium and recommended the puncture technique.[15]

The advantages of the natural ostium technique are (1) absence of injury to the natural structures or bone and (2) there is no tendency to spread infection. The major disadvantage is the difficulty in finding the ostium in some cases.

The direct puncture technique may be performed because of failure of the natural ostium technique or individual preference. Anesthesia is similarly obtained with topical and local agents. A straight trocar is positioned in the central part of the meatus just beneath the inferior turbinate, approximately 1.5 to 2 cm behind its anterior attachment. The tip is aimed midway between the ear lobe and the lateral canthus of the eye. The cannula is then gently advanced and twisted to enter the sinus easily. If there is resistance, the trocar should be removed and repositioned. The obturator is then removed and aspiration performed to avoid injecting a vessel. If blood is aspirated, the cannula is repositioned.[4, 8, 10, 11]

When the cannula is in proper position, the patient is asked to lean forward, a bowl is placed under the chin and instructions are given to breathe through the mouth. Warm saline is then injected slowly, washing the infected material from the sinus. This should be continued until a clear return is obtained.[4]

An antibiotic solution should not be instilled, as it is of no therapeutic value and may produce allergic sensitization of the patient. Goode recommended the temporary placement of an 18-gauge polyethylene cannula for up to 3 weeks to allow irrigation without repeated puncture.[16]

Air should never be injected into the sinus; many fatalities from air emboli have been reported. In 1923, Bacher described the autopsy findings in a patient who died of an air embolism. He cited two other cases from the literature and suggested first aspirating and then injecting saline to avoid this catastrophe.[17] Other complications of irrigation include infiltration or emphysema of the cheek, blindness or proptosis from fluid or air injected into the orbit, and bacteremia with sepsis.

An alternative technique of irrigation is via puncture of the anterior wall of the maxillary sinus through the canine fossa. This method was first reported by Heath in 1889. After topical and infiltrative anesthesia is achieved, the trocar is inserted through the areolar gingiva overlying the canine fossa. The trocar should be positioned above the roots of the premolar teeth and below the exit of the infraorbital nerve. As the trocar is rotated, it will drill itself into the maxillary sinus with slight pressure. After the trocar is in the sinus lumen, the obturator is removed and sinus irrigation can be performed. This technique has good patient acceptance because of excellent regional anesthesia, and it can be performed in the recumbent position. It is also the best way to irrigate the maxillary sinus in children.[18, 19]

When irrigation methods failed, it was clear to the early practitioners that surgical drainage was needed. Dependent drainage seemed most likely to succeed, and early attempts were directed at achieving this. Hunter designed a method in which a maxillary molar tooth was extracted and the alveolar ridge removed until an opening was created into the sinus. This allowed dependent drainage but had the disadvantage of the loss of a tooth and the entrance of food into the antrum.[5] Cowper also described a technique in which either the second premolar or the first molar was removed or a hole was drilled in the edentulous portion of the alveolar ridge. The socket or hole was then enlarged with a Hartmann punch, Chiari hand trephines, or a four-edge hand drill. Immediately after the opening into the sinus was made, the sinus was irrigated. A strip of gauze was then placed into the wound and changed every few days. However, the constant taste of pus and the entry of food into the sinus that resulted led Cowper to employ a dental obturator 8 to 10 days postoperatively, which plugged the hole but could be removed for sinus irrigation.[4]

Hunter also mentions breaking into the antrum through the nose, but considered this method unacceptable as it would fail to provide dependent drainage.[5] Mikulicz described a method for making an opening under the inferior turbinate. He first applied cocaine to the area and then, using a speculum under direct vision, introduced a trocar. The anterior one third of the inferior turbinate was sometimes shaved off to allow better visualization. The cracking of the bone and a sudden toothache were interpreted as an indication of a successful puncture. After the initial hole was created, irrigation could be performed. Curettes and rongeurs were then used to enlarge the hole to preclude closure.[4]

SINUSCOPY

Dionis is credited with developing a nasal speculum in 1714. However, without illumination it was of limited value. Wertheim (1868) developed a "conchoscope," which was a tube with an angled mirror, to examine the deeper structures of the nose. He termed the process *rhinoscopia media*. In 1896, Killian developed a method for deep anterior rhinoscopy, in which he penetrated the middle meatus. Hirschmann, in 1901, introduced a cystoscope into the maxillary antrum (which was termed Highmoreoscopy) via an enlarged tooth socket. This paved the way for sinuscopy as practiced today.[20]

Until recently, it was thought that chronic changes in the mucosa of the maxillary antrum were irreversible. Therefore, the treatment for chronic disease was geared for radical removal. Utilizing telescopic instruments, Messerklinger[21] and others[22] found that some of the changes in the antral mucosa are reversible. If the antral disease then is primarily related to poor ventilation owing to obstruction at the osteomeatal complex, endoscopic decompression of this area should allow for normalization of the antral physiology.

TECHNIQUE

The antral wall is anesthetized and is punctured with a trocar via the inferior meatus or canine fossa. After removal of the stylet, a straight or 30° telescopic instrument is passed through the guide tube to inspect the sinus. Irrigation can be carried out after the initial inspection. Other angled instruments can be passed for examination of all parts of the antrum to evaluate the function of the mucociliary apparatus.

For functional endoscopic surgery (see Chapter 13), a thorough nasal endoscopy should be performed, using a 30° and 70° telescope. The nasal recess and middle meatal area must be examined. Axial and coronal CT scans can be very helpful in evaluating this complex and its relationship to the disease of the maxillary sinus as well as the ethmoid and frontal sinus. A 0°

telescope should be used for the majority of the operation. A decompression is accomplished starting at the anterior inferior attachment of the uncinate process. This is removed to expose the ethmoid infundibulum. The diseased mucosa is removed using upbiting and straight forceps. A KTP laser also has been used to cut the soft tissues bloodlessly via a 400 μ fiber in a bayonette carrier, or special endoscope. After removing the diseased ethmoidal tissue, a middle meatal antrostomy is performed, and diseased mucosa is removed from the maxillary antrum, using a telescope and right-angled forceps.[23, 24]

NASAL ANTROSTOMY

Nasal antrostomy is indicated in patients with recurrent or chronic infection secondary to stenosis or occlusion of the natural ostium. A large opening (1) provides drainage and reduces infections; (2) may be used for frequent sinus irrigation; (3) permits inspection of the interstices of the antrum; (4) allows for drainage or removal of necrotic debris (e.g., patients with tumors receiving radiotherapy); and (5) serves as a route for the removal of foreign bodies.

Historically, Sluder (1919) advocated removal of the entire medial wall of the antrum, and McKenzie (1927) described enlarging the inferior meatus upward into the middle meatus. The usual placement of the nasal antral window is at the inferior meatus, except in children, in whom the meatus has not fully developed.

Many nasal antrostomies fail to drain or to correct the poor ventilation of the maxillary antrum. When good endoscopic visualization and the use of CT scans was achieved, attention was then paid to the osteomeatal complex. Endoscopic nasal surgery is primarily based on treating the infundibular area and opening and decompressing the middle meatus. This allows the maxillary sinus to drain and ventilate in a more physiologic manner. Buiter has added a nasal antrostomy when the major pathology was in the maxillary sinus and not the osteomeatal complex, with a success rate of 92 per cent in almost 400 cases.[22, 25]

TECHNIQUE

The usual technique for creating an inferior meatus nasoantral window begins with the application of topical cocaine and local infiltrative anesthesia. The inferior turbinate is fractured upward and can be packed in this position to allow good exposure of the inferior meatus. An inferiorly based, U-shaped mucoperiosteal flap should be elevated and displaced onto the floor of the nose. A small opening is made into the exposed bone with a trocar and is enlarged with a biting forceps. The bony opening should be as large as the flap that was created. Any intrasinus procedure, such as foreign body removal or biopsy, can be carried out by direct vision. After completion of the antral surgery, the mucosal flap is rotated into the defect to prevent stenosis of the window. The turbinate is returned to its original position, and a small amount of nasal packing is placed for 24 to 48 hours.[26–29]

In the natural ostial method, after regional anesthesia is achieved, the middle turbinate is elevated superiorly. The natural ostium is present in the hiatus semilunaris behind the uncinate process of the middle meatus. The ostium is probed and enlarged using a biting forceps. This window cannot be made as in the inferior meatus because of the limited exposure and surrounding structures. The middle turbinate is returned to its original position, and a small amount of nasal packing is placed.[26]

The complications reported with these procedures are bleeding, closure of the window, and the formation of synechial bands to the septum.[26]

CALDWELL-LUC PROCEDURE

Despite irrigation and trephination procedures, some patients require a more radical operation for removal of chronically infected antral mucosa. Lamarier (1743), Desault (1798), and Weber (1866) described radical methods of sinus opening, but these were all abandoned. In 1899, Kuster reintroduced the radical procedure, describing the Desault-Kuster method of resection of the anterior facial wall of the sinus. After an incision was carried down to bone, flaps were elevated, and an opening of approximately the size of the little finger was made into the anterior wall. A prosthesis was inserted into the opening at 8 to 14 days to maintain its patency. However, the prosthesis was uncomfortable and increased the mucous secretions by acting as a foreign body. In 1892, Robertson described entering the maxillary sinus through a hole in the anterior wall made with a hammer and chisel but did not utilize a nasal antral window. In 1893, Caldwell described a procedure based on Heath's method of making a temporary opening in the canine

fossa area in combination with a nasal antrostomy. Spicer described a similar procedure in 1894 and cited Robertson's work but not Caldwell's. In 1897, Luc reported a similar operation but did not credit Caldwell or Spicer. The operation, termed the Luc procedure in Europe and the Caldwell procedure in the United States, eventually became known as the Caldwell-Luc procedure. This is the most common radical sinus operation performed.[4, 18, 30–32]

The operation is indicated for chronic maxillary sinus disease that appears irreversible, despite conservative therapy with antibiotics and decongestants and repeated irrigation, or that has not responded to antrostomy or other surgical procedures. Patients with bronchiectasis and maxillary sinusitis may need a radical procedure earlier to decrease the potential reservoir of purulent material that may drip into the lungs. Hypertrophic rhinosinusitis with the formation of polyps in the antrum can be treated by this approach. The antrochoanal polyp often tends to recur if simply avulsed through the nose; consequently, a more radical operation will allow removal of the antral portion and prevent recurrence by ostial herniation. This procedure also permits removal of a variety of benign lesions from the sinus.

A recent review of the findings of the Caldwell-Luc procedure showed hypertrophic mucosa in 82 per cent of the cases. Purulent material was found in 8.2 per cent and cysts and mucoceles in 3.4 per cent. A 6.4 per cent negative exploration rate was also reported.[34]

Dome-shaped masses within the antrum are often incidental radiographic findings. These are usually small retention cysts and do not require treatment unless they are symptomatic. Larger masses that may encompass the entire sinus, often causing bulging of the bony wall, are mucoceles. If the mucoceles become large enough, they may cause enophthalmos or proptosis, lower lid distortion, interferences with extraocular motility, diplopia, epiphora, or periocular pain.[35] It has been found that the sinus mucosa plays an active role in the formation of the mucoceles.[36] Postsurgical mucoceles may be related to surgical trauma and may occupy only parts of the maxillary antrum. Therefore, CT scanning is imperative in the evaluation of these cases.[37]

Cysts in the antrum also may have a dental etiology, and evaluation of the dental structures is necessary in establishing a treatment plan. CT scanning also may be very useful in establishing this connection between the dental structures and sinus pathology.[37]

The Caldwell-Luc approach is a superior method for the removal of foreign bodies from the antrum, such as root fragments after exodontia, supernumerary teeth, sinoliths, displaced dental materials, or embedded projectiles.[33] Recent advances in endoscopic sinus surgery have made it possible to approach some of these foreign bodies via an antral puncture or antrostomy and the use of a telescope and forceps. The Caldwell-Luc operation also offers access to the depths of the sinus for exploration and manipulation of complicated facial fractures. This approach allows the harvesting of the anterior wall of the sinus as a free graft for the reconstruction of the fractured orbital floor.

Many oroantral fistulas can be closed via a primary intraoral approach (see Chapter 18). However, pre-existing sinus disease requires débridement of the antrum via the Caldwell-Luc approach, along with a nasal antrostomy and intraoral repair of the fistula. This approach is also useful for the creation of a nasoantral window if a primary nasal procedure has failed.[4, 7, 18, 33, 38]

The Caldwell-Luc procedure also provides access to the ethmoid and sphenoid sinuses through the medial wall (see Chapter 15), to the orbit for orbital decompression (see Chapter 24), and to the pterygomaxillary space via the posterior wall for internal maxillary artery ligation, vidian neurectomy, sphenopalatine ganglionectomy, and sectioning of the second division of the trigeminal nerve (see Chapter 22).[4, 7, 18, 33, 38]

The sublabial approach also can be used for biopsy of suspected malignant neoplasms in the antrum. However, this approach carries the risk of tumorous seeding of the overlying soft tissues of the cheek. Therefore, it may be better to obtain a biopsy via the Canfield-Sturmann modification of Denker's procedure (described in the next section) or a large nasal antrostomy to eliminate buccal contamination.[33]

TECHNIQUE

The procedure can be performed under local or general anesthesia. Local anesthesia has the advantage of decreased operative bleeding and eliminates the risks associated with general anesthesia. Local anesthesia can be supplemented with intravenous sedation. Profound regional anesthesia can be achieved by sphenopalatine nerve block via the greater palatine foramen, infraorbital nerve block, posterosuperior alveolar nerve block, and local infiltration of the gingiva. This may be supplemented by cocaine applied to the anterior ethmoid nerve

intranasally. The head of the patient is elevated 30 degrees to decrease bleeding and swelling.

The incision is made several millimeters above the junction of the attached gingiva and the alveolar mucosa in the maxillary vestibule, which extends from the canine tooth area to the first molar area (Fig. 16–1B). This incision should be carried through the periosteum down to bone. An alternate incision is one made around the necks of the teeth to raise the entire gingiva as a flap. This incision is preferred when it may be necessary to enter the alveolus to remove dental pathology or odontogenic tumors that involve the antrum. It also finds application in revision surgery, in which the amount of residual bone is not known, and when a vestibular incision carries the risk of fistula formation.

Using a periosteal elevator, the superior mucosal flap is raised to the level of the infraorbital foramen, taking care not to damage the neurovascular bundle (Fig. 16–1C). Caution should also be exercised to prevent stretch injury to the infraorbital nerve on retracting the flap. A small gouge can be used to create an opening into the sinus in the area of the canine fossa (Fig. 16–1D). One must be careful not to damage the roots of the teeth or developing tooth buds in children. The opening is then enlarged using a Kerrison rongeur until adequate exposure of the interstices of the sinus has been obtained (Fig. 16–1E). If a free bone graft is needed, the donor area is outlined on the anterior and lateral walls. A small drill or gouge is used to perforate the bone, avoiding injury to the teeth or the infraorbital nerve. The perforations are carefully connected and the graft is removed intact.

Diseased areas within the sinus can now be removed. Gauze packing saturated with an anesthetic solution containing epinephrine can be used to help control bleeding. Meticulous removal of the sinus lining in patients with chronic sinusitis permits replacement and partial obliteration of the cavity with dense scar tissue. Care should be taken in instrumentation of the roof of the sinus to prevent damage to the contents of the infraorbital fissure.

At the end of the procedure, a large nasoantral window should be created. The thin bone of the medial wall is carefully removed with a small chisel, Freer elevator, or rongeur. The nasal mucoperiosteal tissues should be left intact. After the bone is removed, an inferiorly based, U-shaped flap is made from this mucosa and is draped into the antrum. This allows postoperative drainage, irrigation, and inspection of the antrum. Nasal packing is placed into the antrum through the nasoantral window for

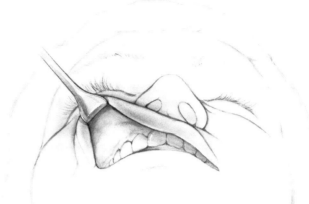

Figure 16–1. Caldwell-Luc procedure.
A, Lip retractor in place exposing the area of the anterior maxilla.

A

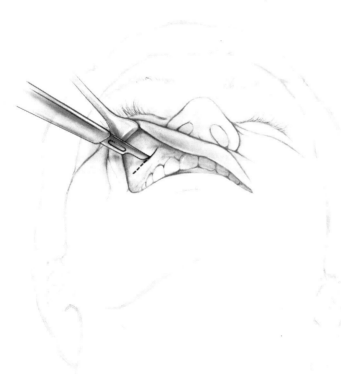

B

Figure 16–1 *Continued*
B, Incision being made several millimeters above the junction of the attached gingiva and the alveolar mucosa in the maxillary vestibule.
Illustration continued on following page

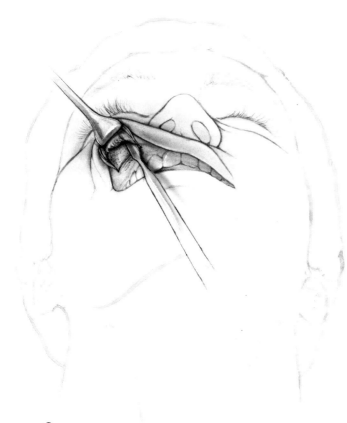

Figure 16–1 *Continued*
C, Using a periosteal elevator, the superior mucosal flap is raised to the level of the infraorbital foramen, taking care not to damage the neurovascular bundle.

C

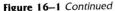

Figure 16–1 *Continued*
D, A small gouge is used to create an opening into the sinus in the area of the canine fossa above the roots of the teeth.

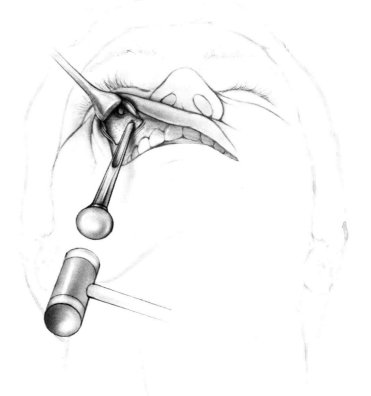

D

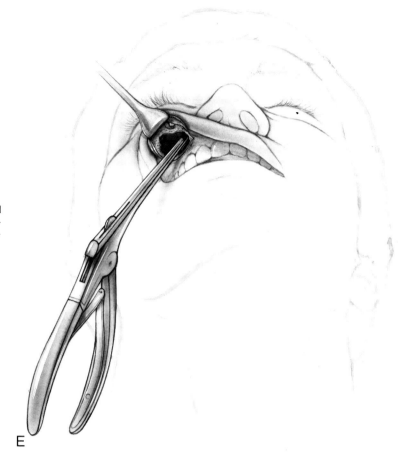

Figure 16–1 *Continued*
E, A Kerrison rongeur is used to enlarge the opening until adequate exposure has been obtained.

E

hemostasis and to hold the mucosal flap in position. The antral cavity can also be lined with Gelfoam, minimizing the amount of packing necessary to control bleeding.[32] Overpacking may lead to bleeding through the anterior wall opening, with increased swelling of the face. The packing should be left in place for 24 to 48 hours. Antibiotic ointment on the packing will help decrease the odor. The intraoral incision is then closed with an absorbable suture material.[3, 4, 10, 11, 18, 31, 33, 38–40]

Denker originally described a modification of this procedure to provide wide exposure of the medial antral wall and the nasal cavity for removal of lesions such as the angiofibroma. In this method, an incision is made in the gingivobuccal fold from the midline to the second molar tooth, and the mucoperiosteum is elevated to expose the face of the maxilla and the piriform aperture. After the antrum is opened, the nasal mucosa is carefully separated from the underlying bone. The bone is then removed from the piriform rim with a chisel. A vertical incision is made in the soft tissues to create a nasal mucosal flap, which is rotated onto the floor of the nasal cavity. The intraoral incision is then closed.[4]

The Denker procedure was later modified by Canfield and Sturmann. In their method, no oral incision was made; the procedure was carried out completely through the nose. This leaves the buccal mucosa intact and avoids a possible oroantral fistula. The crista piriformis was incised down to bone, and the soft tissues were dissected free. The piriform crest was then removed, along with a portion of the canine fossa and lateral wall of the nose. The sinus was explored, and a nasal mucosal flap created and draped into the antrum. This particular approach is good for sinus biopsies, as it leaves the lateral antral wall intact and does not contaminate the buccal soft tissues.[4]

Postoperatively, the patient should be placed on a soft diet and given ice packs to the face; the head of the bed should be elevated to decrease facial swelling. The patient is instructed not to blow the nose or sneeze without the mouth open. The packing is removed in 24 to 48 hours.

The most common complications of radical

antral procedures found in a recent 10-year institutional review of 670 cases was facial swelling in 89 per cent of the cases. This was self-limiting and usually resolved within a week. Recurrent sinusitis was found in 12 per cent of the patients. Paresthesia or anesthesia of the cheek, teeth, and gingiva was found in 9.1 per cent. This complication is usually related to stretch injury of the infraorbital nerve, which may persist for 3 to 6 months. In the same series, recurrent polyps were found in 5.4 per cent of the patients; dacrocystitis in 2.6 per cent; oroantral fistula in 1.1 per cent, and devitalized teeth in 0.4 per cent.[34]

In addition, hemorrhage and massive facial swelling may occur. Care should be taken when working on the medial wall to avoid damage to the lacrimal apparatus.

A cribriform plate injury with cerebrospinal fluid (CSF) leak can result from bone removal superomedially. Blindness from direct injury or secondary to a dissecting hematoma has also been reported. Persistent pain or neuroma formation may arise from damage to neural structures. The formation of an oroantral fistula can occur along the incision line from wound dehiscence. Careful suturing, placement of the incision over bone, and meticulous care of the antrum can avoid this problem. Revision surgery increases the likelihood of all complications, especially injuries to the infraorbital nerve.[1, 38]

Overall, the radical antral operations are safe procedures if performed on the right patient, for the right indications, with meticulous attention to detail.

References

1. Chapnik JS, Bach MC: Bacterial and fungal infections. Otolaryngol Clin North Am 9:44, 1976.
2. Van Alyea OE: Nasal Sinuses: An Anatomic and Clinical Consideration. Baltimore, Williams & Wilkins, 1942, p 13.
3. McMurray J: Intra-antral air pressure incident to the respiratory excursion and its effect on antral drainage. Arch Otolaryngol 14:581, 1937.
4. Hajek M: Pathology and Treatment of the Inflammatory Diseases of the Nasal Accessory Sinuses. St Louis, CV Mosby, 1926, p 145.
5. MacDonald G: A Treatise on Diseases of the Nose and Accessory Cavities. London, McMillan and Co, 1892, p 171.
6. Bell RD, Sone HE: Conservative surgical procedures in inflammatory disease of the maxillary sinus. Otolaryngol Clin North Am 9:175, 1976.
7. Montgomery W: Surgical treatment of sinus infections. In Ballenger JJ (ed): Diseases of the Nose, Throat and Ear. Philadelphia, Lea & Febiger, 1977, p 205.
8. Ritter RN: A clinical and anatomical study of the various techniques of irrigation of the maxillary sinus. Laryngoscope 87:215, 1977.
9. Van Alyea OE: Nasal Sinuses: An Anatomic and Clinical Consideration. Baltimore, Williams & Wilkins, 1951, p 48.
10. Ritter FN: The Paranasal Sinuses: Anatomy and Surgical Techniques. 2nd ed. St. Louis, CV Mosby, 1978, p 89.
11. Montgomery WW: Surgery of the maxillary sinus. In Montgomery WW (ed): Surgery of the Upper Respiratory System. Vol 1. Philadelphia, Lea & Febiger, 1971, p 169.
12. Goldman JL, Blaugrund SM: Complications of surgery of the nasal cavity, sinuses, and pharynx. In Conley J (ed): Complications of Head and Neck Surgery. Philadelphia, WB Saunders, 1979, p 167.
13. Myerson M: The natural orifice of the maxillary sinus. I. Anatomic studies. Arch Otolaryngol 15:80, 1932.
14. Myerson M: The natural orifice of the maxillary sinus. II. Clinical studies. Arch Otolaryngol 15:716, 1932.
15. Mosher HP: Surgical anatomy of the ethmoid labyrinth. Trans Am Acad Ophthalmol Otolaryngol 34:376, 1939.
16. Goode RC: An antral catheter for maxillary sinusitis. Arch Otolaryngol 69:312, 1970.
17. Bacher JA: Fatal air embolism after puncture of the maxillary antrum—Autopsy. Calif State Med J 21:433, 1923.
18. Goodman WS: The Caldwell-Luc procedure. Otolaryngol Clin North Am 9:187, 1976.
19. Peterson RJ: Canine fossa puncture. Laryngoscope 83:369, 1973.
20. Messerklinger W: Endoscopy of the nose. Baltimore, Urban and Schwarzenberg, 1978.
21. Messerklinger W: On the drainage of the normal frontal sinuses of man. Acta Otolaryngol 63:176–181, 1967.
22. Buiter CT: Nasal antrostomy. Rhinology 26:5–18, 1988.
23. Kennedy DW, Zinreich SJ, Shaalan H, Kuhn F, Naclerio R, Loch E: Endoscopic middle meatal antrostomy: Theory, technique, and patency. Laryngoscope 97(Suppl 43):1–9, 1987.
24. Stammberger H, Wolf G: Headaches and sinus disease: The endoscopic approach. Ann Otol Rhinol Laryngol 97(Suppl 134):1–23, 1988.
25. Lund VJ: Inferior meatal antrostomy: Fundamental considerations of design and function. J Laryngol Otol 15(Suppl):1–18, 1988.
26. Hilding A: Experimental sinus surgery: Effects of operative windows in normal sinuses. Ann Otol 50:379, 1941.
27. Lavelle RJ, Harrison MS: Infection of the maxillary sinus: The case for middle meatal antrostomy. Laryngoscope 81:90, 1971.
28. Bryant FI: Conservative surgery for chronic maxillary sinusitis. Laryngoscope 77:575, 1967.
29. Imperatori CJ: The intranasal treatment of suppurative disease of the maxillary sinus. Laryngoscope 40:7, 1930.
30. Stevenson RS, Guthrie D: A History of Otolaryngology. Baltimore, Williams & Wilkins, 1949, p 89.
31. Caldwell G: Diseases of nasal sinuses. NY Med J 527, 1893.
32. Myers EN: Caldwell-Luc operations and extensions. In Goldman JL (ed): The Principles and Practice of Rhinology. New York, John Wiley & Sons, 1987, pp 455–474.
33. Bernstein L: The Caldwell-Luc operation. In English G (ed): Otolaryngology. Hagerstown, Harper and Row, 1980, p 1.

34. DeFreitas J, Lucente FE: The Caldwell-Luc procedure: Institutional review of 670 cases: 1975–1985. Laryngoscope 98:1297–1300, 1988.
35. Weber AL, Rauch SD, Feldon SE: Ophthalmic manifestations of maxillary sinus mucoceles. Ophthalmology 94:1013–1019, 1987.
36. Proto E, Santa Cruz G, Puxeddu P: Histological and ultrastructural findings on mucocele of maxillary sinus. J Otorhinolaryngol 48:345–350, 1986.
37. Som PM, Shugar JMA: Antral mucoceles: A new look. J Comput Assist Tomogr 4:484–488, 1980.
38. Tobin HA: Surgery of the maxilla and mandible. In Paparella M, Shumrick D (eds): Otolaryngology. Vol 3. Philadelphia, WB Saunders, 1973, p 465.
39. Faulkner ER: Radical operation of the antrum. Laryngoscope 40:10, 1930.
40. Macbeth R: Caldwell-Luc operation: 1952–1966. Arch Otol 87:630, 1968.

CHAPTER 17

MANAGEMENT OF DENTAL DISEASE AND ORAL ANTRAL FISTULA

Louis J. Loscalzo, DMD

Chronic oroantral fistulas are much less common than one would suspect considering the compromising anatomy, the high incidence of upper respiratory tract infections frequently involving the maxillary sinus, and the relative nonchalance with which posterior maxillary teeth are extracted.

In a large percentage of adults, the bony floor of the antrum is indistinguishable from the thin cortex that covers the apices of the molars and bicuspids (Fig. 17–1). The sinus frequently descends to occupy a tight space between the buccal and palatal roots of molars to the degree that in attempting to remove a fractured palatal root from the buccal part, beyond the bifurcation, the schneiderian membrane is encountered. This expansion increases with age and often, in the edentulous (whether this be real or the result of marked alveolar bone resorption), the antral outline seems to fill the entire radiograph. Yet, the incidence of this complication remains low indeed.

Maxillary sinusitis, on the other hand, is a common clinical occurrence. Its symptoms are not infrequently localized to the posterior teeth and their resolution sought in the dentist's office. Here, pain in the posterior maxilla and pressure tenderness, particularly in the lateral tuberosity area, could and often does lead to the unfortunate extraction of the suspected tooth. Even though this might result in oroantral fistula, it seldom occurs.

Lack of care in posterior maxillary tooth extraction does exist. It is even measurable by

the paucity of alveolar bone contouring that accompanies the extraction. Nevertheless, in my experience, the incidence of chronic antral fistulas is minimal.

Hence, barring obvious communications that follow trauma or neoplastic surgery, it appears that certain circumstances predispose to the formation of a chronic oroantral fistula. The majority of these are adequately discussed and well illustrated in oral surgery texts. They in-

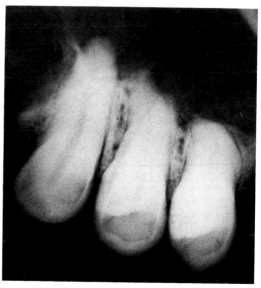

Figure 17–1. Radiograph illustrating a thin layer of bone separating the apices of the teeth from the floor of the antrum.

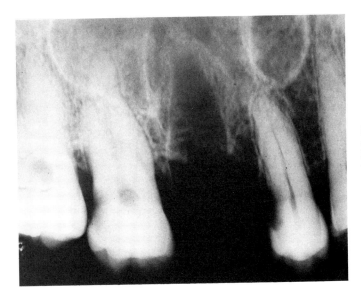

Figure 17–2. Extraction site of a first molar communicating through the antral membrane. No instrumentation is recorded at the apex.

clude (1) immediate surgical penetration of the antral membrane (Fig. 17–2), which constitutes the greatest number and may be anatomically inevitable; (2) periapical pathosis or granulomatous or cystic disease, which on radiographs appears contiguous with the sinus (Fig. 17–3); (3) a retained root tip located near the antral floor (Fig. 17–4); (4) an impacted tooth, generally a third molar, whose surgical exposure is limited and whose delivery is relatively blind (Fig. 17–5); (5) advanced periodontal disease with bi- or trifurcation involvement (Fig. 17–6); (6) maxillary tuberosities requiring reduction for dental prostheses; and (7) large cysts that have distorted anatomy and have grossly encroached on the space normally occupied by the antrum of Highmore.

MANAGEMENT OF PREDISPOSING CONDITIONS

In the case of the immediate penetration after extraction, if there is no suppurative process and the delivery of the tooth is within normal limits, one can proceed with the closure. Packs or absorbable materials placed within the socket are not encouraged, with or without overlying sutures. Instead, a simple and effective means of repair is a buccal mucoperiosteal flap whose intactness and viability have been preserved during the extraction. Therefore, rather than immediately applying a forceps to the tooth, it is expedient to transect both interdental papillae and reflect the mucoperiosteum sufficiently to prevent a tear during the removal. This will quickly permit creation of a small, conventional sliding flap, not unlike one used to retrieve a retained root tip. A wide molar socket or a perforation at the palatal root will require lengthening the vertical incisions and scoring the undersurface of the periosteum. An aperture high at the buccal plate does not require as long a flap or one as tension free when sutured to the palatal margins. The patient is cautioned to avoid increased antral

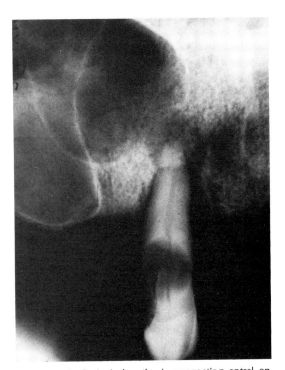

Figure 17–3. Periapical pathosis suggesting antral encroachment.

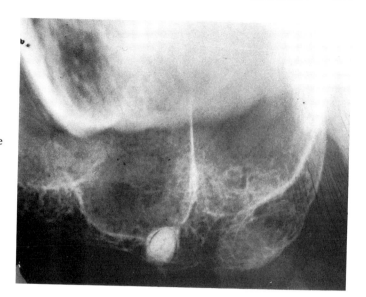

Figure 17–4. A retained root tip at the antral floor.

pressure and is placed on a full fluid or puréed diet during the healing period. Antibiotics, however, are not mandatory.

Periapical pathosis in most instances represents either a granuloma due to chronic dental infection or an inflammatory cyst. Neither of these requires strong instrumentation. In fact, the granuloma will organize by itself, once the source is removed (see Fig. 17–3). In removing the periapical cyst, blunt dissection is effective, and gauze at the end of the curette works well.

Root tips near the antral floor often need not be removed. If indicated, a communication should be anticipated and preparation made for repair. A small buccal mucoperiosteal flap designed for enlargement will generally suffice.

An unerupted maxillary third molar, high and resting on the posterior wall of the sinus, is a challenge if the configuration of the oral cavity does not allow space for direct instrumentation. Here, in particular, a wide flap design is essential.

Advanced periodontal disease may actually destroy the bony floor at a given point. However, the sinus membrane generally remains intact and there is no true penetration. Misplaced vigorous curettage after the extraction will result in a perforation.

The elective maxillary tuberosity reduction, which implies reducing its posterolateral wall as it comes in contact with the anterior border

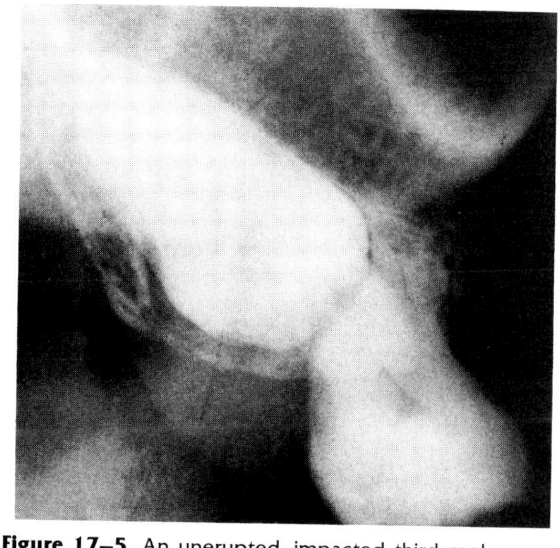

Figure 17–5. An unerupted, impacted third molar contained within the maxillary tuberosity.

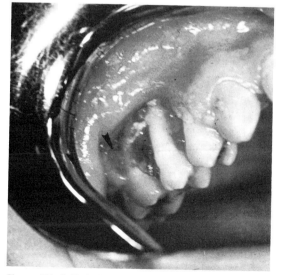

Figure 17–6. Periodontal disease, with destruction up to the apical areas creating an oroantral communication (arrowhead).

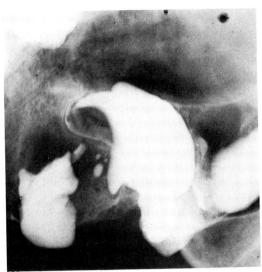

Figure 17–7. Radiograph showing contrast medium within a multiloculated cyst that has displaced but not perforated the maxillary sinus.

of the ascending ramus, will frequently extend to the membrane, not through it. Bone cleaves readily around the sinus membrane. Furthermore, the sinus seldom expands into the posteroinferior boundaries of the tuberosity. Hence a broad, unibeveled chisel angled correctly will move along the cleavage lines and not penetrate the membrane. In removing the bone to increase intermaxillary space, large areas of the maxillary sinus floor may be left without overlying bone, provided the mucoperiosteal flap is solid and intact. This is true even though the bony crest of a totally resorbed alveolus does not regenerate. Instead, cicatrization replaces bone and protects the sinus from the trauma of mastication.

That the antrum of Highmore is resilient, capable of anatomic changes in response to space limitations, is nowhere better demonstrated than in competition with large dental inflammatory or developmental cysts (Fig. 17–7). Continued growth of these cysts gradually resorbs the intervening bone, with the outer connective tissue periphery of the cysts becoming contiguous with the sinus membrane. At this point, an attempt at total enucleation of the cyst will frequently tear the sinus membrane, thus creating a confluency between the antral and cystic cavities. Healing thereafter is no longer predictable. Clot organization, as expected in a cystectomy closed primarily or in one closed by secondary intention, is now disrupted by the semiclosed system of the antrum, and a chronic oroantral fistula ensues. In these cases, it is preferable to decompress the cyst—

enucleate its membrane only up to the area of sinus contact, using packs or obturators in the interim—and await internal bone restructure before reoperating. In many cases, a second operation is not necessary, as the oral defect is minimal.

MANAGEMENT OF CHRONIC OROANTRAL FISTULA

A chronic oroantral fistula differs considerably from the immediate one (Figs. 17–8 and 17–9). The focus is primarily on the antrum, and the implication is that the body has failed to seal both cavities from each other and restore normal physiology. There is, however, a satisfactory system of drainage between the antrum and the mouth, as it utilizes gravity to propel purulence downward rather than through the nasal ostium in the middle meatus, epithelializing the connecting tract. To this investigator it seems reasonable, often enough, to incriminate an infected sinus as the cause of such a complication, even prior to the extraction of the tooth.

Before the era of antibiotics, Berry[7] published a significant study that could well account for the relationship of dentoantral infections and the high probability of their role in the formation of a chronic fistula (Table 17–1).

Presurgical Considerations. Infection must be controlled before closure is attempted. Hence, it is necessary to rule out other possible

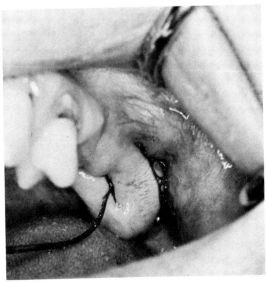

Figure 17–8. Probing a chronic oroantral fistula; the gingival tissues have obliterated much of the defect.

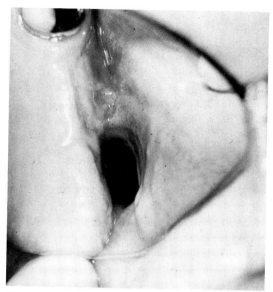

Figure 17–9. A large oroantral communication located lateral to the alveolar crest.

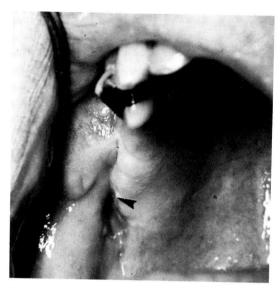

Figure 17–10. The arrowhead indicates a small chronic fistula located lateral to the maxillary tuberosity. Adequate antral drainage is prevented by the fold of buccal tissues.

contributing factors that require consultation with the otolaryngologist, e.g., previous sinus disease, nasal obstruction, malignant neoplasms, osteomyelitis.

An accurate history of the complication must be obtained. The antrum also must be visualized radiographically. Panoramic views are not diagnostically valid. Open-mouth Waters views are preferable for preliminary examination. Tomograms are used if displaced teeth, roots, root canal materials, packs, solid medicaments, and such are suspected.

The efficacy of drainage is ascertained. Too small an aperture or one located off the crest and blocked by the folding buccal tissues will not permit adequate drainage and thus prolong the process (Fig. 17–10). Both can be enlarged by coring or by the removal of surface bone (Fig. 17–11), without the necessity of making a classic flap.

When infection is confined to the communicated sinus, no maneuver gives a more dra-

matic result than irrigation through the oral aperture. A large-gauge, blunted, spinal needle attached to a cannula, which in turn is fitted to a syringe, works well. When the fistula is too large and the sterile water solution refluxes into the mouth, dental compound is used to obliterate the space around the needle (Fig. 17–12). The patient is asked to lower the head below the level of the fistula and hold a kidney basin under the nose. Gentle plunger pressure will fill the sinus and bring the return through the nasal ostium. The return is observed for purulence. Repeating this three or four times a week

TABLE 17–1. Dental Caries as a Contributing Factor in Maxillary Sinusitis*

	Origin in Dental Caries			
	Not Possible	Possible	Probable	Proven
Per Cent of Cases	11	41	30	18

*Read before the American Laryngological Association, May 21, 1929.[7]

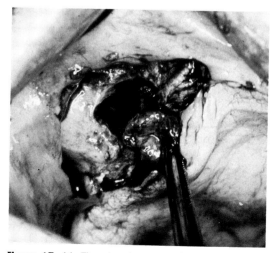

Figure 17–11. The chronic oroantral communication is enlarged to permit adequate drainage in preparation for permanent closure.

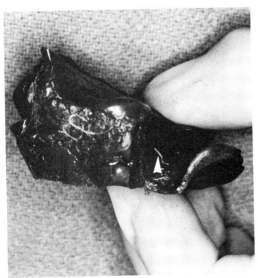

Figure 17–12. Dental compound obturator and irrigating needle *(arrowhead)*.

for about 14 days or less should clear the uncomplicated sinus infection. Irrigating through a nasal ostium is equally effective and preferred by the otolaryngologist. As a working rule, surgery may be performed after clear nasal returns are observed on 3 consecutive days. Antibiotics are administered during this period and continued through the surgical phase.

It is essential here to note that failure to clear the sinus strongly suggests the possibility of other factors. Nasal blockage due to polyps, turbinate disease, and ethmoid or other related infections must be ruled out. Free and open communication with the otolaryngologist is essential.

Sinus Exploration and Curettage. If no cause for the cloudy return is identified, an exploration of the sinus is in order. The procedure can be performed through the fistula, sufficiently enlarged (Fig. 17–11), or in classic Caldwell-Luc fashion. Its purpose is to inspect, curette diseased mucosa or polyps, search for foreign bodies, and remove septal pockets. An attempt at also closing the fistula at this time, however, is not indicated. The sinus is packed open. If the antrostomy is performed via the fistula and there has been minimal soft tissue displacement, the actual closure can be performed in 3 weeks. The gauze pack is retained and changed several times a week. If a Caldwell-Luc approach is used with a nasal antrostomy, the otolaryngologist may follow a routine protocol. In either case, vascular reorganization of the mucoperiosteum must be obtained prior to closure.

Flap Selection. The buccal mucoperiosteal advancement flap as described by Berger,[1] in my opinion, is by far the simplest and most effective in closing an established fistula. A review of 75 such operated cases revealed three failures. One was the result of weak postoperative directions and pipe smoking immediately after surgery; the second, due to an infected septal compartment in the antrum not reached by the irrigation; the third, due to manual interference of the flap by the disturbed schizophrenic patient. These were reoperated 3 months later and successfully closed. The pipe smoker was better motivated; the second case was referred for a nasal antrostomy and preoperative irrigations; for the third, a protective surgical stent (Fig. 17–13) was wired in place at surgery.[5]

Advantages of the Buccal Flap. The buccal flap is a familiar one, routinely used in oral and maxillofacial surgery. The labial and buccal tissues are more elastic than the palatal. The buccal flap can be lengthened and modified as needed during surgery. It permits wide opening into the sinus and thus replaces the Caldwell-Luc approach for the required curettage. It does not leave raw surfaces to heal by secondary intention. Partial denture prostheses are not usually rendered unserviceable.

Disadvantages of the Buccal Flap. A decrease in depth of the mucobuccal fold is an immediate postoperative consequence, which to a large extent is normalized by function in 5 or 6 months. It is important, however, to borrow tissue laterally from the cheek and not infraorbitally.

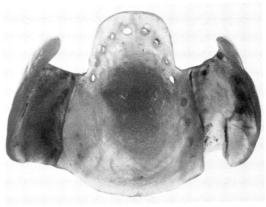

Figure 17–13. An acrylic resin appliance constructed to cover the wound, fixed to the teeth by ligature wires. Care is taken to prevent overcompression of the operated site.

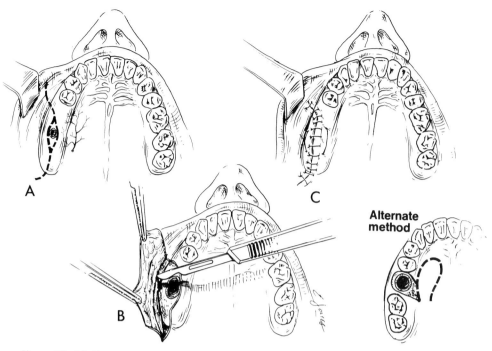

Figure 17–14. The two more commonly used procedures for closure of a chronic oroantral fistula.

TECHNIQUE

Local anesthesia with intravenous sedation is the anesthesia of choice. Complete excision of the fistula is mandatory (Fig. 17–14A). Should the root of a tooth adjacent to the fistula constitute any part of the fistulous tract, it must be extracted. This is generally done at the time of surgery. (In an interesting case, partial removal of a large composite odontoma resulted in a chronic fistula (Fig. 17–15). Two attempts at closure by the referring surgeon failed. The third was successful but was performed only after all the 12 minute denticles lining the tract were removed.) Inspection and curettage of necrotic polypoid antral membrane is considered an integral part of the operation. Antral bleeding is controlled by a gauze pack, which may be left in place until the suturing phase. A nasal antrostomy is not generally required. Sharp edges of bone under the flap are rongeured and filed; abrupt bone margins that cause undue pressure and folding of the flap are reduced and contoured. The length and width of the flap are increased conventionally by lengthening the anterior and posterior incisions. At a given point, when tension becomes considerable, the periosteum is divided (Fig. 17–14B), and thereafter tissue is borrowed laterally from the cheek.

The wound is closed without tension in one layer using 3-0 black silk sutures. A horizontal mattress suture, tied after the interrupted sutures are properly seated, will give a broader adaptation of raw tissues (Fig. 17–14C). If there is a possibility of the lower teeth contacting the operated site, either inadvertently or during sleep, a previously fabricated bite block is inserted (Fig. 17–16). Sutures are removed in about 10 days. Antibiotics and decongestants are routinely administered for about 2 weeks.

Postoperative Care. Postoperative instructions must be meticulous and firm. The patient

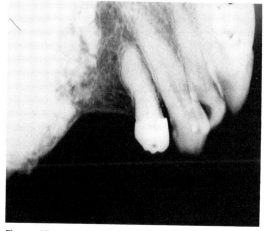

Figure 17–15. Radiograph revealing a composite odontoma adjacent to the fistula.

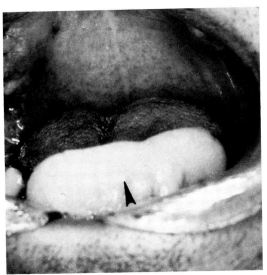

Figure 17–16. An acrylic resin bite block in place *(arrowhead)* over the teeth on the opposite side of the operated site.

should have nothing by mouth for about 6 hours. The patient should limit ambulation and elevate the head when lying down, for the first 24 hours. Increased antral pressure should be avoided; this is aided by not blowing the nose and by opening the mouth to sneeze. A full fluid diet (not using a straw) is taken until sutures are removed; thereafter, the patient should change gradually to a puréed soft and then to a mechanical soft diet for a few weeks. There should be no smoking until sutures are removed. The patient is advised to avoid strenuous physical activity until closure is assured.

Alternative Methods of Closure. The palatal rotating flap (Fig. 17–14) has been and continues to be very popular with some. Aside from the inherent anatomic deficits suggested earlier, it has other disadvantages. Entry into the sinus for curettage is in no way facilitated; an additional buccal approach is required. Once designed, it permits little room for error. Preparing a template on a model, as recommended by Williams,[2] can be useful.

Metal foil and gold plate became popular some time ago because closures could be accomplished with minimal surgery and without the loss of sulcus depth. Budge[3] and others[6] reported their choice to be 36-gauge, 24-karat gold plate. Its neutrality to tissues and easy malleability permitted burnishing onto the bony margins of the aperture. A small mucoperiosteal flap is raised on the buccal aspect, and an accompanying release of the palatal mucosa is made to expose the entire bony margin of the aperture. The flaps are mobilized sufficiently to secure the burnished margins of the plate beneath them. Their margins are not approximated. They are simply held down by sutures. In 2 to 4 weeks granulation tissue forms under the plate and closes the fistula. Once exfoliative motion of the plate is noted, it is literally picked out, and epithelialization is left to secondary intention. This procedure is recommended by most investigators for the immediate perforation. For the chronic fistula, some prefer the plate to be completely covered by the flaps and left in place indefinitely. In neither case is curettage of the sinus a requirement. Crolius[4] and others believe that a metal plate closure always should be tried before resorting to other procedures. I do not share that opinion.

References

1. Berger A: Oroantral openings and their surgical correction. Arch Otolaryngol 30:400, 1939.
2. Williams PE: Diseases of the maxillary sinus of dental origin. *In* Kruger GO: Textbook of Oral and Maxillofacial Surgery. 5th ed. St. Louis, CV Mosby, 1979.
3. Budge CT: Closure of an antraoral opening by use of tantalum plate. J Oral Surg 10(1):32, 1952.
4. Crolius WE: The use of gold plate for the closure of oroantral fistulas. Oral Surg Oral Med Oral Pathol 836, Aug, 1956.
5. Killey HC: An analysis of 250 cases of oroantral fistulae treated by the buccal flap operation. Oral Surg 24:726, 1967.
6. McClung EJ, Chipps JE: Tantalum foil use in closing antral-oral fistulas. US Armed Forces Med J 2:1183, 1951.
7. Berry G: One hundred fifty-two cases of maxillary sinusitis and the possibility of their origin in dental caries, 1929.

CHAPTER 18

LATERAL RHINOTOMY

William Lawson, MD, DDS

Hugh F. Biller, MD

The term *lateral rhinotomy* denotes entry into the nasal cavity through its lateral wall. As Mertz and colleagues[1] stressed, it signifies only an incision and not an operation. Simple incision of the skin and alatomy provide only access to the piriform rim and anterior surface of the inferior turbinates. By modifying the incision, additional exposure enables a variety of procedures to be performed for the extirpation of benign and malignant lesions of the nasal cavity, paranasal sinuses, and nasopharynx. In its broadest form, it includes division of the lip with maxillectomy.[1] It may also be combined with a frontal craniotomy for craniofacial resection of lesions extending through the nasal roof into the anterior cranial fossa. These latter procedures will be discussed in Chapter 26 on Craniofacial Resection. Here, we will consider its use with medial maxillectomy and ethmoidectomy.

HISTORY

The lateral rhinotomy was first described by Michaux[1] in 1848 in France and by Bruns[2] in 1872 in Germany. In the United States, the total rhinotomy was described by Bordley and Longmire[3] in 1949. In 1960, Bordley and Cherry[4] reported 40 patients operated on by this method. In 1968, Doyle[5] described "a modified lateral rhinotomy approach" in which the medial wall of the orbit and anterior surface of the maxilla were exposed and en bloc resection of the ethmoid labyrinth and lateral wall of the nasal cavity was performed.

During the 1970s, numerous reports cited the versatility of the rhinotomy approach in the management of nasal, paranasal, and nasopharyngeal lesions.[6-10] In 1973, Neel and colleagues[8] described the use of the lateral rhinotomy in 56 cases of nasopharyngeal angiofibroma. In their method, the lip was split, with a cheek flap created, and the underlying nasal bone and frontal process of the maxilla were removed. In a later publication, Bremer, Neel, and associates[9] reported its use with another 29 cases.

Vrabec[10] and Suh and colleagues[11] cited the superiority of external rhinotomy over intranasal operation in accomplishing complete extirpation of the inverted papilloma but gave no technical details. The operative method was later reported by Schramm and Myers[12, 13] and by Calcaterra and colleagues.[14] The former workers split the upper lip, whereas the latter left it intact. Schramm and Myers[12] described marsupialization of the transected lacrimal sac to prevent stenosis and stressed attaching the medial canthal ligament to the periosteum of the nasal bone to avoid telecanthus. In 1974, Mabry and Fincher[15] reported the successful use of this procedure in removing melanomas of the lateral nasal wall and ethmoid in three patients.

In 1977, Djalilian and colleagues[7] described a method for the removal of the olfactory neuroblastoma in which exposure of the superior portion of the nasal cavity was gained through a lateral rhinotomy incision. The technique involved excision of the nasal and lacrimal bones, the orbital plate of the ethmoid, the floor and anterior half of the frontal sinus, and the medial half of the orbital floor and anterior wall of the maxilla, along with the soft tissues of the lateral nasal wall. Following this, the tumor was resected along with the cribriform plate. They performed this procedure 19 times in 14 patients.

In the same year, Harrison[16] reported the use of the lateral rhinotomy in 100 cases, the majority of which were melanomas and ethmoid neoplasms. Although he detached the ala, in his method the incision ended below the medial canthus of the eye and did not disturb the medial canthal ligament or the adjacent structures. The anterior portion of the maxilla was removed, but the lesion was generally not resected in a monobloc fashion.

In 1978, Pope[17] modified the procedure to include removal of the posterior wall of the maxillary sinus and ligation of the internal maxillary artery to decrease operative bleeding.

Sessions and Larson[18] coined the term *medial maxillectomy* to describe the en bloc removal of the ethmoid labyrinth, along with the medial aspect of the maxilla and portions of the lacrimal and palatine bones. In their method, the lip was split and a cheek flap created to expose the entire anterolateral aspect of the maxilla; an opening was made into the antrum, with bone cuts designed to preserve the infraorbital rim and anterior crest of the maxilla and nasolacrimal system. Sessions and Humphreys[19] modified their technique by eliminating the lip-splitting incision and transecting the lacrimal sac.

In 1980, Bridger[20] combined the lateral rhinotomy with a frontal craniotomy or transfrontal sinusotomy for the excision of ethmoid malignancies extending to the cribriform plate, or intracranially, in 15 patients. In the same year, Barton[21] reported resection of 32 cases of squamous carcinoma of the lateral nasal wall with a lateral rhinotomy and medial maxillectomy; however, he employed a lip-splitting incision.

In 1984, McGuirt and Thompson[22] utilized a lateral rhinotomy alone for resection of anterior septal tumors and combined it with a sublabial approach for posterior lesions.

In 1988, Biller, Lawson, and colleagues[23] introduced the superior rhinotomy for the en bloc resection of bilateral ethmoid tumors. In this method the bony attachments and overlying soft tissues of the nose superiorly are detached, and the nose is turned downward on its residual alar and columellar attachments. This procedure was used successfully in conjunction with a bifrontal craniotomy in three patients with bilateral ethmoid malignancies that had intracranial extension. One patient succumbed to distant metastasis 1 year later; the other two patients are 1.5 and 2 years postoperative and free of disease.

INDICATIONS

A lateral rhinotomy incision with osteotomy of the nasal bone(s) provides access to the entire nasal cavity and maxillary, ethmoid, and sphenoid sinuses (as well as the frontal sinus if the floor is removed), permitting removal of benign lesions at these sites and en bloc resection of the ethmoid labyrinth and the party wall between the nasal cavity and antrum with infiltrating tumors (Figs. 18–1 and 18–2). The limits of resection are the cribriform plate and fovea ethmoidalis superiorly, the floor of the nose inferiorly, the piriform rim and frontal process of the maxilla anteriorly, and a plane extending from the posterior ethmoid foramen to the face of the sphenoid posteriorly. Invasion of the cribriform plate, roof of the ethmoids, sphenoid sinus, floor of the nose, or any surface other than the medial wall of the maxillary sinus requires more extensive operative procedures.

Among the 26 medial maxillectomies reported by Sessions and Humphreys,[19] there were ten inverted papillomas, five olfactory neuroblastomas, two chondrosarcomas, three adenocarcinomas, two cases of inflammatory polyposis, and one case each of fibrous dysplasia, fibromatosis, mucomycosis, and mucocele.

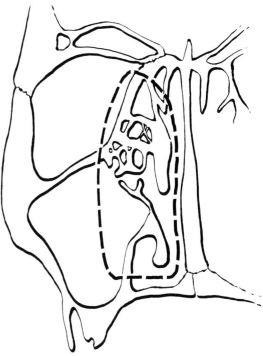

Figure 18–1. Schematic representation of the structures resected by the medial maxillectomy.

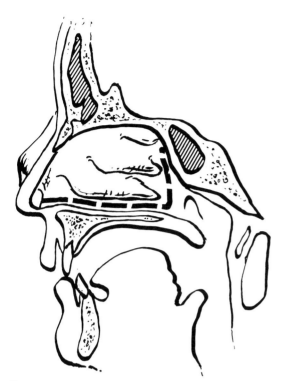

Figure 18–2. Diagram of the intranasal structures encompassed by the medial maxillectomy.

In the review of 226 lateral rhinotomies by Mertz and colleagues,[1] many were extended procedures; these included brow extension in 133, lip splitting in 80, infraorbital incisions in 31, and temporal extension in 6. The ablative procedure ranged from partial maxillectomy to total maxillectomy with orbital exenteration. The lesions were benign in 43 per cent, malignant in 55 per cent, and mixed in 2 per cent of the cases. The benign lesions included papilloma (44 per cent), angiofibroma (19 per cent), cerebrospinal fluid leak (6 per cent), Osler-Weber disease (5 per cent), neurogenic tumors (e.g., glioma, neurilemmoma, meningioma, meningocele) (5 per cent), antrochoanal polyp (4 per cent), and miscellaneous lesions (e.g., osteoma, dental tumor, hemangioma, chordoma, salivary tumor, reparative granuloma) (17 per cent). Among the malignant tumors, 71 per cent were epithelial (carcinoma, melanoma, adenocarcinoma, transitional cell carcinoma) and 29 per cent were mesenchymal (sarcoma, esthesioneuroblastoma, histiocytoma, lymphoma, hemangiopericytoma, ameloblastoma). The spectrum of the lesions excised in these series is representative of that reported by other investigators.[5, 17]

We performed 165 rhinotomies in 151 patients at the Mount Sinai Medical Center, New York, in the period 1974 to 1988. In this series, 142 rhinotomies (86 per cent) were combined with another procedure, which included a medial maxillectomy in 120 patients, a bifrontal craniotomy for a combined craniofacial resection in 15 patients, a median mandibulotomy in 3 patients, bilateral medial maxillectomies in 3 patients, a partial maxillectomy with lip-splitting incision in 2 patients, and a transpalatal approach and a transsphenoidal approach in one patient each.

In this series of 151 cases, 86 patients (57 per cent) had benign lesions. This included 66 inverted papillomas, 4 angiofibromas, 4 angiomatous polyps, 2 schwannomas, 2 benign mixed tumors, 2 aspergillomas, 1 leiomyoma, 1 ossifying fibroma, 1 hemangioma, 1 giant cell tumor, 1 ameloblastoma, and 1 osteoma. There were 62 (41 per cent) malignant tumors; consisting of 13 esthesioneuroblastomas, 9 undifferentiated carcinomas, 9 adenocarcinomas, 8 squamous cell carcinomas, 7 melanomas, 6 adenoid cystic carcinomas, 2 leiomyosarcomas, 2 solitary plasmacytomas, 2 chordomas, 1 hemangiopericytoma, 1 rhabdomyosarcoma, 1 mucoepidermoid carcinoma, and 1 lymphoma. Coexisting benign and malignant lesions were present in three patients (2 per cent), all of which were inverted papillomas associated with squamous cell carcinomas.

The total rhinotomy provides wide access to the nasal cavity and adjacent paranasal sinuses by totally severing the bony attachments of the nasal pyramid and partially severing the overlying soft tissues, permitting the entire external nose to be swung to one side of the face. The increased operative exposure is particularly valuable for the removal of infiltrative and malignant neoplasms. It may be combined with en bloc ethmoidectomy and partial maxillectomy.

In 1960, Bordley and Cherry[4] reported 40 cases treated by total rhinotomy at the Johns Hopkins Hospital (1947–1960). There were 12 benign tumors (pituitary adenoma, cysts, encephalocele, angioma), 17 malignant tumors (carcinoma, sarcoma, plasmacytoma), and 11 inflammatory lesions (osteomyelitis).

The earliest attempt to detach the nose superiorly and hinge it downward was by Proust,[24] in 1908, to provide exposure of the hypophysis. In 1984, Schramm and colleagues[25] employed the same incision but used it to complete a rhinectomy for a recurrent mucoepidermoid carcinoma. In the same year, Hassard and Holness[26] termed it the "crossbow" incision and combined it with a bifrontal craniotomy for the resection of a recurrent adenoid cystic carcinoma involving the ethmoid and frontal sinuses. In a dissection study, these workers showed the rich, reliable blood supply to the nose from the anastomotic arcades derived from the columellar branches of the superior labial and angular arteries.

The superior rhinotomy provides wide exposure to the nasal cavity as well as the maxillary, ethmoid, and sphenoid sinuses. It can be combined with a bilateral medial maxillectomy for bilateral en bloc resection of the ethmoid labyrinth and party wall between the maxillary antrum and nasal cavity. If the superior rhinotomy is combined with a bifrontal craniotomy, en bloc resection of the cribriform plate and both ethmoid labyrinths can be achieved (Figs. 18–3, 18–4, and 18–5). The upper lip can also be divided to perform a radical maxillectomy.

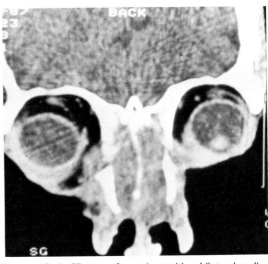

Figure 18–4. CT scan of a patient with a bilateral malignancy extending to the cribriform plate.

TECHNIQUE

LATERAL RHINOTOMY

The skin incision begins beneath the medial aspect of the eyebrow and runs downward, midway between the nasal dorsum and medial canthus of the eye, onto the nasofacial junction and along the nasal alar rim, ending within the nostril (Fig. 18–6A). The incision is deepened in layers, with hemostasis accomplished by electrocautery of the severed blood vessels. The angular vessels should be identified in this part of the dissection and clamped, divided, and ligated to control blood loss. The periosteum along the face of the maxilla and its frontal process is incised and raised with a Freer elevator. Continued elevation of the periosteum in the medial aspect of the orbit results in detachment of the medial canthal ligament from

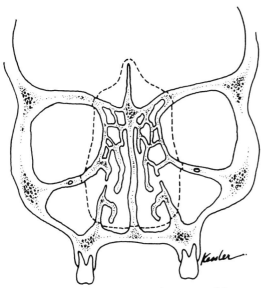

Figure 18–3. Diagram depicting the extent of the resection possible by combining the superior rhinotomy with a frontal craniotomy. Both ethmoid labyrinths, the superior nasal cavity, and the floor of the anterior cranial fossa can be excised en bloc.

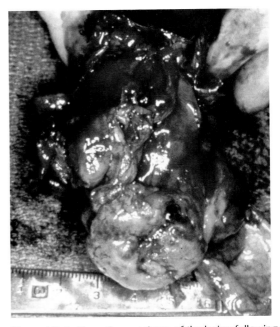

Figure 18–5. Operative specimen of the lesion following craniofacial resection utilizing superior rhinotomy, bilateral medial maxillectomies, and frontal craniotomy.

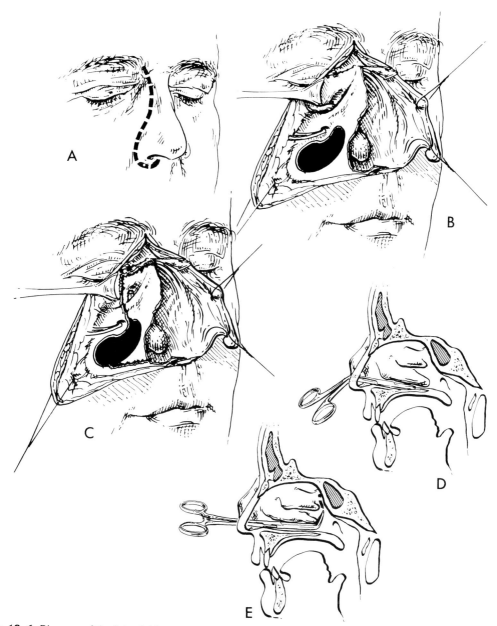

Figure 18–6. Diagram of the lateral rhinotomy procedure. *A,* Skin incisions; *B,* nose reflected, anterior face of maxilla exposed, antrotomy; *C,* orbital and anterior maxillary osteotomies performed; *D,* division of nasoantral party wall in inferior meatus; *E,* division of posterior party wall.

the anterior and posterior crests of the lacrimal fossa. The lacrimal sac is carefully displaced from the fossa and retracted laterally. The periorbita is further elevated and the globe of the eye is displaced laterally with a small malleable ribbon or rigid orbital retractor. This exposes the frontoethmoid suture line, along with the anterior and posterior ethmoid blood vessels passing through it. These structures are the superior boundary of the dissection, as the anterior cranial fossa lies above the suture line. The anterior ethmoid artery is ligated or electrocauterized and divided. The posterior ethmoid artery is exposed but not manipulated because of its proximity to the optic foramen and nerve. The posterior ethmoid artery marks the posterior limit of the dissection. The lacrimal sac may be divided now, splitting and everting the cut lower border with 4-0 chromic catgut sutures to prevent synechia formation and stenosis of the lacrimal outflow. This maneuver permits exposure of the entire medial and inferior portions of the orbit.

The nasal alar rim is detached by dividing the vestibular lining with a scalpel or scissors. A lateral osteotomy of the nasal pyramid is performed with a chisel along the frontal process of the maxilla. The bone is outfractured and retracted to the opposite side, along with the soft tissues of the nose, by a heavy silk suture passed through the alar rim (Fig. 18–6B). The periosteum is now elevated from the anterior face of the maxilla, exposing the infraorbital foramen. Care is taken to preserve and prevent injury to the neurovascular bundle. The antrum is entered with a mallet and gouge through the canine fossa, and the opening is enlarged with a Kerrison rongeur. The antrum is inspected to confirm that there is no extension of disease into its lateral recess, posterior wall, or floor. A bone cut is now made with an osteotome across the piriform rim, at the level of the floor of the maxillary sinus and into the inferior meatus of the nose (Fig. 18–6C). This cut is carried backward within the nose beneath the inferior turbinate with a heavy right-angle scissors or rongeur through the posterior wall of the maxillary sinus (Fig. 18–6D). A cut is also made upward from the opening in the antrum with a chisel, across the infraorbital rim just medial to the infraorbital foramen. A cut is then carried upward posteriorly, just in front of the pterygoid plates, with an angled scissors (Fig. 18–6E). This divides the party wall between the antrum and the nasal cavity behind the posterior margin of the inferior and middle turbinates.

Within the orbit, a superior cut is made along the frontoethmoid suture line (Fig. 18–7). The chisel is angled downward slightly to avoid entering into the anterior cranial fossa or injuring the cribriform plate, which is at a slightly lower level anteriorly. This cut should encompass the upper portion of the ethmoid labyrinth, as well as the middle turbinate, which marks the junction of the lateral wall and roof of the nasal cavity. Anteriorly, the remaining portion of the frontal process of the maxilla is sectioned above the lacrimal fossa to join the lateral nasal osteotomy. Posteriorly, a chisel cut is made downward and forward from the frontoethmoid suture line at the level of the posterior ethmoid artery toward the infraorbital rim cut. The specimen is now engaged with a tenaculum and is removed by rocking it and dividing the remaining soft tissue attachments with a scissors. At this point, brisk bleeding is often encountered posteriorly from torn branches of the internal maxillary artery. These are clamped

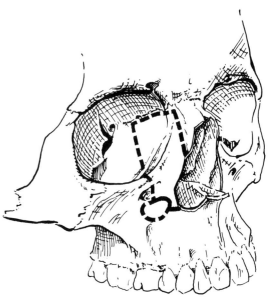

Figure 18–7. Schematic representation of the bone cuts within the orbit and on the anterior face of the maxilla.

and electrocauterized. If there is continuous oozing of blood in the surgical defect, a posterior nasal pack is placed, and the surgical cavity is filled with gauze impregnated with antibiotic ointment. The nose is replaced and the incision is closed in layers. Care is taken to reattach the medial canthal ligament accurately. The nose is then splinted with a plaster cast.

The surgical procedure is designed so that the intraorbital cuts encompass virtually the entire ethmoid labyrinth and permit its en bloc resection, along with the medial portion of the maxilla. The specimen also contains the structures adjoining the common nasoantral wall, including the turbinates and lacrimal fossa, as well as a small portion of the palatal bone (Figs. 18–8 and 18–9).

TOTAL RHINOTOMY

An incision is made across the root of the nose over the frontonasal suture line, is carried down over the nasal bone onto the nasofacial groove, and is continued around the alar margin, similar to that for the lateral rhinotomy (Fig. 18–10A). An upward extension toward the medial aspect of the eyebrow provides additional exposure to the orbital roof and access to the frontal sinus if required. A second incision is made across the base of the columella. Bilateral osteotomies are performed along the frontal process of the maxilla (Fig. 18–10B), and the cartilaginous septum is divided in the plane of

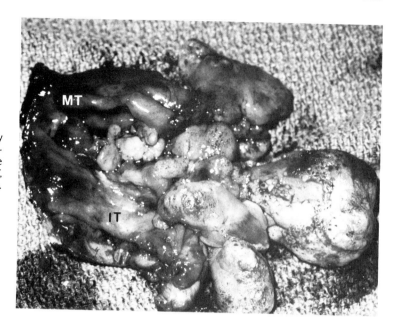

Figure 18–8. Medial maxillectomy specimen from a patient with an inverted papilloma. Note origin of the tumor from the middle meatus. *MT*, middle turbinate; *IT*, inferior turbinate.

the lateral nasal incision (Fig. 18–10C). The nose is swung to the side and a submucous resection of the remaining cartilaginous and bony septum is performed (Fig. 18–10D and E). (Cartilage must be preserved anteriorly to support the nose after it is returned to its normal location, at the end of the procedure.) The sphenoid sinus is widely exposed. Elevation of the periosteum from the medial orbital wall and the face of the maxilla similar to the lateral rhinotomy permits resection of the ethmoid labyrinth and medial portion of the maxillary sinus (Fig. 18–11).

After the lesion is removed, the septum is splinted with mattress sutures, which are placed before the pyramid is replaced to its original position (Fig. 18–10E). The pyramid is further stabilized by the placement of a wire suture superiorly between the nasal bone and the remaining bone.

SUPERIOR RHINOTOMY

A skin incision is made bilaterally along the nasomaxillary groove, beginning superiorly at the medial aspect of the eyebrow and extending downward to the inferior border of the nasal

Figure 18–9. Computed tomography (CT) scan (coronal plane) of the postoperative defect following medial maxillectomy. Note absence of nasoantral party wall, turbinates, and ethmoid labyrinth.

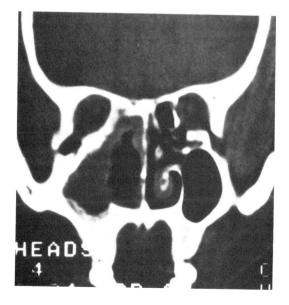

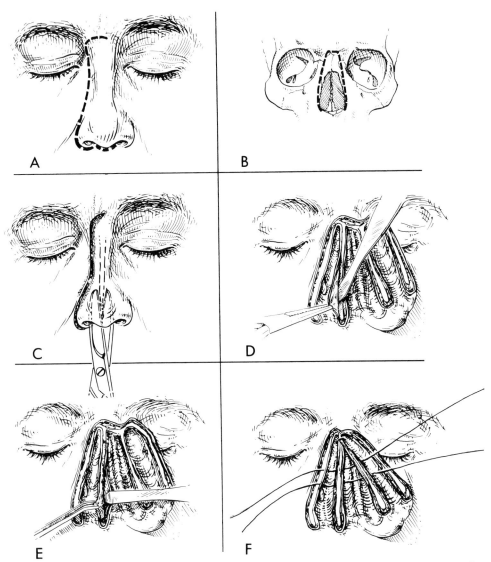

Figure 18–10. Diagram of the total rhinotomy procedure. *A*, Skin incision; *B*, outline of nasal osteotomies; *C*, sectioning of the nasal septum; *D*, submucosal dissection of the septum; *E*, septectomy performed; *F*, repair of the septum.

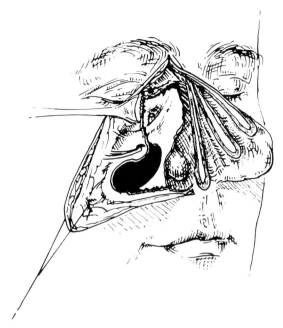

Figure 18–11. Medial maxillectomy combined with total rhinotomy.

a bifrontal craniotomy. The craniotomy is performed through an H-shaped incision in which the upper limb is placed at or behind the hairline and the lower limb transversely above both eyebrows. These two incisions are joined by a vertical limb made in the middle of the forehead, exposing the entire frontal region. The periosteum over the frontal bone is elevated as an inferiorly based flap that is later infolded intracranially to resurface the floor of the anterior cranial fossa (Fig. 18–12C). After the bone flap is removed, the frontal lobes are retracted and the posterior wall of the frontal sinus is removed with a rongeur, so that the anterior bone cut can be made immediately behind the outer table of the frontal sinus. This permits complete resection of the floor of the anterior cranial fossa in an en bloc fashion. Preservation of the nasal process of the frontal bone provides a point of fixation for reattachment of the nasal pyramid, preventing nasal collapse with its attendant functional and cos-

bones. These incisions are joined by a transverse limb made across the glabellar region (Fig. 18–12A).

The periosteum along the medial aspect of the orbit is incised and elevated toward the lacrimal fossa. The medial canthal ligament is detached, and the lacrimal sac is dislocated from its fossa. The sac is sharply transected and the cut end marsupialized. The periorbita is further elevated until the anterior ethmoid artery is identified in the frontoethmoidal suture line, and it is electrocoagulated and divided. The periosteum is then incised along the frontal processes of the maxilla and across the nasofrontal suture line. Lateral osteotomies are made low along the frontal processes of the maxilla. The bony nasal pyramid is completely detached by dividing the nasal bones at the glabella. After the septum is transected, the nose can be reflected downward, hinged inferiorly by its soft tissue attachments (Fig. 18–12B). Care is taken to leave sufficient dorsal cartilaginous septum to serve as a strut as is oncologically feasible. The superior rhinotomy then can be combined with unilateral or bilateral medial maxillectomies, depending on the extent of disease.

With nasoethmoidal tumors that are contiguous with the floor of the anterior cranial fossa or have demonstrable intracranial extension, the superior rhinotomy can be combined with

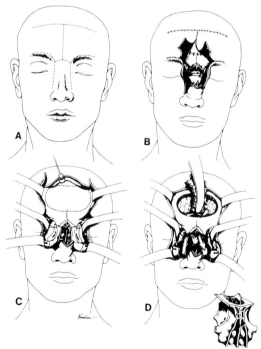

Figure 18–12. Diagram of the superior rhinotomy procedure. *A,* Outline of the incisions made for the superior rhinotomy and craniotomy. *B,* The nasal pyramid is detached and reflected downward, and the medial orbital walls are exposed bilaterally. *C,* The bony cuts of the bilateral medial maxillectomy and frontal craniotomy are outlined. *D,* The frontal lobes have been exposed and are retracted, all the bone cuts have been made, and the detached specimen is delivered downward into the nasal cavity. The resected specimen is represented at lower right.

metic deformities. The lateral and posterior intracranial bone cuts are determined by the extent of the tumor. The superior bone cuts of the bilateral medial maxillectomies are joined to the intracranial bone cuts under direct visualization. The remainder of the medial maxillectomy is performed in standard fashion and the en bloc specimen is delivered downward and outward (Fig. 18–12D). After resection of the tumor, the medial canthal ligaments are sutured to each other with a nonabsorbable (2-0 nylon or proline) suture. The nasal pyramid is wired to the frontal bone. The subcutaneous tissues and skin are carefully reapproximated in layers to complete the closure.

COMPLICATIONS

Despite resection of considerable portions of the lateral nasal cavity and medial aspect of the orbit and maxilla, the cosmetic and functional results of the procedure are generally excellent.[5, 17] Crusting within the nasal cavity is troublesome in the immediate postoperative period but subsides after several months as re-epithelialization of the denuded areas occurs.

Detachment of the medial canthal ligament to expose the lacrimal fossa and medial aspect of the orbit carries the risk of displacement of the inner commissure of the eye. Careful approximation of the orbital periosteum is usually sufficient to anchor the ligament. However, Sessions and Humphreys[19] recommended direct wiring of the ligament to the remaining frontal process of the maxilla.

Although the lacrimal sac is transected, catheterization of the canaliculi is unnecessary and epiphora does not result if the margins of the cut end are everted and the sac is allowed to drain freely into the nasal cavity. Among the ten patients of Sessions and Larson[18] in whom an attempt was made to maintain the integrity of the nasolacrimal system, epiphora developed temporarily in two and permanently in two others. Epiphora occurred in only 1 of 16 subsequent patients undergoing section of the lacrimal sac and placement of a polyethylene tube.[19]

Detachment and loss of bone underlying the trochlea seldom produce permanent diplopia, as reattachment of the orbital periosteum is generally sufficient to provide adequate support and function of the superior oblique muscle. The development of a frontal sinus mucocele

results from interruption and stenosis of the nasofrontal duct.[1, 16]

The incision, if properly placed, usually is barely noticeable. However, operation after high-dosage preoperative radiotherapy is accompanied by impaired healing, regional lymphedema, and even the development of a nasocutaneous fistula.

Increased morbidity accompanies the bilateral nasal osteotomies and septal resection of the total rhinotomy.

The nasal pyramid gains its structural support from its attachments laterally and superiorly to the frontal processes of the maxilla and nasal process of the frontal bone, respectively, centrally from the bony and cartilagenous septum, and caudally from the anterior nasal spine. As these buttresses are disrupted, the tendency to nasal collapse is increased. This may take the form of shift of the nasal pyramid, saddle deformity, septal perforation, columellar collapse, or alar retraction (Fig. 18–13). When a medial maxillectomy is performed, lateral nasal support is lost, and the nasal pyramid and overlying soft tissues tend to collapse into the operative cavity. The lateral osteotomy is made low along the face of the maxilla to preserve as much bone as possible in an attempt to counteract this. When a total rhinotomy is performed, transection of the columella and septum further increase this tendency to collapse, especially when a submucous resection has been performed to increase operative exposure in the posterior nasal cavity. Consequently, when the caudal septum is disarticulated from the anterior nasal spine and the septum divided, it is

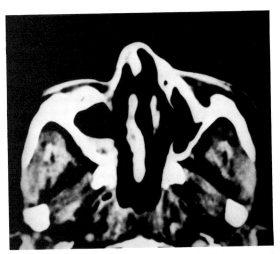

Figure 18–13. CT scan following lateral rhinotomy and medial maxillectomy, revealing collapse of the nasal pyramid into the operative bony defect.

extremely important to leave an adequate dorsal and caudal strut to minimize saddling. In the closure, interosseous wiring of the mobilized nasal pyramid to the frontal bone, suturing the transected septum together, anchoring the caudal end of the septum to the anterior nasal spine, as well as approximating the periosteum and fixing the ala, are essential in achieving nasal stability.

Vestibular stenosis can be avoided by leaving an intact bridge of skin when detaching the ala and dividing the columella in performing the total rhinotomy.

In the series of 220 cases reported by Mertz and colleagues,[1] there was an operative mortality of about 1 per cent. Two patients died of cardiac arrest in the postoperative period. Hemorrhage sufficient to require return to the operating room occurred in two cases. Delayed complications requiring revision surgery arose in 34 patients (15 per cent). Epiphora and ectropion developed in 14 cases, nasal septal abnormalities (adhesions, perforations, deformity) in 8, unsatisfactory scars in 5, cerebrospinal fluid leak in 3, and frontal duct obstruction, frontal mucopyocele, and neuralgia in 1 each.

In our series of 151 cases, 33 patients (21 per cent) developed complications, 17 (11 per cent) of which were early and 24 (16 per cent) occurred late. Among the early complications, 16 patients had blepharitis and marked eyelid edema, 4 had dacryocystitis and epiphora, 3 had cerebrospinal fluid leaks that spontaneously resolved, and 2 had transient diplopia. Among the late complications, ten patients had nasal collapse; six, unacceptable scars; four, persistent crusting and pain; four, dacryostenosis requiring correction; two, vestibular stenosis; two, nasocutaneous fistula; and two developed frontal sinus mucoceles.

The potential complications of the superior rhinotomy are intracranial, orbital, and nasal in nature. We noted a transient cerebrospinal fluid leak in one patient, which spontaneously resolved. Careful repair of dural tears and reconstruction of the floor of the anterior cranial fossa with a pedicled periosteal flap following craniofacial resection reduced the incidence of this complication and meningitis. The potential for orbital complications is greater because, in providing exposure of both ethmoids, the superior rhinotomy places both optic nerves at risk. The posterior ethmoidal artery is in proximity to the optic nerve, and excessive manipulation or electrocoagulation in this area must be avoided. The anterior ethmoidal artery must also be meticulously cauterized or ligated to prevent retrobulbar hemorrhage and visual loss. As with the lateral rhinotomy, the nasolacrimal duct is marsupialized to prevent stenosis and secondary epiphora, only with this procedure it is done bilaterally. Pseudohypertelorism is prevented by attaching the medial canthal ligaments to each other with nonabsorbable suture. The nasal complications include scarring and nasal deformity. Even with careful approximation of the nasal pyramid to the frontal bone with stainless steel wires, nasal collapse may occur.

References

1. Mertz JS, Pearson BW, Kern EB: Lateral rhinotomy; Indications, technique and review of 226 cases. Arch Otolaryngol 109:236, 1983.
2. Bruns P: Eine neue Methode der temporaren (osteoplastichen) Resection der ausseren Nase zur Entfernung von Nasen-Rachenpolypen. Berl Klin Wochenschr 9:137, 149, 1872.
3. Bordley JE, Longmire WP: Rhinotomy for exploration of the nasal passages and accessory nasal sinuses. Ann Otol 58:1055, 1949.
4. Bordley JE, Cherry J: The use of the rhinotomy operation in nasal surgery. Case reports. Laryngoscope 70:258, 1960.
5. Doyle PJ: Approach to tumors of the nose, nasopharynx and paranasal sinuses. Laryngoscope 78:1756, 1968.
6. Devine KD: The rhinologic approach. In Henderson JW (ed): Orbital Tumors. Philadelphia, WB Saunders, 1973.
7. Djalilian M, Zujko RD, Weiland LH, Devine KD: Olfactory neuroblastoma. Surg Clin North Am 57:751, 1977.
8. Neel HB, Whicker JH, Devine KD, Weiland LH: Juvenile angiofibroma. Review of 120 cases. Am J Surg 126:547, 1973.
9. Bremer JW, Neel HB, DeSanto LW, Jones GC: Angiofibroma: Treatment trends in 150 patients during 40 years. Laryngoscope 96:1321, 1986.
10. Vrabec DP: The inverted schneiderian papilloma, a clinical and pathological study. Laryngoscope 85:186, 1975.
11. Suh KW, Facer GW, Devine KD, et al: Inverting papilloma of the nose and paranasal sinuses. Laryngoscope 87:35, 1977.
12. Schramm VL, Myers EN: Lateral rhinotomy. Laryngoscope 88:1042, 1978.
13. Myers EN, Schramm VL, Barnes EL: Management of inverted papilloma of the nose and paranasal sinuses. Laryngoscope 91:2071, 1981.
14. Calcaterra TC, Thompson JW, Paglia DE: Inverting papillomas of the nose and paranasal sinuses. Laryngoscope 90:53, 1980.
15. Mabry RL, Fincher GG: Extended lateral rhinotomy for resection of malignant melanoma. South Med J 67:65, 1974.
16. Harrison DF: Lateral rhinotomy: A neglected operation. Ann Otol 86:745, 1977.
17. Pope TH: Surgical approach to tumors of the nasal cavity. Laryngoscope 88:1743, 1978.
18. Sessions RB, Larson DL: En bloc ethmoidectomy and medial maxillectomy. Arch Otolaryngol 103:195, 1977.

19. Sessions RB, Humphreys DH: Technical modifications of the medial maxillectomy. Arch Otolaryngol 109:575, 1983.
20. Bridger GP: Radical surgery for ethmoid cancer. Arch Otolaryngol 106:630, 1980.
21. Barton RT: Management of carcinoma arising in the lateral nasal wall. Arch Otolaryngol 106:685, 1980.
22. McGuirt WF, Thompson JN: Surgical approach to malignant tumors of the nasal septum. Laryngoscope 94:1045, 1984.
23. Biller HF, Lawson W, Slotnik D, Green R: The superior rhinotomy for the en bloc resection of bilateral ethmoid disease. Arch Otolaryng 115:1463–1466, 1989.
24. Proust R: La chirugie de l'hypophyse. J Chir (Paris) 7:665, 1908.
25. Schramm VL, Myers EN, Maroon JC: Anterior skull base surgery for benign and malignant disease. Laryngoscope 89:1077, 1984.
26. Hassard AD, Holness RO: The "crossbow" incision and nasal flap—its blood supply and clinical application. Head Neck Surg 7:135, 1984.

CHAPTER 19

THE MIDFACIAL DEGLOVING APPROACH TO THE PARANASAL SINUSES AND SKULL BASE

John C. Price, MD

Wayne M. Koch, MD

The surgical approach selected for any operative procedure must provide direct visualization and access for instrumentation. Thorough extirpation of disease is the first priority. Exposure must also be adequate to ensure safe control of major blood vessels and preservation of adjacent vital structures. These things being equal, factors such as cosmesis, operative time, and ease of performance may influence the selection of one approach over another.

Nowhere are concerns for cosmesis, safety, and preservation of vital function more pertinent than with surgery of the nose, skull base, and paranasal sinuses. Located deep to the midface, at the roof of the aerodigestive tract and the base of the skull, surgical procedures in this region offer a unique challenge to the otolaryngologist–head and neck surgeon. The proliferation of surgical approaches, some of which are quite extreme, attests to the inaccessibility of lesions in this area.

The midfacial degloving procedure provides excellent exposure while avoiding facial scars and preserving function, making it a nearly ideal approach for the management of lesions in the paranasal sinuses. The procedure consists of release of the nasal soft tissues as performed in rhinoplasty, combined with bilateral anterior maxillary exposure. Lesions of the nasal cavity; nasal septum; maxillary, ethmoid, and sphenoid sinuses; nasopharynx; and clivus may be managed via this approach. Anterior and middle skull base tumors may be resected using a combined approach of midfacial degloving and anterior or lateral craniotomy.

HISTORICAL BACKGROUND

En bloc maxillectomy had its origin early in the nineteenth century prior to the use of general anesthesia. John Lizars of Edinburgh first attempted the procedure in 1827 but encountered massive bleeding after incising the palate.[1] The next year James Syme performed the procedure successfully.[2] His description is remarkably similar to that of modern total maxillectomy. Both these early procedures involved the use of facial incisions at the oral commissure and the nasal dorsum in order to expose the maxilla.

A benchmark in the development of access to the sinuses was Fergusson's description of the classic (Weber-Fergusson) incision in 1845.[3] The work of George Caldwell was the foundation for the development of the midfacial degloving approach.[4] Prior to his description of a sublabial maxillary antrostomy in 1893, Zeim and Hunter had entered the antrum via the alveolar ridge or a tooth socket. Caldwell attributes the idea for his procedure to Christopher Heath, who described a canine fossa maxillary antrostomy in 1889. Henri Luc later published a report in the French literature of the same procedure described by Caldwell, although apparently independently devised.[5]

In the twentieth century, the per oral approach was expanded for management of extensive inflammatory disease of the paranasal sinuses. Denker and Kahler advocated removal of the piriform margin to provide greater exposure.[6] A radical maxillectomy performed transorally was described a year later by Portmann and Retrouvey.[7]

Lesions located more posteriorly in the nasopharynx and sphenoid require a more extensive approach. Transpalatal incisions have been used to resect nasopharyngeal angiofibromas and other benign tumors since Wilson's report in 1951.[8] Lateral rhinotomy for maxilloethmoidal disease, such as inverted papilloma, was described by Doyle in 1968.[9] In combination with a sublabial incision, these procedures can be used to reach the entire complement of nasal, nasopharyngeal, and paranasal sinus lesions.[10, 11] Midline mandibuloglossotomy, a more radical transoral-transpalatal procedure, has been described by Biller and Lawson.[12]

The lateral skull base approach is an alternative to the midfacial concept for the management of tumors of the nasopharynx. Samy and Girgis described a transzygomatic procedure in 1965.[13] In the next year, Ross and Sukis described a similar transmandibulopterygoid approach.[14] Fisch approaches virtually all lesions of the nasopharynx and posterior paranasal sinuses via the infratemporal fossa approach.[15] A facial degloving procedure was first suggested by Portmann,[7] but the modern technique had its origin in 1974 with the report of Casson, Bonnano, and Converse.[16] Their brief report related the application of the procedure for facial trauma and reconstruction. Conley and Price first suggested the use of the midfacial degloving procedure for excisions of neoplastic disease in 1979.[17] Subsequently, the procedure has been used for the removal of benign lesions, such as inverting papilloma[18] and nasopharyngeal angiofibroma,[19] and for limited malignant disease.[20]

Price employed the midfacial degloving procedure for access of the central and anterior skull base, as reported in 1986.[21] The following year he published a series of cases performed in conjunction with frontal or temporal craniotomy for craniofacial resection.[22] Modifications of the midfacial degloving approach have been suggested by several workers. Paavolainen and Malmberg extended the access to the entire nasal vault by using lateral nasal osteotomies and septal transection to release the entire nasal piriform.[23] Belmont added a LeFort I osteotomy to increase exposure of the clivus.[24]

PREOPERATIVE CONSIDERATIONS

Computed tomography or magnetic resonance imaging is invaluable for surgical planning. The margins of resections can be estimated accurately in many cases. Ophthalmologic and neurosurgical consultations are requested as needed. If partial palatectomy is planned, dental impressions should be made several days prior to surgery so that an obturator is ready at the time of the procedure.

A curved endotracheal tube secured to the midline of the chin is used to administer general anesthesia. The use of a neurosurgical head rest or folded cloth towels as a head rest permits intraoperative adjustments of head position. The nasal mucosa is treated with 4 per cent cocaine solution on cotton pledgets for vasoconstriction. Injection of 1 per cent lidocaine with 1:100,000 epinephrine into planned intranasal and sublabial incisions and the canine fossa further ensures local hemostasis. Bilateral tarsorrhaphies or corneal shields are placed, followed by a standard surgical preparation. A head drape is positioned (taking into account the neurosurgeon's needs in the event of craniofacial resection). The use of a head lamp is essential. A donor site should be selected and draped for skin or dermal graft for intranasal covering of any dural repair.

OPERATIVE PROCEDURE

Using a columellar clamp for retraction, a full standard transfixion incision is carried out (Fig. 19–1). This must extend from high in the tip of the nose onto the nasal floor, sweeping posteriorly near its completion. The inside of the nasal tip is fully exposed with a double ball retractor or alar guard. Intercartilaginous incisions join the superior end of the transfixion incision medially. These incisions extend beyond the lateral margin of the upper lateral cartilages. Full-thickness incision down through the periosteum of the piriform margin and nasal

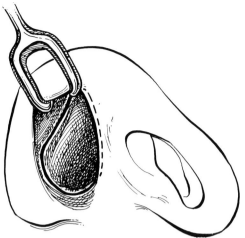

Figure 19–1. Intranasal incisions. A full transfixion incision is connected with intercartilaginous, pyriform, and nasal floor incisions bilaterally.

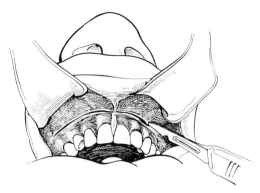

Figure 19–3. The sublabial incision extends to the first molar tooth on each side. Incision placement is such that a cuff of loose labial mucosa remains on the gingival side to facilitate closure.

floor complete the circumvestibular release. These incisions should be placed at the limen vestibuli, the junction of stratified squamous and columnar epithelium. Of course, caudal extension of disease may necessitate modification of incision design.

Dissection through the intercartilaginous incision exposes the dorsum of the upper lateral cartilage that leads to the nasal bones. The periosteum is incised with a curved Joseph knife, and soft tissues are widely elevated (Fig. 19–2). Elevation extends laterally to the nasomaxillary sutures and superiorly to the glabella.

All adhesions between the nasal skeleton and soft tissue must be released to allow full elevation.

The sublabial incision may be made with a No. 10 blade or Bovie electrocautery (Fig. 19–3). The incision is carried down through the periosteum of the canine fossa. It should be designed so as to leave a cuff of loose tissue on the gingival side to allow for closure. The standard incision from one first molar to the contralateral first molar may be extended unilaterally around the maxillary tuberosity and onto the soft palate. This extension provides access to the pterygomaxillary space for palatectomy or total maxillectomy. Soft tissue over the anterior maxilla is elevated in the subperiosteal plane, extending widely to the zygoma and up to the infraorbital rim (Fig. 19–4). The lateral surface

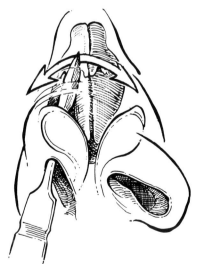

Figure 19–2. Elevation of nasal soft tissue in a subperiosteal plane is carried out through the intercartilaginous incisions bilaterally. Care must be taken not to separate the upper lateral cartilages from the nasal bones.

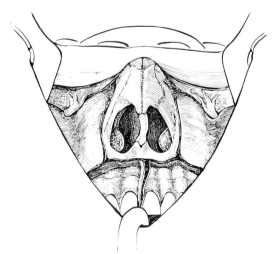

Figure 19–4. Wide subperiosteal dissection permits elevation of the midfacial soft tissues. Adhesions between maxillary and nasal tunnels must be released.

of the maxilla and pterygomaxillary space may also be exposed, although the buccal fat pad is encountered here and will make visualization more difficult. Superiorly, the neurovascular bundle of the infraorbital nerve is visualized and carefully preserved if not involved by malignancy. The nasal floor and sublabial incisions are connected, working through the nose with a spreading motion of Metzenbaum scissors. Army-Navy retractors lift malar and nasal soft tissues, exposing residual periosteal adhesions at the nasomaxillary junction. These are lysed with scissors held firmly against the bone. Full retraction of the facial soft tissues, including the upper lip, intact columella, and nasal tip, is possible up to the level of the medial canthus. Richardson or Jones antrostomy retractors with a self-retaining device, if desired, may be used to maintain exposure during resection of diseased tissue.

Details of the extirpation of disease must be individualized to ensure adequate margins. The anterior wall of the maxilla is resected to expose the lesion. This may be done in a piecemeal fashion with Kerrison rongeurs unless malignant disease fills the antrum. The antrostomy may extend from the zygoma to the nasal aperture, and from the infraorbital rim, sparing the nerve, to the floor of the antrum. Care must be taken to avoid injury to undescended permanent maxillary teeth in children. At the nasomaxillary process, the antrostomy may be extended superiorly to the level of the medial canthus. In the setting of malignancy involving the anterior-inferior maxilla, osteotomies block out the lesion with the anterior wall undisturbed to provide bony margins. Medial or subtotal maxillectomy, complete ethmoidectomy, and sphenoidectomy are accomplished in a sequential fashion.

Removal of the lateral nasal wall exposes the septum in its entirety. After incising the ipsilateral septal mucosa along the nasal floor, releasing the cartilage from the maxillary crest and elevating the mucoperiosteum off the contralateral nasal floor, the septum may be deflected away from the side of the lesion. The septum may be partially or totally removed, although it is highly desirable to preserve a dorsal and caudal strut to provide tip support.

By extending the patient's head 30 degrees, the cribriform plate may be brought into view to facilitate craniofacial resection (done in conjunction with frontal craniotomy) or to inspect the region for dural tears or cerebrospinal fluid (CSF). The maxillary antrostomy, ethmoidectomy, and sphenoidectomy may be repeated on the opposite side, although the maxillary-frontal bony buttress should be preserved on one side to support the midface.

Resection of the posterior wall of the maxillary antrum and the ascending process of the palatine bone affords full access to the nasopharynx and clivus. An otologic drill with large cutting bur is quite useful for this step. Brisk bleeding will be encountered when the palatine artery is disrupted at the greater palatine foramen. Bipolar electrocautery is usually adequate to achieve hemostasis. The pterygoid plates and muscles, posterior wall of the sphenoid sinus, and clivus are thus exposed. A large, coarse diamond bur under microscopic visualization will safely resect the pterygoid plate and the clivus as far as the optic nerve and chiasm. The posterior limit of resection includes these structures, as well as the dura of the pituitary and the posterior cranial fossa. The petrous apex must be reached by a lateral skull base approach. Anterior approach to this area is limited by the carotid arteries laterally and the optic nerve superiorly.

Rough bony contours and spicules are smoothed using a large diamond bur. A temporary pack of gauze soaked in 1 per cent Neosynephrine or 1:100,000 epinephrine diluted 1:10 in normal saline provides initial hemostasis. Meticulous control of bleeding points with bipolar current is then performed. Absorbable thrombostatic powder or sheets may be necessary for areas of diffuse and persistent bleeding.

A dermal or split thickness skin graft is applied to the undersurface of the pericranial flap or dural repair if either has been necessary. A contoured gel-film support is placed beneath the graft and 0.5 inch of antibiotic ointment–soaked gauze is packed firmly into the cavity. The end of the packing strip is passed out through the nostril.

Closure of the nasal incision begins with 3–0 chromic transfixion stitches. The precise placement of this suture is critical in that it determines the final position of the nasal tip. The circumvestibular incisions are carefully reapproximated with three or more 4–0 polyglycolic acid sutures placed at the intercartilaginous, piriform, and nasal floor areas. Closure of the sublabial incision begins with precise reapproximation at the frenulum. It may be completed in a running interlocking or interrupted fashion, using 3–0 chromic or polyglycologic acid material. The skin is washed and dried and benzoin applied, followed by rhinoplastic taping and splinting.

POSTOPERATIVE CARE

Packing is removed in stages, beginning 3 or 4 days postoperatively. The patient should be maintained on antibiotics until all packing is out. Intranasal crusting will occur for several months after surgery until epithelium grows over granulation tissue to line the cavity. Initially, frequent removal of all crusting is necessary. The patient should irrigate the cavity four times a day with a Water-Pic or bulb syringe, starting as soon as the packing has been removed.

COMPLICATIONS

The maxilla and skull base are highly vascular, and operative blood loss often necessitates transfusion. Postoperative nasal dorsum hematomas have developed in patients with a bleeding diathesis. Facial swelling and orbital septal ecchymosis are common in the immediate postoperative period.

The removal of the nasal turbinates and subsequent crust formation might be expected to result in ozena, but this has not been reported thus far. Patients do experience subjective nasal dryness, and some crusting continues for years. Epiphora may occur transiently in the postoperative period while swelling and crusting persist. If the nasal frontal recess and ethmoid or sphenoid ostia have not been widely opened, sinusitis may result.

Anesthesia and paresthesia of the infraorbital and alveolar nerves are the most frequent causes of postoperative complaints. Unless the infraorbital nerve was resected for oncologic purposes, sensation should return within 3 to 6 months.

Excessive scar formation under the nose and maxilla may result in a "sneer" deformity. Polybeak or excessive alar show (snout deformity) is the result of improper transfixion suture position. Vestibular narrowing is commonly seen early during healing but uniformly resolves without treatment. Rare cases of vestibular stenosis have been reported, probably resulting from improper closure of the circumvestibular incision. Other potential problems, such as abnormal facial growth in children and oroantral fistulas, have not been reported.

SPECIAL PRECAUTIONS

Unlike the case in external rhinoplasty, no incision should be made across the columella.

Care must be taken to avoid injury to the delicate lower lateral cartilages and the alar skin margins when making vestibular incisions.

The rich blood supply to the midface (facial, infraorbital, supratrochlear, and transverse facial arteries) allows the surgeon to perform medial orbital, brow, or lip-splitting incisions in addition to midfacial degloving, if necessary. Blood loss may be minimized by the judicious use of topical and injected vasoconstrictive agents. Unnecessary hemorrhage will result if elevation of soft tissues from the facial skeleton is not performed in the proper subperiosteal plane.

The infraorbital nerve, together with the bony foramen and canal, may be released by carefully placed osteotomies on either side, extending up to and along the orbital floor. This improves the mobility of the cheek flap and provides greater access to the orbit.

Lesions involving the anterior ethmoidal labyrinth, nasofrontal recess, and frontal sinus cannot be adequately exposed using the degloving approach alone. A frontoethmoid, brow, or bicoronal incision, in combination with midfacial degloving, or the selection of an entirely different approach is required.

All exposed spicules of bone within the paranasal sinuses should be smoothed at the end of the procedure. Retained fragments serve as a nidus for osteitis. The nasofrontal recess and sphenoid sinus should be widely open to ensure adequate drainage. Postoperative sinusitis owing to edema and crusting is thus avoided. Nasal packing stimulates the development of granulation tissue. After the packing has been removed, multiple daily irrigations with normal saline and application of a eucalyptus-based nasal emollient (such as Ponaris) reduces the amount of crusting. Postoperatively, patients should be seen in the clinic once or twice weekly for endoscopic removal of crusts.

DISCUSSION

Surgical access to the midface and anterior skull base has improved dramatically over the past 30 years, allowing satisfactory extirpation of inflammatory, benign, and malignant neoplastic disease as well as repair of facial fractures and congenital malformations. A major contributing factor has been the development of the midfacial degloving approach. Maxillary operations can now be among the least debilitating and deforming procedures performed in a head and neck practice. The degloving procedure has become a staple in the armamentarium of the otolaryngologist–head and neck surgeon. It offers adequate exposure with rapid, easy access and closure, while sparing vital function and producing no facial scarring. Whereas the lack of a facial incision may be the primary advantage of degloving over other approaches to the region, we find that the overall surgical facility it offers is superior to lateral rhinotomy. Bilateral exposure is provided for larger midline lesions or disease involving multiple sinuses. However, when the zygoma is involved by disease and a far lateral exposure is required, we still would use the Weber-Fergusson incision.

Midfacial degloving is ideally suited for management of benign pathologic conditions, such as inverted papilloma. The lateral nasal wall may be removed en bloc, providing excellent access to the maxillary antrum and ethmoid and sphenoid sinuses (Fig. 19–5). Limited intranasal or antral procedures formerly used for inverted papilloma should be discouraged, because of the propensity for these lesions to recur. Extensive disease involving the frontal sinus, orbit, or skull base cannot be managed via midfacial degloving alone and may require craniofacial resection (Fig. 19–6).

Degloving also has several advantages over alternative approaches for juvenile nasopharyngeal angiofibroma. Bilateral maxillary sinusotomies provide access to both internal maxillary arteries for ligation. Exposure of extension of disease into the paranasal sinuses is more difficult via a transpalatal approach. The site of origin for nasopharyngeal angiofibroma, the pharyngobasilar fascia over the clivus, is widely exposed after medial maxillectomy and ethmoidectomy. Adequate room is provided for the use of the otologic drill, bipolar cautery,

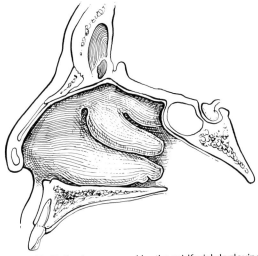

Figure 19–5. Region exposed by the midfacial degloving technique; sagittal view.

and other instrumentation necessary for a safe and complete extirpation of disease. Endoscopic postoperative examination for recurrent disease surveillance is facilitated by the large sinonasal cavity established.

Facial reconstruction, repair of maxillary fractures, and recontouring of the maxilla in cases of fibrous dysphasia are other applications for the degloving procedure. Large, benign neoplasms and small, malignant neoplasms of the paranasal sinuses are appropriate settings as well. With careful attention to detail and proper patient selection, midfacial degloving is employed frequently in our practice with excellent results. We believe it to be the approach of choice for many surgical problems involving the midface.

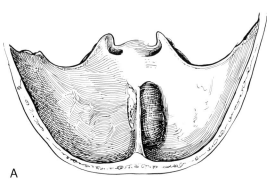

A

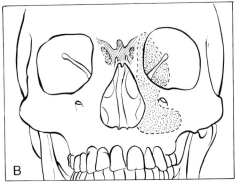

B

Figure 19–6. Craniofacial resection. Tumors at the anterior and midskull base may be approached from below, using the degloving technique, and resected in conjunction with anterior or lateral craniotomy. *A,* Superior resection margins are obtained via the craniotomy exposure. *B,* Tumor in the sinuses is resected by medial or total maxillectomy and complete ethmoidectomy.

References

1. Lizars J: Excision of the upper jaw bones. Lancet 2:54–55, 1829–1830.
2. Syme J: Excision of the upper jaw bone. Lancet 2:677–678, 1828–1829.
3. Fergusson W: Operations of the upper jaw. *In* A System of Practical Surgery. 2nd ed. Philadelphia, Lea and Blanchard, 1845.
4. Caldwell GW: Diseases of the accessory sinuses of the nose and an improved method of treatment for suppuration of the maxillary antrum. NY Med J 58:526–528, 1893.
5. Luc H: Une nouvelle methode operatoire pour la cure radicale et rapide de l'empyeme chronique du sinus maxillaire. Rev Int Rhinol Otol Laryngol (Paris) viii:158–168, 1898.
6. Denker A, Kahler O: Handbuch der Hals-Nasen-Ohren-Heibunde. Berlin, Springer, 1926.
7. Portmann G, Retrouvey H: Le Cancer du Nez. Paris, Gaston Doin et Cie, 1927.
8. Wilson CP: The approach to the nasopharynx. Proc R Soc Med 44:353, 1951.
9. Doyle PJ: Approach to tumors of the nose, nasopharynx and paranasal sinuses. Laryngoscope 78:1756–1762, 1968.
10. Bhatia ML, Mishra SC, Prabash J: Lateral extensions of nasopharyngeal fibroma. J Laryngol Otol 81:99–106, 1967.
11. Butler RM, Nahum AM, Hanafee WJ: New surgical approach to nasopharyngeal angiofibroma. Trans Am Acad Ophthalmol Otolaryngol 71:92, 1967.
12. Biller HF, Lawson W: Anterior mandibular-splitting approach to the skull base. Ear Nose Throat J 65:61, 1986.
13. Samy LL, Girgis IH: Transzygomatic approach for nasopharyngeal fibromata with extrapharyngeal extension. J Laryngol 70:782–795, 1965.
14. Ross DE, Sukis AE: Nasopharyngeal tumors: A new surgical approach. Am J Surg 11:524–530, 1966.
15. Fisch U: Infratemporal fossa approach for extensive tumors of the temporal bone and base of the skull. *In* Silverstein H, Norrell N (eds): Neurological Surgery of the Ear. Birmingham, Aesculapius Publishers, 1977, p 34.
16. Casson PR, Bonnano PC, Converse JM: The midfacial degloving procedure. Plast Reconstr Surg 53:102–103, 1974.
17. Conley J, Price JC: Sublabial approach to the nasal and nasopharyngeal cavities. Am J Surg 38:615–618, 1979.
18. Sachs ME, et al: The degloving approach for total excision of inverted papilloma. Laryngoscope 94:1595–1598, 1984.
19. Terzian AE, Naconecy C: Juvenile nasopharyngeal angiofibroma; Microsurgical approach in 25 cases as unique treatment. *In* New Dimensions in Otorhinolaryngology–Head and Neck Surgery. New York, BV Excerpta Medica, 1985.
20. Maniglia AJ: Indications and techniques of midfacial degloving, a 15-year experience. Arch Otolaryngol Head Neck Surg 112:750–752, 1986.
21. Price JC: The midfacial degloving approach to the central skull base. Ear Nose Throat J 65:46–53, 1986.
22. Price JC: Facial degloving. *In* Goldman JL (ed): Rhinology. New York, John Wiley, 1987, p 1098.
23. Paavolainen M, Malmberg H: Sublabial approach to the nasal and paranasal cavities using nasal pyramid osteotomy and septal transection. Laryngoscope 96:106–108, 1986.
24. Belmont JR: LeFort I osteotomy approach to nasopharyngeal and nasal fossa tumors. Arch Otolaryngol Head Neck Surg 114:751–754, 1988.

CHAPTER 20

TOTAL MAXILLECTOMY

Soly Baredes, MD
Hyun T. Cho, MD
Max L. Som, MD*

The maxillary sinus (antrum of Highmore) is the largest of the paranasal sinuses and the one most frequently involved with malignant tumors. Nearly 80 per cent of sinus malignancies arise in the antrum, 20 per cent in the ethmoid sinuses, and less than 1 per cent in the frontal and sphenoid sinuses.[1-8] The close anatomic relationship of the ethmoid to the antrum often results in early invasion of the ethmoid labyrinth; therefore, many maxillary sinus tumors are, in fact, antroethmoid.[9]

Tumors in this region are not common. Antral carcinoma, for example, is estimated to affect less than 1 of 200,000 people per year in the United States.[10] Malignancies of the maxillary sinus are seen more often in men than in women in a ratio approaching two to one.[1, 11, 12] They are rare before age 30 years, and the majority are noted in the sixth and seventh decades of life.[2, 6, 12] The right and left antrum appear equally susceptible to malignancies.[2, 12, 13]

Cancers of the maxillary sinus are highly lethal, in part because they are often diagnosed at an advanced stage. Effective therapy often depends on close cooperation between surgeon and radiotherapist. The surgical management is based on a thorough understanding of the intricate anatomy of this region.

CLASSIFICATION OF MAXILLARY SINUS TUMORS

A uniform system of classification is important in planning therapy and in evaluating and communicating the results of treatment. Several clinical classifications have been proposed for maxillary sinus malignancies.[5, 14-21] Sebileau[14] first attempted to classify maxillary cancers in 1906. With the floor of the antrum as the dividing line, he separated the maxilla into a suprastructure and an infrastructure and noted that infrastructure tumors were more amenable to therapy. He later also referred to a midportion of the maxilla, or mesostructure, but the exact level of this subdivision was not made clear.[20] Ohngren[15] in 1933 divided the antrum into posterosuperior and anteroinferior segments by a line drawn on lateral section from the inner canthus of the eye to the angle of the mandible. He suggested that this represented a "malignancy plane," with tumors in the posterosuperior segment having a poorer prognosis. No doubt this was because tumors in this region present later and are more intimately related to vital structures such as the orbit, cribriform plate, and pterygoid region.[19]

Huet and Stefani,[16] in 1960 in France, and Sisson and colleagues,[17] in 1963 in America, proposed using the TNM system to classify cancers of the antrum. The extent of the primary tumor (T) was based on tumor location and involvement of particular surrounding structures. Lederman[5] elaborated Sebileau's original classification and adapted it to the TNM system. He separated the maxilla into a suprastructure, mesostructure, and infrastructure by drawing two parallel lines across a frontal section of the skull, with the upper line passing through the floor of the orbit and the lower through the floor of the antrum (Fig. 20–1). Further subdivision was obtained by dropping a vertical line down from the medial wall of the

*Deceased

orbit, separating the ethmoid sinuses and nasal fossa from the antrum.

Only as recently as 1976 did the American Joint Committee on Cancer develop a TNM classification for tumors of the maxillary sinus—Ohngren's line is used to divide the antrum into an infrastructure and suprastructure and the primary tumor classified accordingly. As with previous classifications, the emphasis is on tumor site and degree of involvement of adjacent structures. Early versions of this classification were criticized for failing to relate T categories to clinical experience.[19] The TNM classification published in 1988 (Tables 20–1 and 20–2), however, relates well to clinical experience and is a useful tool in the management and study of maxillary sinus tumors.[21]

We have found Lederman's anatomic subdivisions to be very useful in determining the surgical therapy to be applied in cases of maxillary sinus tumors. Tumors of the infrastructure are almost always amenable to subtotal maxillectomy. Mesostructure tumors require total maxillectomy, but the orbital contents usually can be preserved. Suprastructure tumors usually require total maxillectomy with orbital exenteration, and possibly craniofacial resection.

Topographic classifications such as those described are, of course, limited in that they do not consider tumor histology or the specific host-tumor relationship. Ohngren attempted to include tumor histology in his classification, but the end-result was cumbersome and impractical.

Despite meticulous clinical examination and sophisticated imaging techniques, it is not always possible to determine fully the extent of disease prior to surgery. This is additionally complicated by the multicentric origin of some tumors. In a sense, every maxillectomy is an exploratory procedure in which possible invasion of contiguous structures is evaluated and the surgery modified accordingly.

PATIENT EVALUATION

History. Maxillary sinus cancer tends to be quiescent in its early stages, interfering with no physiologic function. It becomes apparent when it reaches a significant size and affects structures that are contiguous with the bony walls of the sinus—the orbit superiorly, the palate and alveolar ridge inferiorly, the cheek anteriorly, the pterygopalatine and infratemporal fossae posteriorly, and the nose medially. Because these tumors are rare and mimic many benign conditions, and because the early symptoms are nonspecific, there is generally a low index of suspicion for malignancies of the maxillary sinus. It is not unusual, therefore, for a patient with an antral carcinoma to be treated for several months for a presumed benign process by a dentist, ophthalmologist, neurologist, or otolaryngologist.

The usual presenting symptoms are pain and swelling about the cheek.[1, 5, 12] Nasal symptoms, including obstruction, bleeding, and discharge, are also common complaints. Alveolar and palatal swelling and ulceration, proptosis, diplopia, and epiphora are seen less frequently. Involvement of the infraorbital nerve with numbness of the upper cheek is an occasional initial com-

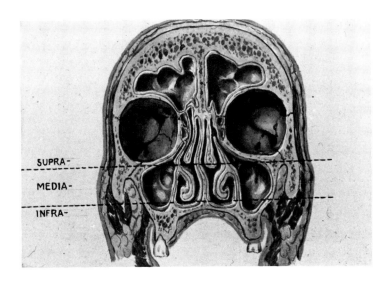

Figure 20–1. Separation of maxilla into suprastructure, meso- or mediastructure, and infrastructure by two parallel lines.

TABLE 20–1. TNM Classifications of Antral Cancer

Primary Tumor (T)

TX Primary tumor cannot be assessed

T0 No evidence of primary tumor

Tis Carcinoma *in situ*

T1 Tumor limited to the antral mucosa with no erosion or destruction of bone

T2 Tumor with erosion or destruction of the infrastructure, including the hard palate and/or the middle nasal meatus

T3 Tumor invades any of the following: skin of cheek, posterior wall of maxillary sinus, floor or medial wall of orbit, anterior ethmoid sinus

T4 Tumor invades orbital contents and/or any of the following: cribriform plate, posterior ethmoid or sphenoid sinuses, nasopharynx, soft palate, pterygomaxillary or temporal fossae, or base of skull

Regional Lymph Nodes (N)

NX Regional lymph nodes cannot be assessed

N0 No regional lymph node metastasis

N1 Metastasis in a single ipsilateral lymph node, 3 cm or less in greatest dimension

N2 Metastasis in a single ipsilateral lymph node, more than 3 cm but not more than 6 cm in greatest dimension, or in multiple ipsilateral lymph nodes, none more than 6 cm in greatest dimension, or in bilateral or contralateral dimension, or in bilateral or contralateral lymph nodes, none more than 6 cm in greatest dimension

    N2a Metastasis in a single ipsilateral lymph node more than 3 cm but not more than 6 cm in greatest dimension

    N2b Metastasis in multiple ipsilateral lymph nodes, none more than 6 cm in greatest dimension

    N2c Metastasis in bilateral or contralateral lymph nodes, none more than 6 cm in greatest dimension

N3 Metastasis in a lymph node more than 6 cm in greatest dimension

Distant Metastasis (M)

MX Presence of distant metastasis cannot be assessed

M0 No distant metastasis

M1 Distant metastasis

(From American Joint Committee on Cancer: Manual for Staging of Cancer. 3rd ed. Edited by Beahrs OH, Henson DE, Hutter RVP, and Myers M. Philadelphia, J.B. Lippincott, 1988.)

plaint. Bleeding appears to be more common when the sinus is involved with a malignant melanoma.[6] In general, however, the anatomic extent of the tumor, rather than the specific type of histology, determines symptoms. The majority of patients will have combinations of symptoms suggesting multiple antral wall involvement.[12]

A history of Thorotrast (thorium dioxide) injection into the sinus is known to predispose an individual to the development of carcinoma.[22, 23] Before its carcinogenic properties were identified, this radioactive, radiopaque material was instilled into the sinus for diagnostic purposes. The latent period for the devel-

opment of carcinoma following exposure is 10 to 20 years. The retained Thorotrast is usually visible on routine sinus radiographs.

Woodworkers in the furniture industry in England have a high incidence of adenocarcinoma of the nose and sinuses.[24] This has been attributed to the chronic inhalation of wood dust. The latency period is usually about 40 years, although wood dust-related cancers have been noted as few as 5 years following exposure. Higher incidences of nasal and sinus carcinoma also have been described among workers in the boot and shoe industry in England,[25] nickel workers in South Wales,[26] and the Bantu of South Africa who are known to use a carcinogenic snuff.[27] Tobacco use may be associated with a higher risk for squamous cell carcinoma of the paranasal sinuses, although this association is not as clear as with other sites in the head and neck.[28]

It has also been suggested that chronic sinusitis can cause a metaplasia of the respiratory epithelium and that antral carcinomas may arise from this altered epithelium.[29] There has been little clinical evidence, however, to support the notion that individuals with chronic inflammatory disease have a higher incidence of maxillary sinus malignancies.

Physical Examination. A careful physical examination will yield much information regarding the extent of the lesion, the required surgery, and chance for cure. Few physical signs are present when the tumor is limited to the antral mucosa. As noted previously, however, few patients are fortunate enough to be identified at such an early stage. The majority of patients will have evidence of tumor beyond the confines of the sinus. By carefully examining areas adjacent to the bony walls of the sinus, the extent of disease is determined.

Rhinoscopy readily reveals extension of tumor into the nasal cavity. The lateral wall of

TABLE 20–2. Stage Grouping of Antral Cancer

Stage 0	Tis	N0	M0
Stage I	T1	N0	M0
Stage II	T2	N0	M0
Stage III	T3	N0	M0
	T1	N1	M0
	T2	N1	M0
	T3	N1	M0
Stage IV	T4	N0, N1	M0
	Any T	N2, N3	M0
	Any T	Any N	M1

(From American Joint Committee on Cancer: Manual for Staging of Cancer. 3rd ed. Edited by Beahrs OH, Henson DE, Hutter RVP, and Myers M. Philadelphia, J.B. Lippincott, 1988.)

the nose (medial wall of the sinus) consists of extremely thin bone and is largely dehiscent in the posterior aspect of the medial meatus. Extension into the nose, therefore, is not uncommon and usually occurs via the middle meatus, an observation made by Sebileau in 1906.[4] Extension of tumor into the nasal cavity should be carefully sought, as it may offer easy access for biopsy material without compromising future surgery.

Anterior wall involvement may cause swelling or asymmetry of the face. This wall is accessible to palpation through the gingivobuccal sulcus; bony defects and palpable tumor may be present despite intact overlying mucosa. Fixation or ulceration of the overlying skin also should be noted.

Alveolar or palatal swelling indicates involvement of the floor of the sinus. Fistulous openings into the gingivobuccal sulcus, alveolus, and palate do occur and may be associated with loose teeth. Patients with tumor in this area may have been seen first by a dentist.

Proptosis or diplopia usually indicates invasion of the orbital floor. Infraorbital nerve anesthesia also implies orbital floor invasion, although occasionally it may result from involvement of the nerve at the infraorbital foramen. The lack of infraorbital nerve anesthesia does not rule out orbital invasion, as significant extension of tumor can occur in the medial aspect of the orbit without disturbing the infraorbital canal, which is laterally located along the floor of the orbit.[30] Epiphora may result from partial or complete occlusion of the nasolacrimal duct and is not necessarily an indication of orbital invasion. When the ocular findings are equivocal, an ophthalmologic consultation can be helpful in elucidating the status of the orbit.

Posterior extension of tumor involves structures in the pterygopalatine and infratemporal fossae. Invasion of the medial aspect of the posterior wall of the sinus may cause hypesthesia or anesthesia along the distribution of the greater palatine nerve (ipsilateral gums and hard palate). Ipsilateral decreased tearing may also be noted with involvement of the sphenopalatine ganglion in the pterygopalatine fossa. Extension into the pterygoid fossa will cause trismus by interfering with the function of the medial pterygoid muscle. The posterior and middle superior alveolar nerves course along the infratemporal surface of the sinus, and invasion of tumor in this area may result in numbness of the molar and premolar teeth, respectively.[30] Advanced lesions may extend posteriorly to involve the nasopharynx and eu-stachian tube. They may be associated with an ipsilateral secretory otitis media.

As with all head and neck cancers, assessment of the neck for evidence of regional metastasis is imperative. The lymphatic drainage of the maxillary sinus is via the retropharyngeal, submandibular, and superior deep jugular lymph nodes. Palpable adenopathy is initially present in 3 to 10 per cent of patients.[2, 12, 19, 31–33] Evidence of retropharyngeal node metastasis is not detectable on physical examination, of course, until it is far advanced. The incidence of neck metastasis has been noted to be higher in patients with tumor extension to the oral cavity, either because breakthrough into the oral cavity generally represents more advanced disease or because of the inherent difference in the lymphatic drainage of the oral cavity.[2]

Radiography. Radiographic studies help confirm the physical examination findings and further define the extent of disease. Standard views of the sinuses do not provide sufficient information. Computed tomography (CT) scanning or magnetic resonance imaging (MRI) always should be performed.[34, 35] If tumor is suspected but tissue is not available for biopsy intranasally or intraorally, these studies are obtained prior to any exploratory procedure. The areas of special interest for surgical planning are the ethmoid sinuses, the cribriform plate, the floor and apex of the orbit, and the pterygopalatine and infratemporal fossae.

Biopsy. Material for histologic examination should be obtained in a way that will not compromise a future resection. The majority of patients will have visible tumor extending into the nasal or oral cavities, and a biopsy specimen should be obtained from these sites. If tumor is not present in these areas, an inferior meatal antrostomy for biopsy is preferred to a Caldwell-Luc approach, as the latter has been associated with a higher incidence of tumor implants to the cheek.[31] If a meatal antrostomy does not provide the desired exposure, the sinus should be explored via a limited Caldwell-Luc procedure (mini-Caldwell-Luc operation[36]). The incision should be placed at the inferior portion of the canine fossa to facilitate its removal with the specimen at the time of definitive surgery. The endoscopic approaches to the maxillary sinus can be used effectively to obtain a biopsy of a suspected tumor. Antroscopy and biopsy via the inferior meatal route again are preferable to the canine fossa approach.[37]

More than 80 per cent of maxillary sinus

malignancies are squamous cell carcinomas.[12, 31, 33] Adenocarcinomas, including adenocystic carcinomas and mucoepidermoid carcinomas, constitute up to 10 per cent of malignancies. The remaining tumors include sarcomas, malignant melanomas, lymphomas, plasmacytomas, malignant schwannomas, malignant histiocytomas, and ameloblastomas.

TREATMENT

Once the extent of disease is delineated and the histology identified, decisions can be made regarding treatment. Surgery is the cornerstone of treatment for squamous cell carcinoma (including variants such as transitional cell carcinoma and undifferentiated carcinoma), adenocarcinoma (including tumors of salivary gland origin), malignant melanoma, malignant schwannoma, malignant histiocytoma, ameloblastoma, and sarcomas arising from mesodermal connective tissues, such as fibro-, chondro- or osteosarcoma. The sarcomas of lymphoid origin and plasmacytomas are primarily managed by radiotherapy, although surgery may at times be helpful.

As previously noted, tumors confined to the infrastructure (Lederman's classification) are generally managed by a subtotal maxillectomy. Mesostructure and suprastructure involvement requires a total maxillectomy. Evidence of pterygopalatine or infratemporal fossa invasion makes it less likely that surgery will completely encompass the tumor but does not contraindicate surgery. When there is involvement of the posterior ethmoid cells, sphenoethmoid recess, cribriform plate, orbital apex, or pterygoid fossa, a craniofacial resection should be considered.[38–42] Tumor in the anteroinferior ethmoid region usually can be encompassed in a total maxillectomy.

It is generally agreed that radiotherapy in addition to surgery offers the patient with antral carcinoma the best chance for cure.[12, 13, 31, 33, 43, 44] Most workers prefer preoperative irradiation, although postoperative treatment may be just as efficacious.[45] We presently administer 6000 rads to the maxilla over a 6-week period preoperatively. The suprastructure is usually included in the field of treatment, with special care being taken to avoid damage to the contralateral eye and lacrimal apparatus. The surgery is performed 4 to 6 weeks following completion of the radiation therapy. Although a greater morbidity has been described with preoperative

irradiation,[45] most surgeons have had few problems with postoperative healing.

Among the more difficult surgical decisions is when to include the orbital contents in the resection. Firm criteria for the preservation of the orbital contents have yet to be developed. When radical extirpative surgery for antral carcinoma became popular in the 1940s and 1950s, the inclination was to consider orbital exenteration as an integral part of total maxillectomy.[46, 47] More recently, however, the value of sacrificing the eye in the majority of patients has been questioned, and many surgeons have adopted a more conservative approach.[31, 43, 48–50] One of us (MLS) has reported his experience with maxillectomy for antral carcinoma in 90 patients who had received 5800 to 6000 rads to the maxilla preoperatively.[31] Radical maxillectomy with orbital exenteration was performed when preoperative evaluation showed involvement of the bony orbital walls or when invasion of the floor or medial aspect of the orbit was evident at the time of surgery. Only 3 of the 27 patients (11 per cent) who had undergone orbital exenteration survived, compared with 27 of the 63 patients (43 per cent) who had a maxillectomy without orbital exenteration. Such disappointing results with orbital exenteration has prompted preservation of the orbital contents unless there is evidence of orbital wall involvement at the time of surgery. This is done despite evidence of orbital floor invasion on preradiation radiographs. Using such criteria for exenteration (i.e., the presence of bony invasion at surgery after a course of radiotherapy), Sisson[43] has been able to greatly reduce the number of exenterations performed without reducing survival. The data reported by Weymuller et al[48] also support such an approach. They noted that the survival of patients with radiologic evidence of orbital bone destruction was not affected by the decision to preserve or sacrifice the eye. Perry and colleagues[50] studied 21 patients with malignant paranasal sinus tumors eroding through the bone of the orbit who did not have orbital exenteration as part of their surgical therapy. Only three of these patients had recurrences in the orbital area, and it was felt that orbital exenteration without more extensive skull base surgery would not have prevented these recurrences. The authors believed that the eyes of all patients with paranasal sinus cancer can be preserved unless, after radiotherapy, the periosteum is extensively involved.

Despite the evidence supporting the present conservative trend in the management of the orbit, the proper role of orbital exenteration has not been fully defined. For example, perhaps the apparent lack of benefit from orbital exenteration in many cases has been a reflection of inability to remove the orbit in a truly en bloc manner. As craniofacial approaches are improved and the orbit can be removed in a truly en bloc manner with the maxilla, exenteration may play a more significant role in improving survival. There is already some evidence that more radical local resections, including orbital exenteration, may lead to improved survival in T3 and T4 carcinoma of the maxillary sinus.[39, 51, 52] Terz and colleagues,[52] for example, have reported a 72 per cent, 3-year disease-free survival in 22 patients with T3 and T4 squamous cell carcinomas of the antrum who had undergone orbital exenteration and combined craniofacial resection of the anterior and middle cranial fossae.

When patients have regional metastasis, the prognosis is extremely poor. Weymuller and colleagues[48] had no survivors among six patients with cervical adenopathy regardless of treatment modality. Schechter and Ogura[33] similarly had no survivors among four patients with cervical adenopathy. Stell[32] has reported on six patients with initial adenopathy; five died within 6 months and one survived for 3 years. Such poor results have prompted Stell to suggest that cervical metastasis be considered a contraindication to surgery. Despite the high failure rate, however, most experienced workers recommend treating cervical metastasis.[13, 31, 43] The neck is usually included in the preoperative irradiation, and a radical neck dissection is performed at the time of maxillectomy.

Using present techniques of radiotherapy and maxillectomy, the 5-year cure rate for antral carcinoma is approximately 25 per cent. The majority of patients will die with persistent or recurrent local or nodal disease.[33, 53] The wider application of craniofacial and chemotherapeutic[54–56] techniques in the future may increase survival.

Maxillectomy has a palliative role in the patient afflicted with cancer in this region. Although more than 70 per cent of these patients will eventually succumb to their disease, many can be made more functional and comfortable by a well-executed combination of surgery and radiotherapy. Significant palliation surgery often can be achieved despite carcinoma being left in situ at the time of surgery. The surgery can free the patient, at least temporarily, of a fungating, odorous tumor and the often associated bleeding, proptosis, and pain of bone erosion.

SURGICAL PROCEDURE

Total maxillectomy is perhaps the oldest of all "monobloc" operations for cancer.[5] It was first performed by Gensoul of Lyons and, independently, by Lizars of Edinburgh in 1827.[57] In the nineteenth century, the anatomic details of the surgical procedures were not unlike those current, but the operative mortality was 30 per cent, and the quality of rehabilitation was poor.[58] For these reasons, alternative treatments, such as electrocoagulation and radiation therapy, largely replaced maxillectomy as primary treatment for maxillary tumors in the early part of this century. In the 1940s, however, advances in anesthetic techniques, blood banking, and antibiotics made possible the safe and effective reapplication of radical surgical techniques.

Preoperative Preparations. Maxillectomy is a major surgical undertaking, with the potential for significant acute intraoperative blood loss. The patient's general status should be carefully evaluated preoperatively, and at least two units of blood should be available at surgery. Consultation with a prosthodontist should be obtained so that dental impressions may be taken and a prosthesis prepared to be inserted at the time of surgery. Such a temporary prosthesis eliminates the need for nasogastric tube feedings postoperatively and enhances patient comfort. Even when exenteration of the eye is not anticipated, the preoperative discussion with the patient should include an explanation of the possible need to sacrifice the eye and consent should be obtained.

TECHNIQUE

TOTAL MAXILLECTOMY WITH ORBITAL PRESERVATION

The patient is placed in the supine position on the operating room table. An oral endotracheal tube is used and taped to the corner of the mouth opposite the side of the tumor. After the field is prepared and draped, the eyelids are sewn together with a 6-0 nylon suture.

An incision is then made along the lateral aspect of the nose, starting at a point midway between the medial canthus of the eye and the dorsum of the nose. The incision is carried inferiorly around the nasal alae to the philtrum. The upper lip is then split vertically in the midline and the superior labial artery is ligated or cauterized. At this point, the surgeon may either choose to extend the superior aspect of the incision transversely along the lower eyelid or superiorly along the medial aspect of the eyebrow. The lower eyelid incision (Fig. 20–2; see also Fig. 20–10) offers good exposure of the lateral aspect of the maxilla and orbit but is often associated with prolonged lymphedema of the lower lid. Another disadvantage of this incision is that material used to reconstruct the floor of the orbit may extrude through it. We prefer extending the incision along the medial aspect of the eyebrow (Fig. 20–3). This approach offers excellent exposure of the medial orbital wall and usually gives adequate exposure of the lateral aspect of the maxilla. An incision is then made in the gingivobuccal sulcus from the point where the lip was split to the maxillary tuberosity. The skin flap is elevated in the supraperiosteal plane, exposing the nasal bone medially and the zygoma and lateral border of the maxilla laterally. The integrity of the anterior maxillary wall is evaluated as the flap is being elevated, so that an adequate soft tissue margin (including skin if necessary) is left on the anterior aspect of the specimen.

The medial aspect of the orbit is now explored. The periosteum along the medial orbital rim is incised, and the medial orbital wall is

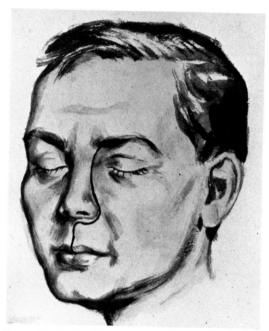

Figure 20–3. Modified incision offers good exposure and avoids complications associated with lower eyelid incision (see text).

exposed by blunt dissection with an elevator. The anterior and posterior ethmoid arteries are identified along the frontoethmoid suture. These are transected and cauterized, keeping in mind that the optic nerve may lie less than 5 mm posterior to the posterior ethmoid artery. Transection of the vessels permits the lateral retraction of the orbital contents. If tumor invasion is noted along the medial orbital wall, no further exploration of the orbit is performed and an exenteration is planned. If the medial aspect of the orbit is free of disease, the floor of the orbit is explored. The lacrimal sac is put on tension by passing a curved clamp deep to it, and it is then transected. The periosteum of the inferior orbital rim is incised and elevated from the orbital floor. The bone is carefully examined for evidence of invasion.

After the status of the orbit has been evaluated and it has been decided to preserve the orbital contents, the maxillectomy is performed in the following manner: An osteotomy is performed, separating the nasal bone from the frontal process of the maxilla. The ethmoid cells are entered, and the level of the cribriform plate and sphenoid sinus is determined. An osteotomy is then performed along the medial orbital wall at a level just inferior to the frontoethmoid suture anteriorly and down to the inferior orbital fissure posteriorly. The zygomatic arch is divided with a Gigli or Stryker

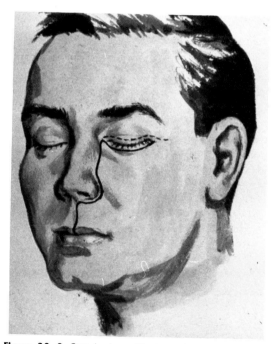

Figure 20–2. Standard maxillectomy incision. An upper eyelid incision *(dotted line)* is performed when sacrificing the orbital contents.

saw. An angled clamp is used to pass a Gigli saw from the inferior orbital fissure to the infratemporal fossa, and the frontal process of the malar bone (lateral wall of the orbit) is divided (Figs. 20–4 and 20–5).

Attention is now directed to the inferior aspect of the maxilla. An osteotome is used to perform a medial palatotomy after extracting the ipsilateral incisor and making the mucosal incision with the electrocautery knife. The soft palate is detached from the hard palate, once again using electrocautery. The final osteotomy to be performed is along the posterior aspect of the specimen. When there is no suspicion of posterior wall involvement with tumor, this cut can be made between the posterior wall of the maxilla and the pterygoid plates. When a fuller posterior margin is desired, the pterygoid plates are included in the specimen by placing a curved osteotome behind the pterygoid plates. Once this osteotomy is completed, the specimen becomes mobile and is held in place only by a few soft tissue attachments. These are easily released, and the specimen is removed. There may be brisk bleeding from the internal maxillary artery when the specimen is released posteriorly. The immediate bleeding usually can be controlled with packing. The branches of the artery can then be individually identified and ligated. The surgical specimen is carefully examined to determine the adequacy of the margins. When there is a doubtful margin, further tissue is removed from the operative field and sent for frozen-section examination.

This standard approach to the resection must be modified to meet the requirements of a

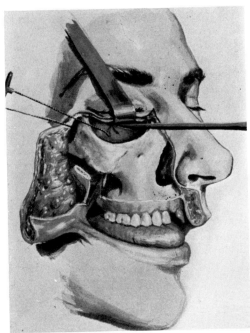

Figure 20–5. The frontal process of the malar bone is divided by passing a Gigli saw from the inferior orbital fissure to the infratemporal fossa.

given situation. When exposure of the infratemporal fossa and pterygopalatine area is of prime concern, for example, the zygomatic arch and coronoid process may be removed and these areas approached directly. The lateral approach described by Dingman and Conley[59] is also useful in obtaining direct access to these areas. In this approach, a lateral skin flap is developed, and the mandible is divided at the angle to expose the posterior aspect of the maxilla. More recently, Attenborough[60] has described a temporal approach, which is also designed to give good exposure to the posterior maxilla. In selected situations, the midface degloving approach can be used to perform a total maxillectomy without facial incisions.[61] The limited access to the orbit via this approach makes its routine use for total maxillectomy impractical.

Reconstruction of the resected orbital floor may be accomplished with Marlex mesh, tantalum mesh, temporalis fascia, nasal septum, dermis, or split-thickness skin graft.[49, 62] We presently favor Marlex mesh, although tantalum mesh has been used with good results. The mesh is made slightly longer than the defect to assure good contact with the lateral and medial bony walls. It is placed under the periosteum, which has been elevated with the orbital contents, and it is sutured to the periosteum of the supporting bone (Figs. 20–6 and 20–7). A split-

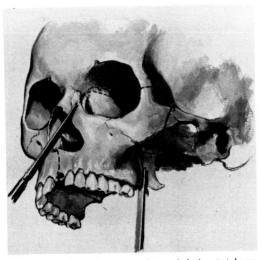

Figure 20–4. Osteotomies performed during total maxillectomy.

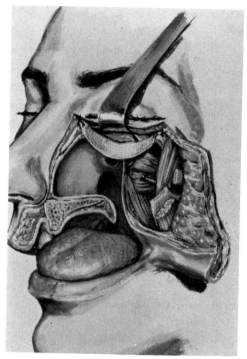

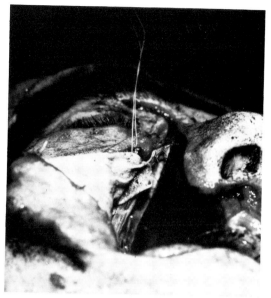

Figure 20–8. Skin graft applied to inner aspect of flap and over mesh supporting orbital contents.

Figure 20–6. The orbital floor can be reconstructed with Marlex mesh, tantalum mesh, temporalis fascia, nasal septum, dermis, or split-thickness skin graft.

thickness skin graft is then sutured to the buccal mucosa on the flap and extended to the roof of the cavity in direct contact with the mesh (Fig. 20–8). The cavity is then packed with bismuth tribromophenate petrolatum dressing (Xeroform gauze), and the palatal prosthesis is inserted and sutured in position (Fig. 20–9). The cheek flap is then replaced, and the nasal cavity is further packed as needed.

Techniques for primary reconstruction of the palatal defect are available but are generally neither necessary nor desirable.[63, 64] Efforts to repair the palate immediately usually prolong the patient's hospitalization and give a less satisfactory result than a well-designed prosthesis. The greatest criticism of this practice, however, is that it precludes adequate inspection of the maxillectomy site for recurrent disease. When reconstruction of the palate is desired, it should be performed after tumor recurrence has been reasonably ruled out.[65] Unlike the palatal defect, it is usually desirable

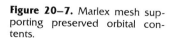
Figure 20–7. Marlex mesh supporting preserved orbital contents.

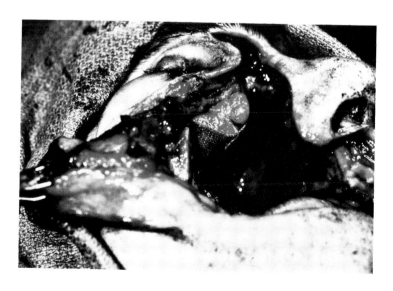

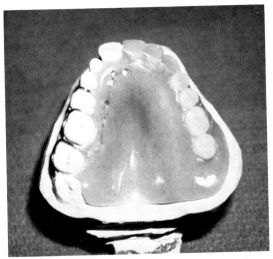

Figure 20–9. Temporary palatal prosthesis prepared preoperatively.

to repair cheek defects with regional flaps at the initial surgery.

TOTAL MAXILLECTOMY WITH ORBITAL EXENTERATION

When an exenteration is to be performed, the incision is extended along the upper and lower eyelids as diagrammed in Figure 20–2. The upper lid incision is deepened to the periosteum of the superior orbital rim but not through this periosteum. The orbital contents are then dissected from the orbital roof back to the apex of the orbit. The bony maxilla is mobilized by performing the osteotomies pre-

viously described. Mobilization of the maxilla permits downward retraction of the orbital contents, thus exposing the optic nerve (Fig. 20–10). The optic nerve is then divided, and the specimen is removed. The cavity is lined with a split-thickness skin graft and packed, and a prosthesis is inserted as previously described (Fig. 20–11).

The eyelids may be preserved by circumferentially incising the conjunctiva and permitting the lids to remain with the skin flap. In our experience, however, few tumors that require orbital exenteration will be sufficiently clear of the lower lid to allow for a comfortable margin when the lids are preserved. When the tumor approaches the cribriform plate, this structure must be removed with the specimen. Small defects in the cribriform plate can be adequately resurfaced with split-thickness skin graft. Larger cribriform defects, however, require regional flaps for coverage.

PARTIAL MAXILLECTOMY (SUBTOTAL MAXILLECTOMY)

Despite its wide usage, the term *partial maxillectomy* encompasses too many surgical approaches. In this chapter, the term describes a subtotal removal of the maxilla with preservation of either the orbital floor (inferior partial maxillectomy) or the hard palate (superior partial maxillectomy). Lateral rhinotomy with medial maxillectomy usually performed for inverting papillomas will not be considered in this chapter.

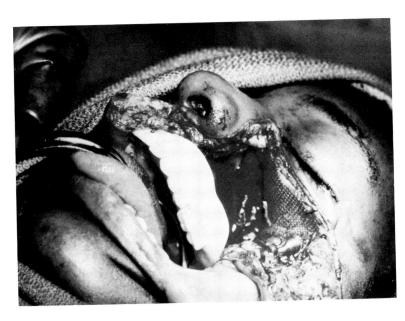

Figure 20–10. Palatal prosthesis inserted following total maxillectomy. Note Marlex mesh supporting orbital contents.

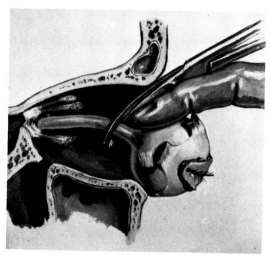

Figure 20–11. Mobilizing the bony maxilla will permit downward retraction of the orbital contents and division of the optic nerve.

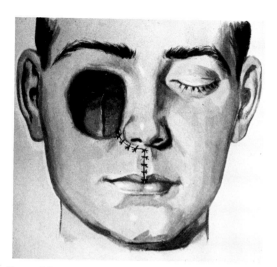

Figure 20–12. Defect following total maxillectomy with orbital exenteration.

INFERIOR PARTIAL MAXILLECTOMY

This procedure is usually performed for tumors confined to the floor of the antrum or the hard palate. The skin incision is similar to that used in total maxillectomy. After exploring the ethmoid and floor of orbit area, an osteotomy is made just below the orbital rim (Fig. 20–12). Laterally, an osteotomy is performed at a level inferior to the zygomatic arch. By releasing the superior aspect of the maxilla in this fashion, the bony floor of the orbit is preserved (Fig. 20–13). The rest of the maxilla is mobilized as described earlier for total maxillectomy, and the defect is lined with a split-thickness skin graft (Figs. 20–14 and 20–15). When it is not necessary to explore the orbit, the procedure may be performed entirely via a sublabial incision or the midface degloving approach.

SUPERIOR PARTIAL MAXILLECTOMY

This procedure is rarely performed but can be considered when there is a small lesion confined to the suprastructure. The technique is similar to that for total maxillectomy except that the hard palate is preserved. This is achieved by performing an osteotomy along the floor of the nasal cavity and floor of the antrum.

COMPLICATIONS

Hemorrhage. Sudden excessive bleeding may occur in the course of a maxillectomy when medium-sized vessels, such as the internal maxillary artery and its branches or the ethmoid arteries, are not adequately controlled. A precise anatomic dissection minimizes the chance of uncontrolled hemorrhaging. The soft tissue dissection of the pterygomaxillary area should always be performed after the bony maxilla has been mobilized. Bleeding in this area can be difficult to localize and control with an immobile bony maxilla.

Cerebrospinal Fluid. A CSF leak may be noted when the dissection is extended along the cribriform plate. When recognized intraoperatively, these leaks can be managed by placing Gelfoam or tissue such as muscle or fat

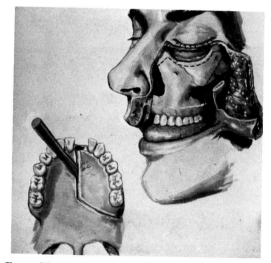

Figure 20–13. Osteotomies for inferior partial maxillectomy.

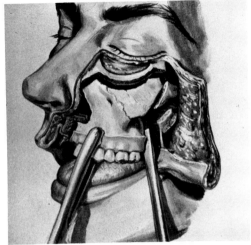

Figure 20–14. Preservation of the orbital floor in partial maxillectomy.

over the defect. The edges of the Gelfoam or tissue should be inserted between the bony margins of the defect and the dura. The majority of these patients will heal uneventfully.

Eye Injury. The cornea may be inadvertently abraded while manipulating and retracting the eye intraoperatively. This complication can be minimized by performing a temporary tarsorrhaphy before beginning the maxillary resection.

The optic nerve may be injured during the dissection in the orbital apex. Careful attention to anatomic landmarks helps avoid this complication. It is important to remember that the

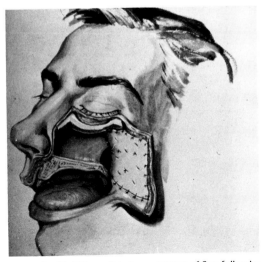

Figure 20–15. Skin graft in inner aspect of flap following partial maxillectomy.

optic nerve may lie less than 5 mm posterior to the posterior ethmoid foramen.

Postoperative Complications. Complications following maxillectomy include infection, skin graft failure, flap contracture or necrosis, and lower eyelid edema. Ocular ptosis, enophthalmos, and epiphora may occur when the eye is preserved.[66, 67]

References

1. Watson WL: Cancer of the paranasal sinuses. Laryngoscope 52:22, 1942.
2. Larsson LG, Martensson G: Carcinoma of the paranasal sinuses and the nasal cavities. Acta Radiol 42:149, 1954.
3. Osborn DA, Winston P: Carcinoma of the paranasal sinuses. J Laryngol 75:387, 1961.
4. Ireland PE, Bryce DP: Carcinoma of the accessory nasal sinuses. Ann Otol Rhinol Laryngol 75:698, 1966.
5. Lederman M: Tumors of the upper jaw: Natural history and treatment. J Laryngol Otol 84:369, 1970.
6. Bennett M: Paranasal sinus malignancies. Laryngoscope 80:933, 1970.
7. Lewis JS, Castro EB: Cancer of the nasal cavity and paranasal sinuses. J Laryngol 86:255, 1972.
8. Conley J: Concepts in Head and Neck Surgery. New York, Grune & Stratton, 1970.
9. Harrison DFN: The natural history of some cancers affecting the head and neck. J Laryngol Otol 86:1189, 1972.
10. Spratt JS Jr, Mercado R Jr: Therapy and staging in advanced cancer of the maxillary antrum. Am J Surg 110:502, 1965.
11. Pourquier H, Dejean Y, Franchebois P, Guerrier Y: Tumeurs du sinus maxillaire. J Radiol Electrol 54(1):27, 1973.
12. Gallagher TM, Boles R: Symposium: Treatment of malignancies of paranasal sinuses: I. Carcinoma of the maxillary antrum. Laryngoscope 80:924, 1970.
13. Lederman M: Cancer of the upper jaw and nasal chambers. Proc R Soc Med 62:65, 1969.
14. Sebileau P: Les formes cliniques du cancer du sinus maxillaire. Ann Mal L'oreille Larynx Nez 32(11):430, 1906.
15. Ohngren LG: Malignant tumors of the maxillo-ethmoid region. Acta Otolaryngol (Suppl) 19:1, 1933.
16. Huet PC, Stefani S: Les Cancers du Massif Maxillaire Superieur. Paris, Masson, 1960.
17. Sisson GA, Johnson NE, Amir CS: Cancer of the maxillary sinus: Clinical classification and management. Ann Otol Rhinol Laryngol 72:1050, 1963.
18. Sakai S, Hamasaki Y: Proposal for the classification of carcinoma of the paranasal sinuses. Acta Otolaryngol 63:42, 1967.
19. Harrison DFN: Critical look at the classification of maxillary sinus carcinoma. Ann Otol 87:3, 1978.
20. Cornet P: La chirurgie des tumeurs malignes du massif facial superieur. Ann Mal L'oreille Larynx Nez 44:573, 1925.
21. American Joint Committee on Cancer: Manual for Staging Cancer. 3rd ed. Edited by Beahrs OH, Henson DE, Hutter RVP, and Myers M. Philadelphia, J.B. Lippincott, 1988.
22. Kligerman M, Lattes R, Rankow R: Carcinoma of the maxillary sinus following Thorotrast instillation. Cancer 13:967, 1960.

23. Buda JA, Conley JJ, Rankow R: Carcinoma of the maxillary sinus following Thorotrast instillation: A further report. Am J Surg 106:868, 1963.

24. Acheson ED, Cowdell RH, Hadfield E, MacBeth RG: Nasal cancer in woodworkers in the furniture industry. Br Med J 2:587, 1968.

25. Acheson ED, Cowdell RH, Jolles B: Nasal cancer in the Northamptonshire boot and shoe industry. Br Med J 1:385, 1970.

26. Morgan JG: Some observations on the incidence of respiratory cancer in nickel workers. Br J Indust Med 15(4):224, 1958.

27. Harrison DFN: The management of malignant tumours affecting the maxillary and ethmoidal sinuses. J Laryngol Otol 87:749, 1973.

28. Hayes RB, Kardaun JWPF, de Bruyn A: Tobacco use and sinonasal cancer: A case-control study. Br J Cancer 56:843, 1987.

29. Larsson LG, Martensson G: Maxillary antral cancers. JAMA 219:342, 1972.

30. Pearson BW: The surgical anatomy of maxillectomy. Surg Clin North Am 57(4):701, 1977.

31. Som ML: Surgical management of carcinoma of the maxilla. Arch Otolaryngol 99:270, 1974.

32. Stell PM: The management of cervical lymph nodes in head and neck cancer. Proc R Soc Med 68(2):83, 1975.

33. Schechter GL, Ogura JH: Maxillary sinus malignancy. Laryngoscope 82:796, 1972.

34. Silver JA, Baredes S, Bello JA, Blitzer A, Hilal SK: CT of the opacified maxillary sinus. Radiology 163:205, 1987.

35. Som PM, Shapiro MD, Biller HF, Sasaki C, Lawson W: Sinonasal tumors and inflammatory tissues: Differentiation with MR imaging. Radiology 167:803, 1988.

36. Sisson GA, Becker SP: Cancer of the nasal cavity and paranasal sinuses. In Suen JY, Myers EN (eds): Cancer of the Head and Neck. New York, Churchill Livingstone, 1981.

37. Pfleiderer AG: Antroscopy via the inferior meatal route under local anesthetic: A practical guide to technique. J Laryngol Otol 101:1035, 1987.

38. Ketcham AS, Wilkins RH, Van Buren JM, Smith RR: A combined intracranial facial approach to the paranasal sinuses. Am J Surg 106:698, 1963.

39. Ketcham AS, Chretien PB, Van Buren JM, et al: The ethmoid sinuses: A re-evaluation of surgical resection. Am J Surg 126:469, 1973.

40. Sisson GA, Bytell DE, Becker SP, Ruge D: Carcinoma of the paranasal sinuses and cranial-facial resection. J Laryngol Otol 90:59, 1976.

41. Terz JJ, Alksne JF, Lawrence W: Craniofacial resection for tumors invading the pterygoid fossa. Am J Surg 118:732, 1969.

42. Wilson JSP, Westerbury G: Combined craniofacial resection for tumor involving the orbital walls. Br J Plast Surg 26:44, 1973.

43. Sisson GA: Symposium III: Treatment of malignancies of paranasal sinuses: Discussion and summary. Laryngoscope 80:945, 1970.

44. Cheng VST, Wang CC: Carcinoma of the paranasal sinuses. Cancer 40:3038, 1977.

45. Jesse RH: Pre-operative versus post-operative radiation in the treatment of squamous carcinoma of the paranasal sinuses. Am J Surg 110:552, 1965.

46. Tabb HG: Carcinoma of the antrum. An analysis of 60 cases with special reference to primary surgical extirpation. Laryngoscope 57:269, 1957.

47. Hilger JA: Maxilloethmoidal carcinoma. Arch Otolaryngol 73:169, 1961.

48. Weymuller EA, Reardon EJ, Nash D: A comparison of treatment modalities in carcinoma of the maxillary antrum. Arch Otolaryngol 106:625, 1980.

49. Larson DL, Christ JE, Jesse RH: Preservation of the orbital contents in cancer of the maxillary sinus. Arch Otolaryngol 108:370, 1982.

50. Perry C, Levine PA, Williamson BR, Cantrell RW: Preservation of the eye in paranasal sinus cancer surgery. Arch Otolaryngol Head Neck Surg 114:632, 1988.

51. Weymuller EA: Carcinoma of the maxillary sinuses. Head Neck Surg 4(1):87, 1981.

52. Terz JJ, Young HF, Lawrence W: Combined craniofacial resection for locally advanced carcinoma of the head and neck. Am J Surg 140:618, 1980.

53. Bridger MWN, Beale MB, Bryce DP: Carcinoma of the paranasal sinuses. A review of 158 cases. J Otolaryngol 7:379, 1978.

54. Yasuo S, Mamoru M, Hiro-omi T, et al: Combined surgery, radiotherapy, and regional chemotherapy in carcinoma of the paranasal sinuses. Cancer 25:571, 1970.

55. Goepfort H, Jesse RH, Lindberg RD: Arterial infusion and radiation therapy in the treatment of advanced cancer of the nasal cavity and paranasal sinuses. Am J Surg 126:464, 1973.

56. Moseley HS, Thomas LR, Everts EC, et al: Advanced squamous cell carcinoma of the maxillary sinus. Results of combined regional infusion chemotherapy, radiation, and surgery. Am J Surg 141(5):522, 1981.

57. Curtin JM: Malignant disease of the ethmoid and maxillary antrum. Ir J Med Sci 6:488, 1957.

58. Devine KD, Scanlon PW, Fiji FA: Malignant tumors of the nose and paranasal sinuses. JAMA 163:617, 1957.

59. Dingman DL, Conley J: Lateral approach to the pterygomaxillary region. Ann Otol Rhinol Laryngol 79:967, 1970.

60. Attenborough NR: Maxillectomy via a temporal approach. J Laryngol Otol 94:149, 1980.

61. Price JC, Holliday MJ, Johns ME, Kennedy DW, Richtsmeier WJ, Mattox DE: The versatile midface degloving approach. Laryngoscope 98:291, 1988.

62. Elkahky M: Orbital floor reconstruction after total maxillectomy. J Egypt Med Assoc 52:313, 1969.

63. Bakamjian V: A technique for primary reconstruction of the palate after radical maxillectomy for cancer. Plast Reconstr Surg 31:103, 1963.

64. Konno A, Togawa K, Iizuka K: Primary reconstruction after total or extended total maxillectomy for maxillary cancer. Plast Reconstr Surg 67:440, 1981.

65. Obwegeser HL: Late reconstruction of large maxillary defects after tumor resection. J Maxillofac Surg 1:19, 1973.

66. Wilder LW, Beyer CK, Smith B, Conley JJ: Ocular findings following radical maxillectomy. Trans Am Acad Ophthalmol Otolaryngol 75:797, 1971.

67. Engzell U, Johnsson G: Epiphora after maxillary resections. Acta Otolaryngol 64:242, 1967.

CHAPTER 21

SURGERY OF THE PTERYGOPALATINE FOSSA

William H. Friedman, MD, FACS

In the past two decades, surgery of the ptery-gopalatine space has become routine. To two generations of otolaryngologists trained in the use of the operating microscope, the pterygo-palatine space is a readily accessible area within which a variety of useful procedures can be accomplished. Ligation of the terminal branches of the internal maxillary artery is probably the most common and urgent reason for surgical access to this space. Vidian neurectomy and sphenopalatine ganglion resection are per-formed less commonly in the United States but are frequently performed for autonomic dys-function in other parts of the world. More recently, surgeons with increased familiarity with the pterygopalatine fossa assist the neuro-surgeon or ophthalmologist because of its close association with the orbit and middle cranial fossa and its relationship to contiguous diseases of these areas. The importance of the pterygo-palatine space is underscored by its central location within the head and the service it provides as a distribution center for the nerves and vessels of the middle third of the face.

ANATOMY

The pterygopalatine fossa is the small space directly behind the posterior wall of the maxil-lary antrum. It is bounded posteriorly by the medial plate of the pterygoid process, postero-laterally by the greater wing of the sphenoid, posteromedially by the sphenoid sinus lateral wall and medially by the ascending process of the palatine bone.[1] The contents of the ptery-

gopalatine space are abundantly surrounded by fat. On the anterior wall separating the posterior wall of the maxillary antrum from the space, a sturdy periosteal membrane acts as a septum between the ascending process of the palatine bone and the maxillary tuberosity. Superiorly, the infraorbital fissure provides an opening in the roof for the fossa. This opening is continuous laterally with the pterygomaxillary fissure, which acts as a conduit for the third division of the internal maxillary artery. Seven foramina open into the pterygopalatine fossa.[2] These are the foramen rotundum high on the posterior medial wall, the vidian canal located slightly medial to and separated from the foramen ro-tundum by a bony ridge on the pterygoid process, the palatine canal located on the floor, the pharyngeal canal, the pterygomaxillary fis-sure laterally, the sphenopalatine foramen lo-cated medially on the palatine process, and the infraorbital fissure, which provides exit ante-riorly and superiorly for the second division of the trigeminal nerve.

There are seven major vessels in the ptery-gopalatine space, including the third division of the internal maxillary artery and its end branches, the posterosuperior alveolar artery, the lesser palatine artery, the infraorbital ar-tery, the nasal accessory and superior pharyn-geal arteries, the artery of the pterygoid canal, the greater palatine artery, and the sphenopal-atine artery. The internal maxillary artery en-ters the pterygopalatine fossa through the pter-ygomaxillary fissure (Fig. 21–1) and provides end branches through tortuous arborization. The posterosuperior alveolar artery leaves the internal maxillary first, descending posteriorly

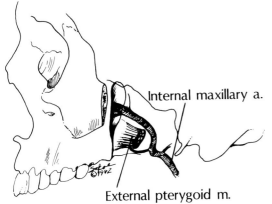

Figure 21–1. The internal maxillary artery entering the pterygomaxillary fissure.

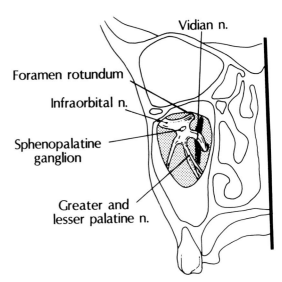

Figure 21–2. The pterygopalatine space showing the foramen rotundum, the vidian nerve, the infraorbital nerve, the sphenopalatine ganglion, and the greater and lesser palatine nerves.

while dividing into numerous branches to the alveolar canal and maxillary sinuses. The greater and lesser palatine arteries descend inferiorly to the hard palate and soft palate through the greater and lesser palatine foramina; the sphenopalatine artery continues medially into the nasal cavity through the sphenopalatine foramen. The infraorbital artery emerges anteriorly and superiorly through the infraorbital fissure; the artery of the pterygoid canal (vidian artery), the artery of the foramen rotundum, and the descending pharyngeal artery exit posteriorly through their foramina.

The nerves of the pterygopalatine space include the second division of the trigeminal, the maxillary nerve, entering posteriorly through the foramen rotundum and continuing anteriorly through the infraorbital foramen (Fig. 21–2). The vidian nerve enters the pterygoid canal posteriorly and medially at the lateral inferior junction of the sphenoid sinus and the pterygoid process of the sphenoid bone, traversing this canal for approximately 1 cm before entry into the pterygopalatine space through a funnel-shaped opening (Fig. 21–3). The pterygopalatine nerve and branches of the greater palatine nerve traverse the sphenopalatine foramen and the foramen of Juvara medially to supply the nasal cavity. The greater and lesser palatine nerves descend inferiorly through the greater and lesser palatine foramina (Fig. 21–2). The infraorbital nerve is the continuation of the maxillary nerve at its exit from the infraorbital fissure. The posterosuperior alveolar nerve connects with the upper jaw through the pterygomaxillary fissure, and zygomatic nerves extend through the pterygomaxillary fissure into the orbit.

Although there is no reliable rule for surgically distinguishing separate planes for nerves and vessels, the surgical plane of the major

vessels is anterior to the plane of the major nerves (Fig. 21–4). If the superiorly exiting vessels are followed to their exits, the maxillary nerve is encountered, along with its connections to the vidian nerve medially. For a surgical approach to the vidian nerve to be successful, visualization must first be achieved either by retracting or ligating and resecting the major branches of the internal maxillary artery.

A tiny vein, the sphenopalatine vein, lies just deep to the anterior periosteum of the pterygopalatine fossa. There are no other veins of importance in this space. A pterygoid venous plexus lies directly lateral to the space, however, on the surface of the internal pterygoid muscle; therefore, it is important that inadver-

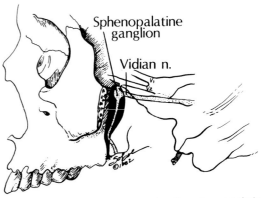

Figure 21–3. Vidian nerve entering the pterygopalatine space through the pterygoid canal and synapsing the pterygoid canal.

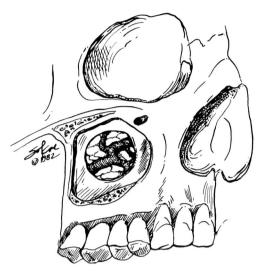

Figure 21–4. The plane of the internal maxillary artery and its branches. Note the surrounding pterygopalatine space fat. The nerves lie deep to this plane.

tent maneuvers outside the immediate field of vision be avoided in operating in this space.

SPHENOPALATINE GANGLION

The sphenopalatine ganglion is a pinkish, 0.5-cm structure located in the upper medial portion of the pterygopalatine fossa between the foramen rotundum and the pterygoid canal (Fig. 21–2). This ganglion serves as a switchboard for the autonomic nervous system and receives the effluent preganglionic fibers of the vidian nerve, which synapse with postganglionic fibers for distribution to nasal and sinus mucosa. Two small postganglionic branches exit the sphenopalatine ganglion and join the maxillary nerve to be distributed to the lacrimal gland. The vidian nerve emerging from the pterygoid canal contains preganglionic parasympathetic fibers originating in the superior salivatory nucleus and traveling with the greater petrosal nerve, and also sympathetic fibers from the carotid plexus originating in the superior cervical ganglia. These fibers join the parasympathetic, ultimately synapsing in the sphenopalatine ganglion, whereas the sympathetic nerves pass through the ganglion, having synapsed close to their ganglia in the neck.

HISTORY

The earliest reported operation on the pterygopalatine space was probably performed by Carnochan[3] in 1858. He reported the successful treatment of trigeminal neuralgia by excising the trunk of the second branch of the fifth nerve via a transpterygomaxillary fissure approach to the pterygopalatine fossa. Segond[4] reported a similar lateral approach to the pterygopalatine fossa in 1890, as did Frazier[5] in 1921 and Braeucker[6] in 1932. In 1928, Seiffert[7] reported a transantral approach to the pterygopalatine fossa for ligation of the internal maxillary artery for epistaxis. Gergely[8] (1935), Hirsch[9] (1936), and Davis[10] (1945) all reported the use of the transantral technique. Finally, the transantral approach for ligation of the internal maxillary artery for epistaxis was popularized in 1965 by Chandler and Serrins[11] and has been reported by many surgeons since. Sewall[12] in 1926 described a transantral approach for sphenopalatine ganglion resection and Auerbaukh[13] in 1935 described the transpalatal approach to the sphenopalatine ganglion. In 1961, Golding-Wood[14] described the vidian neurectomy for chronic vasomotor rhinitis. This operation was originally presented as an alternative to petrosal neurectomy. There have been numerous reports on the subject since.[15–19]

SURGICAL PROCEDURES

INTERNAL MAXILLARY ARTERY LIGATION

Most patients with epistaxis require little or no treatment. By far the most common nasal bleeding is that produced by trauma to the anterior caudal septum, known as Little's area. Kiesselbach's plexus of vessels lies immediately subjacent to the nasal mucosa in this area and can bleed extensively from minor manipulation. This is particularly true in elderly people and very young patients. Most bleeding in this area ceases spontaneously. Persistent bleeding usually can be stopped in the emergency room or the otolaryngologist's office by the use of topical vasoconstrictors, cautery, or nasal packing. Posterior nasal bleeding usually does not cease spontaneously and is most often treated by the use of nasal packing in the form of petroleum jelly–impregnated gauze, inflatable balloons, or Foley catheters, which can apply pressure to the bleeding site for up to 4 days. If the bleeding point is on the septum overlying a posterior maxillary crest spur, a submucous resection is indicated.

Arterial ligation for the control of posterior epistaxis was probably first performed in 1795 by Abernathy, who used common carotid artery ligation. Bartlett and McKittrick[20] in 1917 reviewed 117 ligations of the common carotid for arteriovenous aneurysms, bleeding neoplasms, and head and neck injuries; 33 per cent of these patients failed to survive the procedure. Despite the mortality and morbidity associated with common carotid artery ligation, this procedure persisted until the mid-twentieth century in some areas. In 1908, Barrett and Orr[21] reported external carotid artery ligation for postoperative nasal bleeding. Malcomson[22] reviewed this subject in 1963. Chandler and Serrins[11] reported that external carotid artery ligation was still the most common form of arterial ligation for epistaxis when they began performing internal maxillary artery ligation in the early 1960s. Since that time, external carotid artery ligation has been largely replaced by internal maxillary artery ligation for the control of posterior nasal bleeding. Although anterior ethmoid artery ligation is effective in treating 10 per cent of posterior nasal epistaxis (that arising in the posterior ethmoids), internal maxillary artery ligation has become a standard procedure.

INDICATIONS

Chandler and Serrins[11] initially reported the use of internal maxillary artery ligation for "those patients who ordinarily would require postnasal and anterior nasal packing and hospitalization for control of the bleeding." The procedure did not gain widespread acceptance immediately among otolaryngologists, who were accustomed to the use of anterior and posterior nasal packing. However, complications of posterior nasal packing included failure to control epistaxis and morbidity and mortality related to changes in arterial oxygen tension and pulmonary mechanics.[23, 24] Cook and Komorn[25] demonstrated statistically significant increases in arterial PCO_2 and decreases in arterial PO_2 with nasal packing. This was probably the basis for the sudden death syndrome occasionally seen in patients with posterior nasal packing in place. These changes are pronounced in patients with chronic obstructive pulmonary disease and should be considered a factor in elderly patients and those with underlying heart disease. Thus, internal maxillary artery ligation should be considered in any patient who requires posterior nasal packing.

If patient convenience, discomfort from prolonged packing, and the prolonged hospitalization required for patients with posterior nasal packing in place are considered, internal maxillary artery ligation seems the proper alternative for most patients in whom posterior nasal packing is required. Failure of posterior nasal packing to control epistaxis is an absolute indication for internal maxillary artery ligation. I prefer this technique for all severe posterior nasal bleeding, with the clear understanding that as many as 10 per cent of these patients may require additional ligation of the anterior ethmoid vessels. Although temporary control of posterior nasal bleeding can be obtained with the use of an inflatable balloon catheter, it is convenient and judicious to ligate the internal maxillary artery in most of these patients.

TECHNIQUE

Internal maxillary artery ligation is best performed under local anesthesia, using the operating microscope. A straight eyepiece with a $300\times$ objective lens is preferred, so that the patient may be positioned in slight reversed Trendelenburg position. Three milliliters of 2 per cent lidocaine are then introduced into the greater palatine foramen with a 1.5-inch, 25-gauge needle into the pterygopalatine fossa. Sublabial injections of 2 per cent lidocaine to the anterior cheek are next accomplished. A 6-cm incision from the lateral incisor tooth to the area of the first tricuspid tooth is then made in the gingivobuccal sulcus, taking care not to enter the buccal space nor to injure vulnerable tooth roots (Fig. 21–5). Anterior maxillary antrostomy is achieved with a No. 6 chisel. Most of the anterior maxillary wall is removed, leaving a 1-mm protective rim for the second division of the trigeminal nerve as it emerges from the infraorbital foramen.

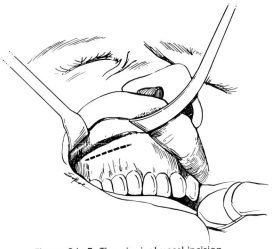

Figure 21–5. The gingivobuccal incision.

The maxillary antrum is then entered and a site on the posterior maxillary wall is selected for entry into the pterygopalatine space (Fig. 21–6). The geographic center of the posterior maxillary wall is located and the posterior maxillary mucosa cauterized to prevent bleeding. A No. 2 chisel is used to outline a circular incision approximately 10 to 15 mm in diameter. When this nickel-sized portion of bone is removed, periosteum of the pterygopalatine space is seen as a grayish white, glistening membrane (Fig. 21–7). There may be a small vein laterally in this membrane. However, the periosteum usually can be incised with a sickle knife and dissected easily from underlying fat within the pterygopalatine fossa. Although it is simple to create a flap of periosteum at this point, it is unnecessary, and periosteum is probably best removed without leaving a remnant to block vision.

The surgeon is now confronted with abundant fat within the pterygopalatine fossa. Nerve hooks are used to locate the terminal branch of the internal maxillary artery entering the fossa laterally. Using a suction tip laterally to medially, the arterial branches can be cleaned of underlying fat until the entire arterial system can be easily visualized (Fig. 21–8). Vascular clips can now be applied to the internal maxillary artery and all its branches (Fig. 21–9). Ordinarily, the internal maxillary artery, the sphenopalatine, and the descending palatine branches are ligated. However, some surgeons prefer to ligate all large branches. At this time, if nasal packing is in place, it is removed. Intranasal suction may be utilized to initiate bleeding if none is seen. There should be no further epistaxis. In 10 per cent of cases, how-

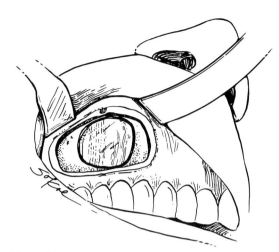

Figure 21–7. The glistening periosteal membrane of the pterygopalatine space is revealed by removing posterior maxillary bone.

ever, epistaxis may continue. If this occurs, ethmoid ligation may be necessary. This is accomplished through an external ethmoidectomy incision with the placement of a vascular clip on the anterior ethmoid artery in the frontoethmoid suture line. I have found this necessary in only 4 per cent of cases. However, persistent anterior ethmoid bleeding has been reported quite commonly following internal maxillary artery ligation.

RESULTS

I am unaware of spontaneous (unrelated to tumor or trauma) unilateral epistaxis that has not been controlled ultimately, either with in-

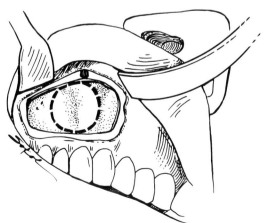

Figure 21–6. The anterior maxillary wall removed. A 10- to 15-mm opening is created in the center of the posterior maxillary wall.

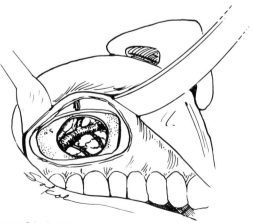

Figure 21–8. The periosteal membrane is removed and branches of the internal maxillary artery are seen along with pterygopalatine space fat.

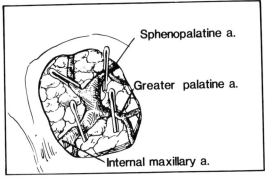

Figure 21–9. Vascular clips on the major branches of the internal maxillary artery.

ternal maxillary artery ligation alone or combined internal maxillary artery ligation and anterior ethmoid artery ligation. Advantages to the patient include early discharge from the hospital, usually within 24 hours of the procedure, less discomfort than that from nasal packing, a permanent result, and the maintenance of normal arterial PO_2 and PCO_2.

The care of the patient following internal maxillary artery ligation is similar to that following Caldwell-Luc antrostomy. In the hypertensive patient, a thorough medical evaluation is indicated. Underlying medical causes of epistaxis should be corrected. There are few disadvantages. Complications are rare. These may include maxillary sinusitis or wound infection, untoward sequelae of injudicous manipulation or cautery, or injury caused by instruments within the pterygopalatine fossa resulting in orbital complications. A thorough knowledge of the anatomy of the area, combined with good surgical technique, prevents these complications.

VIDIAN NEURECTOMY

INDICATIONS

Vasomotor rhinitis resulting in watery rhinorrhea and paroxysmal sneezing is the only indication for vidian neurectomy. Nasal obstruction due to hyperplastic rhinosinusitis, nasal polyps, and other obstructive forms of rhinitis are not indications for this procedure. Case selection is critical in obtaining excellent results with vidian neurectomy. If only those patients with profuse watery rhinorrhea and paroxysmal sneezing are included, the operation should be quite successful (if infrequent). Hiranandani[17] and Golding-Wood[14, 15] have described ex-

panded indications for this procedure. My experience has tended to contraindicate the performance of vidian neurectomy except for paroxysmal rhinorrhea and sneezing.

TECHNIQUE

The transantral approach to the pterygopalatine fossa for vidian neurectomy is identical to that for internal maxillary artery ligation. General anesthesia administered via endotracheal intubation is probably preferable to local anesthesia. Although Golding-Wood[14, 15] prefers a hypotensive general anesthetic for this procedure, hypotensive anesthesia is neither necessary nor particularly desirable.

Vidian neurectomy differs from internal maxillary artery ligation in that it is begun after the internal maxillary artery ligation has been accomplished. All major branches of the internal maxillary artery are ligated with vascular clips. A Y-shaped segment of the arterial system is then resected, cutting the sphenopalatine, descending palatine, and terminal main trunk of the internal maxillary artery to reveal the deeper plane of the pterygopalatine space (Fig. 21–10A). The sphenopalatine ganglion is visualized in the upper medial portion of the pterygopalatine fossa. The foramen rotundum with the emerging second division of the trigeminal nerve can be seen attached to the sphenopalatine ganglion by two slender postganglionic nerve fibers. The ganglion itself is a 1-cm, pinkish soft tissue mass, which may closely resemble surrounding pterygopalatine fat. With careful dissection, however, the fifth nerve connections can be seen and, if the ganglion is displaced cephalad, the vidian nerve can be

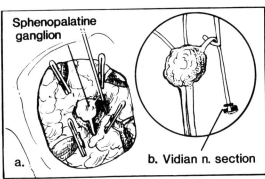

Figure 21–10. A, A Y-shaped segment of the internal maxillary artery and its branches have been removed to reveal the sphenopalatine ganglion. B, A nerve hook is used to stretch the vidian nerve prior to sectioning at the pterygoid canal.

seen attaching to the sphenopalatine ganglion in its medial inferior quadrant. The vidian nerve can be seen emerging from its trumpet-shaped canal and coursing to the ganglion in a supero-lateral fashion. The artery to the pterygoid usually can be seen accompanying it.

The vidian nerve at this time can be severed and allowed to retract into the pterygoid canal (Fig. 21–10B). Although cautery is generally applied to the area, it is important not to insert the cautery tip into the pterygoid canal to avoid damage to structures in the adjacent cavernous sinus. Some surgeons use bone wax to plug the pterygoid canal. This is unnecessary. Once the nerve is severed, the pterygopalatine space can be lightly packed with Gelfoam soaked in anti-biotic solution. Intranasal antrostomy is usually performed. The sublabial incision is closed with interrupted 3–0 chromic catgut sutures.

RESULTS

Vidian neurectomy is an effective method of controlling paroxysmal sneezing and rhinor-rhea. In approximately one third of cases, uni-lateral vidian neurectomy is sufficient to control bilateral rhinorrhea. Bilateral vidian neurec-tomy is not indicated because of this phenom-enon.

Complications following vidian neurectomy include the rare occurrence of partial or total ophthalmoplegia, presumably resulting from the use of cautery or surgical manipulation near the cavernous sinus or the inadvertent entry into the orbit through the inferior orbital fis-sure. These complications should not occur if the anatomy and surgical technique of the area are mastered. Other complications, including occasional maxillary sinusitis or periorbital edema, are rare. These may be treated conser-vatively.

SPHENOPALATINE GANGLION RESECTION

Sphenopalatine ganglion resection is proba-bly useful in the treatment of headaches related to autonomic dysfunction. It has been used to treat the so-called lower half headache, char-acterized by pain in the distribution of the second division of the fifth nerve associated with lacrimation, diaphoresis, erythema of the posterior nostril on the involved side, nasal congestion, and other autonomic disturbances. Sphenopalatine ganglion resection has resulted

in an approximate 50 per cent success rate in treating this disorder. This procedure is not indicated in the treatment of tic douloureux.

In patients with crocodile tears associated with regeneration of the facial nerve in Bell's palsy, sphenopalatine ganglion resection is probably curative. Patients do not require the lacrimal function for maintenance of appropriate lubrication of the conjunctival sac; meibomian glands within the conjunctiva are adequate for this function. Patients may complain because of the loss of emotional tearing, however, follow-ing both vidian neurectomy and sphenopalatine ganglion resection.

References

1. Wentges RT: Surgical anatomy of the pterygopalatine fossa. J Laryngol Otol 89(1):35, 1975.
2. Montgomery WH, Katz R, Gamble JF: Anatomy and surgery of the pterygopalatine fossa. Ann Otol Rhinol Laryngol 79(3):606, 1970.
3. Carnochan JM: Exsection of the trunk of the second branch of the fifth pair of nerves beyond the ganglion of Meckel's for severe neuralgia of the face. Am J Med Sci 69:134, 1858.
4. Segond P: De la resection du nerf maxillaire supérieur et du ganglion sphenopalatin dans la fente pterygo-maxillaire par la voie temporale. Rev Chir 10:173, 1890.
5. Frazier CH: Surgical approach to sphenopalatine gan-glion. Surgery 74:328, 1921.
6. Braeucker W: Klinische Untersuchungen über den Kreislauf beim traumatischen Odem der Extremitaten. Ztschr. f. kreislaufforsch Arch Klin Chir 24:601, 1932.
7. Seiffert H: Ligature of the internal maxillary artery for epistaxis (quoted by Hirsch). Z Hals Nase Ohrenheilk 22:323, 1928.
8. Gergely Z: Transmaxillary ligature of the arteria max-illaris interna. Acta Otolaryngol 22:142, 1935.
9. Hirsch C: Ligation of the internal maxillary artery in patients with nasal hemorrhage. Arch Otolaryngol 24:589, 1936.
10. Davis EDD: Ligation of the internal maxillary artery through the antrum for uncontrollable epistaxis. J Lar-yngol 60:420, 1945.
11. Chandler JR, Serrins AJ: Transantral ligation of the internal maxillary artery for epistaxis. Laryngoscope 75:1151, 1965.
12. Sewall EC: An operation for the removal of sphenopal-atine ganglion. Ann Otol 35:1, 1926.
13. Auerbaukh SS, et al: The palatine access to the ganglion sphenopalatinum and to the second branch of the trifacial nerve. Ann Surg 101:819, 1935.
14. Golding-Wood PH: Petrosal and vidian neurectomy in chronic vasomotor rhinitis. J Laryngol Otol 75:232, 1961.
15. Golding-Wood PH: Cervical sympathectomy in Me-niere's disease. Arch Otolaryngol 97:391, 1973.
16. Agarwal PN: Bilateral vidian neurectomy—Indications and results. J Laryngol Otolaryngol 91(3):235, 1977.
17. Hiranandani NL Jr: Treatment of chronic vasomotor rhinitis with clinico-pathological study of vidian nerve section in 150 cases. J Laryngol 80:902, 1966.

18. Chasin WD, Lofgren RH: Vidian nerve section for vasomotor rhinitis. Arch Otolaryngol 86:129, 1967.
19. Montgomery O, et al: Analysis of pterygopalatine space surgery. Laryngoscope 80:1190, 1970.
20. Bartlett W, McKittrick OF: Ligation of common carotid artery. Ann Surg 65:715, 1917.
21. Barrett JW, Orr WF: Suppuration on the mastoid antrum; von Bezold perforation; tympanum intact. Intercolon. Melbourne, MJ Australasia, 1908, xiii, 203–207.
22. Malcolmson K: The surgical management of massive epistaxis. J Laryngol Otol 77:299, 1963.
23. Unno T, Nelson JR, Ogura JH: The effect of nasal obstruction on pulmonary, airway and tissue resistance. Laryngoscope 78:1119, 1968.
24. Cassisi NJ, Biller HF, Ogura JH: Changes in arterial oxygen tension and pulmonary mechanics with the use of posterior nasal packing. Laryngoscope 81:1261, 1971.
25. Cook TA, Komorn RM: Statistical analysis of the alterations of blood gases produced by nasal packing. Laryngoscope 83(11):1802, 1973.

CHAPTER 22

DACRYOCYSTORHINOSTOMY

Kambiz T. Moazed, MD

William C. Cooper, MD

HISTORY

The initial step in the evaluation of the tearing problem is obtaining the patient's history (Table 22–1).

EYE EXAMINATION

Eye examination is an important part of the evaluation of a patient with tearing problems, as many ocular disorders can cause epiphora. An ophthalmology consultation is indicated, especially if a patient has a history of eye disease or complains of eye discomfort or visual disturbance. On examination, attention should be paid to the position of the eyelids (to rule out entropion or ectropion), absence or stenosis of the puncta, and presence of conjunctivitis, keratitis, corneal foreign body, iritis, undercorrected refractive error, and glaucoma,[1] which all may lead to symptoms of tearing.

NASAL EXAMINATION

It is important to examine the nasal cavity in all patients who complain of tearing. Fractured inferior turbinates, nasal polyps, and nasal carcinomas are some of the possible causes of occlusion of the exit of the nasolacrimal duct into the nasal cavity. In many of these patients, the tearing can be alleviated by nasal surgery.

EVALUATION OF THE LACRIMAL SYSTEM

The evaluation of the lacrimal system is performed in two parts. The first is the testing of the secretory apparatus, and the second is the evaluation of the excretory pathway (Fig. 22–1). The Schirmer I and II and the basic secretion test are used to evaluate the secretory system. The primary and secondary dye tests, the dye retention test, the Hornblass test, and dacryocystography are used to evaluate the excretory system.

The secretory system theoretically can be divided into two parts: basic secretors and reflex secretors. The basic secretions are provided by the accessory lacrimal glands of Wolfring and Krause, the mucin goblet cells of conjunctiva, and the meibomian glands of the lids (Fig. 22–2). Combinations of these secretions keep the external surface of the eye moist during the

TABLE 22–1. Points to Be Addressed in Taking History

1. The severity of the problem: Is the tearing symptomatic to the patient?
2. The extent of the tearing: Is the tearing constant or episodic?
3. The unilaterality or bilaterality of the symptoms: Unilateral tearing is usually associated with excretory obstruction.
4. The role of environmental irritants: Is the problem initiated by wind, smoke, fumes, and so on?
5. History of previous recurrent dacryocystitis: This is usually associated with partial obstruction of the excretory systems.
6. Associated underlying problems:
   a. Underlying eye diseases: iritis, keratitis, conjunctivitis
   b. Underlying systemic problems: thyroid disease, arthritis, menopause
   c. Allergies: allergic rhinitis, sinusitis, conjunctivitis
   d. Previous trauma and operations: facial and nasal fractures, blepharoplasty
   e. Congenital anomalies

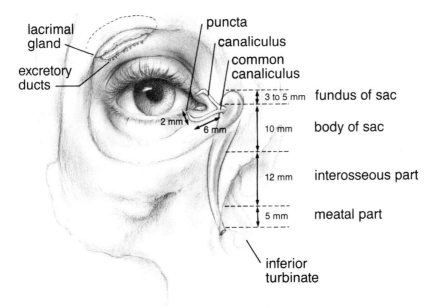

Figure 22–1. Anatomy of the lacrimal excretory system.

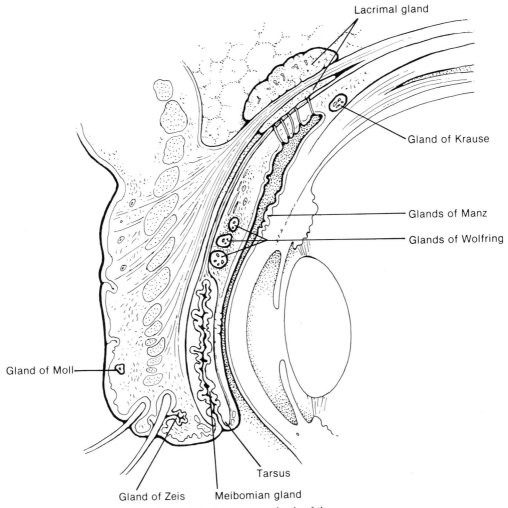

Figure 22–2. Excretory glands of the eye.

day. The lacrimal glands are reflex secretors, providing tears only when stimulated. The reflex secretors may be stimulated by emotional factors or by any irritation of the fifth nerve, such as occurs in keratitis, rhinitis, or sinusitis.

In some conditions the absence of the basic secretion causes dryness of the cornea and results in reflex tearing secondary to stimulation of the fifth nerve. In this case, the basic problem is a hyposecretion of the basic secretors, which leads to the complaint of tearing (pseudoepiphora) and can be associated with eye irritation or foreign body (sandy) sensation secondary to the dry ocular surface.[2]

Schirmer I Test. The first step for evaluation of patients complaining of epiphora is the Schirmer I test.[3] The first 5-mm portion of the Schirmer strip is bent at the notched area. The bent end is then inserted into the lower fornix at the lateral third of the lower eyelid, so that the crease lies over the eyelid margin. The test is done on both eyes, with the patient in a sitting position and the lights dimmed. The patient is instructed to keep the eyelids open, but blinking is allowed while the patient gazes slightly upward at a fixation point. After 5 minutes the strips are gently removed to determine the amount of wetting. The measurement is made from the notch at the bend of the Schirmer strip to the distal end of the wetting on the strip. The Schirmer I test measures both basic and reflex secretions, although the amount of reflex secretion is minimized as much as possible. Less than 10 mm of wetting in 5 minutes indicates a hyposecretion of tears; more than 10 mm of wetting in 5 minutes is compatible with normal secretion or an increased reflex secretory output (pseudoepiphora).

Basic Secretion Test. If hypersecretion or hyposecretion is found to exist, the basic secretion test can be done to obtain more information. The basic secretion test is performed immediately after the Schirmer I test by instillation of several drops of a local anesthetic, such as proparacaine hydrochloride (Alcaine), into each cul-de-sac. The lower cul-de-sacs are then carefully dried with tissue paper, and the Schirmer strips are placed as in the Schirmer I test. The procedure then continues as in the Schirmer I test. The normal basic secretion in 5 minutes is 10 to 15 mm. Less than 10 mm of wetting in 5 minutes indicates hyposecretion of the basic secretions, and the patient's tearing complaint may then be secondary to reflex tearing.

Schirmer II Test. If the basic secretion is normal and the reflex secretion is defective, the Schirmer II test can distinguish between a fatigue block of the reflex secretors and complete lack of function of the reflex secretors. The test is done by placing a cotton-tipped applicator in the nostril and moving it back and forth for 2 minutes. If there is a fatigue block, there will be a marked wetting of the Schirmer strip during this stimulation, whereas there will be minimal or no additional secretion when there is a total failure of the reflux system.[4] Hyperlacrimation must be differentiated from epiphora caused by blockage of the lacrimal passages. This can be accomplished by performing the fluorescein dye excretion tests.

Fluorescein Dye Test. Jones has described the use of fluorescein to test lacrimal outflow functions. In the primary dye test of Jones (I), fluorescein is instilled into the conjunctival sac, and if there is no obstruction, it appears spontaneously in the nose. In the Jones secondary dye test (II), fluorescein does not appear spontaneously in the inferior meatus but can be recovered by irrigation of the lacrimal system.[5]

To perform the fluorescein dye test, the patient should be seated comfortably and the nose sprayed with 4 per cent cocaine. One drop of 2 per cent fluorescein solution is instilled into the conjunctival sac of each eye. In the normal excretory system the fluorescein dye should appear in the inferior meatus of the nose in 1 to 5 minutes and can be identified by inserting a cotton-tipped applicator under the inferior turbinate at 2 minutes and again at 5 minutes after instillation of the dye. Because excessive secretion of tears may affect the results of the fluorescein dye test, excessive stimulation of the lacrimal reflex by frequent insertion and manipulation of applicators should be avoided. If, after 5 minutes, no fluorescein is recovered in this manner, it may be possible to identify the dye in the nasal cavity by having the patient blow into a tissue or by using a cobalt filter light.

If the result of the primary test is negative (i.e., no dye recovered), the secondary dye test should be performed. After instillation of a single drop of topical anesthetic into the conjunctival sac, all the fluorescein remaining in the conjunctiva is flushed out. The puncta are anesthetized by inserting a cotton pledget soaked in topical anesthetic between the puncta for 2 minutes, and the lacrimal system is irrigated with clear saline. The patient's head is tilted forward over a white basin or white towel so that the irrigant emerges from the nose. If fluorescein staining is present, the secondary dye test result is considered positive, whereas if the irrigant is clear or practically clear, the result is negative.

A positive primary dye test result indicates a normal excretory system. It is possible for the excretory system to be normal and for the fluorescein to escape in the nasal cavity and not be seen by the examiner. A positive secondary dye test result confirms that the system is patent and further establishes that the lacrimal pump and the upper lacrimal system (the canaliculi) are normal in patency and function because the fluorescein in the conjunctival sac must have made its way to the lacrimal sac to be flushed into the nose. The secondary dye test does not, however, establish the functional state of the lacrimal sac because the irrigating solution is forced from the lacrimal sac into the nose by means of syringing effort. A positive secondary dye test result indicates only a normal upper outflow system and a patent excretory system.[5] Thus, it is possible to get positive results in a patient with incomplete obstruction of the nasolacrimal duct. If no fluid comes from the nose, a complete obstruction exists. If clear fluid comes from the nose, the secondary test resulted negatively, and the canaliculi are not functioning (no dye has reached the sac).

Fluorescein Dye Disappearance Test.

This test is based on the rate at which the fluorescein color disappears from the conjunctival sac after instillation in the lower cul-de-sac. The fluorescein dye disappearance test consists of simply observing the amount of fluorescein remaining in the conjunctival sac at the end of 5 minutes. This observation is made concurrently with the performance of the primary and secondary dye tests, and the remaining fluorescein is graded in terms of color intensity (from 4+ representing no disappearance of the dye to 0 retention representing complete elimination of the fluorescein dye in a period of 5 minutes). If the fluorescein dye disappearance test result is positive, lacrimal outflow may be considered normal. If the dye disappearance test is abnormal, as indicated by an abnormal retention of fluorescein in the conjunctival sac, the test will not identify whether the abnormality is in the upper or the lower outflow system.[6]

Saccharin (Hornblass) Test.

The saccharin test was first described by Hornblass and is a simple, noninvasive, accurate method for evaluation of nasolacrimal duct patency. The test is performed with the patient erect, and only one eye is tested at a time. After the instillation of proparacaine, 0.4 ml of a 2 per cent saccharin solution (sterilized by ultrafiltration) is put in the lower conjunctival cul-de-sac. The patient reports the moment when the bittersweet solution is tasted. Subjects who do not taste the solution after 20 minutes are again given 0.4 ml of the 2 per cent saccharin solution. After 30 minutes, subjects who do not report tasting the initial saccharin solution have 0.4 ml of saccharin placed on their tongues to determine whether any tasting problems exist. If they have a normal gustatory sense, there is a functional blockage of the lacrimal drainage system.[7]

Dacryocystography.

Dacryocystography[8, 9] is performed by the instillation of a low viscosity, high contrast medium. Isophendylate (Pantopaque) or ethiodized oil (Ethiodol) has been found to be ideal for radiographic contrast studies; it is easy to instill into the lacrimal system and passes through readily. The normal emptying time for the lacrimal sac is 15 minutes and 15 to 30 minutes for the nasolacrimal duct. Only minimal retention of contrast medium is found in the normal system at the end of 30 minutes. Substantial retention after 30 minutes is a highly reliable index of abnormal outflow function. Abnormal retention of the contrast medium after 30 minutes can be found in the systems that are patent, as well as those that are completely obstructed. The term functional block has been used to describe lacrimal systems in which patency can be demonstrated by irrigation and in which abnormal retention of the contrast medium is found after the 30-minute interval. A normal nasolacrimal canal is directed a few degrees medially and posteriorly. The diameter of the nasolacrimal duct increases inferiorly. The outline of the normal lacrimal passage is smooth, except for constrictions that occasionally may be seen in the lacrimal sac (valves of Taillefer and Hasner).

Abnormalities.

A canaliculus that is well outlined by the injected contrast medium indicates some type of abnormality, usually a stenosis of the lacrimal sac or nasolacrimal duct, which causes resistance to the flow of the contrast medium. Irregular distribution of the contrast medium may indicate a lacrimal sac that is filled with soft, cheesy dacryoliths from which fungi frequently can be cultured. Irregularity of outline also may suggest the process of a dacryolith, as may an abnormal shape of the lacrimal sac. The radiographic appearance of lacrimal sac tumors varies greatly, and a shadow on a dacryocystogram only reinforces the clinical impression that a tumor may be present. Dacryocystographic evidence of a mass that extends above the medial canthal tendon strongly suggests a lacrimal sac tumor, even if there is little clinical evidence of infection. Injuries to the lacrimal sac usually reveal irregular radiographic patterns and an enlarged sac or may show extensive scarring from the original injury or from previous attempts to repair the defect. A deviated nasal septum, enlarged turbinates, or nasal polyps may be noted on dacryocystograms, and they should be corrected if they contribute to the lacrimal disorder. The size and position of the ethmoid sinuses should be carefully studied, as an enormously wide ethmoid sinus may make anastomosis of the lacrimal sac into the nose more difficult because of the great distance of the sac from the nasal cavity.[9]

Radioactive Isotope Studies. A technique utilizing the radioactive tracer sodium pertechnetate ^{99m}Tc to outline the lacrimal drainage system by means of scintigraphy has been described by Rossomondo et al.[10] The radiation level to which the patient is exposed is considerably less than with conventional dacryocystography, and because no instrumentation is required, the technique is noninvasive.

LACRIMAL TRACT SURGERY

The treatment of dacryocystitis and tearing problems has been documented in the medical literature since 1800 BC. During the evolution of the surgical techniques, three principles remained the basis of all attempts to improve the lacrimal drainage system: (1) destruction of the sac, (2) drainage into the nose, and (3) restoration of the natural passages.

The decision to treat surgically an obstruction of the lacrimal passage depends on the severity of the patient's symptoms and whether infection of the sac is present. Unlike an eye with pathologic epiphora, an eye that occasionally weeps in the wind or when the person is in a smoky room does not require surgery. Repeated episodes of dacryocystitis that require antibiotic therapy, however, must be considered cause for surgery. In infants, the usual site of obstruction is a mucous membrane closure of the nasolacrimal duct as it enters the nose beneath the inferior turbinate. Tearing is the

first symptom of the condition. In some infants the obstruction disappears spontaneously by the age of 4 to 5 months.[12, 13] In others, massage of the sac may be helpful in opening the tract and preventing infection by keeping the sac empty. If spontaneous reopening does not occur within 6 to 12 months, probing is necessary. If the blockage is complicated by infection, an antibiotic should be used, followed by probing as soon as the infection is under control. Infection is rare before the age of 1 month; however, it sometimes does occur and should be treated with hot compresses and antibiotics.

Massage of the lacrimal sac in children should be carried out by the parent two or three times daily. A finger is placed over the inner canthus to occlude both the upper and lower puncta, and intermittent firm pressure over the sac is then exerted in an inward and downward direction to force the tears into the nose.

The probing procedure consists of breaking the delicate mucous membrane block at the nasal orifice of the duct. This procedure is a good method of investigation of the lacrimal excretory system in adults and is therapeutic in children.

TESTING AND PROBING THE LACRIMAL TRACT

Probing the lacrimal passage was first used by Anel (1713) and popularized by Bowman (1857).[11] Because this procedure failed to obtain or maintain patency in adult cases, it was used as a diagnostic procedure. In adults the probe usually will be inserted as far as the lacrimal sac. Irrigation is usually attempted; if successful, it is not necessary to probe beyond this point. This technique evaluates the patency of the upper portion of the lacrimal drainage system. In adults, obstruction of the nasolacrimal duct (the lower end of the excretory system) is usually not permanently relieved by probing. In children, because of the difference in the etiology of obstruction, probing is therapeutic, and the probe should be passed through the canaliculi, sac, and nasolacrimal duct to enter the nose.

General anesthesia is required in probing children because of the lack of cooperation. In adults, the conjunctiva and punctum should be anesthetized; this can easily be done by placing a cotton-tipped applicator soaked in 4 per cent cocaine solution in the medial canthus for a few minutes. First, the upper punctum is identified. Often it is tiny and may also have an epithelial closure. With good lighting, however, a dimple usually can be seen by magnification. This dimple can then be slightly enlarged by gently dissecting it with the point of a small safety pin so that a slender and rather sharp-pointed punctum dilator can be inserted into the ampulla. This dilator is used to enlarge the punctum slightly and is then replaced by a dilator with a round point that will enlarge the punctum to admit a lacrimal irrigating needle on a syringe.

Irrigation should be attempted before probing. The patency of the lower canaliculus is demonstrated by the appearance of a small spout of fluid from the opposite punctum. The other canaliculus is occluded with a cotton-tipped applicator, and as the pressure is continued, free irrigation indicates that the nasolacrimal duct is mechanically open. In children, if the irrigation does not pass through, a number 00 olive-tipped probe is inserted through the upper punctum and passed nasally through the canaliculus to the common canaliculus as far as the nasal wall of the sac. The tip is then turned downward into the sac. The probe is passed beneath the medial canthal tendon, where it will be at a slightly deeper level than the canaliculus. It is then passed gently inferiorly and nasally, following the funnel-shaped lower portion of the sac, until it is directed into the bony lacrimal canal. When the tip of the probe is engaged, it is much less movable than when it is in the sac. The probe is advanced until it meets the obstruction at the nasal mucous membrane junction. Until this point in the operation, no force should be exerted to make the probe follow the tract. At this stage, a slight push will rupture a congenital membrane and allow the probe to enter the nose, and a little blood will be noticed inside the nose, but if there is a bony obstruction, the procedure will not be successful. It is usually difficult to see the end of the probe in the nose, but often another probe inserted beneath the inferior turbinate will give metal-to-metal contact and indicate that the procedure has been successful. If the first probing has been technically unsuccessful or if symptoms persist, a second probing can be tried in 1 or 2 months. If this attempt fails, or if dacryocystitis is present, a dacryocystorhinostomy may be done.

If dacryocystitis recurs after probing, the probing should be repeated. The second passage through the nasolacrimal duct obstruction should be accompanied by intubation of the lacrimal passages with Silastic tubing to prevent restenosis of the nasolacrimal duct. A vertical cut is made through the internal wall of the upper and lower puncta and canaliculi with a fine, sharp, pointed scissors. This is followed by passing a Quickert probe[17] with attached Silastic through the dilated upper punctum and canaliculus, lacrimal sac, nasolacrimal duct, and nasal cavity, exiting through the external nostril. The probe is pulled through the lacrimal passages after ointment is applied to the junction of the probe and Silastic tube to prevent their separation. The other probe attached to the opposite side of the Silastic tube is passed through the dilated lower punctum, canaliculus, lacrimal sac, and nasolacrimal duct and out through the external nostril. The two ends of the Silastic tubing are connected just internal to the external nostril with 4–0 Dacron suture, and the probes and excess tubing are excised at the nostril (Fig. 22–3). The Dacron suture then passes through the nasal septal cartilage just internal to the external nostrils and is tied. The tubes are removed in 2 to 3 months by cutting the tube between the upper and lower puncta and removing the ends from the nose and the Dacron from the nasal septal cartilage.[18] If dacryocystitis recurs, a dacryocystorhinostomy is performed.

Anesthesia for Lacrimal Drainage System Operations. If the patient's condition is not suitable for general anesthesia, local injections of an anesthetic agent are required. This procedure can be done as follows: The nose is temporarily packed with gauze saturated with 4 per cent cocaine solution above the middle turbinate. The infraorbital nerve then can be blocked by injection of lidocaine below the midpoint of the inferior orbital rim where it emerges from the maxillary bone. Another injection is necessary to block the anterior ethmoid nerves at the point just inferior to the insertion of the medial canthal tendon to the bone (infratrochlear block). Local subcutaneous infiltration of lidocaine at the site of the proposed incision is also necessary to complete the blockage. A posterior nasal pack may be used to prevent aspiration of blood or mucus, but the nose should not be packed in the region of the middle turbinate, which may interfere with the instrumentation of the nasal cavity during the operation.

DACRYOCYSTECTOMY

Excision or destruction of the sac is rarely indicated but may be the procedure of choice in elderly, infirm patients with chronic or recurrent dacryocystitis, who cannot tolerate a

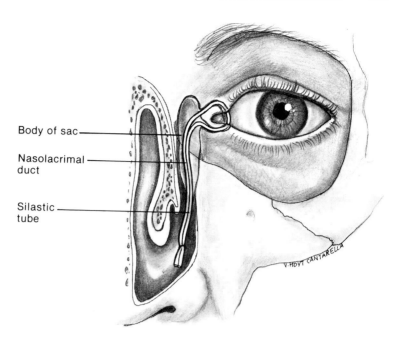

Figure 22–3. Intubation of the nasolacrimal duct, showing a Silastic tube threaded through the canaliculi, through the nasolacrimal duct, and into the nose.

Body of sac

Nasolacrimal duct

Silastic tube

major surgical procedure and who already have decreased tear production due to senile atrophy of the lacrimal glands. Another indication for excision or destruction of the sac is to extirpate a malignant tumor.

The surgical or chemical destruction of the lacrimal sac has the advantage of being a short and easy procedure that demands less technical skill. This was one of the first procedures for dacryocystitis.[15] The elimination of the drainage system may cause persistent epiphora, but postoperative epiphora is rarely a significant complaint in the cases selected for this procedure.

The early method of destruction of the mucous membrane by cautery was replaced by diathermy[15] or by chemical destruction of the mucosa after incision into the sac. Injection of sclerosing agents into the canaliculi has been reported using silver nitrate, zinc chloride, trichloroacetic acid, mercuric chloride, and chromic acid. These procedures, however, are now virtually obsolete with the development of improved surgical techniques.

LACRIMAL BYPASS PROCEDURES

Tear drainage is a relatively complicated process that is susceptible to obstruction at virtually any point. However, significant blockage occurs either proximally in the canalicular system or distally at the lacrimal sac–nasolacrimal duct junction. Bypass procedures aimed at correcting these obstructions must be directed at the site of the blockage (Table 22–2). When the proximal portion of the lacrimal excretory system is occluded, virtually none of the normal drainage apparatus is available for tear excretion, and the entire system must be circumvented. This is referred to as a total bypass. When the distal portion of the lacrimal excretory system is occluded, partial bypass procedures are indicated.

TOTAL BYPASS PROCEDURES

Total bypass procedure was first reported by Jones.[2] He utilized a Pyrex tube that passed from the nasal portion of the conjunctival sac into the nose via a surgical osteotomy.

TABLE 22–2. Nasolacrimal Duct Bypass Procedures

Total Bypass
Jones' Pyrex tube
Reinecke's technique
Wadsworth-Chandler technique
Cooper total bypass
Partial Bypass
Standard dacryocystorhinostomy
Iliff modification
Cooper partial bypass

Indications for Total Bypass Procedures.
Jones[2] has defined the indications for total bypass as follows:

1. Congenital absence, traumatic destruction, or complete closures of both canaliculi in one eye.

2. Closure of 2 mm or more of the nasal ends of the canaliculi.

3. Flaccid canaliculi that are demonstrated to be patent by the primary and secondary dye tests, when all conservative measures for relieving the epiphora have failed.

4. Canaliculi that are patent but nonfunctioning after a dacryocystorhinostomy.

5. Permanent paralysis of the lacrimal pump. Pseudoepiphora and epiphora due to lacrimal hypersecretion are never indications for surgical treatment of the lacrimal excretory system.

JONES' PYREX TUBE TECHNIQUE[20]

After the lacrimal sac is open (see Fig. 22–5 for detail of dacryocystorhinostomy operation), part or all of the caruncle is excised. Care must be taken so that none of the adjacent conjunctival tissue is removed with it. A 23-gauge hypodermic needle (30-mm long) is bent into a curve so that the point of the needle is on the inside of the curve. The needle should be held with the concavity of the curve facing anteriorly, and the point is inserted into the area exactly 2.5 mm posterior to the cutaneous margin of the canthal angle. It is pushed in a direction that will cause its point to emerge just posterior to the anterior flap of the lacrimal sac and slightly below the level of the palpebral fissure. Several attempts may be necessary to get the point to emerge at exactly the right place. It must be anterior to the body of the ethmoid bone and middle turbinate. The anterior end of the turbinate should be resected if it interferes with the tip of the needle. A cataract knife of medium width is inserted from the area through the lacrimal sac, following the guide needle. The needle is removed, and the knife enlarges the passage, superiorly and inferiorly, just enough to allow insertion of a Pyrex tube. The knife is not removed until a number 1 Bowman probe without a handle is inserted along the blade of the knife and into the nose. The knife is removed and a Pyrex tube (about 16-mm long with a 4-mm collar on its distal end) is threaded onto the probe and pushed into place. The remainder of the procedure is as a classic dacryocystorhinostomy. Tubes often can be replaced as an office procedure with the use of local anesthetic.

REINECKE'S TECHNIQUE

This technique uses dacryorhinostomy with silicone tube bypass.[21] Moderate pressure is applied over the area injected with anesthesia so that the swelling is reduced. If available, a scleral shell is applied to avoid corneal abrasions. The incision is made halfway between the center of the nose and the medial canthus. The lacrimal ridge usually can be palpated, and the incision should be just medial to the ridge. The incision is carried down to the bone in one stroke.

The surgeon controls the bleeding by applying small hemostats and cautery to the clamps. The Bovie is also helpful. A retractor is inserted, which exposes the periosteum. A small periosteal elevator raises the periosteum posteriorly. The bone is opened with a trephine, drill, or chisel. The opening is generously enlarged with the Kerrison rongeur. An instrument with a flat handle is inserted, handle first, into the naris so that the handle presses against the mucosa in the area to be incised. A scalpel is used to incise a round piece of mucosa, the handle of the instrument being used in the nose for a cutting block. Annoying bleeding that seems to come from the mucosa of the nose usually can be controlled by pressing the handle of the instrument laterally against the nasal mucosa.

A sharp-pointed scissors is used to make a track from the medial conjunctiva through the lacrimal sac into the surgical incision. The scissors is advanced by spreading until it enters the nose. With the scissors still in place, a small alligator forceps is slid into the track, the scissors is removed, and the end of a number 90 polyethylene tube is grasped and pulled through. The alligator clamp is used to draw the number 90 tube down and out of the nose. The tube is now ready to act as a guide for the silicone tube. It is threaded into the silicone tube. If silicone oil is used, insertion of the number 90 tube becomes easier. Both tubes are maneuvered so that the silicone tube reaches the desired place.

The skin is sutured with interrupted 6–0 silk. The sutures are cut short, and only small bits of skin are taken. The sutures usually fall out unassisted within 1 week. A 5–0 monofilament nylon suture is passed through the flange of the silicone tube and a 3-mm bit of skin at the medial canthus, and the suture is tied. The ends of the suture should be left long so that they will not untie and can be found easily. The suture should remain in place for 1 or 2 months until the silicone tube no longer shows a tendency to move. The number 90 tube is withdrawn from the nose, a drop of antibiotic solution applied to the eye, the scleral shell removed (if present), a small piece of Telfa applied to the wound area, and a mild pressure dressing applied.

WADSWORTH-CHANDLER TECHNIQUE[22]

A flanged polyethylene tube is placed through the inferior conjunctival fornix medially and into the nasolacrimal duct where it enters the nose under the inferior turbinate. This provides a route for tear drainage directly from the conjunctival sac into the nose without the need to create a surgical osteotomy.

This technique has proved to be most successful in our hands with minor alterations. Initially, heat-flared polyethylene tubing was used. Polyethylene is readily available and the end can be flared by holding it close to a lighted match for a few seconds. However, polyethylene is relatively thick walled, so that for a useful inside diameter to be achieved, a large outside diameter is required. In addition, polyethylene is not a wettable substance, thus little or no capillary attraction is developed within the tube. More recently, preformed Teflon tubing has proved to be most effective. Teflon is thin and strong, allowing a maximum inside-to-outside-diameter ratio. It is wettable and has a high tissue tolerance.

COOPER TOTAL BYPASS

If the obstruction is proximal to the nasolacrimal sac, a Teflon tube is placed from the inferior conjunctival sac to the nose via the nasolacrimal canal. This procedure is readily performed under local anesthesia. The nasolacrimal duct can be easily anesthetized by the direct instillation of 1 to 2 ml of 2 per cent lidocaine.

When total obstruction has been present for any length of time, the lacrimal sac frequently atrophies and is difficult to find. Therefore, no attempt to identify the sac is made, hence no skin incision is necessary.

A stab or scissors incision into the lower fornix medially is made (Fig. 22–4A) and carried inferiorly until the orbital floor is encountered near the anterior lacrimal crest. A wire probe similar in size to a number 4 Bowman probe without the flange is inserted into the incision and passed behind the anterior lacrimal crest (Fig. 22–4B). In this manner, the nasal fossa is entered via the nasolacrimal canal. The Teflon

tube is then passed over the probe into the nasolacrimal canal and enters the nose beneath the inferior turbinate (Fig. 22–4C). The probe is withdrawn, and the tube is anchored to the adjacent tissues with a 6–0 mercelene suture (Fig. 22–4D). The Teflon tubes are constructed with a flange, which sets into the conjunctival fornix (Fig. 22–4E). If the caruncle is near the orifice of the tube, as much as is needed is amputated. On occasion, the insertion of the tube meets with resistance. This can be easily overcome by reaming the canal several times with the probe.

PARTIAL BYPASS PROCEDURES

Toti (1904) pioneered the modern operation of external dacryocystorhinostomy.[11] The original external dacryocystorhinostomy of Toti consisted of exposing the sac by an external incision, resecting its inner wall, punching out a corresponding piece of nasal bone with a hammer and chisel, resecting a corresponding area of the nasal mucous membrane, and sewing up the external wound. Its success depended largely on the extensiveness of the resection; even so, the formation of granulations or presence of extensive disease of the walls of the sac frequently resulted in failures from subsequent cicatrization. This led Kuhnt (1914) to suture flaps of the nasal mucosa to the periosteum to limit the formation of granulations. Ohm (1920) sutured the margins of the nasal mucosa to the sac. Dupuy-Dutemps and Bourguet (1921),[11] by incising the posterior wall of the sac without any sacrifice of tissue, sutured the nasal and lacrimal mucous membranes together over the bony margins so that no part of the wound might remain to cicatrize.[15] These operations evolved into the current techniques, which have a high percentage of success.

Indications for Partial Lacrimal Bypass
1. All indications for conventional dacryocystorhinostomy wherein the lacrimal sac is enlarged clinically or radiographically.
2. Patients who are considered poor surgical and/or anesthetic candidates who have distally obstructed nasolacrimal drainage systems.

STANDARD DACRYOCYSTORHINOSTOMY

This technique entails posterior flaps.[16] Both patient and surgeon usually prefer general anesthesia for such major surgical procedures in the facial area.

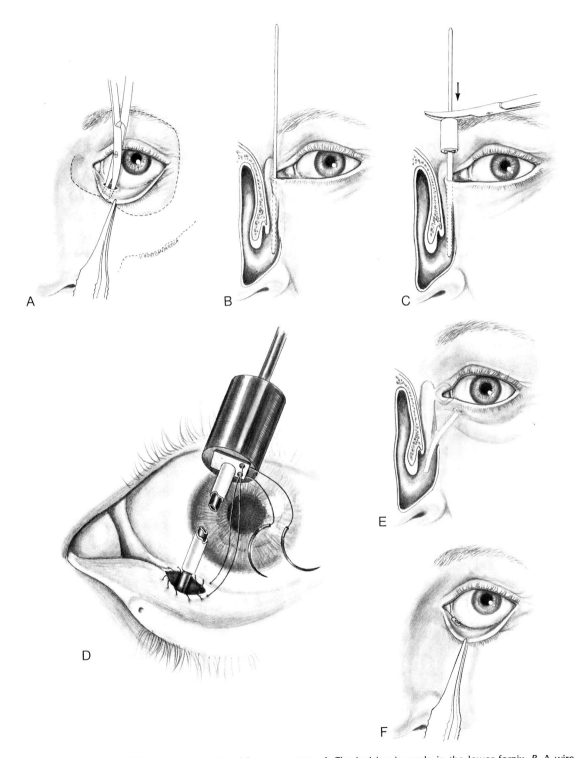

Figure 22–4. Cooper Teflon nasolacrimal total bypass system. *A,* The incision is made in the lower fornix. *B,* A wire probe is inserted into the incision into the nose. *C,* A Teflon tube is placed over the probe. *D,* The 6–0 mercelene sutures are placed to anchor the tube. *E,* Cooper tube in place after the procedure. *F,* View of the orifice of the Cooper tube at the lower fornix.

The approach to the sac is through a skin incision on the lateral side of the nose. The placement of the incision varies with different surgeons. Chandler recommends a slightly curvilinear incision midway between the middle of the bridge of the nose and the medial canthus.[22] Because the angular vein may have a varied course, it may be necessary to vary the site of the incision. If the vein is considered to be a surgical nuisance, it may be cut and tied off without embarrassing the venous circulation in the area.

The incision is taken down to bone, thus dividing the skin, muscle, and periosteum in a clean cut. The periosteum is then separated from the bone, beginning from above downward as far as the anterior lacrimal crest, which is the first landmark sought. Practically no bleed-

ing will occur by following this subperiosteal level incision, except if a nutrient vessel is encountered. Bleeding can be controlled in seconds with cautery or pressure application.

At the level of the anterior lacrimal crest, the periosteum is a little more adherent than on the nasal bone (Fig. 22–5A). The anterior lacrimal crest shelves laterally into a sharp edge, and the lacrimal fossa is deep. The sac lying immediately underneath the crest may be damaged if care is not taken.

It is therefore essential to strip the fascia from the crest and identify the sac before the next step is undertaken. The whole crest is exposed from its upper limit to its lower, where it continues as the lower orbital margin. Once the fascia is separated from the crest, which is the strongest and closest point of adhesion,

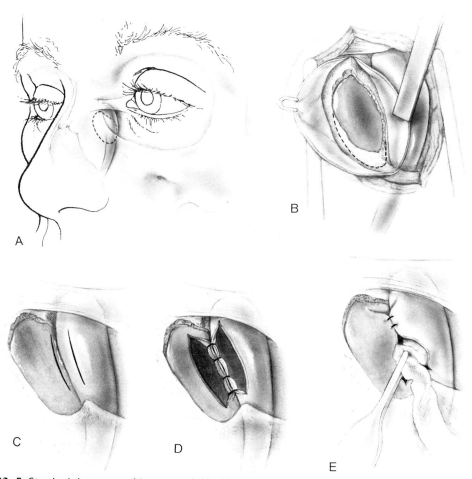

Figure 22–5. Standard dacryocystorhinostomy. *A,* Ideal location for osteotomy. *B,* Bone has been removed, exposing underlying nasal mucosa. *C,* Incisions made through nasal mucosa and lacrimal sac. *D,* Posterior flaps are sutured with an absorbable suture. *E,* Anterior flaps are sutured and the packing is removed.

dislocation of the sac laterally is simple, as it is loosely placed in the lacrimal fossa.

The next step is the removal of the bone that intervenes between the two structures to be anastomosed, namely the lacrimal sac and the nasal mucous membrane. The bone that is involved constitutes the lacrimal fossa, frontal process of the maxilla, and the lacrimal bone.

Removal of the bone can be accomplished by the use of a trephine or by hammer, chisel, and rongeurs (Fig. 22–5B). Some care is required at this stage. An uncontrolled thrust will damage the underlying nasal mucosa and cause massive bleeding. Careful anticipation will avoid such an accident and all its attendant complications. If the trephine is used, the disc of bone can be levered out intact and without difficulty. The site of the trephination is simply a point of entry. Further bone must be removed by rongeurs, down to the level of the posterior lacrimal sac. The temptation to go more posteriorly will lead to unnecessary trouble, as one may encounter anterior ethmoid air cells or, rarely, the anterior ethmoid artery. Not only are these structures unnecessarily exposed, but in the nasal cavity the anterior part of the middle turbinate will be exposed, which will only complicate the anastomosis. The desired position in the nose is anterior to the middle turbinate.

Occasionally, anterior ethmoid cells encroach on the surgical field and it is necessary to remove the cells. It is important to recognize such a cell so as not to confuse its lining with nasal mucosa and effect a useless anastomosis.

When the surgeon has created a bony opening (Fig. 22–5B) correctly placed, the lacrimal sac should be opposite the nasal mucosa. The anatomic arrangement of the structures is such that nasal mucosa slopes downward and laterally, whereas the sac slopes downward and medially.

Entry into the lacrimal sac is undertaken first. This enables nasal mucosal flaps to be fashioned according to the findings in the sac. It also bleeds less than the nasal mucosa and therefore inspection of the interior of the sac is easier.

There are many ways of entering the sac. One is to divide the sac from the nasolacrimal duct at the point where the nasolacrimal duct enters the bony canal. An angled rhinostomy scissors is used to facilitate this maneuver. It is then easy to insert one blade of the angled scissors into the lumen of the sac and simply extend the cut along the medial wall. Two equal flaps result, although the size of the flap could be varied by moving the scissors anteriorly or posteriorly within the sac lumen (Fig. 22–5C).

Direct visualization of the common opening guarantees that the lumen of the sac is entered, because it is possible to divide the outer covering of the sac without exposing the true interior.

The next step is the fashioning of the nasal mucosal flaps, tailored according to the requirements of the already formed sac flaps. The same angled scissors is used for this maneuver. The flap is not hinged unless absolutely necessary, thus avoiding the risk of reducing its blood supply and its viability. Only when apposition is difficult for any reason is hinging performed.

Both anterior and posterior flaps are sutured with an absorbable suture and with a technique selected by the individual surgeon (Fig. 22–5D, E). To ensure separation of anterior and posterior suture lines, an indwelling rubber catheter may be left inside the anastomosis and secured by an absorbable stitch to a point where the fundus of the sac was located. The same effect, of course, can be achieved by securing the anterior flap to the undersurface of the overlying skin-muscle-periosteal block by any appropriate suture. The skin incision is closed by a continuous subcuticular nylon suture. No further subcutaneous sutures are necessary for the underlying tissues.

No postoperative irrigations are carried out. If the operation has been performed correctly and for the proper indications, cessation of epiphora is immediate. A wide-spectrum antibiotic is instilled into the conjunctival sac twice daily for several days. The subcuticular nylon is removed after the fifth day. If a catheter was used to separate the flap suture lines, it is removed at the same time.

ILIFF MODIFICATION

This technique is performed with no flap. The orbital rim (the anterior lacrimal crest) and the medial canthal ligament are palpated to outline clearly the site of the incision, which extends 2 cm from the medial canthal ligament along the rim. A bold incision to the orbital rim is made with a number 15 Bard-Parker knife through skin, subcutaneous tissue, orbicularis muscle, and periosteum. This incision should be placed in the normal skin fold for the best cosmetic result. The reason for insisting on this single bold cut down to the periosteum is that layer-by-layer dissection will often cause the tissues to slide on one another as they are retracted by the assistant, and the direct course to the orbital crest is thus lost. This makes the surgery exceedingly difficult, especially if severe bleeding occurs. The amount of postoperative scarring is minimal. Iliff believes that placing the initial incision closer to the nose, as advocated by some surgeons to reduce the bleeding, is not valid.[19] Moreover, the scar of a more nasally placed incision is more likely to show postoperatively than one in a normal lid crease along the anterior lacrimal crest.

Skin rake retractors (Blair) provide adequate exposure of the anterior lacrimal crest and have proved more satisfactory than a speculum because the retractors can be easily adjusted to control superficial bleeders. The operative field is kept dry by suction, and blood vessels are occluded with cautery.

If the incision of the periosteum along the lacrimal crest has not been complete with the first through-and-through cut, it is deepened to bone with the Bard-Parker knife. A periosteal elevator (Freer) is used to strip the periosteum and sac (to which it is closely adherent) from the bony lacrimal fossa. These tissues are retracted together, thus exposing the anterior lacrimal crest and fossa.

The dacryotrephine of the Stryker saw is placed straddling the anterior crest and is directed nasally, inferiorly, and slightly posteriorly. Slight rotation of the saw increases the cutting action. The bone is cut cleanly, and the plug usually comes out as the trephine blade is withdrawn; if not, it is freed with a periosteal elevator and removed with forceps. Bone wax provides adequate control of any bony bleeding.

Usually the 7-mm trephine hole must be enlarged with a sphenoid punch to provide a more direct passage for the catheter from the nose to the neck of the sac. Any spicules of bone can be removed easily with the punch, and the hole can be enlarged to give a more elliptic opening, the extension being made downward.

A cruciate or H-shaped incision is made in the nasal mucous membrane if it is normal in thickness. If there is marked hypertrophy of the mucous membrane, it is completely excised over the trephine opening.

Often, hypertrophic mucous membrane of the nose will bleed profusely; therefore, by shifting the suction from the operative incision to the nose at the site of the internal opening, the surgical field can be kept dry, and the suction tube will not obscure the work area.

A probe is passed into the sac, usually through the upper punctum. The end of the probe in the sac helps to identify exactly the nasal wall of the sac, which is opened with a number 11 Bard-Parker knife with a vertical incision to expose the end of the probe.

A curved Halsted clamp is passed up through the nose into the nasal trephine window to grasp the tip of a urinary catheter, which is then drawn into the nose and out the external nares. The proximal end of the catheter is cut off, leaving 3 cm projecting from the wound.

A double-armed, 3–0 chromic catgut suture with a small, half-curved, special needle (Ethicon number 748–G) is placed through the wall of the catheter, 1 cm from the cut end. This end of the catheter is grasped with toothed forceps and is pushed gently into the wound past the end of the probe and then is pulled back, threading the catheter over the lacrimal probe that is lying in the sac. Tension on the suture pulls the catheter up into the neck of the sac, with the probe acting as a guide. Care is taken that the cut edges of the sac wall are not caught on the end of the catheter, but lie around it.

The two arms of the suture are then passed through the anterior sac wall and subcutaneous tissue, and as they are being pulled tight and tied, the catheter is forced into the neck of the sac. Placing the suture 1 cm from the end of the catheter (as mentioned) is important in producing this effect.

The probe is then withdrawn, and as the skin rakes are removed, the tissues fall together and the catheter acts as a splint. The cut edges of the medial wall of the sac and the cut edges of the nasal mucous membrane are in contact. Slight tension on the catheter, after it is fastened to the ala of the nose with the 3–0 chromic catgut suture, enhances this tissue approximation and the catheter splinting action. The skin of the incision is closed with 8–0 interrupted but closely placed silk sutures, and the wound is lightly dressed with a nonadherent dressing and an eye pad.

The patient is hospitalized for only 24 hours. The skin sutures are removed after 4 days. The catheter is removed at 10 days by cutting the suture in the ala and giving a short quick tug on the catheter, thus breaking the now friable catgut suture between the catheter and the anterior sac wall.

The conventional surgical approach to restore drainage when the blockage is at the distal end of the nasolacrimal sac is a dacryocystorhinostomy, as was described. A significant number of patients with this problem may be handled in a much simpler and more physiologic manner. This technique is most applicable to those in whom preoperative dacryocystograms reveal an enlarged lacrimal sac.

COOPER PARTIAL BYPASS TECHNIQUE

Local anesthesia is preferred. A curvilinear incision is made over the anterior lacrimal crest as described by Iliff[19] (Fig. 22–6A). The dissection is carried down to the periosteum and then posteriorly until the lacrimal sac is encountered (Fig. 22–6B). The sac is opened vertically and any contents evacuated (Fig. 22–6C). A nonflanged number 4 Bowman probe is then passed into the opened sac and down the nasolacrimal duct (Fig. 22–6D). A funnel-shaped Teflon tube, approximately 20 to 25 mm in length, is then passed over the probe and into the sac and nasal fossa via the nasolacrimal duct. The funnel-shaped proximal end of the tube lodges in the distal end of the lacrimal sac (Fig. 22–6E). The distal end of the tube lies in the nasal fossa. The tube is then anchored by a 6–0 merselene suture into the sac wall (Fig. 22–

6F). The sac is closed with interrupted 5–0 chromic catgut sutures (Fig. 22–6G). The subcutaneous tissues are closed with similar material and the skin with any suture of choice (Fig. 22–6H).

Complications of Dacryocystorhinostomy. Complications are rare if the preceding routine is followed. The following, however, may be encountered: There may be troublesome bleeding from the angular veins if cut. Sometimes an aberrant venous branch is encountered, causing similar problems. The bleeding must be stopped to have a good view of the structures to be identified.

If the nasal mucous membrane is inadver-

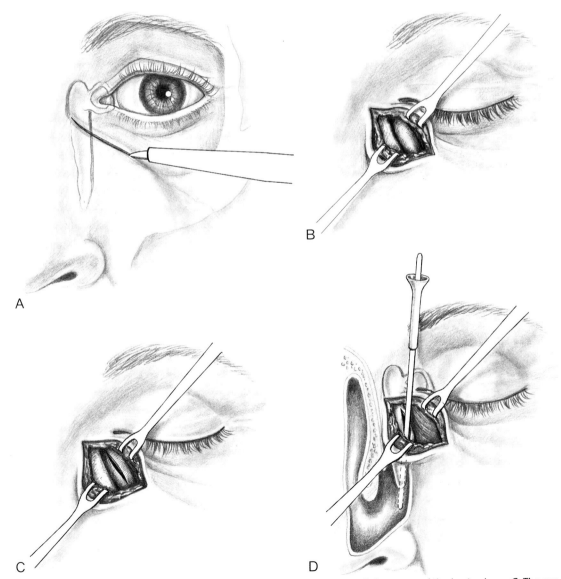

Figure 22–6. Cooper partial bypass technique. *A,* Placement of the incision. *B,* Exposure of the lacrimal sac. *C,* The sac is opened vertically. *D,* A nonflanged Bowman probe is passed into the opened sac and down the nasolacrimal duct.

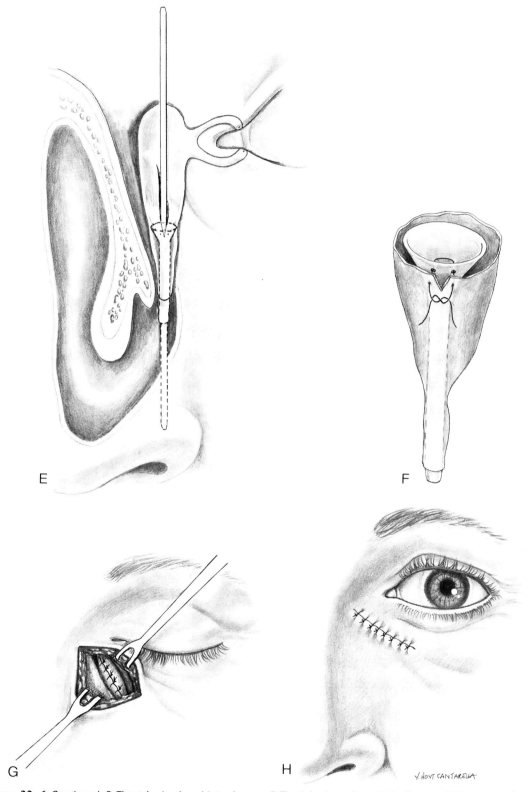

E

F

G

H

V. HOYT CANTARELLA

Figure 22–6 *Continued. E,* The tube is placed into the sac. *F,* The tube is anchored into the sac. *G,* The sac is closed with interrupted sutures. *H,* The skin is closed in a standard fashion.

tently damaged at the time of trephining the bone, repair should be undertaken at that stage. A torn mucosa will make the formation of flaps difficult if not impossible.

Anterior ethmoid air cells must be recognized and removed. If their mucous lining is mistaken for nasal mucosa and used for flap formation, failure is inevitable.

Inspection of the interior of the sac is important. Unsuspected pathologic changes, such as partial occlusion of the common opening, plugs of inspissated mucus, dacryoliths, diverticuli, and tumors, may be seen on inspection when not suspected on clinical investigation. For this reason it should be opened before touching the nasal mucosa.

If flap formation is difficult owing to any mechanical or traumatic incident, the posterior flap is of greater importance than the anterior. A continuous lining of mucosal surface will conduct tears into the nose more easily than if none existed. The roof of the anastomosis is of secondary importance.

Epistaxis is a rare complication, but when it occurs it is troublesome and requires immediate attention. It may be the result of reactionary hemorrhage, infection, or pre-existent nasal "varices."

Failure to relieve symptoms should arouse suspicion of several possibilities: (1) incorrect placing of the bony aperture, (2) incorrect entry into the sac cavity, (3) missed cause in the sac itself, (4) anastomosis of the sac to ethmoid air cell, (5) incorrect selection of the case. In such cases a re-examination of the lacrimal pathway should be undertaken.

References

1. Becker B, Shaffer R: Diagnosis and Therapy of the Glaucomas. St Louis, CV Mosby, 1965, p 219.
2. Jones LT: The lacrimal secretory system and its treatment. Am J Ophthalmol 62:47, 1966.
3. Duke-Elder WS: System of Ophthalmology. Vol XIII, Part II. St Louis, CV Mosby, 1974, p 595.
4. Peyman GA, Sanders DA, Goldberg MF: Principles and Practice of Ophthalmology. Philadelphia, WB Saunders, 1980.
5. Jones LT: The cure of epiphora due to canalicular disorders, trauma and surgical failures on the lacrimal passages. Trans Am Acad Ophthalmol Otolaryngol 66:506, 1962.
6. Zappia RJ, Milder B: Lacrimal drainage function. 2. The fluorescein dye disappearance test. Am J Ophthalmol 74:160, 1972.
7. Hornblass A: A simple test for lacrimal obstruction. Arch Ophthalmol 90:435, 1973.
8. Veirs ER, Duane TD: Clinical Ophthalmology. Vol 4. New York, Harper and Row, 1979.
9. Milder B, et al: Ophthalmic plastic surgery. Am Acad Ophthalmol Otolaryngol 16:168, 1964.
10. Rossomondo RM, et al: A new method of evaluating lacrimal drainage. Arch Ophthalmol 88:523, 1972.
11. Duke-Elder WS: System of Ophthalmology. Vol XIII, Part II. St Louis, CV Mosby, 1974, p 680.
12. Cassady JV: Developmental anatomy of the nasolacrimal duct. Arch Ophthalmol 47:141, 1952.
13. Imre Korchmaros E, et al: Rate of spontaneous opening of congenitally blocked lacrimal pathways. IRCS: The Eye 4:541, 1976.
14. Milder B: Functional Block in the Lacrimal Drainage System, VIII. Balgica, Concilium Ophthalmologicum, 1958, p 1111.
15. Duke-Elder WS: System of Ophthalmology. Vol XIII, Part II. St Louis, CV Mosby, 1974, p 715.
16. Werb A, Yamaguchi M (eds): Recent Advances on the Lacrimal System. Japan, Asahi Evening News, 1978.
17. Quickert MH, Dryden RM: Probes for intubation in lacrimal drainage. Trans Am Acad Ophthalmol Otolaryngol 74:431, 1970.
18. Callahan MA: Silicone intubation for lacrimal canaliculi repair. Ann Plast Surg 2:355, 1979.
19. Iliff C: A simplified dacryocystorhinostomy. Highlights Ophthalmol 13:161, 1971.
20. Jones LT: Conjunctiva-dacryocystorhinostomy. Am J Ophthalmol 59:773, 1965.
21. Reinecke RD, Carroll JM: Silicone lacrimal tube implantations. Trans Am Acad Ophthalmol Otolaryngol 73:85, 1969.
22. Chandler AC Jr, Wadsworth AC: Conjunctival-dacryocystostomy: A modified conjunctival-dacryocystorhinostomy. Trans Am Ophthalmol Soc 71:272, 1973.

CHAPTER 23

ORBITAL DECOMPRESSION

Frank E. Lucente, MD
Hugh F. Biller, MD

Malignant exophthalmos of Graves' disease is a distressing, disfiguring, and hazardous complication of unclear etiology; it poses a threat to the patient's vision and mandates prompt and efficient treatment. The pathogenesis of the ocular changes described over 140 years ago by Graves[1] and von Basedow[2] is poorly understood. The major clinical problem appears to result from the hypertrophy of orbital muscles and fat, which produces increased intraorbital pressure and proptosis.[3] As the disease progresses, changes occur in the lids, conjunctiva and cornea. In severe cases, vision may be lost (Table 23–1).

There is no predictable association between the course of the exophthalmos and the course of the underlying thyroid disorder. In some cases, the exophthalmos antedates the clinical appearance of hyperthyroidism, whereas in other patients it may follow successful treatment of the thyroid disease by either medical or surgical means. It has been suggested by some investigators that the exophthalmos may be of pituitary origin.[4, 5] However, no specific hormone responsible for the exophthalmos has been identified.[6]

The rate of progression of exophthalmos varies. It tends to appear gradually, progressing slowly over a period of several years. However, as the malignant stage is reached, a rapid increase in the proptosis and development of other ocular signs and symptoms may occur over a period of several weeks.

TABLE 23–1. Classification of Eye Changes of Graves' Disease*

Class	Definition
0	No signs or symptoms
1	Only signs, no symptoms (signs limited to upper eyelid retraction and stare with or without lid lag and proptosis)
2	Signs and symptoms of soft tissue involvement (eyelid edema, chemosis, congestion)
3	Proptosis
4	Extraocular muscle involvement
5	Corneal involvement
6	Loss of sight (optic nerve involvement)

Patients in classes 4, 5 and 6 should be considered for decompression and some patients in class 3 are suitable candidates.

(Proposed as a modification of the American Thyroid Association classification by Werner SC: Classification of thyroid disease: Report of the Committee on Nomenclature (letter to editor). J Clin Endocrinol Metab 29:982, 1969, The Endocrine Society.)

PATHOLOGIC CHANGES

In studying the pathologic changes in the orbital tissues and ocular muscles, Kroll and Kuwabara[7] and Riley[8] have demonstrated that the muscles are enlarged and rubbery due to interstitial edema caused by an increase in mucopolysaccharides and round cells (lymphocytes, plasma cells, macrophages and mast cells). This edema also places the orbital fat under increased tension.[9]

The eye has abundant retro-orbital fat, which has the capacity for binding water because of the high content of mucopolysaccharides. The intraorbital pressure increases when intraorbital fat tissue tension rises as a result of a secretion from the thyroid or pituitary gland (such as a long-acting thyrotropic stimulating hormone or some unknown hormone) and an increase in tension causes reduced oxygen supply to extraocular muscle. Extraocular muscle hypertrophy can become pronounced, and the muscles may undergo a Zenker type of degeneration. The superior oblique muscle is usually affected first and later all muscles may be involved. As proptosis becomes pronounced and the lids fail to close, exposure of the cornea predisposes the patient to corneal ulcerations. Subsequent involvement of the anterior chamber and the development of panophthalmitis may lead to progressive loss of visual acuity.[3]

SURGICAL THERAPY

Among the types of therapy currently employed are steroids, radiation therapy, and orbital decompression. A trial of steroids is advised, particularly in patients with mild proptosis. Although others have reported success with the use of radiation therapy to the orbits, we have not used this form of treatment. If the proptosis does not respond or if other eye changes are noted, decompression should be considered.

Walsh and Ogura[11] have listed the following indications for surgical decompression: (1) increasing loss of visual acuity, (2) changes in the corneal epithelium, (3) progressive loss of extraocular muscle function, (4) conjunctival chemosis, (5) orbital edema, and (6) cosmetic disfigurement. In addition, the procedure has been used successfully in patients in whom the exophthalmos presents a social or psychologic handicap rather than a threat to ocular function.

Preoperative Evaluation. Preoperative evaluation includes complete ophthalmologic and endocrinologic evaluation. The severity of the exophthalmos is measured using the Hertel exophthalmometer. Most patients requiring decompression have measurements greater than 23 mm. The visual acuity, extraocular muscle function, and pathologic changes in the ocular adnexa (keratitis, conjunctivitis, and lid abnormalities) are assessed. Candidates for operation should be euthyroid by clinical and biochemical evaluation. Specifically, they should not have elevated levels of long-acting thyroid stimulating hormone (LATS). Optimally, the patient should have clear sinuses by radiographic examination, although mild maxillary sinusitis is

not necessarily a contraindication. Preoperative photographs of the eyes and face are obtained in full face and lateral views.[3]

The computed tomography (CT) scan has also been employed to correlate the clinical and pathologic features of Graves' disease.[12, 13] Although it is not mandatory as a preoperative test, the scan will show swelling of the extraocular muscle bellies and sparing of the tendons. This is in distinction to myositis (idiopathic inflammation of the muscles), which tends to involve the tendons. In addition, the CT scan confirms the enlarged volume of the extraocular muscles, the bowing of the lamina papyracea, venous engorgement, conjunctival and lid swelling, and enlargement of the lacrimal gland. The CT scan also allows objective documentation of the extent of the exophthalmos, a factor that may be important in those patients in whom the tenderness of the periorbital skin and soft tissues precludes adequate recording with the Hertel exophthalmometer. The CT scan is important in the preoperative evaluation and diagnosis in unilateral cases of endocrine exophthalmos.

Evolution of Surgical Decompression. The present surgical approach to orbital decompression has evolved during the past 80 years. In the early part of the twentieth century, Dollinger[14] used the procedure originally described by Kronlein[15]; it involved removal of the lateral orbital rim to allow decompression of orbital contents into the temporal fossa. In 1929, Hirsch[16, 17] treated a 24-year-old man with removal of the orbital floor. He used a transantral approach and local anesthesia. Naffziger[18] later reported his experience with the removal of the orbital roof to allow the orbital contents to be decompressed into the anterior cranial fossa. Unfortunately, this procedure was accompanied by transmission of cranial vascular pulsations to the eyes. In 1936, Sewall[19] demonstrated in the laboratory that removal of the lamina papyracea and ethmoid cells through an external incision in the periorbital skin could allow prolapse of orbital contents into the ethmoid sinus. He also illustrated the feasibility for removing the roof of the maxillary sinus through this external approach and alluded to the potential applicability of this operation in malignant exophthalmos. However, he reported no clinical experience with this procedure. Kistner[20] and Schall and Reagan[21] later confirmed the efficacy of this approach. In 1947, Walsh and Ogura[11] first combined the approaches of Hirsch and Sewall with further modifications to devise the transantral approach to the orbit. Their results were first reported in 1957. Since that time, others[22, 23, 24] have confirmed the applicability of this technique.

Objectives. Walsh and Ogura[11] have stated the following to be the objectives of the transantral orbital decompression: (1) restoring threatened vision, use of extraocular muscles, and ability to close both eyelids; (2) relieving increased orbital tension by allowing periorbital tissue to herniate into an actual space; (3) obtaining a satisfactory cosmetic result; (4) avoiding unnecessary incisions on the face or scalp; (5) avoiding surgical trauma to a damaged eye; and (6) avoiding serious immediate or late postoperative complications.

TECHNIQUE

The procedure is performed under general anesthesia. The patient is placed in a semisitting position with the head at a 45-degree angle. To prevent venous stasis in the legs and subsequent venous embolism, the legs are wrapped with elastic bandages from ankle to midthigh. After the patient is intubated, the endotracheal tube is secured with tape around the head so that it will not be dislodged. Sterile ophthalmic lubricant drops are placed in the eyes frequently to prevent desiccation from exposure to the air.

The first stage of the procedure involves performing a Caldwell-Luc maxillary antrotomy (Fig. 23–1) through the standard buccogingival sulcus incision (Fig. 23–2A). After the antrum is entered with an osteotome, a rongeur is used to enlarge the opening by complete removal of the anterior wall (Fig. 23–2B). It is important to remove the superior and medial portions of the wall to provide access into the ethmoid cells.

Entry into the ethmoid cells is facilitated by identifying the points at which the superior, posterior, and medial walls of the maxillary sinus join and the superior, anterior, and medial walls join. Midway between these points, one enters the ethmoid cells with a forward bone-biting forceps. The anterior cells are removed with forward and backward biting forceps. Removal of the ethmoid cells proceeds posteriorly to the previously noted junction between the superior, medial, and posterior walls (Fig. 23–2C). A bony ridge is encountered posteriorly and is removed with a chisel or mastoid curette to allow exposure of the posterior cells to the anterior face of the sphenoid sinus (Fig. 23–2D). The surgeon must be careful to avoid injuring the cribriform plate. This plate slopes inferiorly from anterior to posterior when the head is upright. When the head is extended for the surgical procedure, the plate assumes an almost vertical position. Therefore, the surgeon must be constantly aware of the distance between the anterior nasal spine and the face of the sphenoid, as well as the position of the head.

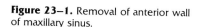

Figure 23–1. Removal of anterior wall of maxillary sinus.

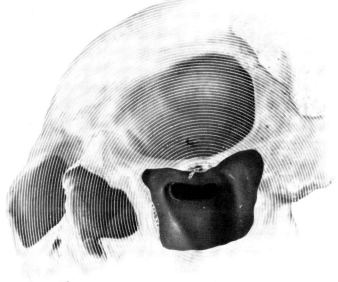

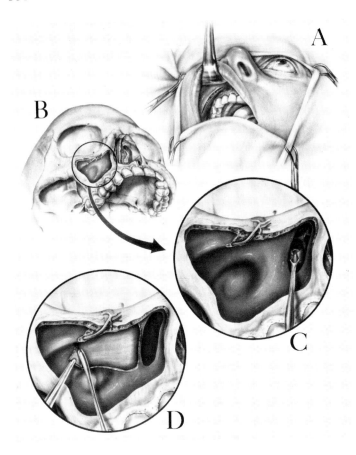

Figure 23–2. *A,* Buccogingival sulcus incision with cheek retracted. *B,* View of floor of orbit after removal of anterior wall of maxillary sinus. *C,* Removal of ethmoid cells with curette. *D,* Removal of floor of orbit with preservation of infraorbital nerve.

Next, the bony floor of the orbit is removed from medial to lateral, using a Kerrison bone rongeur. Care is taken to avoid injuring the infraorbital nerve and artery, which travel through the floor to exit at the infraorbital foramen. Removal of the floor extends laterally to the zygoma, anteriorly to the orbital rim and posteriorly until the bone becomes thick and does not include the region of the optic nerve. The orbital periosteum is preserved as the bone is removed, because premature lacerations of the periosteum allow orbital fat to herniate into the field of vision. Next, the lamina papyracea is removed by fracturing it with a Freer elevator. Again, the periosteum is preserved.

Some reduction of the proptosis is generally noted simply from removing the bony floor and medial wall of the orbit. However, maximal decompression is obtained by controlled incision of the periosteum. Shallow incisions are made with the otologic sickle knife in a posterior to anterior direction (Figs. 23–3 and 23–4). The first incisions are made in the medial aspect (ethmoid region) progressing from superior to inferior. Subsequent incisions proceed across the floor. If the decompression is inadequate,

crosshatching incisions are made to achieve the desired result. The surgeon must be careful to avoid grasping and removing fat; injury to the inferior rectus and inferior oblique muscles will occur.

Intraoperative measurements with the Hertel exophthalmometer allow the surgeon to assess the amount of decompression achieved and the symmetry of the eyes. If the eyes are not balanced, the adequacy of bone removal should be checked. Additional periosteal incisions with removal of periosteum can be performed.

After the desired result is obtained, bilateral nasal-antral windows are created (see Chapter 16) and the buccogingival sulcus incisions are closed with running sutures of 3–0 chromic catgut. Sterile antibiotic ophthalmic ointment is placed in the conjunctiva, and the eyes are dressed with light dressings. Oral or parenteral antibiotics are not usually required. The patient's ability to perceive light is checked postoperatively. If the patient experiences severe pain or has no light perception, intraorbital hematoma or optic nerve damage should be suspected and further studies undertaken.

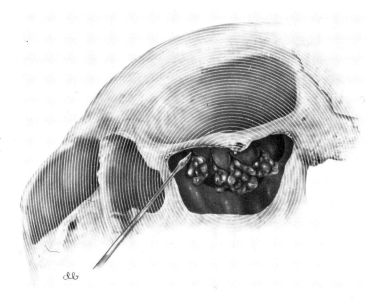

Figure 23–3. Incisions in orbital periosteum with sickle knife, allowing herniation of orbital fat.

MANAGEMENT OF UNILATERAL EXOPHTHALMOS

Hyperthyroidism is the leading cause of unilateral exophthalmos, but other causes to consider include intraorbital tumor, infection, and vascular malformation. When other causes have been excluded, the patient may be considered for surgical correction. There are several important differences between correcting unilateral and correcting bilateral exophthalmos. Removing the medial orbital wall and the orbital floor with slitting of the periosteum allows the intraocular contents to drop inferiorly, with correction of the proptosis. In the unilateral case, the result would be one eye at a lower level than the unoperated eye. This would produce double vision and also a poor cosmetic result. To avoid these complications, the decompression must be modified. The lateral half of the floor is not removed—only the medial bony wall and the medial half of the floor are removed. Periosteal slits are likewise confined to these areas. This precludes maximum decompression, and, therefore, in severe cases a Kronlein procedure may have to be performed as well.

RESULTS

Ogura and associates[3, 25–29] have reported the largest series of orbital decompressions, most recently the treatment of 252 patients who ranged in age from 16 to 80 years.[3] The male to female ratio was 66 to 186. One hundred eleven patients had undergone thyroid surgery, and 141 patients had been treated with radioactive iodine. Three patients had no history of hyperthyroidism. Preoperative exophthalmometer readings ranged from 22 to 36 mm. The recession results ranged from 2 to 12 mm. Proptosis had been present for less than 1 year in 30 per cent of patients, 1 to 2 years in 27 per cent, 2 to 5 years in 17 per cent, and over

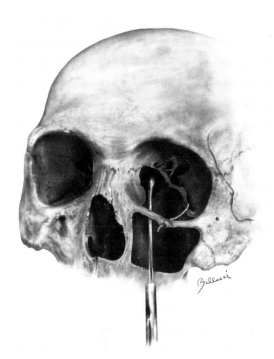

Figure 23–4. View of extent of bone removal from medial and inferior walls of orbit.

5 years in 26 per cent. Postoperatively, 42 per cent of patients showed equal exophthalmometer readings, 39 per cent showed the readings to be within 1 mm, 11 per cent had readings of 2 mm difference, 5 per cent had 3 mm difference, and 3 per cent had greater than 3 mm differences.[3]

Preoperative visual acuity was almost always preserved after decompression except in those four patients with panophthalmitis who progressed to total loss of vision. Many patients noted improved visual acuity immediately following surgery. Of the 252 patients, 172 had extraocular muscle impairment and 80 had no normal eye movement. Although some patients experienced improvement in extraocular function, many others required muscle-balancing procedures. Because many patients returned to their local hospital for the eye muscle surgery, it was not possible to obtain a complete estimate.

Postoperative Muscle Balancing-Surgery.

The correction of residual or ocular muscular imbalance following the decompression procedure requires great skill. Often several procedures are required. The inflammatory nature of the myopathy and subsequent postoperative scarring make the correction extremely difficult. The ophthalmologic surgeon attempts to achieve binocular vision in the primary and reading positions. It is often not possible to obtain full rotation.[30]

In some patients with mild proptosis, ocular muscle surgery is performed before decompression becomes necessary. However, if the proptosis is more than 22 to 23 mm (on the exophthalmometer), Dyer[9] recommends that decompression be performed before the muscle surgery, even if vision does not appear to be threatened. Patients with extraocular muscle imbalance before decompression almost always require muscle surgery later. Patients in whom the procedure is done more for cosmetic than for functional indications are less likely to require subsequent muscle balancing procedures. The inferior and medial rectus muscles are those most often requiring recession. Dyer[9] also recommends that a period of 4 months or longer be allowed to elapse between the decompression and the ocular surgery. This interval allows for the maximum effects of the decompression to be appreciated and for the extent of the muscle imbalance to be assessed accurately.

The orbital decompression does not correct lid retraction. This cosmetically distracting process can be corrected by levator tenotomy with or without grafting. Among the other ophthalmologic procedures sometimes required after decompression are release of prior tarsorrhaphy, blepharoplasty, and repair of entropion or ectropion of the lower lid.

Complications. In most large series of patients, this procedure has been remarkably free of complications. Among the few reported complications are postoperative sinusitis, oroantral fistula, postoperative pain requiring surgical division of the maxillary division of the right trigeminal nerve, bleeding from an aneurysm of the anterior cerebral artery, and meningitis from cerebrospinal fluid leakage.[3]

Secondary procedures are sometimes required for patients with suboptimal results. At the secondary procedure, further cross-hatching of the periosteum or more extensive removal of the lateral and posterior bony floor of the orbit may be required. Several patients have required Kronlein procedures (resection of the lateral orbital wall) to reduce proptosis further.

Finally, it should be noted that the patient with malignant exophthalmos has undergone a psychologically traumatic experience as the proptosis has progressed. Considerable preoperative and postoperative psychologic support is often required to achieve maximal benefit for the patient.

References

1. Graves RJ: Clinical lectures. London Med Surg J 7:516, 1835.
2. Von Basedow KA: Exophthalmos durch Hypertrophie des Zellgewebes in der Augenhohle. Wchnschr Heilk Berl 6:197, 220, 1840.
3. Ogura JH, Thawley SE: Orbital decompression exophthalmos. Otolaryngol Clin North Am 13:29, 1980.
4. McCullagh EP: Comments on the exophthalmos of Graves' disease—an editorial. J Clin Endocrinol Metab 13:818, 1953.
5. Dobyns BM, Steelman SL: The thyroid stimulating hormone of the anterior pituitary as distinct from the exophthalmos producing substance. Endocrinology 52:705, 1953.
6. Adams DD: The presence of an abnormal thyroid stimulating hormone in serum of some thyrotoxic patients. J Clin Endocrinol 18:699, 1958.
7. Kroll AJ, Kuwabara T: Dysthyroid ocular myopathy: Anatomy, histology, and electron microscopy. Arch Ophthalmol 76:244, 1966.
8. Riley FC: Orbital pathology in Graves' disease. Mayo Clin Proc 47:975, 1972.
9. Dyer JA: Ocular muscle surgery in Graves' disease. Trans Am Ophthalmol Soc 76:125, 1978.
10. Werner SC: Classification of thyroid disease: Report of the Committee on Nomenclature (letter to editor). J Clin Endocrinol Metab 29:982, 1969.

11. Walsh TE, Ogura JH: Transantral orbital decompression for malignant exophthalmos. Laryngoscope 65:544, 1957.
12. Kriss JP, Marshall WH Jr, Enzmann DR, Rosenthal AR: Computed axial tomography of the orbit in patients with Graves' ophthalmopathy. Excerpta Medica International Congress Series 378:621, 1975.
13. Trokel SL, Jakobiec FA: Correlation of CT scanning and pathologic features of ophthalmic Graves' disease. Ophthalmology 88:553, 1981.
14. Dollinger J: Die Drickentlastung der Augenhohle durch Entfernung der ausseren Orbitalwand bei hochgradigen Exophthalmus und konsekutwer Hornhauterkrankung. Dtsch Med Wochenschr 37:1888, 1911.
15. Kronlein: Practice of Surgery. Dean Leuis IV: 1–203. Alan V. Woods.
16. Hirsch O, Urbanek: Behandlung eines excessiven Exophthalmus (Basedow) durch Entfernung von Orbitalfett von der Kieferhohle aus. Monatsschr. Ohrenh 64:212, 1930; Zentralbl Hals Nasen Ohrenh 16:59, 1931.
17. Hirsch O: Malignant exophthalmos. Arch Otolaryngol 51:325, 1950.
18. Naffziger HC: Progressive exophthalmos following thyroidectomy: Its pathology and treatment. Ann Surg 94:582, 1931.
19. Sewall EC: Operative control of progressive exophthalmos. Arch Otolaryngol 24:62, 1936.
20. Kistner FB: Decompression for exophthalmos: Report of three cases. JAMA 112:37, 1939.
21. Schall LA, Reagan DJ: Malignant exophthalmos Ann Otol Rhinol Laryngol 54:37, 1945.
22. DeSanto LW, Gorman CA: Selection of patients and choice of operation for orbital decompression in Graves' ophthalmopathy. Laryngoscope 83:945, 1973.
23. Calcaterra TC, Hepler RS: Antral-ethmoidal decompression in Graves' disease; Five year experience. West J Med 124:87, 1976.
24. Baylis HI, Call NB, Shibata CS: The transantral orbital decompression (Ogura technique) as performed by the ophthalmologist: A series of 24 patients. Ophthalmology 87:1005, 1980.
25. Ogura JH, Walsh TE: The transantral orbital decompression operation for progressive exophthalmos. Laryngoscope 72:1078, 1962.
26. Ogura JH: Transantral orbital decompression for progressive exophthalmos. Med Clin North Am 52:399, 1968.
27. Ogura JH, Pratt LL: Transantral decompression for malignant exophthalmos. Otolaryngol Clin North Am 4:193, 1971.
28. Ogura JH, Lucente FE: Surgical results of orbital decompression for malignant exophthalmos. Laryngoscope 84:637, 1974.
29. Ogura JH: Surgical results of orbital decompression for malignant exophthalmos. J Laryngol Otol 92:181, 1978.
30. Miller JE, van Heuven W, Ward R: Surgical correction of hypotropias associated with thyroid dysfunction. Arch Ophthalmol 74:509, 1965.

CHAPTER 24

JUVENILE ANGIOFIBROMA

H. Bryan Neel, III, MD, PhD

The term *juvenile angiofibroma* is more accurate than juvenile nasopharyngeal angiofibroma, because the tumors almost always extend beyond the nasopharynx, often quite extensively. Microscopically, the tumor has two striking features: a fibrous stroma and a rich vascular network (Fig. 24–1). The fibrous stroma within a tumor is not uniform. In some areas, the cells resemble young fibroblasts and are spindled, plump, and stellate. In other areas, the stroma is less cellular, and the cells may be replaced by collagen. The vascular channels are sometimes small, of a capillary size, but are usually large and lined by endothelial cells. The tumor more appropriately could be called a hemangiofibroma. The endothelial cells lie directly against the stroma cells. There is no intervening smooth muscle, which explains the propensity of these tumors to bleed. The portion of the tumor within the nose, sphenoid, and nasophar-

ynx is covered with mucosa. The lobulations that extend laterally through the pterygomaxillary fossa have a firm, fibrous pseudocapsule, and manipulation of these lobules is less likely to cause troublesome bleeding than is manipulation of the portion of the tumor within the nasopharynx and nasal cavity.

Bleeding at operation and when a biopsy specimen is taken, as well as the troublesome symptom of spontaneous epistaxis, has been a source of interest since the time of Hippocrates and Celsus.[1] Angiographic studies have established that the main blood supply comes from an enlarged internal maxillary artery.[2] The venous plexus that drains the tumor consists of a tangle of numerous small, irregular vessels. The blood supply can come from both sides of the neck, particularly when the external carotid artery has been ligated. Often, arterial vessels to the tumor are identified from dural, sphe-

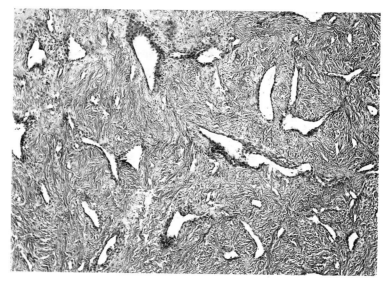

Figure 24–1. Typical juvenile angiofibroma. Hematoxylin and eosin; × 60. (From Neel HB III, Whicker JH, Devine KD, Weiland JH: Juvenile angiofibroma. Review of 120 cases. Am J Surg 126:547, 1973.)

TABLE 24–1. Primary Treatment of
Juvenile Angiofibroma*

Treatment	Percentage 1945–1971 (n = 120)	1972–1983 (n = 30)
Surgical removal	49	100
by lateral rhinotomy	47	97
Radon seed implantation and electrocoagulation	42	0
External irradiation	5	0
Biopsy only	4	0

*Two Mayo Clinic series.

noid, and ophthalmic branches of the internal carotid artery and the vertebral artery and thyrocervical trunk. The tumor may actually be pulsating, but it is compressible and spongelike.

Much of the material in this chapter is based on study of 150 patients at the Mayo Clinic who had microscopically confirmed juvenile angiofibromas and were seen from January 1, 1945, through December 31, 1983. From 1945 to 1955, treatment consisted primarily of interstitial irradiation with radon seeds, which were most commonly inserted by way of a transantral approach through a Caldwell-Luc incision (Table 24–1). From 1955 through 1971, the primary method of treatment consisted of removal of the tumor, although, early in that era, electrocoagulation and implantation of radon seeds were sometimes employed; lateral rhinotomy was used to expose the tumor and its extensions.[3] From 1972 through 1983, all the tumors were removed surgically: 29 by the lateral rhinotomy approach and 1 by a transpalatal approach (Table 24–2).[38]

The typical patient with a juvenile angiofibroma is a young boy who has had nosebleeds intermittently and whose nose has become obstructed, more commonly on one side. He may have bulging of the face or eye. An examination shows a pale, bluish, smooth mass in the nasopharynx. All the patients in this study were Caucasian males from 7 to 29 years old, with a mean age of 15 years (Fig. 24–2). Most had the triad of nasal obstruction, epistaxis, and nasal drainage.

TUMOR LOCATION AND ORIGIN

The tumor was usually located on one side in the nasopharynx. Occasionally, it filled the nasopharynx. Ulceration was unusual, unless the patient had had a previous biopsy or treatment. The large surgical experience has permitted identification of a specific point of origin. As noted, the tumor is most commonly lateralized and always obstructs or fills to some degree one nasal cavity. The origin is somewhere in the posterior portion of the nasal cavity and not in the nasopharynx. The specific point of origin is on the *posterolateral wall of the roof of the nose*, where the sphenoid process of the palatine bone meets the horizontal ala of the vomer and the root of the pterygoid process of the sphenoid. This junction forms the superior margin of the sphenopalatine foramen. The ethmoid crest, or attachment of the posterior end of the middle turbinate, lies on or above the foramen (Fig. 24–3).

Embryologically, this site represents the approximate location of the attachment of the buccopharyngeal membrane, which is the boundary between the stomatodeal ectoderm and the foregut endoderm.[4] This site is also the junction of the membranous viscerocranium, represented by the palatine, vomer, pterygoid lamina, and sphenoid bone, which is formed in the cartilaginous neurocranium.

TABLE 24–2. Routes of Tumor Removal
in Juvenile Angiofibroma*

Procedure	Number of Patients 1955–1971	1972–1983
Lateral rhinotomy	56	29
Transpalatal	1	1
Nasal-oral	2	0

*Two Mayo Clinic series.

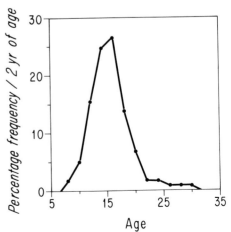

Figure 24–2. Age distribution of patients with juvenile angiofibroma. (From Neel HB III, Whicker JH, Devine KD, Weiland JH: Juvenile angiofibroma. Review of 120 cases. Am J Surg 126:547, 1973.)

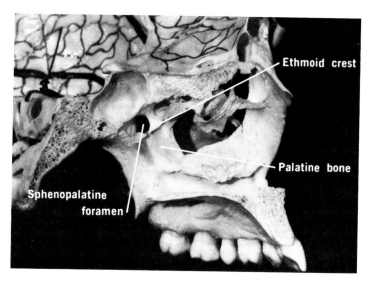

Figure 24–3. Left nasal cavity showing the point of origin, which lies near the superior margin of the sphenopalatine foramen at the attachment of the posterior end of the middle turbinate. (From Neel HB III, Whicker JH, Devine KD, Weiland JH: Juvenile angiofibroma. Review of 120 cases. Am J Surg 126:547, 1973.)

At one time, it was believed that the tumor originated in the vault of the nasopharynx in the fibrocartilage of Tillaux[5] or the fascia basilaris of Brunner[6] or at the spheno-occipital synchondrosis. Holman and Miller[7] noted roentgenographic evidence of destruction of the body of the sphenoid in 19 of 36 patients, but in all patients, the destruction occurred in front of the spheno-occipital synchondrosis. Earlier, others proposed that the primary site of origin was the back of the nose at the margin of the choana.[8–10]

As the tumor enlarges from its point of origin, it insinuates under the mucosa just inside the posterior choanal margin on the roof laterally. It extends under the mucosa along the roof, reaching the posterior border of the septum and extending downward along this margin. At operation, the tumor almost always must be separated from the posterior margin of the septum and from the roof of the posterior nasal cavity. It also extends anteriorly to fill the posterior nasal cavity, displacing the septum into the opposite nasal cavity and flattening the turbinates. The tumor protrudes out of the posterior choana and may fill the nasopharynx, displacing the soft palate, and may be visible below the free edge. The tumor enlarges laterally into the sphenopalatine foramen and expands the posterior end of the middle turbinate, which becomes continuous with the tumor—a constant finding at operation.

Once the tumor enters the pterygomaxillary fossa through the sphenopalatine foramen, it exerts pressure on the surrounding bony walls and displaces the anterior wall of the pterygomaxillary fossa, which is the posterior wall of the maxillary sinus, anteriorly (Fig. 24–4). It is important to recognize that the tumor does not enter the maxillary sinus through the lateral wall of the nose but rather enters by displacing the posterior wall anteriorly. At operation, if the posterior wall of the maxillary sinus is carefully removed, the tumor often can be found in the pterygomaxillary fossa. The tumor may destroy the root of the pterygoid process of the sphenoid bone posteriorly. If the tumor continues to enlarge, it extends into the infratemporal fossa through the pterygomaxillary fissure, where it expands and induces the classic facial fullness and actual bulging of the cheek (Fig. 24–5). Further enlargement leads to extension into the lower part of the temporal fossa, which results in swelling above the zygoma. When this occurs, the tumor usually extends into the inferior orbital fissure; the inferior orbital fissure opens into the upper anterior part of the pterygomaxillary fossa and is an entrance into the lower end of the superior orbital fissure, which meets the inferior (lateral) orbital fissure in the posterosuperior wall of the pterygomaxillary fossa (Fig. 24–6).

When the tumor reaches this site, it may destroy the great wing of the sphenoid bone, forming the characteristic widening along the lower lateral margin of the superior orbital fissure (Fig. 24–7). This leads to proptosis. If the tumor enlarges in the infratemporal and pterygomaxillary fossae, it can destroy the bone that forms the base of the pterygoid process where the body and great wing of the sphenoid bone meet; the tumor then rests against the dura of the middle fossa, anterior to the foramen lacerum but lateral to the cavernous sinus.

Sometimes the tumor pushes straight up from its point of origin through the floor of the

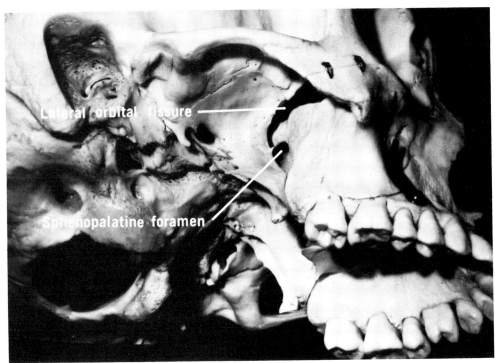

Figure 24–4. Right side of skull showing infratemporal, temporal, and pterygomaxillary fossae and their relationships to the sphenopalatine foramen, pterygomaxillary fissure, and posterior wall of the maxillary antrum. (From Neel HB III, Whicker JH, Devine KD, Weiland JH: Juvenile angiofibroma. Review of 120 cases. Am J Surg 126:547, 1973.)

sphenoid sinus. Although the sphenoid sinus is commonly involved (Table 24–3), the tumor does not often expand intracranially in this area, fortunately. However, if the tumor does expand, fill the sinus, and push through the top of the sphenoid, it displaces the pituitary gland to one side and appears in the sella turcica, where it can cause blindness by pressure on the optic chiasm. Here, the tumor is closely associated with the cavernous sinus and branches of the internal carotid artery.

Therefore, the tumor can enter the cranial cavity by one or both of two routes: by way of the middle fossa anterior to the foramen lacerum and lateral to the cavernous sinus and carotid artery, or through the sella medial to the carotid artery and lateral to the pituitary gland. Intracranial extension is seen in less than 10 per cent of patients.[3, 3a, 37, 38]

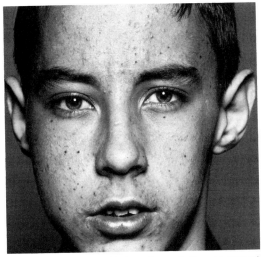

Figure 24–5. Patient with juvenile angiofibroma extending into infratemporal fossa, causing bulging in right cheek. (From Neel HB III, Whicker JH, Devine KD, Weiland JH: Juvenile angiofibroma. Review of 120 cases. Am J Surg 125:547, 1973.)

TABLE 24–3. Roentgenologic Evaluation of Sinus(es) in Patients Undergoing Lateral Rhinotomy for Juvenile Angiofibroma*

Sinus(es)	Number of Patients
Maxillary, ethmoid, sphenoid	16
Maxillary, sphenoid	4
Ethmoid, sphenoid	2
Maxillary only	2
Sphenoid only	2
Maxillary, ethmoid	1
Ethmoid only	1
Total	28 (96%)

*Mayo Clinic series (1972–1983).

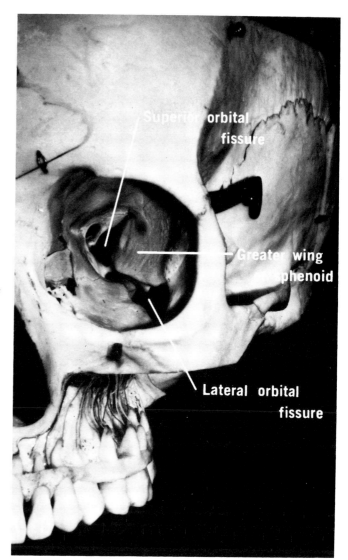

Figure 24–6. Left side of skull showing relationships of the superior orbital fissure, lateral (inferior) orbital fissure, and greater wing of sphenoid. Note proximity of optic foramen.

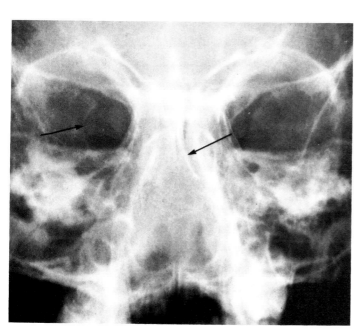

Figure 24–7. Enlargement of superior orbital fissure *(arrows).* (From Holman CB, Miller WE: Juvenile nasopharyngeal fibroma: Roentgenologic characteristics. Am J Roentgenol 94:292, 1965.)

Tumors may be safely removed from the middle fossa dura (Fig. 24–8). However, those that are intimately associated with the branches of the internal carotid artery and the cavernous sinus are difficult to manage surgically, because massive and uncontrollable hemorrhage may ensue. Probably this latter group of patients with central tumor extension into the cranium should be managed either by a combination of surgery and irradiation or by external irradiation alone.

A recent study by McGahan et al. reviewed 15 patients; of these, 11 had middle cranial fossa involvement and 10 had cavernous sinus involvement. Ten of the 15 patients were treated with radiation therapy. Recurrence was treated with surgical resection or further radiation. The researchers concluded that a total dose of greater than 40 Gy may provide better control in advanced lesions.[3b] A contrary opinion was voiced by Close et al., who reported 6 patients with cavernous sinus involvement who were treated with a midline extracranial surgical approach.[3c]

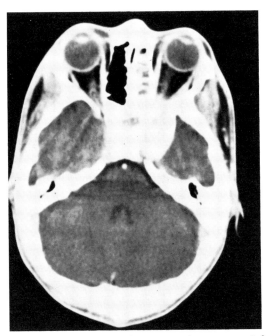

Figure 24–9. CT scan with contrast shows an angiofibroma in the right posterior nasal cavity and in the pterygomaxillary region. The posterior wall of the antrum has been pushed anteriorly—a common finding.

ROENTGENOGRAPHIC EVALUATION

The capability to localize the extensions of the tumor specifically has been improved immensely with the development of computed tomography (CT), supplemented with contrast medium. Because the tumor is vascular, it takes up the contrast medium and is clearly visualized in CT scans (Fig. 24–9).

More than 90 per cent of patients have definite roentgenographic abnormalities on plain sinus films (Table 24–3). Generally, there is obvious opacity involving one or more sinuses and bone displacement or erosion (or both); frequently there are both opacity of sinus(es) and bone involvement. The maxillary sinus was most commonly involved; next in frequency was the combination of the maxillary, ethmoid, and sphenoid sinuses in the second Mayo Clinic surgical series (1972–1983).[38] In 1965, Holman and Miller[7] had described the roentgenographic manifestations of 46 Mayo Clinic cases. They found bony erosion of the body of the sphenoid in 30 patients, anterior bowing of the posterior wall of the maxillary in 40, erosion of the hard palate in 18, and enlargement of the superior orbital fissure in 16. The characteristic anterior bowing of the posterior wall of the maxillary antrum is virtually pathognomonic of juvenile angiofibroma in young male patients (Fig. 24–10). However, there have been rare false-positive interpretations owing to the presence of benign fibrous inflammatory polyps.

Holman and Miller[7] emphasized not only the characteristic anterior bowing of the posterior

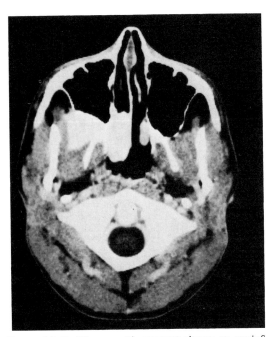

Figure 24–8. CT scan with contrast shows an angiofibroma in the base of the middle fossa. The tumor was separated and removed from the middle fossa dura by way of a lateral rhinotomy approach.

wall of the maxillary sinus (Fig. 24–10) but also the enlargement of the superior orbital fissure (Fig. 24–7) and the characteristic bone erosion of the adjacent structures.

Tomograms of the paranasal sinuses and nasopharynx are rarely used now. With the development of CT, the indications for and use of tomography have become much less frequent.

Angiography can sometimes supplement the other roentgenographic studies. Currently, it is used primarily in patients with very large tumors and intracranial extension to identify precisely the blood supply to the tumor in preparation for embolization procedures.[37] Super selective embolization of the internal maxillary artery, the accessory meningeal artery, the ascending pharyngeal artery, and branches of the internal carotid artery was reported by Wilms et al.[10a] Some surgeons have the impression that embolization reduces the blood loss at surgery.[10b, 10c] If embolization is undertaken, it is advisable to do it a day or two before the surgical procedure so that if any neurologic sequelae should occur after the embolization, they will be recognized before surgery is undertaken. Angiograms are also helpful in detecting residual tumor and the site of bleeding, should this occur after irradiation or surgical treatment (or both). These studies are not without risk, as shown by the report of a death 10 hours after angiographic studies for angiofibroma,[11] permanent transverse myelitis in another patient in a series of 16 patients,[12] the development of transient hemiplegia in one of two patients[13] and the notation of another patient in whom hemiplegia developed but who recovered most of his function in 90 days.[14] In a recent Mayo Clinic series (1972–1983), one patient developed a right retinal artery infarction and some residual optic atrophy after angiography alone.[38] Holman and Miller[7] emphasized that the roentgenographic features are so characteristic that only in unusual circumstances would angiography be necessary. This opinion was given before CT scanning was available and still is currently true. The presence of a nasopharyngeal mass with pneumocephalus depicts intracranial extension, as shown in a recent report by Chrys et al.[14a]

It is recognized that not every boy with nasal obstruction, nosebleed, and a polypoid tumor in the nasopharynx has juvenile angiofibroma. Diagnosis can be difficult. Conventional roentgenograms of the sinuses, CT scans, perhaps an MRI scan (which will "light up the flow voids"), a thorough physical examination, and knowledge of the natural history and point of origin do help in making the appropriate diagnosis and determining the extent of tumor. If doubt remains about the nature of the lesion in a patient with a symptomatic tumor after the physical examination and standard roentgenographic studies, the patient should be examined under anesthesia; a biopsy specimen should be taken if there is still doubt and the tumor should be removed by way of a lateral rhinotomy. (A limited rhinotomy incision, which does not transect the upper lip, gives excellent exposure for removal of sphenochoanal polyps or similar fibromyxomatous polyps involving the sphenoid

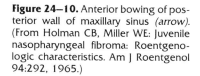
Figure 24–10. Anterior bowing of posterior wall of maxillary sinus *(arrow)*. (From Holman CB, Miller WE: Juvenile nasopharyngeal fibroma: Roentgenologic characteristics. Am J Roentgenol 94:292, 1965.)

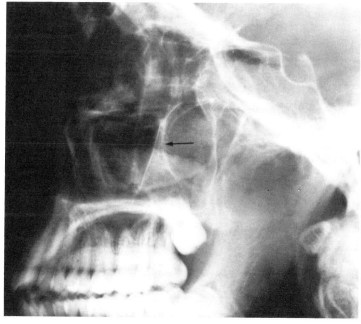

or nasopharynx, eliminating the tumor and the distressing symptoms and at the same time confirming the diagnosis.)

SURGERY

In 1834, Chelius[15] emphasized that the danger of hemorrhage was always less if the tumor could be extirpated in its entirety, with all its extensions. The surgeon must decide which approach, preferably a single one, will provide excellent exposure not only of the point of origin but also of the extensions of the tumor. In 1911, Hellat[16] surveyed 55 different approaches, and in 1957, Wilson[17] described an approach to the nasopharynx by way of lateral rhinotomy that had been practiced 100 years previously. Surgeons have recommended eight approaches. Except for the lateral rhinotomy, none gives satisfactory exposure to all of the extensions. A summary follows:

In the *natural orifice approach*, a portion of the tumor is avulsed with a special clamp that is introduced through the mouth to relieve nasal obstruction.[18] The *transpalatal approach* can be used for removing small tumors that are limited to the nasopharynx and the posterior part of the nose. Cocke[19] believed that the transpalatal approach was not practical for any tumor larger than 5 cm. In our series, this approach was used in two patients with very small tumors. The *transmandibular*[20] and *transzygomatic approaches*[21] are used to expose the extension of the tumor into the infratemporal and temporal fossae but are not satisfactory for removing the other more common extensions of the tumor. The *transhyoid approach* could be used for small tumors limited to the nasopharynx, but it is inadequate if there are other extensions, which is true for most tumors. The *transantral (Denker) approach*[22] is often used in combination with the transpalatal approach. Figi and Davis[10] used the Caldwell-Luc incision and the transantral operation almost exclusively, which was sometimes modified into a Denker operation. This approach is also inadequate, which is the reason that electrocoagulation and radon seeds are commonly used to treat the residual tumor. The *craniotomy-rhinotomy approach* is recommended by Krekorian and Kempe[23] for any patient who has definite or suspected intracranial extension. Unfortunately, even this approach may not be satisfactory if the extension into the middle cranial fossa or pituitary is great and impacted.

Standefer and colleagues[24] emphasized that recent advances in surgical and anesthetic techniques, transfusion capabilities, pharmacologic agents, and radiographic techniques have contributed to the improved surgical cure rates for angiofibromas, including those that have extended intracranially. They advocate a combined approach by an otolaryngologist and a neurosurgeon, using a midfacial degloving procedure, a bifrontal craniotomy, or a transantral or transpalatal (or both) approach. Initially, the intracranial portion of the operation is carried out to define the margins of the tumor and to resect the portion of the tumor within the cranium. This is followed by resection of the extracranial components. The internal and external carotid arteries are exposed in the neck initially to assist in the control of bleeding. Surgical removal of the tumor is generally preceded by arteriography, embolization with Gelfoam into the tumor and instillation of tufted wire coils into the large proximal feeding vessels. They cite the study of Roberson and colleagues,[25] who reported that embolization decreased the loss of blood in their series from 2400 ml to approximately 800 ml for each patient. Embolization cannot be used on the feeding vessels from the internal carotid artery because of the risk of stroke.

The *lateral rhinotomy approach*[3, 26–28] provides access to the extensions upward into the sphenoid sinus, the pterygomaxillary fossa, the temporal and infratemporal fossae, the middle fossa and the "roots" of the tumor in the lateral wall of the nose.

LATERAL RHINOTOMY

TECHNIQUE

The skin incision begins just beneath or within the medial aspect of the brow and curves downward and forward to within 5 mm of the inner canthus (Fig. 24–11). The portion of the incision in the brow should parallel the hair follicles, and the portion near the depression of the inner canthus should be curved so that a web of scar does not form over the depression in the region of the medial canthus. The incision is extended along the side of the nose midway *between* the dorsum and the nasal-maxillary crease. The fullness of the midface in this area may be lost if the incision is placed within the nasal-maxillary crease, because the underlying bone is removed, leading to the formation of an unsightly depression or notch. The incision must be above the nasal-maxillary crease. The

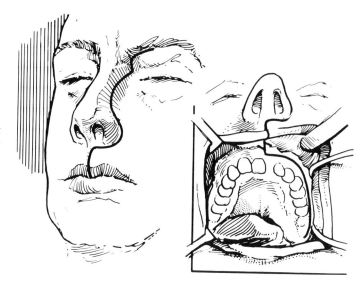

Figure 24–11. The skin incision most commonly used in treatment of juvenile angiofibroma.

incision may be terminated at the level of the ala, but for the treatment of angiofibromas, the incision usually is continued around the base of the nose to the base of the columella and down the center of the philtrum of the upper lip, because most angiofibromas extend beyond the nose and nasopharynx. The alar part of the incision is best placed in the alar sulcus. Before the lip is divided, the vermilion border is marked to help ensure proper realignment of the closure. The incision on the mucosal surface of the upper lip has a Z incorporated into it. The incision is carried down to the level of the alveolobuccal sulcus and continues in the sulcus to the maxillary tuberosity. Important structures encountered in making the incision are the angular vein and the facial artery.

Underlying bone must be adequately removed to get good exposure of the tumor and its extensions, and this should be completed *before the tumor is touched.* The nasal bone is removed almost to the midline and to its junction with the frontal bone. The frontal process of the maxilla and the facial surface of the maxilla are removed, but a small margin of bone around the infraorbital nerve at the inferior orbital foramen is preserved. This opens the antrum and allows inspection of the posterior wall. If the tumor is pushing the posterior wall of the antrum forward, this is apparent and more exposure is usually needed. This is accomplished by removing the infratemporal surface of the maxilla, and the eggshell of bone on the posterior wall of the maxilla is gingerly removed from the surface of the tumor. Usually, the terminal branches of the internal maxillary artery or the artery itself can be identified and ligated, clipped, or electrocoagulated.

The tumor can be extricated from the ptery-

gomaxillary, infratemporal, or temporal fossa and pushed medially with packing. The fat pad of the cheek usually partially obstructs this area and it is teased out of the operative field.

The frontal process of the maxilla is removed. The nasolacrimal sac and duct are exposed. The bone surrounding these structures should be carefully removed so that the sac and duct are standing free. The nasal antral wall below the inferior turbinate is removed from front to back. Removal of bone is continued backward along the floor of the nose. The inferior turbinate is divided posteriorly, and the posterior end of the middle turbinate is divided anterior to the portion that is incorporated into the tumor. If the bone has been removed thoroughly around the nasolacrimal sac and duct, the remnants of the two turbinates and the middle meatus can be lifted from the wound or pushed out of the line of sight. With the inferior turbinate mobilized as a pedicle on the nasolacrimal duct, the posterior nasal cavity and choana are exposed. The tumor often pushes the posterior septum to the opposite side, but the septum can be mobilized and also pushed out of the field.

The periosteum of the medial wall of the orbit is carefully elevated to avoid tearing and releasing the periorbital fat. The medial canthal ligament is detached in the process of sharp elevation of a clean and thorough periosteal incision. As the periosteum is elevated posteriorly, the anterior ethmoid artery is identified and coagulated or clipped. At the completion of the operation, the periosteum is carefully reattached; this repositions the ligament in the absence of the underlying frontal process of the maxilla. The canthus tends to slide inferiorly, so the lateral periosteum is reapproximated 1 or 2 mm higher than it was in its original state.

The lacrimal bone and lamina papyracea of the ethmoid bone are removed and, at the same time, the ethmoid cells are removed along the cribriform plate. As the surgeon proceeds posteriorly, the tumor may be in the posterior ethmoid cells but it is usually not encountered until the sphenoid sinus is reached. The tumor usually can be pushed and packed downward out of the sinus.

The attachment of the tumor to the posterior margin of the septum is then separated with a finger and the tumor is pushed laterally with packing to its point of origin; there never is any attachment along the floor of the nose.

All the lobulations of the tumor should now be free and be seen to communicate with each other and with the body of the tumor, where it is attached in the roof and lateral wall of the posterior nasal cavity. All intervening bone that can interfere with removal of the tumor should be excised. Most large angiofibromas extend under the adenoid pad and lift it posteriorly in the vault and posterior base of the nasopharynx on the side of the lesion. It is necessary to use an index finger to aid in avulsion of the tumor. The tumor is firmly grasped with a strong forceps and removed.

Once the tumor is removed, a search is made for any residual lobules of tumor remaining in the body of the sphenoid and in the operative field. The cavity is packed with petroleum jelly–impregnated gauze packing, which is removed 1 week later with the patient under general anesthesia. Tracheotomy tubes and feeding tubes are unnecessary.

It should be clear that the lateral rhinotomy is not an operation but rather an incision along the side of the nose. The incision can be extended down the center of the upper lip, when lateral exposure is required beyond the infraorbital foramen.[3, 29] *The incision with its extensions allows wide access to the nose, some elements of the skull base, the nasopharynx, the paranasal sinuses, the temporal fossa and infratemporal fossa.* Mertz and colleagues[29] recently reviewed 226 consecutive patients who required a lateral rhinotomy for various diseases and concluded that excellent surgical exposure is assured by this approach and that minimal postoperative complications are attributable to the incision. An understanding of the several extensions may help the surgeon to tailor the approach to the individual patient.[3, 37, 38]

RESULTS

Of the 89 patients in whom surgical approaches were used, 85 underwent lateral rhin-

otomy. These were analyzed in two separate series: 56 patients from 1955 to 1971 and 29 patients from 1972 to 1983 (see Table 24–2). In the earlier surgical series, the tumor was completely removed in 40 patients and incompletely removed in 7 (in the opinion of the surgeon); in 9 cases, the outcome was not stated. Fifteen patients required two or more secondary procedures after lateral rhinotomy. Twelve patients had electrocoagulation or implantation of radon seeds in residual tumor (or both). One patient had external irradiation, one had secondary ligation of the external carotid artery, and three patients had repeated lateral rhinotomies for excision of residual tumors. In the later surgical series (1972–1983), the surgeon noted incomplete removal in one of the patients, and this patient had external irradiation postoperatively.

Of the 56 patients in the earlier surgical series (1955 to 1971), 45 were alive without disease at the time of the last report.[3] The nine patients for whom the surgeon did not state whether all the tumor was removed are alive and free of tumor. Of the seven patients with known incomplete removal, two are alive without disease, three have small asymptomatic masses in the nasopharynx, and two have died as a result of the tumor. Three others have died, and one was lost to follow-up study. In the later series, 29 patients are alive: 27 without disease and 2 with disease. None has died, and none has been lost to follow-up. Longer follow-up is needed for some of the patients in the later surgical series.[37, 38] There were no deaths in the later surgical series; however, in the earlier series (1955–1971), five patients with lateral rhinotomies died. All five had extensive involvement of the maxillary, ethmoid, and sphenoid sinuses. In one patient, the tumor extended into the upper part of the neck and around the trachea from beneath the mandible. Three patients had had surgical procedures previously, and one had been treated with radon seeds. Preoperatively, four of the patients had facial deformities, exophthalmos, palatal displacement, a mass in the neck, or a combination of these. Three of the patients had large intracranial extensions of tumor involving the cavernous sinus and adjacent structures. Only one patient died at operation; death was due to a cardiac arrest, presumably from hypovolemia. This patient had been operated on before referral, yet all the tumor was removed without difficulty by way of the lateral rhinotomy approach.

Blood Replacement. In the earlier series, the mean volume of blood replacement was

TABLE 24–4. Blood Replacement in Patients
Undergoing Lateral Rhinotomy for Juvenile
Angiofibroma

Series	Mean Replacement (ml)	Patients (%)
1955–1971	1280	88
1972–1983	1464	96
Hypotension	1167	
No hypotension	1588	

1280 ml. Seven patients did not require transfusion. In the later surgical series, mean blood replacement was 1464 ml; one patient did not require transfusion. Hypotensive anesthesia reduced the blood loss by about 400 ml, but the difference was not significant (Table 24–4). Seven patients had embolization procedures preoperatively. The mean blood loss was not reduced; however, the number of patients was too small to make any firm statements about the value of the procedure.

Complications. The postoperative and late complications in 150 patients are shown in Table 24–5. Irradiation delivered interstitially approximately doubled all the complications, compared with the incidence of complications after excision. One patient who had had external irradiation before lateral rhinotomy had hemifacial atrophy, and several patients had obvious skin changes. Eleven patients had had external irradiation before treatment was undertaken. After lateral rhinotomy and removal, only three patients had unsightly cosmetic results. In most patients, the lateral rhinotomy incision, with or without division of the upper lip, led to a satisfactory cosmetic result. Any cosmetic aberrations must be weighed against the excellent exposure of the tumor and its extensions, which

TABLE 24–5. Postoperative and Late
Complications in 150 Patients with Juvenile
Angiofibroma

Complication	Number of Patients		
	Interstitial Irradiation (1945–1955)	Surgery (1955–1971)	Surgery (1972–1983)
Nasal crusting or sequestrum (or both)	39	12	6
Hemorrhage requiring transfusion	11	6	3
Eye symptoms or deafness (or both)	9	5	5
Unsightly scar	0	2	1
Meningitis	2	0	0

can be routinely obtained using the lateral rhinotomy approach.

EXTERNAL RADIATION THERAPY

In recent years, most students on the subject of angiofibromas have advocated surgical treatment; however, some have employed radiation therapy, primarily for the treatment of recurrences and intracranial tumor. An outstanding exception has been the series of patients from the Princess Margaret Hospital in Toronto.[30] Otolaryngologists and radiotherapists there have stressed the value of external radiation therapy for most of their patients. In their most recent review of 35 patients treated for the first time, irradiation controlled the tumor both clinically and radiologically from 2 to 20 years in 28 (80 per cent). Ten patients who were initially treated by surgery had radiation for recurrence, and in seven the tumor was controlled. Overall, 10 of 45 tumors (22 per cent) were not controlled by the first course of radiotherapy; seven of these were controlled by a second course, and three were treated by surgery. A dose of 3000 rads in 3 weeks induced thrombosis, fibrosis, and tumor regression, although a latent period of up to 2 years may elapse before final disappearance of the tumor. Fitzpatrick and colleagues[30] also pointed out that radiation damage is minimized by using sophisticated radiotherapeutic techniques and protecting radiosensitive tissues.[30a] The 3000-rad dose in 3 weeks that they recommend is much lower than that reported by most authorities. They believe that this dose is unlikely to initiate neoplastic change. Other authors believe that radiation therapy should be reserved for disease extending intracranially.[30b]

The incidence of iatrogenic radiation-induced tumors is unknown, but it is a source of concern, especially because the legal risk is ongoing after treatment of children and because lifetime follow-up would be necessary. One would be particularly concerned about thyroid cancer and bone and soft tissue sarcomas. Another consideration is the cost, inconvenience, and anxiety of lifelong follow-up.[31] Malignant transformation of angiofibromas has been reported by several authors.[31a, 31b] There also may be potential cosmetic and functional problems associated with irradiating the facial skeleton in patients who have not reached skeletal maturity. One would be concerned about cataract formation, hearing loss, and eustachian tube dysfunction at higher doses of radiation therapy. Nevertheless, the radiotherapist is a member of the team managing the treatment of patients with this most difficult tumor (Fig. 24–12).

Cummings[32] mathematically assessed the relative cumulative risks of surgery compared with radiation therapy. He concluded that the rates of potentially fatal complication for the two methods of treatment (surgery and radiation) were equivalent. He estimated that the cost of radiation therapy is likely to be considerably less than that of surgery in Canada for a course of 3000 to 3500 rads in 3 weeks.[33] An assessment of cost at the Mayo Clinic indicates that the cost for 3000 rads or surgical removal would be essentially the same if the duration of hospitalization for surgery is 7 days; inpatient hospital care during surgery is a major cost factor.

TREATMENT TRENDS

There has been a trend toward surgical therapy as the primary form of treatment for patients with juvenile angiofibromas, including those with intracranial extension.[10b, 30b, 33b, 33c] The lateral rhinotomy approach, in one procedure, allows exposure of all the extensions of the tumor and may be used with a craniotomy as a combined otolaryngologic-neurologic-surgical effort. Large lateral transfacial approach

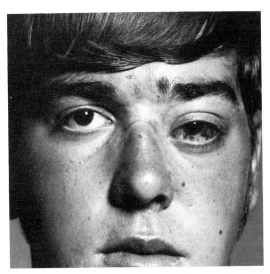

Figure 24–12. Patient with intracranial extension, progressive proptosis, and the loss of vision in the left eye after partial excision of angiofibroma. There was no tumor in the nose or nasopharynx. The patient was treated with ^{60}Co, causing arrest of the tumor. (From Neel HB III, Whicker JH, Devine KD, Weiland JH: Juvenile angiofibroma. Review of 120 cases. Am J Surg 126:547, 1973.)

has recently been advocated for massive angiofibromas that may involve the parotid gland and infratemporal fossa.[33a] It is important to remove overlying bone before the tumor is touched. Once this is accomplished, tumor in the pterygomaxillary fossa and infratemporal, temporal, antral, sphenoid, nasal, and nasopharyngeal regions can be removed. The tumor can be compressed, pushed toward its point of origin, at the posterior end of the middle turbinate and avulsed. There has been a trend toward more ligations of the internal maxillary artery at the time of operation. There has been increasing use of adjunctive procedures—hypotensive anesthesia and embolization 12 to 48 hours preoperatively. Hormones,[34, 34a] cryotherapy,[35] or external carotid artery ligation appears to be of no value in the control of hemorrhage at operation, and it is doubtful that hypotensive anesthesia is beneficial. A clear definition of the extent of the angiofibroma can be obtained with CT scanning, which enhances well with intravenous contrast material because of the luxuriant blood supply of the tumor.[36] Presently, CT scanning is used to establish the diagnosis and define the extent of the tumor prior to biopsy and to determine whether angiography is needed. Skull and plain roentgenograms have limited appeal as screening examinations, but they are still considered useful in some technical aspects of diagnosis and surgical planning. There has been a trend toward more complete removal at the time of operation and fewer recurrences postoperatively. In recent surgical series, mortality has been virtually zero.

References

1. Härmä RA: Nasopharyngeal angiofibroma: A clinical and histopathological study. Acta Otolaryngol (Stockh) (Suppl) 146:1, 1958.
2. Rosen L, Hanafee W, Nahum A: Nasopharyngeal angiofibroma, an angiographic evaluation. Radiology 86:103, 1966.
3. Neel HB III, Whicker JH, Devine KD, Weiland JH: Juvenile angiofibroma: Review of 120 cases. Am J Surg 126:547, 1973.
3a. Sarpa, JR, Novelly, NJ: Extranasopharyngeal angiofibroma. Otolaryng Head Neck Surg 101:693, 1989.
3b. McGahan RA, Durrance FY, Parke RB, et al: The treatment of advanced juvenile nasopharyngeal angiofibroma. Int J Radiat Oncol Biol Phys 17:1067, 1989.
3c. Close LG, Schaefer SD, Mickey BE, Manning SC: Surgical management of nasopharyngeal angiofibroma involving the cavernous sinus. Arch Otolaryngol Head Neck Surg 115:1091, 1989.
4. Hamilton WJ, Mossman HW: Human Embryology: Prenatal Development of Form and Function. 4th ed. Baltimore, Williams & Wilkins, 1972.
5. Tillaux P. Cited by Härmä RA: Nasopharyngeal angiofibroma: A clinical and histopathological study. Acta Otolaryngol (Stockh) (Suppl) 146:1, 1958.

6. Brunner H: Nasopharyngeal fibroma. Ann Otol Rhinol Laryngol 51:29, 1942.

7. Holman CB, Miller WE: Juvenile nasopharyngeal fibroma: Roentgenologic characteristics. Am J Roentgenol 94:292, 1965.

8. Sebileau P: Considérations sur les fibromes naso-pharyngiens. Ann Mal l'Oreille Larynx 42:553, 1923.

9. Jacques D: Insertion and seat of rhinopharyngeal fibromata. Ann Otol Rhinol Laryngol 20:881, 1911.

10. Figi FA, Davis RE: The management of nasopharyngeal fibromas. Laryngoscope 60:794, 1950.

10a. Wilms G, Peene P, Baert AL, et al: Pre-operative embolization of juvenile nasopharyngeal angiofibromas. J Belge Radiol 72:465, 1989.

10b. Roberts JK, Korones GK, Levine H, et al: Results of surgical management of nasopharyngeal angiofibroma. The Cleveland Clinic experience, 1977–1986. Cleveland Clin J Med 56:529, 1989.

10c. Garcia–Cervigon E, Bien S, Rufenacht D, et al: Preoperative embolization of naso-pharyngeal angiofibromas. Report of 58 cases. Neuroradiology 30:556, 1988.

11. Fitzpatrick PJ: The nasopharyngeal angiofibroma. Can J Surg 13:228, 1970.

12. Wilson GH, Hanafee WN: Angiographic findings in 16 patients with juvenile nasopharyngeal angiofibroma. Radiology 92:279, 1969.

13. Thomas ML, Mowat PD: Angiography in juvenile nasopharyngeal haemangiofibroma. Clin Radiol 21:403, 1970.

14. Butler RM, Nahum AM, Hanafee W: New surgical approach to nasopharyngeal angiofibromas. Trans Am Acad Ophthalmol Otolaryngol 71:92, 1967.

14a. Chrys RA, Pribram HF, Strelzow V, Fritts H: Juvenile angiofibroma: a unique case presenting with intracranial air. Otolaryngol Head Neck Surg 97:572, 1987.

15. Chelius JM. Cited by Härmä RA: Nasopharyngeal angiofibroma: A clinical and histopathological study. Acta Otolaryngol (Stockh) (Suppl) 146:1, 1958.

16. Hellat P: Die sogenannten fibrösen Nasenrachenpolypen: Ort und Art ihrer Insertion und ihre Behandlung. Arch Laryngol Rhinol 25:329, 1911.

17. Wilson CP: Observations on the surgery of the nasopharynx. Ann Otol Rhinol Laryngol 66:5, 1957.

18. Furstenberg AC, Boles R: Nasopharyngeal angiofibroma. Trans Am Acad Ophthalmol Otolaryngol 67:518, 1963.

19. Cocke EW Jr: Transpalatine surgical approach to the nasopharynx and the posterior nasal cavity. Am J Surg 108:517, 1964.

20. Kremen AJ: Surgical management of angiofibroma of the nasopharynx. Ann Surg 138:672, 1953.

21. Samy LL, Girgis IH: Transzygomatic approach for nasopharyngeal fibromata with extrapharyngeal extension. J Laryngol Otol 79:782, 1965.

22. Denker A: Zur operativen Behandlung der typischen Nasenrachenfibrome. Z Ohrenheilkd 64:1, 1912.

23. Krekorian EA, Kempe LG: The combined otolaryngology-neurosurgery approach to extensive benign tumors. Laryngoscope 79:2086, 1969.

24. Standefer J, Holt GR, Brown WE Jr, Gates GA: Combined intracranial and extracranial excision of nasopharyngeal angiofibroma. Laryngoscope 93:772, 1983.

25. Roberson GH, Biller H, Sessions DG, Ogura JH: Presurgical internal maxillary artery embolization in juvenile angiofibroma. Laryngoscope 82:1524, 1972.

26. Witt TR, Shah JP, Sternberg SS: Juvenile nasopharyngeal angiofibroma: A 30 year clinical review. Am J Surg 146:521, 1983.

27. Biller HF: Juvenile nasopharyngeal angiofibroma. Ann Otol Rhinol Laryngol 87:630, 1978.

28. Waldman SR, Levine HL, Astor F, et al: Surgical experience with nasopharyngeal angiofibroma. Arch Otolaryngol 107:677, 1981.

29. Mertz JS, Pearson BW, Kern EB: Lateral rhinotomy: Indications, technique, and review of 226 patients. Arch Otolaryngol 109:235, 1983.

30. Fitzpatrick PJ, Briant TDR, Berman JM: The nasopharyngeal angiofibroma. Arch Otolaryngol 106:234, 1980.

30a. Robinson AC, Khoury GG, Ash DV, Daly BD: Evaluation of response following irradiation of juvenile angiofibromas. Br J Radiol 62:245, 1989.

30b. Economou TS, Abemayor E, Ward PH: Juvenile nasopharyngeal angiofibroma: an update of the UCLA experience, 1960–1985. Laryngoscope 98:170, 1988.

31. Jafek BW: Risk factors in angiofibroma (editorial comment). Head Neck Surg 3:26, 1980.

31a. Haughey BH: Malignant angiofibromas. Otolaryngol Head Neck Surg 99:607, 1988.

31b. Makek MS, Andrews JC, Fisch U: Malignant transformation of a nasopharyngeal angiofibroma. Laryngoscope 99:1088, 1989.

32. Cummings BJ: Relative risk factors in the treatment of juvenile nasopharyngeal angiofibroma. Head Neck Surg 3:21, 1980.

33. Cummings BJ: Juvenile nasopharyngeal angiofibroma: Control rates and treatment costs (editorial). Head Neck Surg 3:169, 1980.

33a. Haughey BH, Wilson JS, Barber CS: Massive angiofibroma:surgical approach and adjunctive therapy. Otolaryngol Head Neck Surg 98:618, 1988.

33b. Amedee R, Klaeyle D, Mann W, Geyer H: Juvenile angiofibroma: a 40 year surgical experience. ORL J Otorhinolaryngol Relat Spec 51:56, 1989.

33c. Mahara D, Fernandes CM: Surgical experience with juvenile nasopharyngeal angiofibroma. Ann Otol Rhinol Laryngol 98:269, 1989.

34. Johnsen S, Kloster JH, Schiff M: The action of hormones on juvenile nasopharyngeal angiofibroma: A case report. Acta Otolaryngol (Stockh) 61:153, 1966.

34a. Brentani MM, Butugan O, Oshima CT, et al: Multiple steroid receptors in nasopharyngeal angiofibromas. Laryngoscope 99:398, 1989.

35. Smith MFW, Boles R, Work WP: Cryosurgical techniques in removal of angiofibromas. Laryngoscope 74:1071, 1964.

36. Sessions RB, Bryan RN, Naclerio RM, Alford BR: Radiographic staging of juvenile angiofibroma. Head Neck Surg 3:279, 1981.

37. Jones GC, DeSanto LW, Bremer JW, Neel HB III: Juvenile angiofibromas: Behavior and treatment of extensive and recurrent tumors. Arch Otolaryngol Head Neck Surg 112:1191, 1986.

38. Bremer JW, Neel HB III, DeSanto LW, Jones GC: Angiofibromas: Treatment trends in 150 patients during 40 years. Laryngoscope 96:1321, 1986.

CHAPTER 25

CEREBROSPINAL FLUID RHINORRHEA

Peter W. Carmel, MD, DMedSci

Arnold Komisar, MD, DDS, FACS

Leakage of cerebrospinal fluid (CSF) from the nostrils is now regarded as an abnormal and alarming sign. However, this recognition is fairly modern. The Greek view, epitomized by Galen, was that the nose was the normal excretory pathway for cerebrospinal fluid. The cerebrospinal fluid was thought to be distilled in the region of the pituitary gland, and this "pituita" was then discharged through the nose.

Thompson[1] credits Schneider[2] with showing that there was no free communication between the nose and the ventricles of the brain; the membranous barrier is known as the schneiderian membrane.[2] Willis (1676)[4] and Morgagni (1762)[5] both recognized that CSF passing through the nose was an abnormal condition. The first case in which autopsy findings were fully described was that of Miller.[6] His patient had communicating hydrocephalus in which the leak was through the cribriform plate.

A number of classifications of spinal fluid leak have been proposed, principally by Cairns,[7] Ommaya and associates,[8] and Cole and Keene.[9] The number of different classifications of this entity highlights its multietiologic nature. CSF leaks may be either traumatic or nontraumatic in origin. The traumatic leaks are generally related to head or facial injury and may appear immediately following trauma or may be delayed. The trauma also may be iatrogenic, associated with either otorhinologic or intracranial surgery.

Nontraumatic cases may be caused by tumors, may be due to congenital anomalies (usually in the bones of the base of the skull), or may be related to focal atrophy of the brain.[10] Osteomyelitic erosion of the skull may also cause CSF leak. Both obstructive and communicating hydrocephalus may cause CSF rhinorrhea. Tumors may lead to leakage by erosion of the skull base or by obstruction of CSF pathways, which induces a high intracranial pressure.

TRAUMATIC CEREBROSPINAL FLUID RHINORRHEA

Trauma is by far the most common cause of cerebrospinal fluid rhinorrhea. It is most often seen following motor vehicle or biking accidents, generally in the adolescent and young adult. In most cases the cerebrospinal fluid leak is noted within 24 to 48 hours after the accident. However, leakage at times remote from the trauma has been reported. The interval between inciting injury and appearance of leakage may be many years or even decades.[11]

Data in larger series reported by Robinson[11] and Lewin[12] suggest that the vast majority of these leaks stop spontaneously within 1 week. The patient is generally positioned in bed with the head upright. If leakage continues in the upright position, a supine posture may stop the leak. A period of attempted postural control of CSF rhinorrhea is advocated for traumatic cases, and most leaks are likely to be stopped in this fashion.

In addition to fractures of the calvarium or base of the skull, facial fractures commonly accompany CSF rhinorrhea, and these may be quite complex. Patients with fractures in the nasofrontal-ethmoid region, or those with LeFort III fractures, are most at risk to develop cerebrospinal fluid rhinorrhea.

The sites of CSF fistula in traumatic rhinorrhea are (in order of frequency) the frontal sinus, the ethmoid sinuses, directly into the nasal cavity, the sphenoid sinus, and the eustachian tube.[12, 13] Lewin and Cairns have shown that fractures of the sphenoid sinus causing cerebrospinal fluid rhinorrhea are the least likely to close.[14] This peculiar persistence occurs because the sphenoid sinus underlies large CSF-containing cisterns around the chiasm, providing a large CSF volume and preventing arachnoideae from covering the leak. Fractures through the mastoid bone may drain into the middle ear either through the floor of the middle fossa or through the posterior fossa. CSF will then drain through the eustachian tube and leak through the nose.

Spinal fluid rhinorrhea may follow nasal, craniofacial reconstructive, or trans-sphenoid surgery. These leaks are far less likely to stop spontaneously than those following accidental trauma.

NONTRAUMATIC CEREBROSPINAL FLUID RHINORRHEA

A number of different etiologies have been reported for nontraumatic CSF rhinorrhea. Cole and Keene have reviewed 196 cases reported in the literature in which the etiology could be established by surgical observation, histology, or postmortem examination.[9] Of this group, less than half (43 per cent) were due to neoplasm (17 per cent pituitary tumors, 26 per cent nonpituitary tumors). The largest group of CSF leaks was related either to congenital malformations or focal atrophy, which respectively caused 31 and 15 per cent of the cases. Congenital anomalies included encephaloceles, meningoencephaloceles, bony or dural defects, and bony dehiscences. Minor trauma or a sudden rise in intracranial pressure may open an anatomic defect not previously apparent. Focal atrophy of brain substance may expose the base

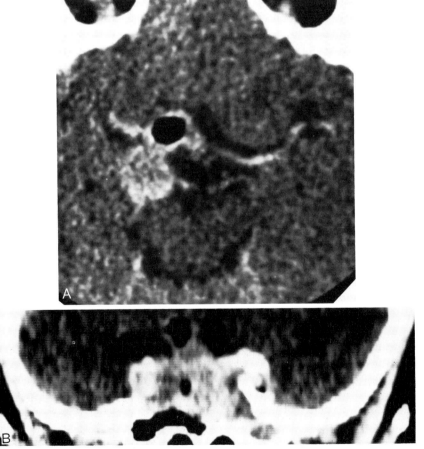

Figure 25–1. A large pituitary tumor with extension to the right temporal region. *A*, Axial enhanced CT scan. There is a large air collection (dark area) within the anterior portion of the tumor. *B*, Coronal reconstruction. The tumor has eroded the entire sellar floor and fills the upper sphenoid sinus. Air is seen in the mid and upper portions of the tumor. The patient had an intermittent rhinorrhea for almost a year before this scan.

of the brain to the constant pulsations of cerebrospinal fluid. Thus, when there is atrophy of the olfactory bulb or the pituitary gland, a meningeal pouch may form where these structures have atrophied.[46] As the meningeal pouch expands, it may erode bone and eventually may rupture to leak through the bone. Surprisingly, hydrocephalus accounts for only 5 per cent of nontraumatic CSF leaks; osteomyelitis accounts for 6 per cent.

Direct neoplastic erosion of bone at the base of the brain that causes spinal fluid leakage occurs relatively rarely. Such tumors include osteomas of the frontal sinus, pituitary tumors (Fig. 25–1), nasopharyngeal carcinomas, and cholesteatoma in the cerebellar pontine angle.[15] Other tumors may cause leakage by obstruction of CSF pathways, which leads to increased intracranial pressure. Pressure may subsequently cause erosion and leakage through bone defects.

CSF rhinorrhea has been associated with the empty sella syndrome. Ommaya and associates pointed out the relationship between elevations of CSF pressure and the empty sella.[8, 16] These investigators felt that CSF leaks from an empty sella might result from persistence of a cranio-pharyngeal duct that was secondarily forced open by increased intracranial pressure. Accurate figures on the incidence of CSF leak in patients with primary empty sella are not readily available. However, relatively few cases of trans-sellar leakage have been reported, whereas there is a substantial incidence of empty sellas in autopsy reports. Weisberg and associates had two patients with rhinorrhea in their group of 25 empty sella cases.[17] In cases of nontraumatic CSF rhinorrhea, the sella is a far less frequent site of leakage than the cribriform plate. In addition, CSF leakage has been reported in patients who have been taking long-term bromocriptine for the treatment of macroprolactinomas.[18, 18a] The case illustrated by Figure 25–2 shows that finding an empty sella is not sufficient; rather, the actual site of leakage must be identified.

In some cases the relationship between the bony opening in a sinus and the dural tear may cause a ball-valve effect, which will let air in but still not leak CSF. Air may be forced intracranially with cough or sneeze, which elevates the sinus pressure.[19] This collection may expand over a period of time as new air is pushed into it, causing the signs and symptoms

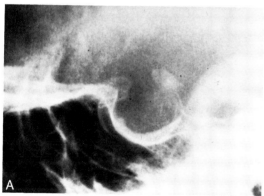

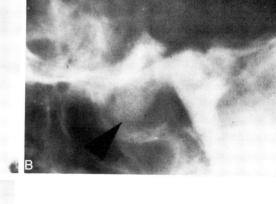

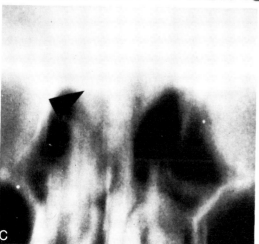

Figure 25–2. A 58-year-old woman with a CSF rhinorrhea of 10 months' duration. The patient, who was hypertensive and obese, denied significant head injury. Two bouts of meningitis had been treated with antibiotics without sequelae. *A,* Lateral radiograph. The sella is large and ballooned, but the clinoids are not eroded. *B,* Intrathecal metrizamide study, lateral view. The CSF space fills most of the sella *(arrowhead),* with the remnant gland pushed downward and posteriorly. Although the sella is large and empty, there is no evidence of leakage. *C,* Frontal tomogram during an intrathecal metrizamide study. Contrast material drains from the skull at the lateral cribriform area and is seen in the right ethmoid sinus *(arrowhead).*

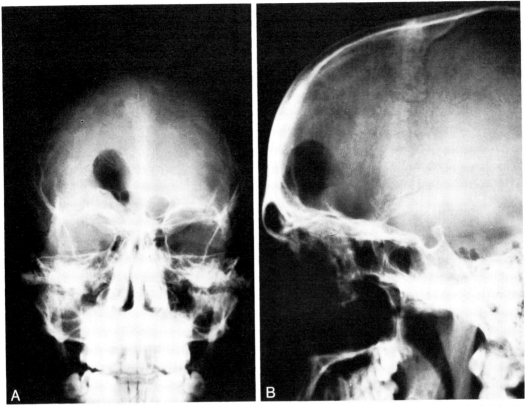

Figure 25–3. A 14-year-old boy had been in a motor vehicle accident 3 days earlier. He complained of right frontal headache and developed mild weakness in his left arm. *A,* Anterior radiograph. Air is seen extending into the right frontal lobe and appears to arise at the frontal sinus. *B,* Lateral radiograph. Air is seen behind the frontal sinus and pushing into the brain. A fracture of the posterior wall of the sinus and a dural/arachnoidal laceration are seen.

of a mass lesion (Fig. 25–3*A, B*). Pneumoceles of this type have the same significance as rhinorrhea in risk of infection but may require emergency surgery because of increased intracranial pressure or shift of brain structures.

An unusual group of patients are those in whom an opening to CSF spaces from outside the skull is found only after shunting for hydrocephalus.[19] In cases reported by Pitts and associates[20] and Steinberger and associates,[21] patients developed pneumocephalus after shunting. It is less surprising when patients with a pre-existing CSF rhinorrhea develop pneumocephalus after shunting. In these patients the opening to the subarachnoid space allowed air to enter the skull through a defect in the wall of a neighboring sinus. In the case of Steinberger and associates, the patient developed pneumocephalus (Fig. 25–4*A, B*), and the shunt was ligated.[21] The patient then developed a CSF leak through an opening in the posterior wall of the frontal sinus (Fig. 25–4*C*).

In these cases it is necessary to correct the opening from the sinus to the subarachnoid space as the initial operative procedure. In patients with hydrocephalus and increased pres-

sure, the shunt should remain functional, which may make sealing the sinus defect more difficult. However, ligation of the shunt in shunt-dependent patients may carry considerable risk. An on-off valve system may be useful under these circumstances.

Diagnosis of cerebrospinal fluid fistulas may be quite difficult. It is useful first to establish that the leaking fluid is indeed CSF. Because the spinal fluid has a much higher sugar content than mucinous secretions, testing the leaked fluid for sugar is widely employed. However, most of the commercially available sticks and tapers are now quite sensitive to even the low levels of sugar present in mucous secretions. Therefore, a quantitative determination is preferable, which usually requires collection of at least 0.5 ml of leaked fluid. Because CSF glucose levels may fluctuate, it is best to obtain a sample of blood or lumbar CSF simultaneously with collection of leaked fluid. The glucose content of the leaked CSF sample should be similar to that of the specimen obtained by lumbar puncture and 40 to 60 per cent of the blood level.

All efforts then should be aimed at correctly

localizing the site of leakage prior to operation. Operative data indicate that almost 30 per cent of surgically treated rhinorrhea patients require additional procedures for control of recurrent leakage.[22, 23] Of patients who have had inadequate control of their CSF leak, almost 15 per cent develop meningitis before control is finally secured.[16] Although intraoperative localization of a spinal fluid fistula is possible, the better procedure by far is identification of the defect before operation.

Radiographic techniques used for identifying CSF fistulas have included skull radiography, multidirectional polytomography, radionuclide or fluorescein cisternography, and pantopaque CSF studies.[3, 24, 25]

In a study by Lantz and associates, the site of leak was identified on only 21 per cent of preoperative plain radiographs.[26] With the use of polytomography, almost 53 per cent of the leakage sites were correctly identified. Both radionuclide and fluorescein cisternography have been successfully employed for localizing CSF fistulas. In these methods, small pledgets of cotton are placed in the nasal cavities at the outlet sites of the sinuses. By observing the density of material on these pledgets, it is possible to identify the site of greatest leakage. In addition, during isotope cisternography the head can be scanned at frequent intervals after injection and the site of leakage may possibly be identified. In the series of Lantz and associates, CSF radioisotope cisternography helped localize the site of leak in 50 per cent of patients and was suggestive of the site of leakage in another 25 per cent.[26] Pantopaque CSF studies are far less likely to reveal the dural defect owing to the viscosity of this contrast material.

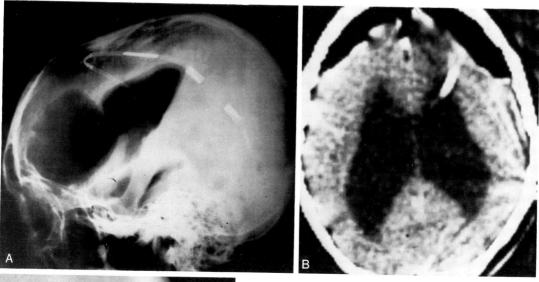

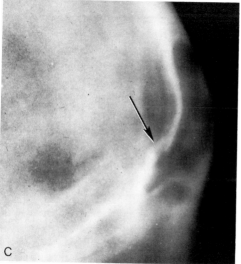

Figure 25–4. A woman with a chronic hydrocephalus had undergone a shunting procedure several days earlier. Ambulation was followed by acute neurologic decompensation. *A,* Lateral radiograph. *B,* Axial CT scan showing pneumocephalus and shunt. *C,* Lateral radiograph showing dehiscence in the posterior wall of the sinus *(arrow).* The dural opening was treated with a patch graft, and the shunt ligature was removed several days later.

Use of Pantopaque for basal cisternography has gradually been replaced, in part because of the possibility of postexamination arachnoid reactions.

It is likely that all these methods have been made obsolete by the introduction of metrizamide cisternography. A dilute solution of metrizamide may be injected by lumbar or cisternal tap and allowed to diffuse through the CSF. The Trendelenburg position with the head extended may help bring the dye to the floor of the cranium. Metrizamide cisternography can be used in conjunction with high-resolution computed tomography in the coronal plane. In many institutions the incidence of correct identification of CSF leaks with this method is over 90 per cent. More recently, water-soluble iohexol has been used to identify leaks in conjunction with CT scanning.[25, 25a]

TREATMENT

Treatment of CSF rhinorrhea may be either conservative or operative. Operative correction employs transcranial, trans-sphenoid, or transethmoid approaches. The choice will be determined by the site of the leakage, the cause of the leak, and the presence of associated injuries.

The great majority of post-traumatic CSF leaks will stop spontaneously within a week. The patient is placed in a position in which leakage does not spontaneously occur. The patient is then kept at strict bed rest in this position until all evidence of CSF leak has been absent for several days. It is a matter of continued controversy as to whether these patients should be treated with prophylactic antibiotics during the period of leakage.[27] We generally do not treat these patients unless the CSF leak persists for more than 3 days. If treatment with antibiotics is to be started, it is necessary to obtain a culture of the CSF. Antibiotic should be given in sufficient doses to treat, rather than obscure, intercurrent infection.

The use of spinal drainage via an indwelling catheter to control CSF leak was introduced in the early 1960s.[28] Since that time a number of investigators have described the use of continuous spinal drainage in treating both postoperative and post-traumatic CSF leaks.[29] This method is dependent on draining more fluid than is normally produced by the choroid plexus. The normal rate of CSF production in the adult is approximately one third of a milliliter per minute, or approximately 450 to 500 ml per day. The rates of therapeutic CSF drainage have varied considerably in different reported series, ranging from 60 to 600 ml per day. Patients undergoing continuous external drainage are treated with intravenous antibiotics. The antibiotic chosen should be effective against gram-positive cocci and the usual skin flora.

Continuous spinal drainage is not without occasional complication.[30] Serious, even life-threatening, complications may occur and are most frequently caused by pneumocephalus. The air that is aspirated through the CSF fistula into the head is at room temperature but rapidly heats to body temperature and expands accordingly. The staff must be alert to this complication, often marked by headache, restlessness, vomiting, and progressive stupor. Several ingenious methods have been described to prevent excessive pressure gradient between the intracranial space and the drainage apparatus. These work most often by regulating pressure or by regulating flow.[29]

NEUROSURGICAL INTERVENTION

Neurosurgical intervention is reserved for CSF leaks that are not controlled by positioning and conservative therapy. Two types of treatment plans are used. The first involves those patients who have CSF rhinorrhea due to increased intracranial pressure.[3] Here the therapy is directed at lowering the intracranial pressure by CSF drainage. This can be done on a trial basis by repeated lumbar punctures or an externalized lumbar catheter. For leaks that are persistent despite these measures, an internalized shunting procedure may be required. If obstructive hydrocephalus is enlarging the ventricles, a ventriculoperitoneal shunt may be performed. However, in many cases decompression of the spinal fluid through the leak is sufficient to prevent ventricular enlargement. For these patients a lumboperitoneal shunt, utilizing the lumbar cistern, may be worthwhile. Shunting procedures may not be indicated if the patient has either a tumor obstructing CSF pathways or meningitis. In these cases attention must be paid to the primary pathology.

Creating low pressure within the head has two inherent risks. The first is risk of meningitis by reflux of bacteria backward into the intracranial cavity through the fistula. The actual incidence of this is rare.[23] The other problem, creation of pneumocephalus by shunting, already has been discussed.[21]

Shunting procedures are probably not useful

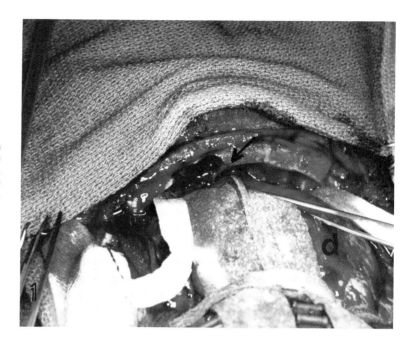

Figure 25–5. Dural herniation through the posterior wall of the frontal sinus after trauma *(arrow)*. The patient has a fracture of the posterior wall of the frontal sinus. *d,* Dura.

if the leak is profuse. It is likely that the size of the opening will result in failure of shunting to stop the leak and a greater possibility of pneumocephalus. For high volume leaks, direct operation may be required. After a short period to allow the repair to fibrose into position, a shunting procedure may be performed.

For leaks from the sella, parasellar regions, and sphenoid sinus, a repair via the transsphenoid approach is useful.[18, 31] Once the sphenoid sinus is entered, the operating microscope is used to try to visualize the leak site. The fistula is closed with either bone wax, muscle,

Gelfoam, or acrylic cement. The entire sinus, including its lateral extension, is then packed with fat taken from either the anterior portion of the abdomen or the thigh. The floor of the sinus is then reconstituted, using bone, cartilage, or cement.

Leaks from the base of the frontal fossa or from the posterior wall of the frontal sinus are best treated by direct intracranial repair via craniotomy.[13, 32] If the operative site is well identified, the choice may be between an intradural or extradural approach (Figs. 25–5 and 25–6). In general, most of the leaks in the floor

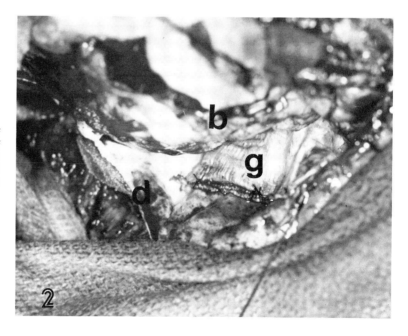

Figure 25–6. Intradural repair of a CSF leak through the floor of the anterior cranial fossa. g, fascia lata and muscle graft; d, dural flaps; b, brain. (Courtesy of Martin Camins, MD.)

of the frontal fossa are best treated by an intradural approach, whereas those on the posterior wall of the frontal sinus may be treated extradurally.

When the leak is through the cribriform plate or elsewhere above the ethmoid sinus, the tract must be obliterated. Often there is a "funnel" sign indicating the area of leakage (see Fig. 25–5A). This tract must be stuffed with bone wax, muscle, Gelfoam, or other obliterating materials. Grafts of fat and fascia are then placed over the top of the funnel and sutured to the basal dura (see Fig. 25–5B).

For patients with a paradoxic CSF leak coming from a fracture extending into the middle ear (Fig. 25–7), the choice of operation depends often on whether the hearing is impaired. When hearing is intact, an intracranial approach in the middle fossa is preferable. However, for those who have already lost hearing, an endaural repair may be preferable.

Despite the most elaborate attempts at diagnosis, the precise site of CSF leak may escape detection. In these cases the operation becomes exploratory. It is often necessary to expose the floor of both frontal fossae and to inspect both cribriform regions, as well as the rest of the frontal fossa floor. A large piece of freeze-dried dura, fascia lata, or dural substitute may be used to cover the entire floor. It is sutured into position along the sphenoid ridges bilaterally and the anterior base of the frontal fossa. Inspection of these cases must include the lateral extension of the sphenoid sinus where the leakage may be coming through the pterygoid recesses of the sinus.[33] Exploratory repairs have the unenviable distinction of a high rate of surgical failure and the concomitant complication of a permanent anosmia.

RHINOLOGIC APPROACHES

For many years the rhinologic procedure employed when craniotomy was contraindicated was transnasal cauterization of the site of leakage with silver nitrate.[34] This was sometimes augmented with serial lumbar punctures and bed rest. Dohlman was perhaps the first to describe a rhinologic operative procedure to control CSF rhinorrhea from the skull base.[35] His exposure was via frontoethmoidectomy and used a flap from the middle turbinate, which bolstered a free muscle graft and was held in position with nasal packing. Recurrent leakage required re-exploration, and a septal flap of mucoperiosteum successfully controlled the leak.

Hirsch, a pioneer of trans-sphenoid surgery, reported endonasal control of CSF leakage into the sphenoid sinus utilizing a septal mucosal flap.[36] This operation employed his classic endonasal trans-sphenoid approach. McCoy expanded the experience of Hirsch, adding a lateral rhinotomy for increased exposure.[36] Montgomery[37] used the external ethmoidectomy for exposure but utilized mucosal flaps similar to those described by Hirsch and Dohlman. Finally, McCabe described an osteomucoperiosteal flap that utilized the posterior septum.[38] This was constructed so that a flap of perpendicular plate and attached mucosa was swung into position against the dural dehiscence.

All these procedures are useful for control of isolated leaks involving the fovea ethmoidalis and cribriform plate area and somewhat less useful for sphenoid leaks. Each procedure allows a limited exposure, operates in a contaminated field, and cannot be employed for leaks of the frontal sinus.

ETHMOID

The rhinologic approach currently favored is a compilation of the aforementioned techniques (Fig. 25–8). If the site can be pinpointed to one side, then an external ethmoidectomy is performed, with the following modifications: After the incision is made and the orbital contents retracted, the ethmoid labyrinth is opened and some of the inner mucosa and attachments of the middle turbinate are preserved. The site of leakage is identified, and any brain herniating through the defect is amputated. The mucosa around the fistula is stripped so that the bone of the cribriform plate or fovea ethmoidalis is exposed, and the mucosa is preserved so that it may be reflected into the site of leakage. If bone is absent, healthy dura is exposed. A determination as to whether to use a septal or a middle turbinate flap is made. If a septal flap is used, a long mucoperiosteal flap (which may or may not include cartilage or bone) is fashioned from the nasal septum. This is reflected up to the area of the leak. Nasal packing is used to keep the flap in position. It sometimes is possible to place an anchoring suture through the flap to other nasal tissue for retention. If a middle turbinate flap is used, the entire middle turbinate may be swung into position after the leak site is suitably prepared. The mucosa of the flap may be denuded where it comes in contact with the site of leakage. The middle turbinate bone may be removed to lengthen the flap. This flap is held in position with nasal

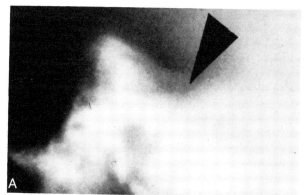

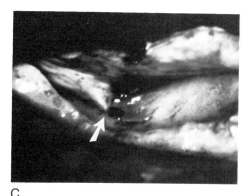

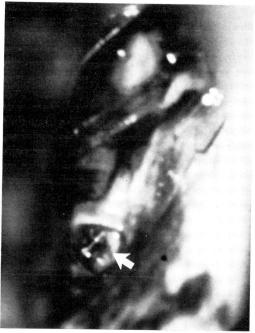

Figure 25–7. An 8-year-old boy with rhinorrhea following a fall. Hearing was decreased but not absent on the right. Radiographs of the frontal fossa and cribriform region were negative. *A,* Anterior tomogram of right petrous bone. The fracture *(arrowhead)* extends to the floor of the middle fossa beneath the temporal lobe. *B, C,* Operative photographs. An extradural approach has been made beneath the right temporal lobe. The dura has been pinched into the fracture *(arrow),* and CSF leaks directly into the middle ear. *D,* Photograph of repair. The hole was plugged with bone wax and covered with fat; and then fascia was sutured into place, successfully closing the leak.

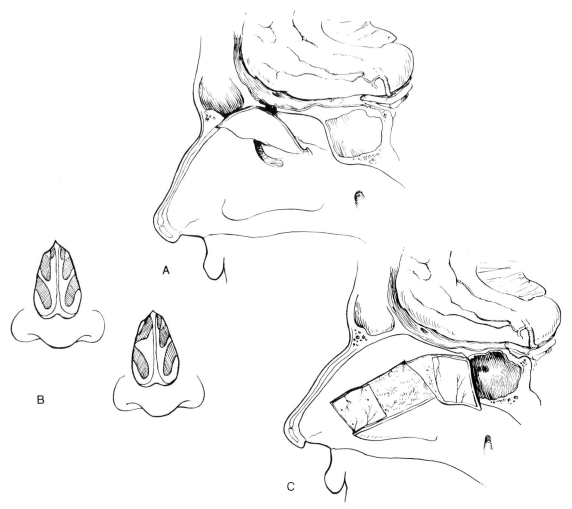

Figure 25–8. *A*, Lateral view of nose, showing incisions made along the inferior and anterior aspects of the turbinate. The flap has been elevated from the medial surface of the turbinate bone and rotated into the area of the cribriform plate. *B*, Frontal views showing the rotation of the turbinate flap to the area of the cribriform plate. *C*, Lateral view of the nose showing the elevation of a septal flap, including perichondrium and cartilage, which is reflected posterosuperiorly toward the area of the leak.

packing. A lateral rhinotomy may sometimes be added to increase exposure. The ethmoidectomy is closed in a usual manner.

A recent study of the use of an osteomucoperiosteal flap at the University of Iowa revealed a very favorable success rate in fistula closure.[39] Fibrin glue also has been reported as a successful method of stopping CSF leaks through the cribriform plate and anterior fossa. The fibrin glue has been used with muscle plugs, as well as with bone chips, fascia, and plaster of Paris.[40, 41]

The nasal endoscope has also added a new dimension to the ability to diagnose the site of leakage, as well as closure of the leak by various techniques, including the use of fibrin glue and muscle or fascia.[42, 43]

FRONTAL

The anterior osteoplastic approach to the frontal sinus was first described for chronic disease of the frontal sinus at the turn of the century (see Chapter 10). Beck was the first American to describe this approach for sinus disease.[44] The operation was greeted with much skepticism and fell into disfavor until introduction of the concept of sinus obliteration with fat.[37, 45]

The anterior osteoplastic approach may be used for control of leakage through the posterior wall of the frontal sinus. If there is a dural tear, it is exposed by removing posterior table bone until viable dura is seen circumferentially. If primary repair of the dural dehiscence is possible, this is accomplished with fine silk suture. When there is too much disruption to effect a primary repair, a graft may be laid against the dura, usually fascia bolstered by Gelfoam. The mucosa of the sinus is removed and the sinus obliterated with adipose tissue. In cases in which the posterior table is extensively destroyed, the sinus may be cranialized following repair of the dural dehiscence. In cases with extreme comminution of both the anterior and posterior tables, the sinus may be removed and the dura repaired and permitted to come in contact with the coronal flap.

References

1. Thompson St C: The Cerebrospinal Fluid: Its Spontaneous Escape from the Nose. London, Cassell, 1899.
2. Schneider: Über de Osse Cribriform. Witten bergae (quoted by St C Thompson), 1655.
3. Schechter MM, Rovit RL, Schachter JM: Rhinorrhea and hydrocephalus: Observations on spontaneous cerebrospinal fluid fistulae in patients with increased intracranial pressure. Acta Radiol 9:101, 1969.
4. Willis T: Opera Omnia. Cerebri, Anatomia, Nervorumqui. Descriptio et Usus. Geneva, 1676.
5. Morgagni JP: De Sedibus et Causis Morborum. Liber 1. epxv art 21 (quoted by St C Thompson), 1762.
6. Miller C: Trans Med Chir Soc Edinburgh 2:243, 1826.
7. Cairns H: Injuries of the frontal and ethmoid sinuses with special references to cerebrospinal rhinorrhea and aeroceles. J Laryngol Otol 52:589, 1937.
8. Ommaya AK, Di Chiro G, Baldwin M, Pennybacker, JB: Nontraumatic cerebrospinal fluid rhinorrhea. J Neurol Neurosurg Psychiatry 31:214, 1968.
9. Cole IE, Keene M: Cerebrospinal fluid rhinorrhoea in pituitary tumours. R Soc Med J 73:244, 1980.
10. Som ML, Kramer R: Cerebrospinal fluid rhinorrhea: Pathological findings. Laryngoscope 50:1167, 1940.
11. Robinson RG: Cerebrospinal fluid rhinorrhea, meningitis and pneumocephalus due to non-missile injuries. Aust NZ J Surg 39:328, 1970.
12. Lewin W: Cerebrospinal fluid rhinorrhoea in closed head injuries. Br J Surg 42:1, 1954.
13. Jamieson KG, Yelland JDN: Surgical repair of the anterior fossa because of rhinorrhea, aerocele, or meningitis. J Neurosurg 39:328, 1973.
14. Lewin W, Cairns H: Fractures of the sphenoidal sinus with cerebrospinal rhinorrhoea. Br Med J 1:1, 1951.
15. Shugar JMA, Som PM, Eisman W, Biller HF: Nontraumatic cerebrospinal fluid rhinorrhea. Laryngoscope 91:214, 1981.
16. Ommaya AK: Spinal fluid fistulae. Clin Neurosurg 23:363, 1976.
17. Weisberg LA, Housepian EM, Saur DP: Empty sella syndrome as complication of benign intracranial hypertension. J Neurosurg 43:117, 1975.
18. Carmel PW: The empty sella. In Wilkins R (ed): Neurosurgery. New York, McGraw-Hill, 1984.
18a. Bronstein MD, Musolino NR, Benabou S, Marino R: Cerebrospinal fluid rhinorrhea occurring in long-term bromocriptine treatment for macroprolactinomas. Surg Neurol 32:346, 1989.
19. Little JR, Macarty CS: Tension pneumocephalus after insertion of ventriculoperitoneal shunt for aqueductal stenosis: Case report. J Neurosurg 44:383, 1976.
20. Pitts LH, Wilson CB, Dedo HH, Weyand R: Pneumocephalus following ventriculoperitoneal shunt: Case report. J Neurosurg 43:631, 1975.
21. Steinberger A, Antunes JL, Michelsen WJ: Pneumocephalus after ventriculoatrial shunt. Neurosurgery 5:708, 1979.
22. Ray BS, Bergland RM: Cerebrospinal fluid fistula: Clinical aspects, techniques of localization, and methods of closure. J Neurosurg 30:399, 1969.
23. Spetzler RF, Wilson CB: Management of recurrent CSF rhinorrhea of the middle and posterior fossa. J Neurosurg 49:393, 1978.
24. Di Chiro G, Ommaya AK, Ashburn WL, et al: Isotope cisternography in the diagnosis and follow-up of cerebrospinal fluid rhinorrhea. J Neurosurg 28:522, 1968.
25. Naidich TP, Moran CJ: Precise anatomic localization of atraumatic sphenoethmoidal cerebrospinal fluid rhinorrhea by metrizamide CT cisternography. J Neurosurg 53:222, 1980.
25a. Chow JM, Goodman D, Mafee MF: Evaluation of CSF rhinorrhea by computerized tomography with metrizamide. Otolaryngol Head Neck Surg 100:99, 1989.
26. Lantz EJ, Forbes GS, Brown ML, Laws ER: Radiology of cerebrospinal fluid rhinorrhea. Am J Radiol 135:1023, 1980.
27. MacGee EE, Cauthen JC, Brackett CE: Meningitis following acute traumatic cerebrospinal fluid fistula. J Neurosurg 33:312, 1970.
28. Vour'ch G: Continuous cerebrospinal fluid drainage by indwelling spinal catheter. Br J Anaesth 35:118, 1963.
29. Swanson SE, Kocan MJ, Chandler WF: Flow-regulated continuous spinal drainage: Technical note with case report. Neurosurgery 9:163, 1981.
30. Graf CJ, Gross CE, Beck DW: Complications of spinal drainage in the management of cerebrospinal fluid fistula: Report of three cases. J Neurosurg 54:392, 1981.
31. Weiss MH, Kaufman B, Richards DE: Cerebrospinal fluid rhinorrhea from an empty sella: Transsphenoidal obliteration of the fistula: Technical note. J Neurosurg 39:674, 1973.
32. Rengachary SS: Surgical repair of cerebrospinal fluid fistula: A modified technique. Am Surgeon 47:268, 1981.
33. Morley TP, Wortzman G: The importance of the lateral extensions of the sphenoidal sinus in post-traumatic cerebrospinal rhinorrhea and meningitis. Clinical and radiological aspects. J Neurosurg 22:326, 1965.
34. Fox N: Cure in a case of cerebrospinal rhinorrhea. Arch Otolaryngol 17:85, 1933.
35. Dohlman G: Spontaneous cerebrospinal rhinorrhea case operated by rhinological methods. Acta Otolaryngol (Suppl) 67:20, 1948.
36. Hirsch O: Successful closure of cerebrospinal fluid rhinorrhea by endonasal surgery. Arch Otolaryngol 56:1, 1952.
37. Montgomery WW: Cerebrospinal rhinorrhea. In Montgomery WW (ed): Surgery of the Upper Respiratory Tract. Vol 1. Philadelphia, Lea & Febiger, 1971.
38. McCabe BF: The osteo-mucoperiosteal flap in repair of cerebrospinal fluid rhinorrhea. Laryngoscope 86:536, 1976.
39. Yessenow RS, McCabe BF: The osteo-mucoperiosteal flap in the repair of cerebrospinal fluid rhinorrhea: A 20 year experience. Otolaryngol Head Neck Surg 101:555, 1989.

40. Nishihira S, McCaffrey TV: The use of fibrin glue for the repair of experimental CSF rhinorrhea. Laryngoscope 98:625, 1988.
41. Olofsson J, Bynke O: Transantral repair of cerebrospinal fluid fistulas using bone chips, Tisseel, fascia, and plaster of Paris. Acta Otolaryngol Suppl (Stockh) 449:89, 1988.
42. Papay FA, Maggiano H, Dominguez S, Hassenbusch SJ, Levine HL, Lavertu P: Rigid endoscopic repair of paranasal sinus cerebrospinal fluid fistulas. Laryngoscope 99:1195, 1989.
43. Thumfart W: Personal communication, 1990.
44. Beck JC: A new method of external frontal sinus operation without deformity. JAMA 51:6, 1908.
45. Calcaterra TC: External surgical repair of cerebrospinal rhinorrhea. Ann Otol Rhinol Laryngol 89:108, 1980.
46. Applebaum EL, Desai NM: Primary empty sella syndrome with CSF rhinorrhea. JAMA 244:1606, 1980.

CHAPTER 26

CRANIOFACIAL RESECTION

Andrew Blitzer, MD, DDS
Kalmon D. Post, MD
William Lawson, MD, DDS

Cancers of the paranasal sinuses generally have a poor prognosis. They have been difficult to diagnose owing to their insidious onset and vague symptoms. All of the paranasal sinuses, with the exception of the maxillary sinus, share a wall with the orbit and intracranial cavity. This easily allows extension of the tumors into the cranium.[1, 2]

In the past, en bloc resection of these sinuses was thought to be too hazardous, and local partial resections were performed. These often allowed local recurrence at the cribriform plate and skull base, producing an overall 5-year survival rate of 0-8 per cent, with only 10 per cent dying from distant metastases.[2, 3]

Historically, the early management of cancer of the paranasal sinuses included drainage, electrocauterization, and radiation therapy. This approach was well described by Ohngren, in 1933,[4] and Watson, in 1942.[5] In 1948, Martin described the surgical excision of frontoethmoid and sphenoid cancers as being hazardous, with complete removal impossible, because surgery would involve the skull base.[6] He suggested using surgery initially to remove as much tumor as possible and to provide adequate drainage, to facilitate radiotherapy later. However, by this method, tumor control was poor. His reported series had a 13 per cent 5-year survival, but it included numerous cases accidentally discovered on nasal polypectomy. The surgery he advocated violated the basic oncologic principle of en bloc resection with wide margins because of the proximity of the skull base.

Skull base resection was first attempted for the removal of orbital tumors with extension intracranially. In 1934, Adson and Benedict described the transcranial excision of an orbital hemangioendothelioma.[7] In 1938, Cushing reported a transcranial approach for orbital tumors,[8] which was elaborated on by Dandy in 1941.[9] Dandy realized from his experience with intracranial pituitary surgery that the access to the skull base (orbital roof), exposure of the orbital contents (globe, muscles, ophthalmic vein, and artery), and exposure of the brain were best achieved from above. He stated that anything short of a combined approach offered no surgical solution, as most of these tumors extended intracranially. Dandy also acknowledged the limitations of using ether as an anesthetic because of the resultant brain swelling.

In 1943, Ray and McLean published their combined intracranial and transorbital approach for retinoblastoma. They considered this the optimal approach as these tumors tended to spread intracranially along the optic nerve.[10] Smith and associates[11] in 1954 were the first to report a combined craniofacial approach for the management of advanced frontoethmoidalorbital cancer. They were able to salvage one of the three patients so treated. This initiated the use of this technique of removing the skull base in continuity with sinus tumors. In 1959, Malecki described his technique of combined craniofacial resection, including the cribriform area.[12] He reconstructed the area with fascia, iliac crest bone, or nasal cartilage to prevent brain herniation.

The anesthetic, neurosurgical and infectious

problems were great, and many surgeons did not embrace this new technique. Ross, in 1959, described a procedure in which the cribriform plate and the floor of the anterior cranial fossa were resected from below without a formal craniotomy.[13] The controversy continued. In 1962, Pool and associates considered the frontal sinus approach to the anterior fossa to be inadequate and hazardous.[14] One year later, Frazell and Lewis warned that removal of the entire cribriform plate could rarely be performed without cerebral complications.[15]

The relative safety and propriety of the combined craniofacial resection was well established by the work of Ketcham and associates.[16] In 1963, they evaluated the results obtained in 30 patients with advanced paranasal sinus, nasal, and orbital cancers treated at the National Institutes of Health, most of whom were failures of other modalities. After careful evaluation, 19 of these patients were found to be candidates for combined resection. With the exception of one perioperative mortality related to infection, the other patients did well. In 1968, they reviewed their 10-year experience, reporting an approximate 30 per cent cure rate in an otherwise unsalvageable group of patients, which by 1973 rose to a 56 per cent determinate 5-year survival.[17]

Despite this work, some investigators considered a craniotomy to be unnecessary, producing an additional morbidity. Ross and associates suggested that en bloc resection of the ethmoids could be performed via a lateral rhinotomy approach.[18] This was based on an experience with 11 cases, with 5 cures; however, this series included a number of small tumors.

Development of reconstructive surgery for craniofacial malformations added to the advancement of the craniofacial resection technique.[19-21] In 1975, Westbury and associates reported using a frontal sinus osteoplastic flap as an approach for combined resection.[22] Sisson and associates used a frontal craniotomy and described methods of skull base reconstruction employing bone and cartilage.[23] Shah and Galicich strongly recommended the use of a bifrontal craniotomy because it provided additional exposure, permitted better assessment of tumor resectability, and facilitated dural resection and repair.[24] Schramm and associates, in 1979, expanded the role of the frontal bur hole and described the use of a frontotemporal flap for cases with greater involvement of the skull base.[25] Clifford[26] and Terz and associates[3, 27, 28] described the use of a temporal craniotomy for resection of lesions involving the middle cranial fossa and a combined frontal and temporal approach for removal of the anterior and middle fossae.

Resection of the middle fossa skull base has been used independently and in conjunction with anterior skull base resection. The middle fossa can be resected with extension of the anterior craniotomy along the lateral and inferior walls. Donald[28a] and Sehkar and associates[28b] have shown the efficacy of this technique for managing large tumors involving the skull base. Fisch[28c] has popularized infratemporal fossa approaches to tumors of the infratemporal fossa, nasopharynx, and parasellar area. Biller and associates[28d] and Krespi and associates[28e, f, g] have approached medial and lateral compartment middle skull base lesions via a mandibular split and an inferior approach. At times, several of these approaches are necessary, as dictated by the tumor involvement. Carotid ligation or bypass allows complete resection of tumors of the infratemporal and middle fossae.[28h, i, j] Techniques have also been developed for management of tumors that involve the cavernous sinus. The sinus and its contents have been successfully resected, encouraging more work in this area.[28k, l, m]

PREOPERATIVE EVALUATION

A thorough history and physical examination, with special attention to neurologic deficits, are of paramount importance. An ophthalmologic examination should be performed to detect minimal oculomotor or visual field defects. Preoperative dental consultation should be obtained to evaluate the status of the teeth and help in the construction of a prosthesis, if the palate or eyes are to be sacrificed.

Radiographic examination should include standard sinus radiographs, including a submental vertex projection, to detect erosion of the lesser wing of the sphenoid and middle cranial fossa extension. Clouding of the sphenoid should not contraindicate surgery, as this may be inflammatory in nature. The limitations of resection are involvement of the optic chiasm and cavernous sinus superiorly, and the carotid canal inferiorly. Tomography of the skull base is also useful to evaluate erosion of the sphenoid bone. Angiography may demonstrate the presence of invasion or compression or displacement of the carotid artery or jugular venous system. It will also give information regarding the vascularity of the tumor (tumor blush) and demonstrate major feeding vessels. Embolization of feeding arteries may be considered in order to make subsequent surgery easier and safer.

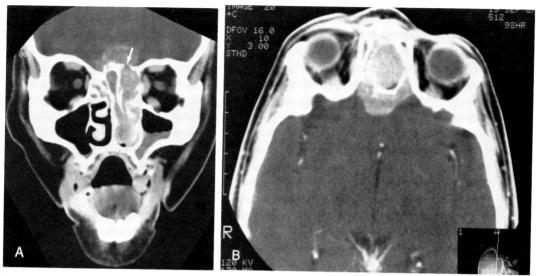

Figure 26–1. *A,* Axial enhanced CT scan demonstrating the tumor through the cribriform plate. *B,* Coronal enhanced CT scan showing the tumor and the bone destruction at the right cribriform plate *(arrow).*

The computed tomography (CT) scan with bone algorithms and magnetic resonance imaging (MRI) with gadolinium enhancement are excellent for evaluating the extent of the lesion. They show dural or intracranial involvement, displacement or invasion of orbital structures, cavernous sinus involvement, and the erosion or invasion of bone. Axial, coronal, and sagittal views are needed for surgical decisions (Figs. 26–1A, B and 26–2A, B). A recent study by Lund and associates found that CT alone offered 78 per cent accuracy in depicting tumor extent compared with operative and histologic findings.[28n] The addition of MRI increased the ac-

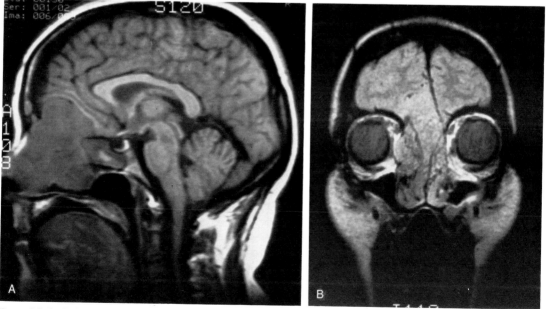

Figure 26–2. *A,* A 41-year-old woman had a history of epistaxis and a mass in the right nasal cavity. Biopsy showed a esthesioneuroblastoma. Thereafter, she received 5400 rad over 47 days; subsequent MRI scans failed to show shrinkage. CSF rhinorrhea developed, and she developed pneumococcal meningitis. Sagittal MRI demonstrated a large subfrontal and intranasal esthesioneuroblastoma. It has extended through the dura on the right side. *B,* Coronal MRI demonstrating the same tumor. The orbital contents have not been invaded.

curacy to 94 per cent, and adding MRI with gadolinium increased the accuracy to 98 per cent. The MRI with gadolinium is better able to distinguish inflamed, swollen mucous membranes and retained tumor secretions. Because the MRI does not image bone, the CT should also be used to analyze the integrity of the bony skull base.[28n, o]

These studies are of paramount importance in making therapeutic decisions, because prior reports have shown a 31 per cent likelihood to underestimate the extent of paranasal sinus tumors. CT and MRI scans are also useful postoperatively for the evaluation of recurrences and bone flap viability.

Studies such as cerebrospinal fluid (CSF) chemistry and cytology, electroencephalography (EEG), and pneumoencephalography are of little value.[3, 16, 17, 25–29]

Preoperative studies assessing the status of the carotid artery blood flow are important, particularly in the lateral and posterior approaches, in which the carotid artery may be involved. The surgeon should know the status of the collateral circulation via the circle of Willis to determine if the carotid artery can be ligated or if it needs to be bypassed. The effect of carotid occlusion can be studied preoperatively with balloon occlusion followed by a xenon/CT cerebral blood flow (CBF) study. If the flow is inadequate, the surgery may be aborted or a bypass performed prior to resection.[28r]

INDICATIONS

The combined craniofacial resection is indicated in patients who are good surgical risks and who have malignant tumors of the superior nasal cavity, ethmoid sinus, frontal sinus, and orbit. Radiotherapy alone for these lesions has been found to be hazardous, causing bone necrosis and sequestration, panophthalmia and cataracts.[30] This combined technique has also been employed for benign but locally aggressive tumors of this region, such as esthesioneuroblastomas,[31, 32] meningiomas, fibro-osseous lesions,[32a] melanomas, sarcomas, basal cell carcinomas,[28a] chordomas, and osteomas. Juvenile angiofibromas with intracranial extension can also be managed via this approach.[25, 33] Patients with maxillary or oropharyngeal carcinomas that extend into the pterygopalatine fossa have an extremely high recurrence rate (80 per cent) and a correspondingly diminished 5-year survival (3 per cent). Radiotherapy is ineffective in

this region, and so en bloc resection with the floor of the middle cranial fossa can be utilized.[27]

Patients with systemic diseases who are in poor condition or who have metastases are not candidates for craniofacial resection. Intractable pain, trismus, serous otitis media, and cranial nerve paralyses are not necessarily contraindications for craniofacial resection. Demonstration by CT or MRI scanning of involvement of the nasopharynx, superior or posterior sphenoid; sphenoid ridge, invasion at the optic chiasm; vertebral bodies and/or clivus; foramen lacerum; prevertebral space extension; or significant intracranial or intracerebral extension contraindicate these procedures[16, 17] for cure, but may not contraindicate surgery for palliation (especially for intractable pain). In these cases the patient and family should be informed about the extent of disease, the low curability rate, the extent of surgery, the functional and/or cosmetic deficits expected, and the goals of surgery.[28g, 28o]

TECHNIQUE

The key to the successful management of tumors involving the skull base is a two-team collaborative effort by the head and neck surgeon and the neurologic surgeon. Because infections are life-threatening, the patients receive preoperative and intraoperative antibiotics. Central venous pressure and arterial lines are generally placed. A bladder catheter to accurately measure urine output aids in the management of fluid balance. Often a cooling blanket is used. A leg should also be shaved, prepared, and draped, for harvesting a fascia lata, muscle, or split-thickness skin graft, if needed. Although several workers recommend a preliminary tracheostomy,[16] this is rarely necessary, as airway compromise is uncommon in midface cancer resection.[34] Other workers have created a cervical esophagostomy;[28] however, a feeding tube is not needed unless the palate is sacrificed. Even in these cases, the fabrication of a surgical prosthesis permits the patient to begin oral feedings early in the postoperative course. If feedings are delayed, a fine nasogastric tube often will provide an uncomplicated method of alimentation.[24, 35]

A spinal drain is placed via a lumbar puncture to allow relaxation of the brain and postoperative diversion of CSF. The patient is then placed in a supine position and the head is shaved. The skin of the head and face are prepared and draped in a sterile fashion. The neurosurgical team makes a wide coronal incision (Fig. 26–3). A forehead crease or brow incision can also be made if a frontal sinus approach or low anterior bur hole is to be utilized. The scalp flap is raised in the subgaleal plane and retracted anteriorly. We advise raising a separate pericranial flap for use later in the cranial reconstruction.[2, 3, 24–26] Many authors have also advocated the use of a vascularized pericranial flap for reconstruction of the skull base (Fig. 26--4)[26a–d, 28o]

The approach to the anterior fossa has varied from an osteoplastic frontal sinus flap or a frontal bur hole to a bifrontal craniotomy with a bone flap. The bifrontal flap is preferred because of the wide exposure, easier assessment of tumor extension, and better control of intracranial CSF leaks or hemorrhage.

Spinal drainage facilitates the extradural dissection by the reduction of intracranial pressure. Other workers administer mannitol 20 per cent (1.0 to 1.5 g/kg) to produce cerebral decompression.[26] We employ a combination of both methods. Once the bone flap is removed, cerebral decompression is achieved by removing 20 to 60 ml of CSF through the spinal drainage system, as well as by administering mannitol, to allow blunt dissection of the dura. In the region of the cribriform plate, the olfactory nerves with their dural sleeves must be cut. Each small hole is closed immediately with a 4–0 silk suture to prevent a CSF leak.[2, 24]

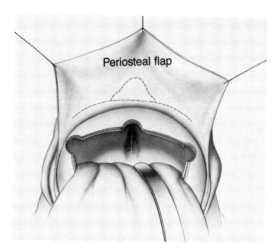

Figure 26–4. Schematic drawing demonstrating the periosteal flap based along the frontal ridge, leaving the blood supply intact.

If the tumor is found to invade to the dura, the dura should be opened to inspect the intracerebral area. If the tumor contacts the dura but does not invade it, the dura can be split so that the outer part can be taken with the specimen. If the dura is invaded, it should be resected along with the specimen. After the dura is removed, repair is accomplished with fascia lata or preserved dura. Meticulous closure is imperative.[28o, 29]

The blunt dissection of the dura is carried back to the planum sphenoidale. The brain is retracted with soft, malleable retractors and cottonoids. The sphenoid sinus is entered from above and biopsied. If the sphenoid is involved with tumor, the resection is terminated. Drainage of the sinus is performed to facilitate palliative radiotherapy.[2, 3]

If the tumor is resectable, the area of the skull base removal is outlined with a high speed drill and osteotome. This should include the ipsilateral ethmoid labyrinth, superior and lateral walls of the sphenoid, anterior cranial fossa, and the cribriform plate. The resection can be extended to include the orbital roof, the opposite ethmoid, or the frontal sinus (Figs. 26–5 and 26–6). Some workers prefer to defer the skull base cuts until the facial resection is performed.[2, 3, 24]

A wet lap pad is then placed in the anterior cavity, and the retractors are removed from the brain. The head and neck surgical team now performs the resection from below. A lateral rhinotomy or Weber-Ferguson incision is usually employed (Fig. 26–3), and a medial maxillectomy (see Chapter 20) or a total maxillectomy (see Chapter 21) is performed, with or without

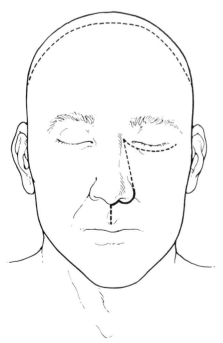

Figure 26–3. Drawing showing the coronal incision for the anterior craniotomy and the Weber-Ferguson incision for the facial resection.

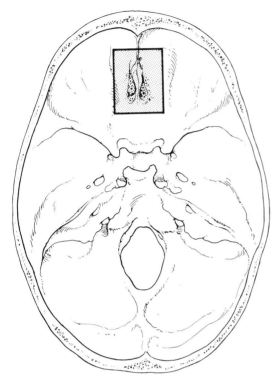

Figure 26–5. View of the skull base from above, showing the area resected in standard fashion. This can be expanded depending on the location of the tumor (see text).

orbital exenteration. After the facial resection is completed, the brain is again retracted and, working from above and below, the entire specimen is delivered through the facial opening

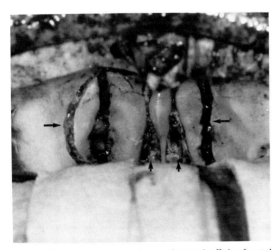

Figure 26–6. The dura has been elevated off the frontal floor and protected with cottonoids. The olfactory nerves have been transected and the dural sleeves have been cut and sutured closed. The olfactory grooves are well seen *(arrowheads)*. The cuts in the skull base are evident *(arrows)*. Because the initial cut on the left side was not lateral enough to pass the tumor, a second cut was made.

(Figs. 26–7 and 26–8). The facial incision can be modified for excision or access as dictated by the pathology. Cocke and associates have reported and extended maxillotomy or subtotal maxillectomy for exposure from the roof of the sphenoid sinus to the fifth cervical vertebra, and from the eustachian tubes to the carotid canals. These incisions are performed in a similar fashion to maxillectomy; however, the maxilla can be left hinged to the facial skin and swung out of the way, giving access to the more posterior structures. At the end of the procedure the maxilla can be replaced and fixed into position.[28q]

With frontal sinus and orbital carcinomas, the initial craniotomy permits assessment of extension along the optic nerves or infiltration into the frontal lobes.[37] If these areas are not involved, external incisions can be made to expose the frontal sinus. The ethmoid sinus is also explored to assess the necessity for its resection. The orbit similarly is explored and possibly included in the resection.

After the resection has been completed and the specimen removed, repair of the anterior cranial fossa is begun, utilizing the pericranial flap raised at the beginning of the procedure. The pericranium is draped over the defect and

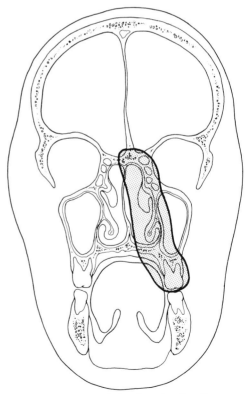

Figure 26–7. A coronal drawing showing the area resected in standard fashion. This can be enlarged depending on the location of the tumor.

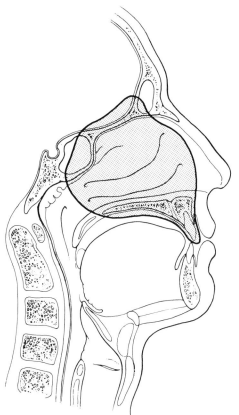

Figure 26–8. A lateral drawing showing the area resected in standard fashion. This can be enlarged depending on the location of the tumor.

The anterior craniotomy is closed by replacement of the bone, which is wired back into position. Reconstruction of frontal bone defects should be delayed, as primary repair with autogenous and alloplastic materials carries a high failure rate because of contamination and increases the risk of meningitis.

The coronal incision is then closed. A split-thickness skin graft is placed over the pericranium and is held in place with a bolus of xeroform gauze. The remaining facial incisions are then closed. If there is a palatal defect, a surgical stent is inserted and wired into position. This greatly facilitates the rehabilitation of the patient.

In cases in which the tumor involves the infratemporal fossa or extends more posteriorly, access for complete exposure can be achieved with an extension of the anterior approach. The temporalis muscle is detached from the cranium and dropped inferiorly along with the middle segment of the zygomatic arch. The craniotomy can then be extended. The dura is reflected, and the middle meningeal artery and second and third divisions of the fifth cranial nerve can be divided for exposure, if necessary (Fig.

the remaining floor of the anterior cranial fossa. The technique of dural patching and use of a periosteal sling is most important in the prevention of CSF leakage and possible meningitis. The frontal periosteal sling is brought beneath the frontal lobes and is sutured to the basal dura over the posterior planum. The periosteal flap is also sutured to the edges of the skull base resection. This suturing has been facilitated by drilling holes for additional sutures along the resected posterior edge of bone (Fig. 26–9). Placing sutures through these holes assures that the flap will cover the entire skull base opening and will not slip forward (Fig. 26–10A, B). For larger defects, regional myocutaneous flaps and distant microvascular free flaps have been used for repair and coverage of the defect in the skull base (Fig. 26–11).[25a, b] A split-thickness skin graft is later placed over the pericranium via the facial defect. We have not needed any other materials for skull base reconstruction, although others have described using cartilage, nasal septal flaps, bone grafts, or metal or alloplastic materials.[2, 23]

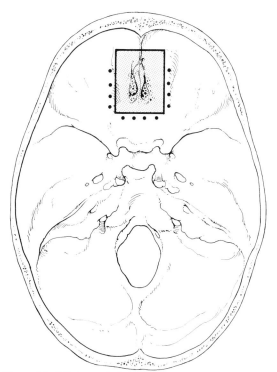

Figure 26–9. Schematic drawing demonstrating the holes drilled along the edge of the bone defect to facilitate periosteal sutures.

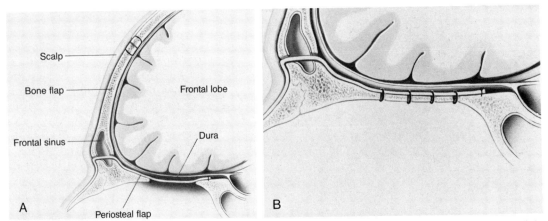

Figure 26–10. *A*, Drawing depicting the midline sagittal plane with the periosteal flap rotated beneath the frontal dura and across the bone defect, and sutured to the dura at the level of the planum. This periosteal flap supports the frontal lobes. *B*, Drawing depicting a more lateral sagittal plane with the periosteal flap sutured to the holes in the bone edge, as well as to the dura.

26–12A, B).[27, 28, 28a, 28g] A drill is then used to connect the foramen spinosum, foramen ovale, and foramen rotundum. The bone incision is extended posterolaterally in a line anterior to the petrous ridge and through the temporomandibular joint. The bone incision then curves anteriorly through the sphenoid bone. This intracranial portion delineates the superior limits of the pterygoid space through the orbital fissure and includes an orbital exenteration. The pterygomaxillofacial complex is then removed.

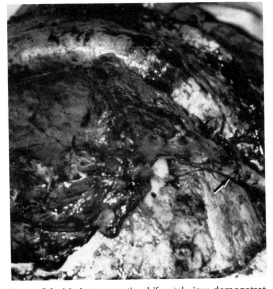

Figure 26–11. Intraoperative bifrontal view demonstrating a latissimus dorsi free graft with a microvascular anastomosis filling the subfrontal and anterior defect. Note the superficial temporal artery and vein anastomoses *(arrow).*

The reconstruction is performed with a forehead flap alone or with bone or alloplastic materials.

A lateral skull base resection can also be performed using a transcervical-transmandibular approach, as described by Biller and associates[28d] and Krespi and associates.[28e–g] This technique allows maximal exposure of the cranial nerves and excellent vascular control. The medial compartment allows approach to the clivus, nasopharynx, and cervical spine. The lateral compartment allows approach to the lateral pharynx and infratemporal fossa. Combined with a temporal or anterior-lateral craniotomy, massive resections can be performed with complete control of vascular and neural structures. The transmandibular approach is accomplished with release of the digastric muscle from the hyoid bone and retraction and release of the sternocleidomastoid muscle for exposure of the carotid artery. The external carotid artery is ligated distal to the lingual artery. All of the cranial nerves are identified and isolated in the neck. A midline mandibulotomy is performed unless part of the mandible is to be resected. The dissection proceeds along the lingual gutter with division of the styloid and pterygoid muscles. This allows the mandible to swing laterally to expose the parapharyngeal space. If the middle compartment is to be reached, the incision is extended onto the soft palate and follows the upper dentition anteriorly, exposing the nasopharynx.

Fisch and Pillsbury[28c] reported several lateral approaches to the infratemporal fossa. Type A is achieved via a lateral parotidectomy with identification of the stylomastoid foramen and facial nerve. The ear canal is resected and closed

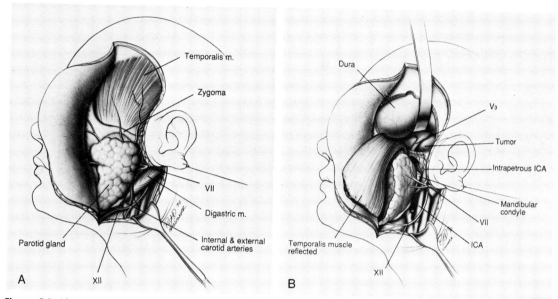

Figure 26–12. *A,* Schematic drawing of the "question mark" incision used to achieve initial operative exposure for middle cranial fossa and infratemporal fossa surgery. This incision is combined with a neck exploration to identify the internal and external carotid arteries, the jugular vein, and cranial nerves IX, X, XI, XII. The VII nerve is identified from the stylomastoid foramen into the parotid gland. *B,* Schematic drawing showing the exposure of a jugular foramen tumor after craniotomy, resection of the zygomatic arch, and reflection of the temporalis muscle. V2 and V3 have been exposed in their canals. The intrapetrous carotid artery is exposed and mobilized anteriorly.

in a blind pouch. The facial nerve is skeletonized and released, the tympanic bones are removed, mastoid tip is resected, and the sigmoid sinus and jugular vein area are ligated. The infratemporal fossa is now in direct view for tumor resection. In the type B approach for the clivus and nasopharynx, in addition to the steps in type A, the temporalis muscle is reflected, and the zygomatic arch is cut and flapped inferiorly. The mandibular condyle is resected, and from above the middle meningeal artery and third division of the fifth nerve are resected, along with the petrous apex. The carotid artery is now fully exposed, with adequate exposure for tumor removal or carotid bypass. The type C approach, described for parasellar lesions, involves additional removal of the lateral and inferior orbital rims and section of the second and third division of the fifth nerve.

ADVANTAGES

The craniofacial resection permits accurate evaluation of the intracranial extension of tumor. It permits protection of the brain during the resection, avoids unnoticed or unrepaired CSF leaks, and affords better control of intracranial hemorrhage. Even for palliation, it significantly reduces pain related to tumor invasion

of the base of skull. Adequate soft tissue is available for a cosmetically acceptable reconstruction. It facilitates en bloc resection for better cancer control and possible cure in patients who otherwise would have little hope.[1, 16, 38]

COMPLICATIONS

Infection is the most common complication of craniofacial surgery. The incidence is even higher in patients who have received preoperative radiotherapy. Ketcham and associates reported 27 infectious complications (13 significant) in 31 patients undergoing craniofacial resection.[39] These included cellulitis, incisional infection, graft slough, bur hole infection, osteomyelitis (2 cases), and subdural infection (2 cases). Of four patients who developed meningitis, two died. All the patients with meningitis had CSF leaks and postoperative infections. Ketcham recommended meticulous dural leak closure and antibiotic coverage before, during, and after surgery. Most workers recommend prophylaxis with broad-spectrum antibiotics.

Infection and CSF leakage are the most common complications of craniofacial surgery. The patients who have had dural resection have the highest possibility of leakage. The incidence of CSF leakage is also higher in patients who have had prior radiation therapy. The best solution is prevention of leakage by meticulous intraoperative dural closure. If a leak occurs postoperatively, the patient's head should be elevated and spinal drainage continued. In Ketcham's series, all the leaks closed in 2 to 17 days.

Ophthalmologic complications occur in patients with and without orbital exenteration. These consist of diplopia, paralytic ptosis, and monocular or binocular blindness.

Cerebral complications include headache, acute brain syndrome (abnormal behavior or somnolence), pneumatocele, meningocele or encephalocele, hemiplegia, transient confusion, or coma. The causes of coma in Ketcham's series were subdural hematoma in one case and cerebral edema in two cases, which cleared in 5 days.

The endocrine complications were related to pituitary insufficiency, diabetes insipidus, and hypothalamic damage.

Hepatitis has been reported secondary to blood replacement. The average blood replacement required for this surgery is 3 to 6 units. Bleeding may also occur postoperatively after packing removal but rarely needs operative intervention.

In bifrontal approaches, all the patients developed permanent anosmia. This should be explained in detail to the patients preoperatively.

In our last 20 craniofacial resections, there were no cases of CSF leakage, meningitis, blindness, hemiparesis, or other neural deficits. Two patients developed infection, one requiring removal of the bone flap and the other requiring removal of the bone flap and necrotic soft tissue.

In Donald's series[28a] of 35 patients, he reported two cases of infection, one with meningitis and one with CSF leakage. He also reported two deaths associated with carotid artery ligation.

Snyderman and associates reported 30 patients who underwent craniofacial resection, with three cases of CSF leakage, one bone flap infection, and no cases of meningitis.[26a] David and Cooter,[39a] in a series of 170 transcranial resections over 10 years, found a 6.5 per cent infection rate in children and 23.5 per cent infection rate in adults. This is similar to findings by Sundaresan and Shah, who reported a 23 per cent infection rate.[39b] This is in contrast to some authors, including Cheesman and associates,[39c] who reported no complications in a series of 60 patients.

Lund and Harrison[39d] in a 9-year experience with 92 patients reported two cases with frontal abscesses and encephalitis. They also had two patients who had CVAs, two deaths, three cases of CSF leakage, two cases of epiphora, and two cases with hemorrhage.

The alternative to surgical resection, full-course radiotherapy, is not curative and has a considerable morbidity (74 per cent). The ophthalmologic complications of radiotherapy are common and include retinal degeneration, progressive ocular wasting leading to blindness, a dry painful eye, glaucoma, cataracts, and nasolacrimal duct obstruction. The otologic complications include vertigo and hearing loss. Patients also develop nasal synechia, septal perforations, necrosis of bone and cartilage, and sinusitis. Others have developed aseptic meningitis, hemiparesis, headache, and lethargy.[40]

Although the morbidity of craniofacial resection is significant, its impact is diminished when the morbidity of alternate treatments and the natural history of the disease are considered.

RESULTS

The published results of craniofacial resection are encouraging, as these patients often are failures of other treatment modalities and have advanced disease with a near zero per cent survival. Early reports were of single cases with short follow-up, which did not permit meaningful conclusions to be drawn. In 1972, Ross and associates reported 11 en bloc ethmoidectomies: two patients died of distant metastases, three died of other causes, and five were without disease for more than 2 years.[18] In 1976, Sisson and associates reported eight cases, of which three died and three were without disease for longer than 2 years.[23]

In 1973, Ketcham and associates published the results of operations on 54 patients over 16 years.[36] There was a 52 per cent 3-year survival and a 49 per cent 5-year survival. There was a significant recurrence rate (32 per cent in Terz's series[3]). Schramm and associates, in 1979, reported a 75 per cent 4-year survival and an 8 per cent recurrence rate.[25] In 1980, Terz and associates described a 72 per cent 3-year survival and a 32 per cent recurrence rate with 10.7 per cent mortality.[3]

In 1988, Lund and Harrison[39d] reported a 45 per cent 5-year survival in their first 26 patients. In 1990, Snyderman and associates[26a] reported on 47 patients operated on from 1987 to 1989. In their series, eight patients (17 per cent) died of disease; two patients (4 per cent) died of unrelated causes; 11 (23%) are alive with the disease; and 25 (53%) are without evidence of disease with a mean follow-up of 13 months.

It therefore appears that craniofacial resection in the appropriate patients can offer not only good palliation but also an opportunity for cure. These patients otherwise have a negligible survival with all other treatment methods. The recurrence rates, morbidity, and mortality should continue to decrease as more experience is gained with these procedures.

References

1. Miller HS, Petty PG, Wilson WF: A combined intracranial and facial approach for excision and repair of cancer of the ethmoid sinuses. Aust NZ J Surg 43:179, 1973.
2. Donald PJ: Recent advances in paranasal sinus surgery. Head Neck Surg 4:146, 1981.
3. Terz JJ, Young HF, Lawrence W: Combined craniofacial resection for locally advanced carcinoma of the head and neck. II—Carcinoma of the paranasal sinuses. Am J Surg 140:618, 1980.
4. Ohngren L: Malignant tumors of the maxillo-ethmoidal region. Acta Otol 19:1, 1933.
5. Watson WL: Cancer of the paranasal sinuses. Laryngoscope 52:22, 1942.
6. Martin H: Cancer of the head and neck. JAMA 137:1306, 1366, 1948.
7. Adson AW, Benedict WL: Hemangioendothelioma of the orbit: Removal through a transcranial approach. Arch Ophthalmol 12:484, 1934.
8. Cushing H: Meningiomas. Springfield, Ill., Charles C Thomas, 1938.
9. Dandy WE: Orbital tumors: Results following the transcranial operative attack. New York, Oskar Piest, 1941, p 1; 154.
10. Ray BS, McLean JM: Combined intracranial and orbital operation for retinoblastoma. Arch Ophthalmol 30:437, 1943.
11. Smith RR, Klopp CT, Williams MM: Surgical treatment of cancer of the frontal sinus and adjacent areas. Cancer 7:991, 1954.
12. Malecki J: New trends in frontal sinus surgery. Acta Otolaryngol 50:137, 1959.
13. Ross DE: Radical en bloc ethmoidectomy for cancer. SGO 108:109, 1959.
14. Pool JL, Polanos JN, Kruegar EG: Osteomas and mucoceles of the frontal paranasal sinuses. J Neurosurg 19:130, 1962.
15. Frazell EL, Lewis JS: Cancer of the nasal cavity and accessory sinuses. A report of the management of 416 cases. Cancer 16:1293, 1963.
16. Ketcham AS, Wilkins RH, VanBuren JM, Smith RR: A combined intracranial facial approach to the paranasal sinuses. Am J Surg 106:698, 1963.
17. VanBuren JM, Ommaya AK, Ketcham AS: Ten years' experience with radical combined craniofacial resection of the malignant tumors of the paranasal sinuses. J Neurosurg 28:341, 1968.
18. Ross DE, Sakis AE, Chiang TM, Wharton CF: En bloc ethmoidectomy for cancer. Laryngoscope 82:682, 1972.
19. Tessier P: The definitive plastic surgical treatment of the severe facial deformities of the craniofacial dysos-

toses: Crouzon's and Apert's diseases. Plast Reconstr Surg 48:419, 1971.
20. Derome PJ: Craniofacial surgery. In Schmidek HP, Sweet WH (eds): Current Techniques in Operative Neurosurgery. New York, Grune & Stratton, 1971, p 233.
21. Jackson IT, Munro IR, Salyer KE, Whitaker LA: Atlas of Craniomaxillofacial Surgery. St. Louis, CV Mosby, 1982.
22. Westbury G, Wilson JSP, Richardson A: Combined craniofacial resection for malignant disease. Am J Surg 130:463, 1975.
23. Sisson GA, Bytell DE, Becker SP: Carcinoma of the paranasal sinuses and craniofacial resection. J Laryngol Otol 90:59, 1976.
24. Shah JP, Galicich JH: Surgical approach to carcinoma of the nasal cavity and paranasal sinuses with extension to the base of the skull. Clin Bull 8:61, 1978.
25. Schramm VL, Myers EN, Maroon JC: Anterior skull base surgery for benign and malignant disease. Laryngoscope 89:1077, 1979.
25a. Schuller DE, Goodman JH, Miller CA: Reconstruction of skull base. Laryngoscope 94:1359, 1984.
25b. Jones NF, Schramm VL, Sekhar LN: Reconstruction of the cranial base following tumor resection. Br J Plast Surg 40:155, 1987.
26. Clifford P: Transcranial-facial approach for tumors of superior paranasal sinuses and orbit. J Soc Med 73:413, 1980.
26a. Snyderman CH, Janecka IP, Sekhar LN, Sen CN, Eibling DE: Anterior cranial base reconstruction: Role of galeal and pericranial flaps. Laryngoscope 100:49–56, 1990.
26b. Schaefer SD, Close LG, Mickey BE: Axial subcutaneous scalp flaps in the reconstruction of the anterior cranial fossa. Arch Otolaryngol Head Neck Surg 112:745–749, 1986.
26c. Jackson IT, Adham MN, March WR: Use of the galeal frontalis myofascial flap in craniofacial surgery. Plast Reconstr Surg 77:905–910, 1986.
26d. Price JC, Loury M, Carson B: The fericranial flap for reconstruction of anterior skull base defects. Laryngoscope 98:1159–1164, 1988.
27. Terz JJ, Alkane JF, Lawrence W: Craniofacial resection for tumors invading the pterygoid fossa. Am J Surg 118:732, 1969.
28. Terz JJ, Young HF, Lawrence W: Combined craniofacial resection for locally advanced carcinoma of the head and neck. I—Tumors of the skin and soft tissues. Am J Surg 140:613, 1980.
28a. Donald PJ: Craniofacial surgical resection: New frontier in advanced head and neck cancer. Aust N Z Surg 59:523–528, 1989.
28b. Sekhar LN, Janecka IP, Jones NF: Subtemporal and basal subfrontal approach to extensive cranial base tumors. Acta Neurochir (Wein) 92:83–92, 1988.
28c. Fisch U, Pillsbury HC: Infratemporal approach to lesions in the temporal bone and skull base. Arch Otolaryngol Head Neck Surg 105:99–107, 1979.
28d. Biller HF, Shugar JM, Krespi YP: A new technique for wide-field exposure of the skull base. Arch Otolaryngol 107:698–702, 1980.
28e. Krespi YP, Sisson GA: Skull base surgery in composite resection. Arch Otolaryngol 108:681–687, 1982.
28f. Krespi YP, Sisson GA: Transmandibular exposure of the skull base. Am J Surg 148:534–538, 1984.
28g. Krespi YP, Levine TM, Sisson GA: Tumor surgery of the skull base. In Johnson JT, Blitzer A, Ossoff R, Thomas JR (eds): Instructional courses—Am Acad Otolaryngol Head Neck Surg. St. Louis, C.V. Mosby, 1989, pp. 279–289.

28h. Urken ML, Biller HF, Haimov M: Intratemporal carotid artery bypass in resection of a base of skull tumor. Laryngoscope 95:1472–1477, 1985.

28i. Sekhar LN, Schramm VL, Jones NF, Yonas H, Horton J, Latchaw RE, Curtin H: Operative exposure and management of the petrous and upper cervical internal carotid artery. Neurosurg 19:967–982, 1986.

28j. Sekhar LN, Sen CN, Jho HD: Saphenous vein graft bypass of the cavernous internal carotid artery. J Neurosurg 72:35–41, 1990.

28k. Sekhar LN, Moller AR: Operative management of tumor involving the cavernous sinus. J Neurosurg 64:879–889, 1986.

28l. Sekhar LN, Sen CN, Jho HD, Janecka IP: Surgical treatment of intracavernous neoplasms: A four-year experience. Neurosurg 24:18–30, 1989.

28m. Sekhar LN: Operative management of tumors involving the cavernous sinus. In Sekhar LN, Schramm VL (eds): Tumors of the Cranial Base Mt, Kisco, Futura, 1987, pp. 393–419.

28n. Lund VJ, Howard DJ, Lloyd GA, Cheesman AD: Magnetic resonance imaging of paranasal sinus tumors for craniofacial resection. Head Neck Surg 11:279–283, 1989.

28o. Post KD, Blitzer A: Surgery of the skull base. In Goodrich JT, Argamaso RV, Post KD (eds): Plastic Techniques for Neurosurgery. New York, Thieme Med. Pub., 1990.

28p. Robin PE, Powell DJ: Diagnostic errors in cancer of the nasal cavity and paranasal sinuses. Arch Otolaryngol 107:138–140, 1989.

28q. Cocke EW, Robertson JH, Robertson JT, Crook JP: The extended maxillotomy and subtotal maxillectomy for excision of skull base tumors. Arch Otolaryngol Head Neck Surg 116:92–104, 1990.

28r. Ebra SM, Horton JA, Latchow RE: Balloon test occlusion of the internal carotid artery with stable xenon/CT cerebral blood flow imaging. AJNR 9:533–538, 1988.

29. Saunders WH, Miglets A: Surgical techniques for eradicating far advanced carcinoma of the orbital-ethmoid and maxillary areas. Trans Am Acad Ophthalmol Otolaryngol 71:426, 1967.

30. Gibb R: The treatment of carcinoma of the maxillary antrum and ethmoid by radiation. Proc R Soc Med 50:534, 1957.

31. Shah JP, Galicich JH: Esthesioneuroblastoma—treatment by combined craniofacial resection. NY State J Med 79:84, 1979.

32. Chapman P, Carter RL, Clifford P: The diagnosis and surgical management of olfactory neuroblastoma: The role of craniofacial resection. J Laryngol Otol 95:785, 1981.

32a. Blitzer A, Post K, Conley J: A craniofacial approach to resection of extensive osteomas and ossifying fibromas of the ethmoid and frontal sinuses. Arch Otol 115:1112–1116, 1989.

33. Tanner SB, Shaw J, Clifford P: Massive chordoma of the skull base. J R Soc Med 72:615, 1975.

34. Guggenheim P, Kleitsch WP: Combined craniotomy-rhinotomy for ethmoid cancer. Ann Otol Rhinol Laryngol 75:105, 1967.

35. Shah JP, Galicich JH: Craniofacial resection for malignant tumors of ethmoid and anterior skull base. Arch Otol 103:514, 1977.

36. Ketcham AS, Chretien PB, VanBuren JM, et al: The ethmoid sinuses: A re-evaluation of surgical resection. Am J Surg 126:469, 1973.

37. Adelglass JM, Samara M, Cantor JO, et al: Thoratrast-induced frontal sinus carcinoma—A case report. Bull NY Acad Med 56:453, 1980.

38. Bridger GP: Radical surgery for ethmoid cancer. Arch Otol 106:630, 1980.

39. Ketcham AS, Hoye RC, VanBuren JM, Johnson RH: Complications of intracranial facial resection for tumors of the paranasal sinuses. Am J Surg 112:591, 1966.

39a. David DJ, Cooter RD: Craniofacial infection in 10 years of transcranial surgery. Plast Reconstr Surg 80:213–223, 1987.

39b. Sundaresan N, Shah JP: Craniofacial resection for anterior skull base tumors. Head Neck Surg 10:219–224, 1988.

39c. Cheeseman AD, Lund VJ, Howard DJ: Craniofacial resection for tumors of the nasal cavity and paranasal sinuses. Head Neck Surg 8:429–435, 1986.

39d. Lund VJ, Harrison DFN: Craniofacial resection for tumors of the nasal cavity and paranasal sinuses. Am J Surg 156:187–190, 1988.

40. Ellingwood KE, Million RR: Cancer of the nasal cavity and ethmoid/sphenoid sinuses. Cancer 43:1517, 1979.

CHAPTER 27

ANCILLARY NASAL PROCEDURES

Fred J. Stucker, MD, FACS
Gary Y. Shaw, MD

SEPTAL AND TURBINATE SURGICAL THERAPY

Surgical therapy of the septum dates from Loyall's initial description of surgical correction of septal deformities in 1882. Freer, in 1902, and Killian, in 1904, independently advanced the submucous resection (SMR). This approach, with various modifications, served as the benchmark for septal operations for the ensuing 60 years. A paucity of scientific work relative to the physiology of nasal breathing contributed to the long reign of this standard for nasal operation. The variations and minor changes in techniques that did occur generally proved to be of questionable benefit. The submucous resection was successful in relieving the nasal obstruction in a large percentage of patients, which explains its wide acceptance and utilization, but the basic premise of the procedure was flawed. The submucous resection is clearly contraindicated in most instances. Its inordinate morbidity, which includes septal perforation, saddle deformity, and collumellar retraction, far overshadows its benefits. These complications are avoidable with contemporary septal techniques.

The fundamental purpose of septal surgical therapy, in most instances, is to provide a reasonably straight septum by orienting it in the center relative to the nasal pyramid. The technique is far more sophisticated in its surgical demands than simple mucoperichondrial flap elevation and resection of the deformed and gnarled portion of the quadrangular cartilage (submucous resection) and septal bones. Just as a myriad of septal deformities are possible, so too a myriad of surgical corrections are possible. The type of surgery is determined by the magnitude, type, and location of the various abnormalities.

It is reasonable to establish consistency and regular patterns in solving problems. Unfortunately, a single-technique approach when managing a wide variety of deformities often results in either excessive aggressiveness or too timid a solution. It is prudent to temper one's approach to septal surgery in accord with the magnitude of the problem.

A successful technique entails a sequence of surgical maneuvers aimed at correcting the abnormal anatomy without undermining function and stability. Each step must be undertaken with the foresight to allow progression to the subsequent steps without jeopardizing the structural integrity of the nose. Successive reconstructive steps tend to destabilize the nose increasingly, which can frustrate the overall reconstructive effort. For this reason, intranasal packing is avoided; it may give the surgeon an artificial sense of success in accomplishing alignment and support, as well as causing the patient extreme discomfort and potentially life-threatening sequelae. Basic to septal surgery is preserving maximal structural support while correcting the deformity. Stabilizing the septal integrity with quilting sutures, while coapting the mucosal flaps of the cartilage septum, optimally achieves septal fixation without lending false support.

Some maneuvers that improve the airway do not compromise the structural integrity. Spur resection and turbinectomy are two; since they do not jeopardize stability, they require no compensatory stabilization. On rare occasions, a loss of support occurs such that no meaningful maneuver for structural integrity is possible without the use of grafts. Autogenous tissue, such as septal or conchal cartilage or iliac crest or cranial bone, is the only legitimate choice with which to reconstruct the nose.

Reconstructive nasal surgical therapy is not to be confused with augmentation rhinoplasty. Ignoring the need to re-establish architectural support as a procedure progresses increases the likelihood of a surgical misadventure and failure. A nose that results from the additive effects of a succession of ill-advised destabilization maneuvers without compensatory maneuvers is a potential disaster.

A geometrically perfect endonasal correction is usually unnecessary and often impossible to achieve routinely. The goal of surgery is realignment, through functional and structural measures that result in a pleasing external nasal appearance and a normal airway. The correction must not be complicated by untoward sequelae, such as atrophic rhinitis or a septal perforation.

In this chapter, we present the more common endonasal deformities, with recommendations for a rational surgical approach. Combinations of deformities are usually present in patients, and surgeons must adjust or modify as they see fit the various corrective suggestions as they apply to the abnormalities in a given patient.

GENERAL PRINCIPLES OF ENDONASAL SURGICAL THERAPY

The management principles that follow concerning septal operations for airway problems will serve to amplify the descriptions in this chapter of the anatomic corrections recommended for specific problem areas.

1. Endonasal (septal and turbinate) problems are routinely corrected at a single procedure.

2. Adequate septal cartilage must be retained or replaced to provide necessary support.

3. Unilateral septal mucosal flaps are preferred when possible to ensure safety, stability, and surgical expediency. One should acquire equal facility in elevating the septal mucosa from either side. This experience will pay great dividends when it is not possible for the flap to be developed from a side that has become a surgeon's routine procedure.

4. Nasal surgery in children, while conservative, should not be eschewed.

5. Surgical resection of spurs is important only as it relates to esthetics or function.

6. Skeletal (bony or cartilage) carving and fashioning are as critical to nasal operation as are strategic resections and repositioning.

SEPTAL SURGICAL THERAPY

All possible maneuvers in septal operations for all specific abnormalities cannot possibly be chronicled here. Some procedures are arbitarily omitted, but it is hoped that assimilation of the principles described in this chapter will allow a course of surgical action for most deformities encountered.

BONY SEPTUM

Before any incisions are made, the perpendicular plate and vomer are fractured and completely mobilized by means of a Sayer elevator. The instrument is placed first in one nostril and guided into the apical junction of the bony vault between the perpendicular plate and nasal bone. The Sayer elevator is rocked back and forth in a lateral-to-medial fashion to fracture the bony septum (Fig. 27–1). The instrument is then repositioned more inferiorly and rocked back and forth to mobilize the vomer. Following this, the same maneuvers are carried out on the opposite side. This fracturing of the bony septum usually improves even the most severe of septal deflections. In 10 per cent or more patients, this maneuver corrects the septal de-

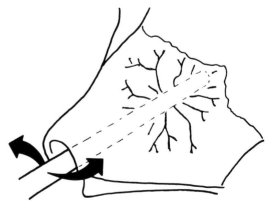

Figure 27–1. Fracture and mobilization of the bony septum as an initial maneuver in septal surgery. (From Stucker FJ: Management of the scoliotic nose. Laryngoscope 92(2):128, 1982.)

formity, and no further septal operation is required. Another gain from this bony mobilization is that it clearly demonstrates whether augmentation of local anesthesia is required. If the patient experiences discomfort, that portion of the bony septum that perhaps prevented proper access for injection prior to mobilization now can be properly anesthetized by topical or local anesthesia. Contrary to older textbook teaching, cerebrospinal fluid rhinorrhea has not been evident in over 3000 septoplasties in which this technique was employed.

The next step is placement of the incisions for gaining access to the supportive structures of the septum. The unilateral transfixion and the complete septal transfixion are two approaches used. An external rhinoplasty also affords excellent surgical access to the septum. Whatever the approach, a unilateral mucoperichondrial flap elevation is preferred. Occasionally bilateral flaps are necessary to free the attached cartilage and bone. Strategic portions of the septum are then resected to allow midline positioning. The running septal whipstitch is used routinely for coapting the flaps. This suturing technique affords stability, prevents hematoma, and circumvents the use of nasal packing (Fig. 27–2).

ANTERIOR NASAL SPINE

Malposition or hypertrophy or both of the anterior nasal spine can contribute to an esthetically displeasing abnormality that often obstructs the nasal airway. Lateral displacement additionally deviates the caudal septal cartilage, often completely blocking the nares on the involved side. Frequently, there is a concomitant bowing of the quadrangular cartilage and a compromised airway posteriorly in the opposite nasal passage. Anterior or caudal nasal spurs are often the sequelae of nasal spine injuries.

A retracted columella can result from injudicious resection of the caudal septum and spine. This overzealous management of the anterior nasal spine substitutes one deformity for another that is far more difficult to correct. This complication has led many nasal surgeons to avoid any resection of the anterior spine.

A displaced anterior nasal spine is rather easily mobilized. It is uncommon, however, for a spinal deformity not to require at least a partial resection. The approach we prefer is to use an osteotome along the lateral aspect of the spine on the obstructed side and routinely resect 50 per cent or more of the displaced bone. The osteotome, imbedded in bone that acts as a fulcrum, is then rotated to the opposite side, which forces the remaining spine and caudal septum to the midline (Fig. 27–3). Whether these structures must be fixed to the midline position depends on the spine's stability and the associated septal and nasal deformities. Mobilization should allow midline placement without disrupting the substantial fibrous attachment. Should suture fixation be required, the fibrous attachment of the anterior spinal remnant can be anchored to the opposite side with buried nonabsorbable suture.

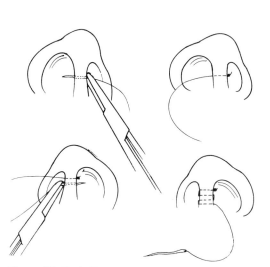
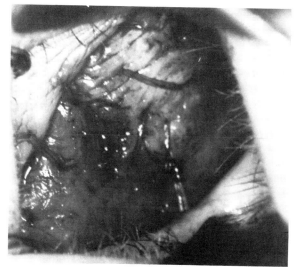

Figure 27–2. A, Sequence in placement of septal whipstitch. (From Stucker FJ: Management of the scoliotic nose. Laryngoscope 92(2):128, 1982.) B, Placement of running chromic septal suture.

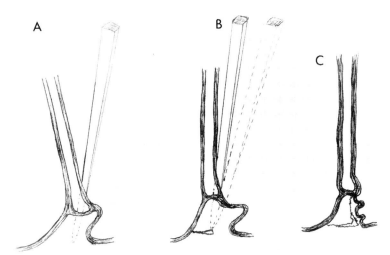

Figure 27–3. *A*, Osteotomy of displaced anterior nasal spine. *B*, Osteotome rocked laterally to mobilize displaced spine. *C*, Result after resection and realignment.

Partial resections of the spine may result in a palpable spicule, which, if unattended, can be quite annoying postoperatively to the patient. The spicule is readily removed with a rongeur.

An intraoral sublabial incision can be an alternative approach to the anterior nasal spine. Rarely, this may be considered when more complete visualization is needed or when compromising scars with antecedent grafts or flaps contraindicate the standard transfixion incision. The open rhinoplasty affords an extraordinary access to the anterior nasal spine. However, access to the spine should never be the sole determinant for employing this approach.

COLUMELLAR RETRACTION

Prior to the popularization of the open rhinoplasty technique, the results of correcting a retracted columella were far less predictable. The etiology of this condition is often related to previous surgical misadventure or trauma resulting in a tissue deficit. A retracted columella may be the result of tissue deficiency or loss of structural support at the caudal base of the septum. The anterior nasal spine, medial crura, and quadrangular cartilage contribute to the proper inferior projection of the columella and an acceptable nasolabial angle. The usual columellar retraction results from tissue deficiency and dislocation of the leading edge of the septum (and often the anterior nasal spine) from the midline.

The correction of the retracted columella is most effectively managed through an external rhinoplasty. Excellent exposure of the caudal septum and medial crura is obtained by splitting the lower lateral cartilages and allowing bilateral elevation of mucoperichondrial and periosteal flaps. The deformity can then be corrected by the most appropriate method. This may be as simple as mobilization and caudal advancement of the septal cartilage, with fixation, using a continuous running suture (Fig. 27–4). This fixation is accomplished by placement of a continuous through-and-through septal suture coapting the bilateral mucosal flaps to the quadrangular cartilage. The flaps afford unusual stabilization because the medial crura of the lower lateral cartilages serve as battens to reinforce the structural support.

For the columellar retraction that cannot be managed with advancement or repositioning of

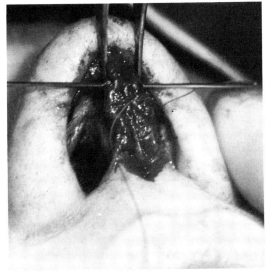

Figure 27–4. Caudal advancement of the septal cartilage with fixation, using a through-and-through running septal suture.

local tissue, it is necessary to use an autogenous graft. The choices in order of preference are septal cartilage, septal bone, and conchal cartilage. The implant is shaped as necessary and placed between and cephalad to the medial crura of the lower lateral cartilage. The open rhinoplasty offers unparalleled exposure and flexibility in positioning the graft. Splitting the mucosal flaps with their lower lateral cartilage battens provides marked stability of cartilage implants when a running through-and-through whipstitch is utilized to resecure the flaps (Fig. 27–5). The thin, perpendicular plate of the ethmoid requires three or four holes to be drilled through it so that a continuous suture can be passed. A small stapes footplate drill works well for this. A running suture prevents areas of undue pressure and the potential for necrosis inherent in individual mattress sutures or intranasal splints. This has proved to be a most propitious method of managing the retracted columella and is easily combined with correction of tip ptosis, which often is associated with the retraction.

CAUDAL DEFLECTION OF THE SEPTUM

The correction of a deflected caudal septum can be managed through various surgical approaches. Among these are a hemitransfixion, a complete transfixion, or an open rhinoplasty technique. The surgical correction is tailored to the deformity, using the simplest technique that is consistent with the septal reconstruction. Our

method entails straightening the septal (quadrangular) cartilage by strip excision after a unilateral flap elevation and fixation in a midline position by using the running septal whipstitch. Mobilization of the septum along the floor is necessary, as well as appropriate management of any spurs contributing to the deformity (Fig. 27–6). Straightening the septum often requires carving and shortening the caudal margins, always preserving an adequate strut to maintain support and to avoid columellar retraction. Resection of up to 75 per cent of an eccentric nasal spine has not been associated with retraction or other untoward sequelae if proper bony and cartilage support is maintained. However, retraction is a common finding in the non-Caucasian nose, in which there is a congenital deficiency in this area. It is important to emphasize that some bony spine must remain at the base of the cartilaginous septum to avoid the potential of a retracted columella.

PTOSIS OF THE TIP

Tip ptosis is the result of a combination of anatomic findings. These include a short columella, columellar retraction, and supratip prominence. It is perhaps easier to conceptualize tip ptosis as too little tip projection to accommodate the remaining nose esthetically. This makes the problem easier to understand and aids in forming a rationale for subsequent correction, regardless of whether the defect is real or apparent. An extremely large cartilaginous or bony hump can easily produce an

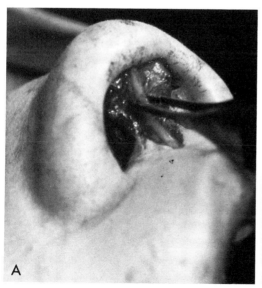 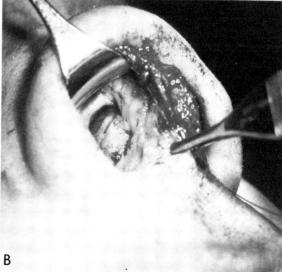

A   B

Figure 27–5. *A*, Placement of cartilage graft in columella. *B*, Graft stabilized with running septal suture.

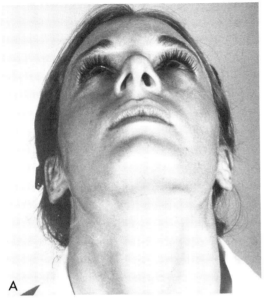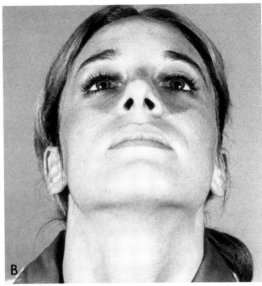

Figure 27–6. *A,* Submental view of preoperative caudal deflection of septum. *B,* Three years postoperative following the described corrective technique.

apparent as well as a real tip ptosis. An acute nasolabial angle always accentuates the appearance of the ptotic tip.

Management of supratip prominence is by resection of soft tissue and cartilage in the supratip area. Columellar struts of autogenous cartilage best correct the short columella. Plumping grafts, tip rotation, and shortening the nose all help correct tip ptosis. Surgical management focuses on modifying the structures involved, regardless of whether the correction is for functional or cosmetic reasons.

HANGING COLUMELLA

This particular deformity is a disproportionate show of the columella when viewed from the side. It is rarely of functional significance and most often is an indication of previous nasal surgery in which rotation of the tip and the resulting cephalic positioning of the alae produce the disproportionate columella show. It is especially evident postoperatively in the very large nose when the three-dimensional reduction is technically complex. This columellar defect also can be produced by trauma, but most result from failure to shorten the septum or an inordinate cephalic rotation of the alae secondary to surgery.

A hanging columella usually can be corrected by resecting a full-thickness, fusiform segment of tissue from the caudal end of the septum.

The columella is generally not violated with the resected tissue, which includes the skin and septal cartilage just cephalic to the columella. The medial crura are usually left intact, and enough membranous columella must remain to allow normal mobility. The closure of the bilateral flap is accomplished with a running 4-0 chromic suture. In rare situations, either or both margins of the medial crura require surgical attention to manage the hanging columella.

REDUPLICATION AND THICKENED SEPTAL CARTILAGE

The thickened and foreshortened septum is most often the late sequela of a telescoping nasal injury. The width of the septum is decreased by carving one or both sides. If one side or the other is reasonably straight, the incremental shaving can be carried out via a unilateral mucoperichondrial flap elevation. Most often the deformity dictates cartilaginous recontouring on both sides, and bilateral flaps must be elevated. The open rhinoplasty technique offers excellent exposure, and the reconstruction has greater stability via this approach by virtue of the medial crural battens in the flaps. Regardless of the exposure, the reconstructive effort utilizes the continuous septal whipstitch to coapt the mucosal flaps (Fig. 27–7).

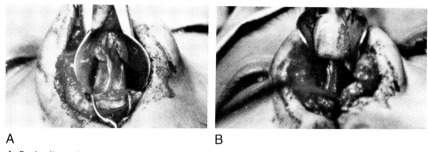

Figure 27–7. *A*, Reduplicated septal cartilage exposed through open rhinoplasty. *B*, Result after cartilage contouring to narrow the septum. (From Stucker FJ: Management of the scoliotic nose. Laryngoscope 92(2):128, 1982.)

CAUDAL SPUR

Caudal spurs are often of little functional or cosmetic consequence, and their presence in the absence of other abnormalities is not an indication for operation. Spurs require surgical attention only if they are responsible for obstructive symptoms, if they produce a visible deformity, or when removal aids in the overall endonasal correction.

Much has been written about septal spurs, most of it far more complicated than need be. The mucoperichondrial flap is developed using hemitransfixion, complete transfixion, or open rhinoplasty technique. The flap development is aided by the local infiltration of anesthetic solution, especially inferiorly where there is firm, fibrous attachment of the soft tissues to the bone and cartilage. The mucoperichondrial flap is meticulously elevated from the superior aspect, where the dissection is markedly easier to start, and progresses inferiorly until the apex of the spur is reached. In this area fibrous decussation occurs, and the plane of relatively facile elevation of the mucoperichondrial flap rather abruptly ends. After the mucoperichondrial flap is elevated inferiorly to the spur, the flap is incised along its dependent border.

The inferior incision has many practical advantages. It allows the spur to be removed without danger of tearing the flap, provides dependent drainage of any blood accumulation, thus decreasing the likelihood of hematoma formation, and permits much greater visibility and surgical access compared with the restrictive exposure of working within the flap.

The spur, which includes bone, cartilage, fibrous tissue, and mucosa, is resected with a sharp osteotome and mallet. Since the mucosal flap is reflected laterally and is completely detached from the spur, the danger of avulsion or inadvertent tearing is avoided. Any attached segments can be resected by the appropriate instruments. Concomitant deformities are managed appropriately at this time. If the spur is the only area to be corrected, the mucosal flap is replaced and coapted with a running 4-0 chromic septal whipstitch. In most instances, the mucoperichondrial flap has a more than adequate superior-inferior length to cover the area of a resected spur. By virtue of its redundancy, which results from the mucosa covering the hypertrophic spur, the resulting stretched mucosa invariably covers the exposed tissues after the spur has been avulsed (Fig. 27–8). The nose is not packed, which decreases the

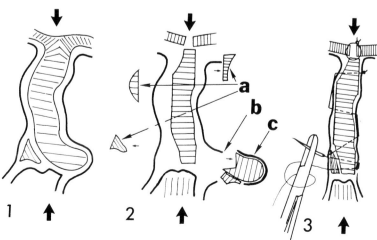

Figure 27–8. *1*, Diagram of preoperative deformity. *2*, Mucosal flap elevation and spur resection: (a) resected cartilage; (b) inferior border of elevated mucosal flap; (c) resected spur. *3*, Completion of surgical correction with coapted mucosal flaps by whipstitch. (From Stucker FJ: Management of the scoliotic nose. Laryngoscope 92(2):128, 1982.)

incidence of infection and results in more rapid healing and greater patient comfort.

SEPTAL PERFORATIONS

Until quite recently, the successful repair of a septal perforation depended upon its size. Perforations of 1 cm or less were rather predictably closed surgically, but in many instances these small perforations lacked symptoms other than an occasional whistle and did not require surgical attention in the first place. Septal perforations do not need to be repaired if they are not symptomatic. Prior to the popularization of the external rhinoplasty, the small perforations either were successfully closed or were often enlarged as a result of the surgical trauma. Perforations of greater than 2 cm in diameter were frequently associated with futile correction attempts. Prior to 1981, when the senior author adopted the open rhinoplasty technique, successful results in septal perforation closure were rare.

The open rhinoplasty has revolutionized the technique for managing septal perforations greater than 2 cm. As with any surgery, the degree of success is directly correlated to exposure, and the older, closed techniques were very restrictive. The open rhinoplasty allows the lower lateral cartilages to be divided, incorporating them as battens in the mucoperichondrial flaps. There are alternative ways of using the upper lateral cartilages, depending on the size of the perforation, its location, and the needs of the repair. The mucosa can be elevated from the undersurface of the upper lateral cartilage and then mobilized inferiorly to a suitable position. One or both upper lateral cartilages may be severed from the quadrangular cartilage, but the mucoperichondrial tissue is elevated from the septum intact and in continuity with that beneath the upper lateral cartilage. The most common sequence is the development of a unilateral flap after severing the upper lateral cartilage from the side of the flap elevation. The open rhinoplasty provides excellent exposure and accessibility to the perforation, allowing ease of elevation of the mucoperichondrial flaps circumferentially around the perforation. The rolled cuff of mucosal epithelium around the margin of the perforation is elevated from the septal cartilage on the opposite side and is excised.

If support is required, mobilized septal cartilage or bone is brought into the defect and stabilized by fixation sutures. Three points are available for fixation: (1) inferiorly, to the fibrous soft tissue along the floor of the nose; (2) superiorly, to the upper lateral cartilage; and (3) caudally, by utilizing the batten stability of the lower lateral cartilages in the mucosal flaps. In the absence of adequate septal cartilage, conchal cartilage is easily fashioned to support and bridge the dehiscence. More commonly, structural support is not required in the repair of a septal perforation, and only an autogenous soft tissue bridge is needed. Temporalis fascia is our preference, but periosteum also may be utilized.

The mucosal flaps are elevated, as described earlier, and the fascia is sandwiched between the mucosal flaps. The mucosa is mobilized, and the flaps are advanced or rotated in an attempt to close the perforation on both sides. The septal flaps and autogenous graft are coapted with a continuous whipstitch of 0000 chromic. The fascia is stabilized with the quilting suture. It is usually possible to obtain enough mucosal tissue from beneath the upper lateral cartilage on the side not severed from the septum and from the floor of the opposite side. The repair is more secure if both sides are covered by the mucosal flaps, but incomplete bilateral flap coverage has occurred in several instances with ultimate successful closure of the perforation. To date we have closed 16 of 17 perforations greater than 1.5 cm with this technique. Successful closure is determined by bilateral mucosal epithelialization, with no evidence of a perforation at 6 months.

UNDULATED, GNARLED, BUCKLED, SCOLIOTIC SEPTUM

A unilateral mucoperichondrial flap is developed following fracture and mobilization of the bony septum as previously described. The mucosal flap, after elevation, is incised inferiorly in a horizontal fashion along the floor, where there is a firm, fibrous adherence of the mucoperichondrial flap. This incision is along the junction of the quadrangular cartilage and the maxillary crest, where the inferior decussation of the tissue from the two sides occurs. With the flap based and hinged superiorly and cephalad, it is then reflected laterally. The exposure is superb for excising strips of cartilage in strategic places to allow midline realignment of the septum. The quadrangular cartilage is routinely separated from the perpendicular plate of the ethmoid, and the thickened superior section is commonly removed with Takahashi forceps. Depending on the deflection, either one or both upper lateral cartilages may require separation from the septum to attain midline positioning. The mucoperichondrium is not incised and is essential for stability, which is obtained by sutures passing through the mucosal flaps and the cartilage to fix the structures following straightening. The sutures reattaching the upper lateral cartilages and the septum are interrupted 4-0 chromic; septal fixation is achieved by running whipstitch of the same suture material.

SEPTAL DEFLECTION ASSOCIATED WITH EXTERNAL NASAL DEFORMITY

The scoliotic septum is most often associated with a bony vault deformity, and the correction of both is interdependent. The septal repair is essentially the same as just described. It is imperative to preserve as much of the soft tissue attachment in the septoplasty as possible. It is wise to re-establish structural continuity with sutures prior to repair of the external nasal deformity. For a detailed discussion of the external crooked nose, consult Stucker.[6]

THICKENING OF THE POSTERIOR SUPERIOR SEPTAL CARTILAGE

A unilateral flap is elevated, but it may not be necessary to make a horizontal incision along the entire inferior border of the flap. A drainage incision of at least 1 cm along the floor at the most dependent part of the septal flap is essential if the drainage is to be adequate without a complete anteroposterior incision. An oblique incision with a scalpel is made through the cartilage just caudal to the thickened portion. The incision is angled and the depth controlled so that it does not cut through the perichondrium on the opposite side. A Cottle elevator elevates the opposite flap just over the cartilage to be resected. The thickened cartilage is then removed with Takahashi forceps. A running septal whipstitch coapts the flaps and obliterates the dead space.

COLLAPSE OF LATERAL NASAL WALL

Collapse of the lateral nasal wall should not be excluded from a discussion of nasal obstruction. The involved upper lateral cartilage or nasal bone or both are separated from the septum with a knife and an osteotome. Often the collapse of the upper lateral cartilage is secondary and totally dependent on its firm attachment to a depressed nasal bone. The correction involves freeing the midline attachment of the depressed nasal wall, with lateral mobilization of the depressed nasal bone. A 6-mm, curved osteotome is used for the medial osteotomy, and a prying motion elevates the nasal bone. There is no need to treat the upper lateral cartilage as a separate entity if the entire lateral nasal wall can be mobilized. A lateral osteotomy is not necessary, as the bony nasal wall is hinged laterally by fibrous connections but not fused at the old fracture site. A bony depression occurs as a result of a fracture dislocation, which then heals by a fibrous union. By avoiding an osteotomy, the entire complex is more stable after elevation because of this lateral fibrous attachment, and there is no additional surgical trauma. The contralateral nasal bone is most often deflected away from the depression; it routinely requires a lateral osteotomy for relocation to the midline and impaction against the opposite nasal bone.

A more difficult deformity to correct is the depressed upper lateral cartilage when it is avulsed or separated from its usual firm, bony attachment to the undersurface of the nasal bone by trauma or surgery. Nasal surgical therapy is more often responsible than is trauma for this type of deformity. Cosmetic correction can be achieved by employing a cartilage onlay graft in the depressed region, but this does not eliminate the obstruction in the valve area. In some instances, surgical correction can be achieved by mucosal preservation and amputation of the prolapsed scar and cartilage. More often, though, isolation of the upper lateral cartilage and repositioning to achieve a normal anatomic relationship with the nasal bone are required.

It is imperative that sufficient endonasal mucosa be preserved for resurfacing. The cartilage and surrounding scar are carved and trimmed to duplicate the shape of the upper lateral cartilage. To hold the newly positioned cartilages in place, a mattress suture of 4-0 nylon on a double-armed Keith needle is utilized. The mattress suture is passed through the cartilage approximately 4 to 5 mm from its cephalic border and as close to the edge of the nasal bones as possible. The mattress suture is placed through the mucosa, upper lateral cartilage, and skin, carefully oriented parallel to the relaxed skin tension lines. If this corrective maneuver is done in conjunction with a rhinoplasty, all other technical aspects are first completed, and it is done just before applying the external cast. The cartilage is fixed in place by the mattress suture and is sandwiched between the mucosa and the skin. The 4 to 5 mm of cartilage-bone overlap provides enough contact to assure fixation by fibrosis. The splint and suture are removed 5 to 7 days after surgery.

ALAR COLLAPSE

Any one or a combination of anatomic abnormalities can produce an alar collapse. Loss of cartilage support and the subsequent convex bowing produced by the lateral crura of the lower lateral cartilage can cause this deformity, as can excessive resection of the lower lateral cartilage. Incisions or excisions injuring the muscles that tense or dilate the nares cause the alae to fall or bow inward. Injudicious surgery of the alar base or in the region of the lateral margins of the lower lateral cartilage can injure the dilator nasi or lateral nasalis muscles or their attachments. Little can be accomplished by surgical manipulation or resection along the lateral margins of the lower lateral cartilage, and this area should be avoided in rhinoplasty surgery. Incisions along the lateral alar crease or across the base are also discouraged. Another common cause of alar collapse is related to a generous hump removal associated with severing most of the soft tissue attachments to the lateral nasal wall. When a lateral osteotomy is performed, the lateral nasal wall is very unstable and falls inwardly, producing a complete collapse of the nasal wall. In a rhinoplasty, this situation is one of the infrequent indications for the postoperative use of endonasal packs to

support the unstable structures until adequate fixation from fibrosis can occur.

Prevention of alar collapse is far preferable to correction by a secondary procedure. Certain guidelines should be followed to avoid this surgical disaster. Preservation of as much lower cartilage as is consistent with the desired result is paramount. Routine rhinoplasties do not require resection or dissection of lateral margins of the lateral crura of the lower lateral cartilage, and operation in this region should be avoided. The incision for lateral osteotomy should be at a right angle to the incision used to gain access to the lower lateral cartilages and nasal dorsum. If one uses an unguarded osteotome, it easily can be pushed through the mucosa without an incision any larger than the width of the osteotome. Use of a 2- or 3-mm osteotome without periosteal elevation for the lateral osteotomy is preferred so that significant investing soft tissue is left intact, preventing the bone from collapsing following the bony cut.

Management of an alar collapse is at best difficult. The reconstruction must be directed toward the underlying problem. This may be the inward bowing that results from loss of the cartilage support, the inward collapse of the lateral nasal wall, or a combination of these. Management of the inward bowing of the ala is best corrected with autogenous cartilage grafts. Either septal or conchal cartilage can be used. Perichondrium is left attached to one side, the cartilage is shaved to the thickness of the lower cartilage, and the edges are feathered with a diamond rasp. A pocket is developed using a marginal incision. The cartilage batten graft is

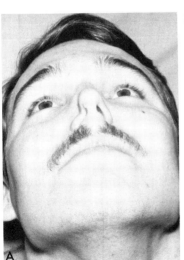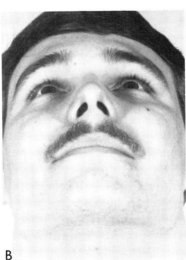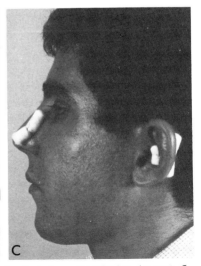

Figure 27–9. *A,* Preoperative alar collapse. *B,* Postoperative result employing the technique described in the text. *C,* Bolster dressing in place on another patient.

sized and placed in the pocket. The perichondrium is in contact with the dermis and is fixed with a mattress suture encompassing the mucosa, graft, and skin. The suture is tied with an orientation in the direction of the relaxed skin tension line (Fig. 27–9).

A collapsed lateral wall requires repositioning of the nasal process of the maxilla and nasal bone, with fixation until stability occurs from the fibrous tissue. This generally necessitates both medial and lateral osteotomies to allow proper realignment. Intranasal packing for approximately 1 week is necessary to maintain stabilization and proper realignment until fixation occurs.

TURBINATE SURGERY

It is not the intention to argue the philosophy or indications for inferior turbinate surgery in this chapter. It is sufficient to say that surgery on the hypertrophic inferior turbinate is necessary and more likely essential in many cases. The problem with turbinate surgery in combination with septal surgery is the potential for synechiae formation.

When a patient's septum is significantly deflected to one side, a contralateral compensatory turbinate hypertrophy usually occurs. This is nature's mechanism to decrease the endonasal space and increase the nasal resistance essential for normal nasal air flow. Unfortunately, the air currents are usually so markedly altered and normal laminar flow so disrupted that a normal physiologic state does not exist. It is essential to resect a portion of the inferior turbinates in order to anatomically move the septum to the midline.

Three principles of turbinate surgery markedly improve the likelihood of success in this operation. First, it is essential to evacuate the engorged vascular tissues before any type of surgery. This is easily accomplished with topical applications and local infiltration of vasoconstrictive agents. This mucosal shrinkage profoundly aids any subsequent surgical modification. Second, there is rarely a need to resect more posteriorly than the caudal third of the inferior turbinate, and it is strongly recommended that routine resections be limited to this region. Complications—primarily bleeding both immediate and late—are the result of blind resections deep posteriorly in the nose. Third, if the first two tenets are followed, turbinate surgery is conveniently combined with nasal septal reconstruction, and the two

procedures are not only compatible but inseparable from one another.

The overall goal in turbinate surgery is to improve the airway in an expeditious manner with the least possible morbidity. Our desire to combine septal and turbinate surgery, plus a fundamental aversion to the use of nasal packing, led to an evaluation of nontraditional surgical techniques. Experience with cryosurgery, with its lack of predictable destruction and occasional late sloughing and late hemorrhage, prompted abandonment of this as a sole therapeutic approach. Also, freezing is not consistent with simultaneous use in those anatomic situations when the turbinectomy must precede repositioning the septum in the midline, since occasionally swelling is marked. Electrocautery also results in extensive swelling and edema and frequently results in late hemorrhage; in addition, synechiae formation is common when electrocautery is combined with simultaneous septal surgery. Sharp surgical amputation would appear to be an attractive method of removing the anterior turbinate, allowing the midline positioning of the septum. Unfortunately, packing is required for homeostasis, which interferes with and then precludes the septal operation. When the turbinate operation does not necessarily precede the septoplasty, packing is still required postoperatively; removal of the packing often predisposes the two raw surfaces (secondary to the surgery and the packing) to synechiae formation. Steroids and sclerosing agents have no immediate effect and an unpredictable long-term effect upon a hypertrophic turbinate.

The procedures we have found valuable when combined with septal operation are submucous resection, out-fracturing, and lasering the caudal one fourth to one third of the inferior turbinate. We use one or a combination of these three procedures for management of the turbinates, employing whatever is best for a particular situation.

To decrease the likelihood of failure or complications in inferior turbinate operations, we have developed three tenets that warrant repeating. First, it is prudent to obtain maximal vasoconstriction prior to turbinate reduction by any method. This engorged organ is emptied by utilizing topical vasoconstriction (usually cocaine) and an infiltration of epinephrine mixed with the local anesthetic agent. Second, an important consideration is to make certain that the caudal one quarter of the inferior turbinates maximally clears the airway. Third, the posterior portion of the inferior turbinates contains large vessels that can cause catastrophic bleeding and may be difficult to control. Hemorrhage at the time of surgery is often brisk; but hemorrhage days after operation can be alarming. These considerations should provide the prudent nasal surgeon an incentive to avoid indiscriminate avulsion of the posterior portion of the inferior turbinate. It has been our experience, based upon thousands of nasal procedures, that the posterior portion of the inferior turbinate rarely requires surgical modification or resection to improve the airway.

SUMMARY

Techniques are described that are a compilation of procedures assimilated in formal training programs, from the literature, through personal observation of many outstanding nasal surgeons, and firsthand experience gained in over 6000 nasal procedures. Many of the important tenets and subtleties of nasal surgical therapy that we describe result from borrowing liberally from others. It is the sincerest form of flattery to copy another person, and this chapter is meant to flatter a great many people.

References

1. Ballenger JJ: Disease of the Nose, Throat and Ear. 12th ed. Philadelphia, Lea and Febiger, 1977.
2. Beekhuis GJ: Nasal septoplasty. Otolaryngol Clin North Am 6(3):693, 1973.
3. Beekhuis GJ: Saddle nose deformity: Etiology, prevention and treatment; Augmentation rhinoplasty with polyamide. Laryngoscope 84:3, 1974.
4. Kern EB: The phenomenon of paradoxical nasal obstruction. Arch Otolaryngol 103:669, 1976.
5. Saunders WH: Septal dermoplasty—its several uses. Laryngoscope 80:1342, 1970.
6. Stucker FJ: Management of the scoliotic nose. Laryngoscope 92(2):128, 1982.
7. Stucker FJ, Ansel DG: A case against nasal packing. Laryngoscope 88:1314, 1978.
8. Stucker FJ, Smith TE: Pitfalls in management of defects of bony dorsum and cartilaginous vault. Arch Otolaryngol 102:695, 1976.
9. Stucker FJ: Nasal and sinus surgery: Septoplasty, operative challenge. In Pillsbury H, Goldsmith MM (eds): Otolaryngology/Head and Neck Surgery. Chicago, Year Book Medical Publishers, 1990.

CHAPTER 28

RHINOLOGIC MANIFESTATIONS OF ACQUIRED IMMUNODEFICIENCY SYNDROME

Frank E. Lucente, MD

Lawrence Z. Meiteles, MD

William Lawson, MD, DDS

AIDS (acquired immunodeficiency syndrome) is one of the most significant diseases to emerge in the last 100 years. Although this disorder has been recognized since 1981, it has become pandemic; it is estimated that by 1991, there will be 50 to 100 million persons infected with the AIDS virus worldwide. This disease is important to the otorhinolaryngologist because of the frequency of involvement of the head and neck and the devastating impact of the disease on the health care system.

Presently, the disease principally involves homosexual or bisexual males and intravenous drug abusers; however, other affected groups include the sexual partners of this primary group, children of infected mothers, and the recipients of blood and blood products (e.g., hemophiliacs).

Clinically, the AIDS syndrome is generally recognized by the occurrence of one or more opportunistic diseases that indicate an underlying cellular immunodeficiency in the absence of another established cause of immunodeficiency. This clinical condition correlates markedly with the serologic presence of the human immunodeficiency virus (HIV) antibody.

Epidemiologically, 93 per cent of affected persons are male and 7 per cent are female. Sixty-eight per cent are between 20 and 39 years of age and 31 per cent are 40 years old or over. About 1 per cent are under the age of 20 years; this group consists primarily of infants born to infected mothers. Ethnically, 61 per cent are white, 25 per cent are black, and 14 per cent are hispanic. Currently, approximately 74 per cent of cases have been reported in homosexuals or bisexuals, 16 per cent in drug abusers, and 10 per cent in heterosexuals, including infants.[1]

The three principal modes of transmission are (1) sexual contact, (2) through contaminated blood or blood products, and (3) perinatal. The inapparent-to-apparent disease ratio with the AIDS virus is not completely known. It has been estimated that there may be as many as 50 times more HIV infections as there are actual cases of AIDS. These estimates are complicated by the long incubation period of AIDS, which spans 4 years or longer until opportunistic infections and other clinical manifestations of the disease appear. At present, it appears that AIDS will develop in approximately 35 per cent of

HIV-infected persons. This percentage of conversion will probably increase as clinicians gain more experience with this disease and the actual incubation period is better defined. In addition to the 35 per cent who develop AIDS, approximately another 25 per cent develop other signs of HIV infection, such as the AIDS-related complex (ARC). This is characterized by lymphadenopathy, fever, night sweats, or those diseases directly related to HIV infection, such as encephalopathy or cardiomyopathy. Some but not all ARC patients eventually will develop the full-blown AIDS syndrome. The ultimate prognosis of the remaining 40 per cent of HIV-positive patients who do not currently have AIDS or ARC is not yet known.[1]

It has been reported that more than 40 per cent of AIDS patients present with lesions of the head and neck (Table 28–1). Accordingly, it is essential that the otorhinolaryngologist be knowledgeable of the various clinical manifestations of AIDS, understand its primary and supportive therapy, and implement the optimal methods of protecting health care personnel from infection with HIV.

CLINICAL MANIFESTATIONS

Rhinosinusitis. The mucosa of the nose, paranasal sinuses, and nasopharynx represents a potential portal of entry for pathogenic organisms. Although a wide spectrum of opportunistic infections of the nose and paranasal sinuses is possible in hosts having only cell-mediated immunity, a limited number of organisms have been reported to cause sinusitis in the AIDS patient (Table 28–2).

A case of cytomegalovirus (CMV) rhinitis was reported by Kotler and coworkers in a patient with a concomitant *Pneumocystis carinii* pneumonia.[2] The patient had purulent rhinitis, with normal sinus radiographs. The nasal mucosa

TABLE 28–1. Rhinologic Manifestations of AIDS

Rhinosinusitis
Nasal septal abscess
Kaposi's sarcoma
Candidiasis
Seborrheic dermatitis
Nasopharyngeal lymphoid proliferation
Lymphoma of the nasal cavity and sinuses
Herpetic lesions

was erythematous and granular; biopsy revealed multiple CMV inclusions within endothelial cells, squamous metaplasia of the mucosa, and scattered areas of acute and chronic inflammation. Viral inclusions were not found in rectal biopsy specimens. CMV infection can be identified histologically by intranuclear inclusion bodies in vascular endothelial cells.

Legionella pneumophila rhinosinusitis was reported by Schlanger and colleagues in a patient with disseminated CMV disease.[3] Open lung and liver biopsy specimens revealed the intranuclear inclusion bodies of CMV. The patient had purulent nasal discharge, and maxillary sinus air fluid levels were seen on sinus radiography. A Caldwell-Luc procedure was performed; culture revealed only a few colonies of *Staphylococcus epidermidis*. However, direct immunofluorescence staining using group 1 *Legionella pneumophila* antiserum demonstrated bright fluorescent bacilli. Direct immunofluorescence of the lung and hepatic biopsy specimens were negative. Treatment with oral erythromycin for 10 days resulted in resolution of the drainage. *Legionella pneumophila* is a facultative intracellular pathogen and represents a potential infectious agent in the immune-deficient host.

Rhinosinusitis caused by *Acanthamoeba castellanii* was reported by Gonzalez and colleagues in a patient with concomitant *Pneumocystis carinii* pneumonia.[4] The patient presented with the complaints of progressive

TABLE 28–2. Reported Sinonasal Infectious Agents

Cytomegalovirus	1 case	Kotler et al[2]
Legionella pneumophila	1 case	Schlanger et al[3]
Acanthamoeba castellanii	1 case	Gonzalez et al[4]
Pseudomonas aeruginosa		
Staphylococcus aureus	1 case	Poole et al[5]
Streptococcus pneumoniae		
Haemophilus influenzae		
Streptococcus pneumoniae	12 patients	Sooy[6]
Pseudoallescheria boydii		
Alternaria alternata	1 case	Wiest et al[7]
Cryptococcus neoformans	1 case	Choi et al[8]
Staphylococcus aureus	1 case	Henry et al[9]

nasal obstruction, epistaxis, nasal tenderness, and frontal headache. Physical examination revealed nasal obstruction, with crusted mucosa covering the turbinates. Computed tomography revealed mucosal swelling of the turbinates, soft tissue swelling in the maxillary sinuses, and partial opacification of the ethmoid sinuses. Biopsy of the left inferior turbinate revealed a granulomatous inflammation containing *Acanthamoeba castellanii.* Despite treatment with rifampin and ketaconazole, the patient died 3 months later from salmonella sepsis. Autopsy revealed a pale, edematous, yellow mucosa with focal areas of hemorrhage present in all the sinus cavities. The patient also had a right leg mass that represented an abscess cavity containing *Acanthamoeba* bacteria, most probably the result of hematogenous spread of nasal infection. *Acanthamoeba* has been isolated from the nasopharynges of healthy individuals, and the transition from colonization to infection probably occurs only in the immunocompromised host.

Poole and colleagues reported a case of sinusitis in a patient with central nervous system toxoplasmosis and mucosal candidiasis.[5] The patient had purulent nasal discharge and opacified paranasal sinuses on radiologic examination. Culture of an antral aspirate revealed *Pseudomonas aeruginosa, Staphylococcus aureus,* and *Streptococcus pneumoniae.* Surgical drainage resulted in cessation of symptoms. The authors of this report commented that AIDS patients with fungal and parasitic infections respond poorly to antimicrobial therapy, and they recommended early surgical intervention.

Among 12 AIDS patients with sinusitis, Sooy found *Hemophilus influenzae* and *Streptococcus pneumoniae* to be the most common bacterial organisms and *Pseudallescheria boydii* the most common fungal pathogen.[6] He recommended early sinus irrigation for both diagnosis and therapy, particularly in the toxic patient. He also noted that tumor should be included in the differential diagnosis of sinus opacification and listed Kaposi's sarcoma and lymphoma as possible causes.

Rhinosinusitis secondary to *Alternaria,* a ubiquitous filamentous fungus recognized as a plant pathogen and soil saprophyte, was described in a patient with AIDS by Wiest and colleagues.[7] Two months prior to diagnosis, the patient had been treated for *Pneumocystis carinii* pneumonia and esophageal candidiasis. While the patient was on ketaconazole and oral acyclovir for herpes zoster of the right second branch of the trigeminal nerve, he complained of tenderness over the right side of his nose

and persistent clear discharge. Sinus radiographs revealed mucosal thickening of the right maxillary sinus. CT scan confirmed the presence of a right antral soft tissue density. Physical examination disclosed a 0.5-cm well-circumscribed, black necrotic lesion on the right nasal septum. Culture and biopsy of the septal lesion revealed *Alternaria alternata.* A biopsy specimen of the maxillary sinus through a Caldwell-Luc procedure showed only chronic inflammation. Treatment was instituted with amphotericin B. However, because of persistent pain, the patient underwent repeat biopsies of the right antrum, but no evidence of fungal infection was found. The patient died 8 months later; autopsy revealed no evidence of fungal infection. For this patient to develop *Alternaria* rhinitis while receiving ketaconazole for mucosal candidiasis is explained by the fact that the average reported serum concentration of ketaconazole achieved with 400 mg/day is 3.32 mg/ml, which is a level well below the mean inhibitory concentration (MIC) needed for *Alternaria.*[7]

Two distinct histologic patterns are encountered with *Alternaria* infection.[7] In the first, broad hyphae with occasional branching and chains of conidia are present, along with a granulomatous or suppurative tissue reaction. In the second, a granulomatous inflammation with numerous giant cells is seen. The giant cells contain periodic acid–Schiff–positive rounded fungal forms, hyphae, or chains of conidia. Treatment of *Alternaria* rhinosinusitis should include surgical excision and the intravenous administration of amphotericin B.

Choi and colleagues reported systemic cryptococcosis secondary to cryptococcal sinusitis in an AIDS patient.[8] The patient presented with complaints of frontal headache, intermittent fever, and nausea and vomiting of 2 weeks' duration. The patient also noted the onset of malaise and anorexia and a 14-pound weight loss 3 months prior to admission. Physical examination was significant for oral thrush and diffuse, shotty cervical lymphadenopathy. A CT performed prior to lumbar puncture revealed an air-fluid level in the right frontal and maxillary sinuses, as well as bilateral opacification of the sphenoid and left maxillary sinuses (Fig. 28–1). India ink preparation of the cerebrospinal fluid was positive for *Cryptococcus neoformans,* which was confirmed by cultures. Despite therapy with amphotericin B and 5-flucytosine, the patient did not improve and underwent bilateral intranasal sphenoethmoidectomies, bilateral antrostomies, and a right frontal sinus trephination. Biopsies from

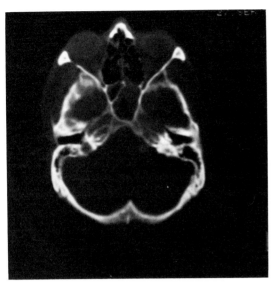

Figure 28–1. CT scan revealing sphenoid opacification in an AIDS patient with disseminated cryptococcosis. Biopsy of the sinus revealed *Cryptococcus neoformans.*

all sinuses were positive for *Cryptococcus neoformans.* After 8 weeks of amphotericin B and 5-flucytosine therapy, the patient was discharged on intermittent amphotericin B and 5-flucytosine treatment for 6 months. The patient was followed for 14 months without relapse.

The diagnosis of cryptococcosis is made by India ink preparation and culture of appropriate body fluids.[8] Another useful test is a latex agglutination procedure for detection of the cryptococcal antigen. The treatment of disseminated cryptococcosis consists of intravenous amphotericin B with or without oral 5-flucytosine.[8]

A nasal septal abscess due to *Staphylococcus aureus* in a patient with concomitant *Pneumocystis carinii* pneumonia was reported by Henry and colleagues.[9] The patient presented with nasal obstruction, marked maxillary tenderness, and purulent posterior nasal drainage. Computed tomography revealed a large mass in the nasal septum, from which 10 ml of purulent material were drained. Cultures revealed *Staphylococcus aureus.* The patient recovered fully after treatment with pentamidine and cephalexin.

In the cases of rhinosinusitis, a variety of infectious agents were encountered, which included bacteria, fungi (Fig. 28–2), protozoa, and viruses. The gram-positive and gram-negative bacteria isolated are organisms indigenous to the upper respiratory tract and also are often pathogenic in the noncompromised patient. In the AIDS patient, the infections are often mul-

tibacterial and fail to respond to medical therapy alone because of the impaired host defenses. Invasive procedures serve both as diagnostic maneuvers to obtain culture and histologic material and as therapy by providing debridement and drainage. The exotic nature of the other causative agents cited is characteristic of the opportunistic infections that occur in AIDS patients and underscores the value of obtaining fresh diagnostic material (cultures, smears, aspirates, biopsies), since these individuals may have concurrent infection of other organ systems with different organisms. Consequently, therapy must be aggressive, employing appropriate systemic antibiotics as well as regional surgery.

Kaposi's Sarcoma. In the pre-AIDS era, Kaposi's sarcoma was a rare neoplasm that arose primarily in distinct ethnic groups comprised principally of elderly men of Italian ancestry and Eastern European Jews. The usual clinical presentation was cutaneous lesions of the lower extremities. With AIDS patients, the disease often assumes a more fulminant form.[10] Although Kaposi's sarcoma rarely affects the respiratory tract, pulmonary involvement has been reported in as high as 47 per cent of AIDS cases at autopsy.[10] Isolated cases of Kaposi's sarcoma have been reported to involve the upper respiratory tract. Sooy reported a case of paranasal sinus involvement with Kaposi's sarcoma.[6] This tumor has been found to arise in the nasal cavity, in the nasal vestibule, on the nasal septum, and in the nasopharynx.[6, 11] We have seen a case of Kaposi's sarcoma in an AIDS patient in which a palatal lesion eroded into the nasal cavity to form an oronasal fistula. In the report by Patow and colleagues of 13 AIDS

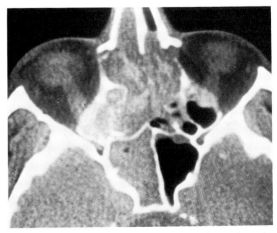

Figure 28–2. Extensive aspergillosis involving the ethmoid and sphenoid sinuses.

patients with Kaposi's sarcoma, 11 had facial cutaneous lesions, of which at least 2 involved the nasal skin.[12]

Patients with nasal Kaposi's sarcoma generally complain of nasal obstruction, drainage, and epistaxis. On physical examination discrete nodular violaceous tumors are seen. The diagnosis is confirmed by excisional biopsy of such a cutaneous nodule. Microscopically, fascicles of spindle cells surrounding cleftlike spaces containing extravasated erythrocytes are seen. Some areas show hemosiderin deposition, plasma cell and polymorphonuclear leukocyte clusters, and dilated lymphatic and capillary channels. The histologic findings are identical in lesions at all anatomic sites.[13] Chemotherapy and radiation therapy are the treatments of choice. In a study by Schenk,[14] virus particles ultrastructurally identical to those of HIV were identified within Kaposi's sarcoma of the oral mucosa.

Candidiasis. Oral candidiasis is often a presenting symptom in ARC and the forerunner of the development of AIDS. Candidiasis generally can be diagnosed clinically by its typical pseudomembranous appearance, with the cheesy white plaques wiping off and leaving an erythematous base. Other variants have been described, which include a hyperplastic form that does not scrape off, an erythematous or atrophic form, and a form that presents as angular cheilitis.[15] Oral candidiasis also may be a marker for esophageal candidiasis in AIDS patients.[16] Oral candidiasis can spread caudally into the hypopharynx and esophagus and cephalad into the nasopharynx. The diagnosis of nasopharyngeal candidiasis can be confirmed by making smears and cultures. Oral and oropharyngeal candidiasis usually can be successfully treated with mycostatin mouth rinses. However, the nasopharynx cannot be treated topically, and candidiasis in this region is generally best managed systemically with oral ketaconazole.

Seborrheic Dermatitis. Seborrheic dermatitis in AIDS patients has been reported to range from 22 to 83 per cent.[17] The head and neck is the most common site of involvement, with a malar rash often present over the nose and cheeks.[18, 19] Other sites of involvement include the chest, back, groin, and extremities. The skin eruption is characterized by indurated, erythematous, scaly plaques. Soeprono and colleagues demonstrated that the seborrheic dermatitis of AIDS is a histologically distinct entity separate from ordinary seborrheic dermatitis.[19]

Histologically, the lesions show spotty keratinocytic necrosis, leukoexocytosis, and superficial perivascular infiltrates of plasma cells and neutrophils.[19] These histologic features are not encountered in the common form of seborrheic dermatitis, despite the fact that they are clinically indistinguishable. Other differences of the AIDS variant are its occurrence in a younger population, its greater severity, and its involvement of the extremities and chest—sites not usually affected by ordinary seborrheic dermatitis. The appearance of seborrheic dermatitis may serve as a marker for AIDS or ARC. It tends to be somewhat refractory to treatment with topical corticosteroids.[18]

Nasopharyngeal Lymphoid Proliferation. In a recent report by Stern and colleagues, nasopharyngeal lymphoid proliferation was found to be a presenting sign of HIV infection.[20] Affected patients complained of nasal obstruction and also of hearing loss from serous otitis media. Flexible fiberoptic nasopharyngoscopy revealed large submucosal nasopharyngeal masses that occluded the posterior choana and torus tubarius. Biopsy specimens showed histologic evidence of benign lymphoid hypertrophy. While all the patients tested positive for HIV, they were asymptomatic for AIDS or ARC. Adenoidectomy provided symptomatic relief. Accordingly, the authors of the report recommended adenoidectomy and HIV testing of high-risk patients who have nasal obstruction secondary to benign lymphoid hypertrophy.

Lymphoma. Leess and colleagues reported a case of high-grade, undifferentiated, large cell lymphoma involving the nasal cavity and maxillary antrum in an AIDS patient.[21] The patient presented with nasal obstruction, persistent foul left nasal discharge, and a history of a 20-pound weight loss. On physical examination, a large necrotic mass was found to fill the left nostril and cause flaring of the ala. Computed tomography (CT) revealed a soft tissue density in the left nasal cavity and maxillary sinus but with no bone destruction. Follow-up CT showed enlargement of the sinus mass and the presence of a right temporo-occipital lesion. The patient had a poor response to chemotherapy and was lost to follow-up. Leess and colleagues also reported a case of a high-grade, small, noncleaved B cell lymphoma involving the palate and antrum.[21] The patient presented with an enlarging lesion of the left maxillary molar region. CT demonstrated bone destruction with extension of the mass into the antrum. The patient responded well to chemotherapy, with complete resolution of the mass. These authors noted a high incidence of central nervous system involvement in association with non-Hodgkin's lymphomas of the head and neck and recommended lumbar puncture and brain CT to aid in the diagnosis. They also recommended aggressive radiation and chemotherapy as the treatment of choice. We have seen an AIDS patient who was diagnosed as having medically refractory pansinusitis, with biopsy-proved B cell lymphoma diffusely in the ethmoid sinuses (Fig. 28–3).

Herpes Zoster and Herpes Simplex. Herpes zoster infection represents reactivation of latent varicella-zoster virus in the dorsal root ganglia of patients previously infected. Localized herpes zoster is usually seen as a disorder of elderly and immunocompromised patients and is thought to be secondary to deficient cell-mediated immunity.[22, 23] It has been well-documented that herpes zoster infection arising in asymptomatic individuals at high risk for AIDS may be the presenting sign of HIV infection.[22, 23] Friedman-Kien and colleagues found that, among 48 patients with herpes zoster who were in high risk groups for AIDS, 35 (73 per cent) were seropositive for HIV.[23] Seven patients subsequently became HIV-positive 1 to 28

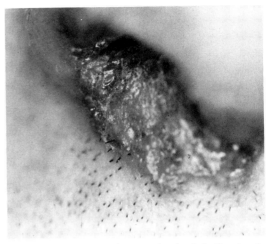

Figure 28–4. Fulminate herpes simplex infection involving the floor of the nostril and extending onto the perinasal skin.

months after their zoster infection was diagnosed. The herpes zoster infections seen in HIV-positive and AIDS patients are of greater severity and tend to become generalized.[18] It has been observed at the New York Eye and Ear Infirmary that high-risk individuals with herpes zoster ophthalmicus often are later found to be HIV-positive. Treatment is with acyclovir. The incidence or severity of postherpetic neuralgia in AIDS patients is no greater than that seen in the general population.

A new entity of giant herpetic nasal ulcers also has been reported in AIDS patients.[6] The ulcers begin in the vestibule and may extend onto the face or septum, achieving a size as great as 3 cm in diameter (Fig. 28–4). Treatment is with acyclovir.

We have also encountered an AIDS patient with extensive molluscum contagiosum involvement of the skin of the nose and midface. The lesions were well-circumscribed and elevated and had central umbilication.

PRECAUTIONS FOR HEALTH CARE WORKERS

The unknown carrier of HIV is a greater risk to the health care worker than the known AIDS sufferer, as optimal precautions are observed in the care of the latter. However, the overall risk to the health care worker appears to be minimal. To date, only 33 cases of AIDS have been reported to have developed through occupational exposure, the majority in housekeeping

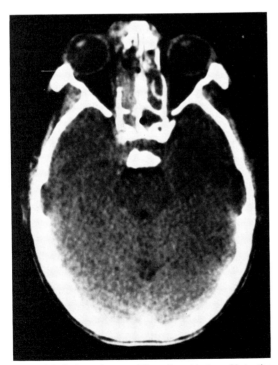

Figure 28–3. Lymphoma of the ethmoid sinus. Note the presence of an enhancing lesion destroying the lamina papyracea.

and other support personnel.[1] However, because the time interval for seroconversion following inoculation may be as long as 6 months, all patients must be considered as being potentially infected. Accordingly, it is necessary to practice those measures that will reduce the hazards of any virus infection by percutaneous or mucous membrane inoculation. The following precautions are recommended:

In the office, when treating *any* patient, frequent handwashing before and after examining patients remains the most important precaution. Since viruses do not traverse intact skin, there is no reason to avoid shaking hands with a patient or touching the ear, nose, face, or neck of *any* patient.

—Gloves should be worn when touching mucous membrane surfaces, blood and body fluids, and nonintact skin of *all* patients.

—Change gloves after contact with each patient, or if torn.

—Avoid unprotected patient contact if you have broken skin.

—Wear masks and protective eyewear or face shields when aerosol spray is a risk. This may be during routine office examination, endoscopic procedures, the induction of local or general anesthesia, or the performance of surgery under local anesthesia.

—Wear gloves when performing venipuncture.

—Do not recap needles—discard them into protective containers designed for medical waste disposal.

—Lay out instruments before beginning an examination or procedure rather than reaching into the instrument drawer with contaminated hands.

—Reduce the number of sharp objects present in any operative field and allow only one person to handle a scalpel at any time.

—Clean all instruments thoroughly and disinfect them in a dilute solution of sodium hypochlorite or glutaraldehyde.

—Communicate infection control facts to staff members and patients even if they seem unnecessary, or frightening. They will respect us for our cautiousness.

—Try to convey to all patients that these are the necessary precautions that a prudent physician should observe and that they should introduce these measures into their own lifestyle to reduce the danger of hematogenous or transmucosal inoculation of infectious agents.

The AIDS epidemic poses a serious challenge to the rhinologist, who needs to remember three important watchwords: *vigilance* (to recognize manifestations of AIDS as early as possible), *prudence* (to protect the self and all health care workers) and *compassion* (to continue to render the highest standards of care to all patients).

References

1. Lucente FE, Dull HB, Pincus RL: Acquired immunodeficiency syndrome. *In* Cummings CW, et al (eds): Otolaryngology—Head and Neck Surgery. St. Louis, CV Mosby, 1988.
2. Kotler DP, Scholes JV, Jacob AL, Edelheit W: Disseminated CMV infection. JAMA 253:3093, 1985.
3. Schlanger G, Lutwick LI, Kurzman M, Hoch B, Chandler FW: Sinusitis caused by *Legionella pneumophila* in a patient with the acquired immune deficiency syndrome. Am J Med 77:957, 1984.
4. Gonzales MM, Gould E, Dickinson G, Martinez AJ, Visvesvara G, Cleary TJ, Hensley GT: Acquired immunodeficiency syndrome associated with *Acanthamoeba* infection and other opportunistic organisms. Arch Pathol Lab Med 110:749, 1986.
5. Poole MD, Postma D, Cohen MS: Pyogenic otorhinologic infections in acquired immune deficiency syndrome. Arch Otolaryngol 110:130, 1984.
6. Sooy CD: The impact of AIDS in otolaryngology—head and neck surgery. Adv Otolaryngol Head Neck Surg 1:1, 1987.
7. Wiest PM, Wiese K, Jacobs MR, Morrissey AB, Abelson TI, Witt W, Lederman MM: *Alternaria* infection in a patient with acquired immunodeficiency syndrome: Case report and review of invasive *Alternaria* infections. Rev Infect Dis 9:799, 1987.
8. Choi SS, Lawson W, Bottone EJ, Biller HF: Cryptococcal sinusitis: A case report and review of literature. Otolaryngol Head Neck Surg 9:414, 1988.
9. Henry K, Sullivan C, Crossley K: Nasal septal abscess due to *Staphylococcus aureus* in a patient with AIDS. Rev Infect Dis 10:428, 1988.
10. Zibrak JD, Silvestri RC, Costello P, Marlink R, Jensen WA, Robins A, Rose RM: Bronchoscopic and radiologic features of Kaposi's sarcoma involving the respiratory system. Chest 90:476, 1986.
11. Marcusen DC, Sooy CD: Otolaryngologic and head and neck manifestations of acquired immunodeficiency syndrome (AIDS). Laryngoscope 95:401, 1985.
12. Patow CA, Steis R, Longo DL, Reichert CM, Findlay PA, Potter D, Masur H, Lane HC, Fauci AS, Macher AM: Kaposi's sarcoma of the head and neck in the acquired immune deficiency syndrome. Otolaryngol Head Neck Surg 92:255, 1984.
13. Hymes K: Kaposi's sarcoma in AIDS. *In* Wormser GP, Stahl RE, Bottone EJ (eds): Acquired Immune Deficiency Syndrome and Other Manifestations of HIV Infection. Park Ridge, NJ, Noyes Publications, 1987, pp 747–766.
14. Schenk P: Retroviruses in Kaposi's sarcoma in acquired immune deficiency syndrome (AIDS). Acta Otolaryngol (Stockh) 101:295, 1986.
15. Lucente FE, Meiteles LZ, Pincus RL: Bronchoesophageal manifestations of acquired immunodeficiency syndrome. Ann Otol Rhinol Laryngol 97:530, 1988.
16. Tavitan A, Raufman JP, Rosenthal LE: Oral candidiasis as a marker for esophageal candidiasis in the acquired immunodeficiency syndrome. Ann Intern Med 104:54, 1986.

17. Matis WL, Triana A, Shapiro R, Eldred L, Polk BF, Hood AF: Dermatologic findings associated with human immunodeficiency virus infection. J Am Acad Dermatol 17:746, 1987.
18. Cockarell CJ: Cutaneous manifestations of AIDS other than Kaposi's sarcoma. *In* Wormser GP, Stahl RE, Bottone EJ (eds): Acquired Immune Deficiency Syndrome and Other Manifestations of HIV Infection. Park Ridge, NJ, Noyes Publications, 1987, pp 808–811.
19. Soeprono FF, Schinella RA, Cockarell CJ, Comite SL: Seborrheic-like dermatitis of acquired immunodeficiency syndrome. J Am Acad Dermatol 14:242, 1986.
20. Stern J, Lin PT, Lucente FE: Symptomatic Benign Nasopharyngeal Lymphoid Proliferation and Human Immunodeficiency Virus (HIV) Infection. Presented at the Second International Conference on Head and Neck Cancer, Boston, Aug 1, 1988.
21. Leess FR, Kessler OJ, Mickel RA: Non-Hodgkin's lymphoma of the head and neck in patients with AIDS. Arch Otolaryngol Head Neck Surg 113:1104, 1987.
22. Cone LA, Schiffman MA: Herpes zoster and the acquired immunodeficiency syndrome. Ann Intern Med 100:462, 1984.
23. Friedman-Kien AE, Lafleur FL, Gendler E, Hennessey NP, Montagna R, Halbert S, Rubinstein P, Krasinski K, Zang E, Poiesz B: Herpes zoster: A possible early clinical sign for development of acquired immunodeficiency syndrome in high-risk individuals. J Am Acad Dermatol 14:1023, 1986.

CHAPTER 29

SINUSITIS IN INFANTS AND CHILDREN

Blair Fearon, MD, FRCS(C), FACS, FAAP
Beverly Denise McMillin, MD

DEVELOPMENTAL ANATOMY

The nose and sinuses are essentially a single structure in children. The ethmoid air cells begin development in the fourth fetal month as evaginations from the nasal chambers. They are present at birth as separate recesses that grow into a honeycomb of cells, each with its own opening into the meatus from which it originated. (These are the inferior, middle, and superior meatus.) These cells vary in shape and size, with small cells occurring anteriorly and larger cells posteriorly. The air cells enlarge until they reach adult size between the ages of 12 and 14 years (Fig. 29–1). The ethmoid sinuses are bounded by the anterior cranial fossa superiorly, the sphenoid sinus posteriorly, the lamina papyracea laterally, and the nasal chamber and inferior turbinate inferomedially (Fig. 29–2).

The maxillary sinuses evaginate early in the second trimester from the lateral walls of the ethmoid infundibulum. All the sinuses are said to be slitlike at birth, with the floor at the level of the inferior turbinate, but the antrum can be at least a centimeter in size. Eruption of the teeth determines inferior growth and therefore the level of the sinus floor. By the age of 8 years the floor is at the level of the inferior meatus and reaches the level of the nasal floor between the ages of 8 and 12 years. The maxillary sinus reaches adult size by 15 years of age, except for growth that can occur after the eruption of the third molar tooth. In the adult,

the floor of the antrum can be 5 to 7 mm below the nasal floor, and the volume reaches 12 to 15 cc (Fig. 29–3).[4, 6, 7, 10]

The frontal sinuses develop as evaginations from the anterior end of the middle meatus at about the fourth fetal month. The sinus is a small pit at birth and is not distinguishable from the ethmoids until 6 or 8 years of age (Fig. 29–2). They do not reach adult size until puberty. They are seldom symmetrical, vary greatly in shape and size, and indeed occasionally may not develop at all. The development of the sphenoid sinus also starts around the fourth fetal month in the dome of the cartilaginous nasal capsule. Growth and pneumatization start in the fourth year with resorption of the nasal capsule, bringing the sinus into contact with the sphenoid bone. Posterior lateral growth precedes ventral growth so that there is an early relationship between the sphenoid sinus and the cavernous sinus. Growth is slow and sporadic, although the sphenoid reaches adult size before the other paranasal sinuses. The position of the ostium is high in the nasal cavity, and for this reason infections of the sphenoid sinuses are less frequent than those of the other sinuses.

PATHOGENESIS

The lining of the sinus cavities is respiratory mucous membrane that is continuous with the mucosal lining of the nasal cavity. Cilia in the sinuses beat toward the ostia and help expel

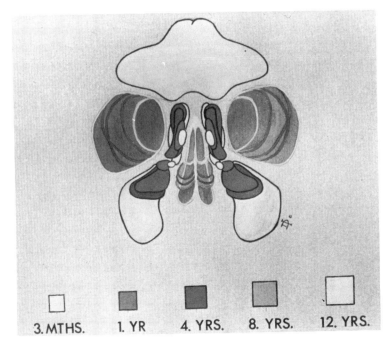

Figure 29–1. Comparative sizes of paranasal air sinuses and nasal and orbital cavities at different ages. (From Fearon B, Edmonds B, Bird R: Orbital-facial complications of sinusitis in children. Laryngoscope 89:947, 1979.)

3. MTHS.   1. YR   4. YRS.   8. YRS.   12. YRS.

material from the antrum into the nose. Ciliary dysfunction or obstruction of the sinus ostia impairs drainage and results in retained secretions.

Hyperemia, edema, and thickened mucous membrane, as well as thick mucous secretions, cause obstruction of the sinus ostium during acute sinusitis. Overgrowth of organisms in the retained secretions may lead to infection, increasing the number of inflammatory cells and

causing superficial erosion of the lining epithelium. In the presence of infection, oxygen tension and pH are reduced, while the carbon dioxide content is increased. These changes impair ciliary and phagocytic activity.[4, 7, 15]

Children are prone to frequent upper respiratory infections, and the resultant mucosal congestion can narrow the sinus ostia, causing secretions to be retained in the involved sinus or sinuses. This results in the development of

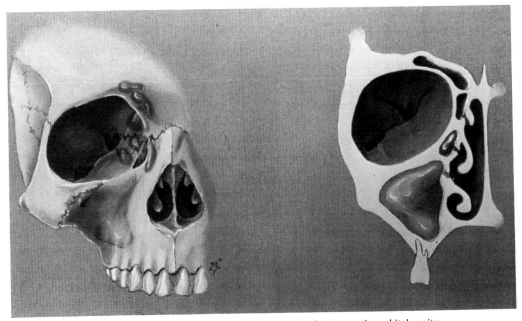

Figure 29–2. Relationship of sinuses and internal nares to the orbital cavity.

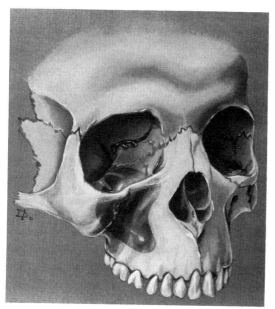

Figure 29–3. Anatomy of the medial wall and floor of the orbital cavity.

sinusitis. Edema and secretory changes also occur in the nasal mucosa and sinuses in allergies without bacterial infection, and therefore there may be opacification of the sinuses on radiologic studies. The appearance of the nasal mucosa should make it possible to differentiate between inflammatory and allergic changes in the nasal mucosa.

In infants and younger children, adenoiditis is either a cause of sinusitis or, at least, a most commonly associated problem. Unfortunately, adenoiditis as such is seldom recognized. Adenoid hypertrophy can be readily evaluated by soft tissue lateral x-ray films of the nasopharynx, but only direct vision of the adenoid (nasopharyngeal tonsil) can determine the degree of infection in the adenoid tissue. Furthermore, the eustachian tube cushions occasionally can be so hypertrophied that they project an image of adenoid enlargement even when there is no adenoid tissue present. Unfortunately, acute, as well as chronic, adenoiditis is commonly overlooked as a source of fever and malaise in the child. Indeed, the diagnosis of acute sinusitis is often made clinically when the adenoid alone is the source of the illness, and acute adenoiditis is commonly overlooked in the evaluation of pyrexia.

Although most authorities agree that the adenoid is a predisposing factor in sinusitis, tonsil disease also is an important factor in sinus disease, especially in older children. Other entities that may cause sinusitis in children include nasal foreign bodies, nasopharyngeal tumors, allergy, and the immotile cilia syndrome. A deviated septum that impinges on the middle meatus may interfere with sinus drainage. (In approximately 95 per cent of individuals with deviated septum, the deviation is to the left side. In the patients we studied, there was no predominant localization of the sinusitis to the left side; consequently, deviation of the septum per se cannot be a significant cause of sinusitis.[6])

SIGNS AND SYMPTOMS

The clinical features of acute sinusitis in children differ considerably from those in adults, and the younger the child, the more the symptoms and signs differ, as does the location of the sinuses involved. Because the maxillary and ethmoid sinuses are the first to develop, it follows that maxillary and ethmoid involvement is most prominent. Pain, for example, is a relatively uncommon symptom in the child, and indeed children under 6 years of age rarely complain of pain or headache, even in severe acute infections. The pain of sinusitis in the older child is described as a dull ache in the frontal, parietal, or occipital areas or behind one or both eyes. In acute maxillary sinusitis, there may be pain like a toothache in the upper teeth of the involved side, and these teeth may be sensitive to pressure or percussion. More commonly, the signs of sinusitis are nasal congestion, purulent or mucopurulent rhinorrhea associated with a foul odor, persistent cough, anorexia, and general malaise. These are much the same as those signs found in children with any acute upper respiratory tract infection, except that they are more severe and protracted. Chronic rhinorrhea may be due to sinusitis but also may be caused by an uncomplicated rhinitis or chronic adenoiditis.

In the very young child, the first evidence of sinus infection, other than the rhinitis, may be a complication. Orbital cellulitis or signs of intracranial infection should arouse the suspicion of sinus involvement even without prior history of sinus infection. Complications may occur at a very early age (for example, we have treated a 3-week-old baby with an orbital abscess secondary to maxillary sinusitis).[6]

In children, the differentiation between acute and chronic sinusitis is difficult. Purulent discharge from the nose or evidence of a complication relative to the sinuses is usually indicative of an acute infection or an aggravation of chronic infection. An opaque sinus (with or without an air-fluid level) on radiography, along with other symptoms of an acute infection, usually denotes acute sinusitis. Opacification of the sinus may also be noted in chronic sinusitis.

Mucosal thickening tends to occur with chronic infection. This, in turn, may lead to mucous cysts in the antra, although standard x-ray views are not always diagnostic. A radiographic abnormality does not necessarily signify sinusitis in the young child. Mucosal changes can occur with an uncomplicated upper respiratory tract infection or with nasal allergy because of the continuity of the nasal and sinus mucosal lining. Radiographic interpretation is also made difficult by the variation in sinus development. Ultrasonography is considered a reliable method of detecting secretions in the sinus and thus a means of following the status of the sinus infection to resolution.[14]

Acute sinusitis may be diagnosed on the basis of localized and systemic signs and symptoms in conjunction with radiographic abnormalities. Chronic sinusitis may be suspected if there are localized manifestations and radiographic abnormalities with few consistent systemic signs. However, chronic sinusitis must be considered in children with recurrent upper respiratory tract infections and in those with intractable asthma. There is a high prevalence of sinusitis in children with asthma, and the sinus disease may contribute to its severity. Several theories account for this relationship.[16] One is that bacterial seeding of the lung from the sinuses may cause secondary bronchitis, resulting in exacerbations of the asthma. Another postulates that inflammation in the sinus stimulates the nasal ganglia and thus induces reflex bronchospasm via the vidian nerve and stellate ganglion.[3]

The sphenoid and frontal sinuses have little clinical significance in the young child. In the older child, the signs and symptoms are similar to those in adults. In the sphenoid, the pain tends to be described as deep in the head, and there is no localized tenderness. With frontal sinus involvement, the pain is over the forehead, and there may or may not be tenderness over the involved sinus.

Transillumination can be helpful in the diagnosis of maxillary and frontal sinusitis but also may be misleading. If both maxillary sinuses do not transilluminate, it does not necessarily mean that the antra are diseased. However, it is significant if one antrum is opaque and the other clear. Transillumination can be useful in following the clearing of the involved sinus. If both antra or frontal sinuses transilluminate clearly, one can assume that the sinuses are clear or the disease is minimal.[1, 4, 7, 15]

Another modality that may be useful in the diagnosis of maxillary sinus disease is ultrasonography. This painless, noninvasive test is based on transmitted (reflected) ultrasonic waves. An air-filled sinus will not reflect the waves, whereas fluid and/or thickened tissue in the antrum will. Ultrasonography's effectiveness in aiding a diagnosis has been controversial, however; Rohr and associates suggested that it may be useful in following the course of therapy once a positive diagnosis has been established.[15a]

Computed tomography (CT) scanning has also added a new dimension to making a diagnosis of sinus disease. The CT scan is useful for inspecting fine bony detail as well as soft tissue. Magnetic resonance imaging (MRI) also has become useful in the evaluation of sinus disease. It has the advantage of not involving any radiation exposure and it allows excellent soft tissue detail, but it shows any bone and is very expensive. More information about the advantages and disadvantages of CT and MRI can be found in Chapter 4.[15b, 15c]

TREATMENT

Oral antimicrobial therapy is generally the appropriate initial treatment for bacterial sinusitis. The prevalence of *Haemophilus influenzae* or *Streptococcus pneumoniae* makes ampicillin or amoxicillin the appropriate first choice.[4a] Other effective antimicrobials are trimethoprim-sulfamethoxazole, cefaclor, erythromycin, cloxacillin, dicloxacillin, cephalexin, or erythromycin-sulfonamide combinations. However, in the severely and acutely ill child, especially with extension of the inflammation beyond the sinuses, intravenous antibiotics such as ampicillin, chloramphenicol, gentamicin, methicillin, or cephalothin may be advisable.

In the acute phase of sinusitis, topical decongestants, such as 0.25 per cent phenylephrine or 0.05 per cent xylometazoline hydrochloride solutions, introduced intranasally, may provide symptomatic relief and probably help in the drainage of the sinuses. In infants and young children, the solution may be applied by dropper, or in older children by dropper or spray. The objective is to reduce the swelling of the nasal mucosa. The value of oral decongestants is controversial, but in many instances they do seem to promote aeration of the sinuses. This is particularly true if there is an underlying allergic factor.[13, 16]

When response to medical therapy is ineffective, surgical drainage is advisable. Impairment of ciliary activity and phagocytosis from the infection tend to prevent resolution of sinusitis, even in the presence of an adequate level of an appropriate antibiotic. Purulent sinus secretions are proteolytically active, and if not inactivated by a proteinase inhibitor, the enzymes cause tissue damage to the sinus mucosa. Aspiration or lavage removes the proteinase-containing secretions along with the debris, bacteria, and granulocytes.[4]

Exudate can be removed from the maxillary antrum by aspiration, lavage, or Proetz displacement. The latter, however, is difficult to achieve in a child and may spread infection to uninvolved sinuses.[5]

Antral puncture with an antral trocar and cannula through the nasoantral wall can be accomplished in even the youngest patient unless there is a structural abnormality (e.g., septal deviation, stenosis of nares) obstructing the meatus. Wherever possible, the puncture should be made through the inferior meatus, but if this is impossible, puncture through the middle meatus or canine fossa may be resorted to. It is important to introduce the tip of the trocar and cannula as high under the midportion of the inferior turbinate as possible, where the nasoantral wall is thinnest or membranous. The tip of the trocar and cannula is directed toward the outer canthus of the eye. Care must be taken to avoid puncturing the floor of the orbital cavity or the lateral wall of the antrum. The trocar is withdrawn from the cannula and a syringe containing normal saline solution is attached to the cannula. The barrel of the syringe should always be withdrawn first to evacuate air or secretion from the antrum before introducing the solution into the antrum for lavage. Too much pressure in injecting the solution must be avoided, because, in the young child especially, the solution can readily be forced into the orbital space through a dehiscence in the bony floor of the orbit. If the antrum is found to be completely blocked, it is preferable to use a second cannula to irrigate the antrum thoroughly or to perform an intranasal antrostomy.[5, 5a, 5b]

In treating antral disease, we are always prepared to carry out an antrostomy whenever the antrum cannot be thoroughly cleared by syringing. If care is taken, an antrostomy is a benign and effective procedure that permits the antrum to drain thoroughly, enabling the mucosa to recover from the inflammatory process. The antrostomy opening usually closes in a matter of weeks but, should the sinusitis recur, the antrostomy may be repeated if necessary.

In performing an antrostomy, the opening of the nasolacrimal duct must be scrupulously avoided by keeping the anterior margin of the antrostomy posterior to the anterior and middle thirds of the inferior turbinate. In a child, the Caldwell-Luc operation is seldom necessary to treat inflammatory disease of the maxillary sinuses, but when it is performed, great care must be taken to avoid damaging unerupted teeth.

In the infant and younger child, ethmoid sinusitis is virtually always accompanied by and probably caused by maxillary sinusitis. Consequently, in treating ethmoiditis in the young patient especially, it is imperative to provide adequate drainage to the maxillary sinus on the involved side. However, the maxillary sinus should not be overlooked in treating ethmoiditis in the older patient.

Ethmoidectomy may be needed if there are intracranial complications or if the ethmoiditis fails to resolve. Middle turbinectomy alone may suffice, especially if there is involvement of the frontal sinus. Ethmoidectomy may also be important when intranasal polypectomy fails to control the recurrence of nasal polyps or to eradicate effectively a mucocele involving ethmoid sinuses. (Recurrent nasal polyposis is usually associated with cystic fibrosis.)[6, 6a, 6b]

The addition of the fiberoptic telescope has dramatically changed the approach to sinus surgery. Nasal endoscopy with magnification and bright light has aided in the diagnosis of many sinus conditions in both adults and children. In addition, surgery of the osteomeatal complex to decompress the maxillary, ethmoid, and frontal sinuses may be performed with direct visual control. Maxillary antrotomies via a puncture technique allow the passage of an endoscope into the maxillary sinus for direct inspection and biopsy or removal of soft tissue under direct vision.[6c]

The treatment of disease of any of the sinuses must include the correction of intranasal deformities (such as a severe deviation of the nasal septum) that clearly obstruct the drainage of one or more of the sinuses. Furthermore, as mentioned earlier, chronic infections, such as those of the adenoid and tonsils, and dental infections that involve the maxillary antrum must be attended to. In reviewing the cases of complicated sinusitis we treated over a 25-year period, it was found that none of the patients had adenoid and tonsil removal prior to the onset of the sinusitis.

At the onset of treatment for an acute upper respiratory tract infection, if possible, cultures should be obtained from the nose and the throat in an effort to identify the causative organism or organisms. Sensitivity tests on the bacteria cultured can be carried out to determine which antibiotic or antibiotics will be most effective. The most significant cultures are those obtained from aspiration of the involved sinus. If the patient with maxillary sinusitis is not making satisfactory progress on the treatment instituted, antral aspiration is indicated to obtain a specimen for culture and sensitivity tests to choose an antibiotic that is likely to be more effective.[8, 11, 15]

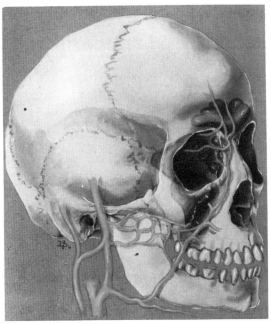

Figure 29–5. Venous drainage of orbital space and sinuses.

COMPLICATIONS

Orbital (Periorbital) Cellulitis. In children, the commonest orbitofacial complication of sinusitis is orbital cellulitis. There are numerous modes of spreading infection from the sinuses to the orbital space, including direct extension via the dividing bony wall from pressure necrosis of the bone; venous spread by direct invasion of the vessel wall via the communicating veins between the sinus and the orbit; a retrograde thrombophlebitis or periphlebitis; natural pathways, such as the anterior and posterior ethmoid vessel openings; or congenital bony dehiscences in the open suture lines, fascial planes, lymphatics, and perineural lymphatics (Figs. 29–3 through 29–5). In children under 1 year of age, direct extension from the maxillary sinus occurs, often without any ethmoid sinus involvement.

The clinical course of orbital cellulitis is fairly consistent. The cellulitis is preceded for several days by a suppurative rhinosinusitis, which rather quickly may proceed to an intensely red, inflammatory swelling and edema of the eyelids, completely closing the involved eye (Fig. 29–6). When the cellulitis originates in the ethmoids, the swelling is most pronounced in the upper eyelid, and the eyeball is pushed downward and forward (Fig. 29–7). If the maxillary sinus is the primary source, the lower lid is more swollen, and the eyeball is pushed upward and forward (Fig. 29–8). Proptosis of a variable degree is characteristic, and there can be a mild limitation of movement of the eyeball or a complete ophthalmoplegia. Pain is not a complaint, and the swelling is not usually tender. There may be a high fever, malaise, and an elevated white blood cell count. The majority of the cases of orbital cellulitis respond to the conservative measures described earlier.

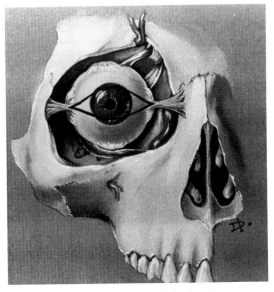

Figure 29–4. Contents of orbital cavity.

Orbital (Periorbital) Abscesses. An orbital cellulitis may advance to suppuration either because of delayed treatment or because of inadequate or ineffective management. In 75 per cent of our patients, the source was the ethmoid air cells, whereas in the other 25 per cent, the source was the maxillary sinus. Although the frontal sinus may be involved as part of the generalized sinus infection, it is unlikely to involve the orbital space directly.

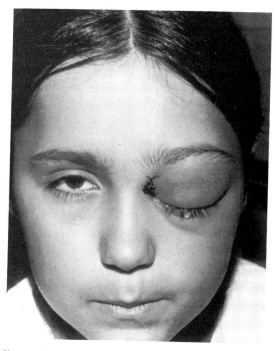

Figure 29–6. Appearance of orbital (periorbital) cellulitis.

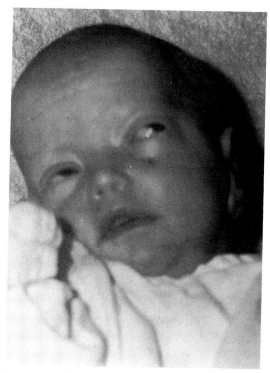

Figure 29–8. Orbital abscess in an infant causing upward displacement of the eye.

The periorbital inflammation may subside on treatment, but one must not assume that there may not be infection still in the periorbital space. Any residual proptosis indicates that there may be an abscess behind the orbit (Fig. 29–8).

When an abscess has formed in the orbital space, surgical drainage is imperative to prevent further complications and, in particular, optic atrophy due to prolonged proptosis secondary to the abscess. It is vitally important that the patient's vision be checked regularly and, if there is any deterioration in the visual acuity in the affected eye, drainage should be considered a surgical emergency. (We have seen three patients who became permanently blind in the involved eye when the drainage was delayed for more than 10 days.) Once complete optic atrophy has developed, the recovery of vision is unlikely.

In the infant, it is not usually necessary to make an incision into the orbital space to drain an orbital abscess. It will usually suffice to perform an antrostomy on the affected side. To drain an orbital abscess in the older patient, an incision of about 15 mm in length is made through the eyebrow over the superior orbital margin (Figs. 29–9 through 29–13). The incision is continued through periosteum to the inferior aspect of the supraorbital ridge, avoiding the supraorbital nerve. The periosteum of the roof of the orbit is elevated with a Freer elevator until purulent exudate is located. Usually it is found medially in the orbit, but occasionally it may be localized quite laterally. After the exudate has been evacuated, a 15-mm Penrose drain is introduced into the abscess cavity and retained with a suture through the margin of

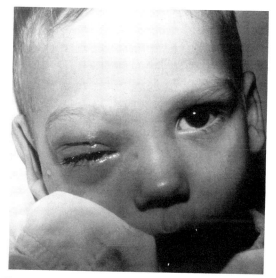

Figure 29–7. Orbital abscess causing downward displacement of the eye.

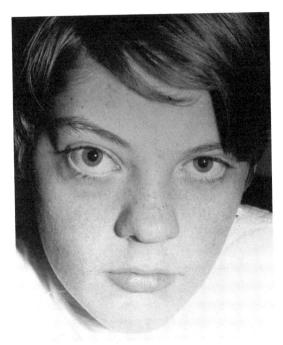

Figure 29–9. Proptosis from orbital abscess after apparent resolution of orbital inflammatiion.

the skin incision. If the eyelid itself is abscessed, it must be incised independently. If the frontal sinus is involved, it may be drained through the same incision.

In the young child, adenoidectomy may be carried out at the same time as drainage of the

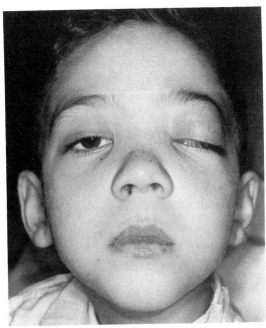

Figure 29–10. Orbital abscess before surgery.

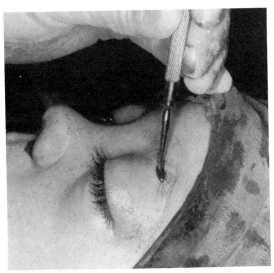

Figure 29–11. Exploring the abscess cavity in the patient in Figure 29–10.

orbital abscess and the maxillary sinus. In the older patient, we advocate removal of adenoid and tonsils when the child is fully recovered from the acute sinus process, usually before he or she leaves the hospital.[6]

Osteomyelitis. Osteomyelitis of the maxilla is considered a rather common complication of staphylococcal infection of the maxillary antrum, but in our experience, complete resolution has occurred after the maxillary sinus and orbital space have been drained. Osteomyelitis of the frontal bone from frontal sinusitis is not uncommon, and there may be an associated

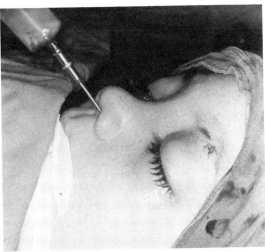

Figure 29–12. Aspiration of pus from the antrum (same patient as in Figures 29–10 and 29–11).

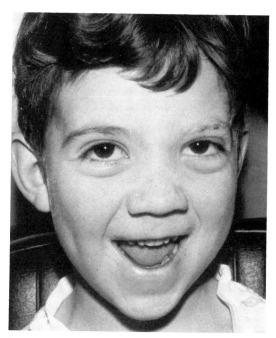

Figure 29–13. Same patient as in Figures 29–10 to 29–12, 5 days after surgery.

subdural empyema or brain abscess (Fig. 29–14). In such cases, in addition to intensive antimicrobial therapy, the diseased bone must be completely eradicated (see Chapter 10).

Cavernous Sinus Thrombosis. Fortunately, cavernous sinus thrombosis is relatively rare today, but when a patient with sinusitis develops bilateral orbital signs, the possibility must be considered. The cavernous sinuses are valve-less venous channels adjacent to the sphenoid sinus and the pituitary fossa. The lateral sinus wall contains the second, third, fourth, and fifth cranial nerves. The carotid artery, sympathetic plexus, and abducens nerve are related to the medial wall. Normally blood flows through the cavernous sinus slowly because of the relatively large size of the venous channels, combined with the fine trabecular network, which also impedes flow. As a result, bacterial organisms and emboli have a greater opportunity to initiate thrombosis in the cavernous sinus. Infection in the cavernous sinus is followed by a septic thrombophlebitis of the associated venous drainage apparatus. Obliteration of the lumen of the vein quickly follows, with subsequent expulsion of septic clots that pass to the cavernous sinus via venous drainage pathways of the nasal sinuses and orbit. Damage to the endothelium of the vessel wall by diffusion of toxins along the perivascular lymphatics may contrib-

ute to thrombosis of the anastomotic venous channels.[17]

The clinical picture is characterized by bilateral exophthalmos, chemosis, edema of the lids, and intraorbital congestion secondary to venous obstruction. The cranial nerve involvement accounts for proptosis, fixation of the eyeball, supraorbital headaches, and decreased vision. Generalized sepsis with meningeal irritation completes the picture.

Treatment consists of high doses of antibiotics given intravenously. The usefulness of anticoagulants has not been established; although heparin is reported to prevent propagation of a thrombus, it does not lyse the organized clot. Urokinase intravenously may prove to be effective in clot dissolution and recanalization. Surgical drainage of the source of the infection must be carried out as a part of the treatment.

One complication found in a patient with posterior ethmoiditis and sphenoiditis was an aneurysm of the internal carotid artery in the cavernous sinus (Fig. 29–15). This was not apparent on CT scan but was evident on a carotid angiogram. The patient, a 9-year-old girl, had a complete optic atrophy on one side and a partial optic atrophy on the other from a previous untreated sinus infection. She subsequently developed an abscess in the posterior fossa, which did not show on the initial CT scan. Along with the antibiotic treatment, the right carotid artery was occluded surgically, and eventually the brain abscess

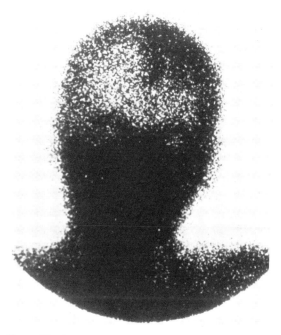

Figure 29–14. Gallium scan showing acute inflammatory reaction caused by frontal sinusitis and osteomyelitis of the frontal bone.

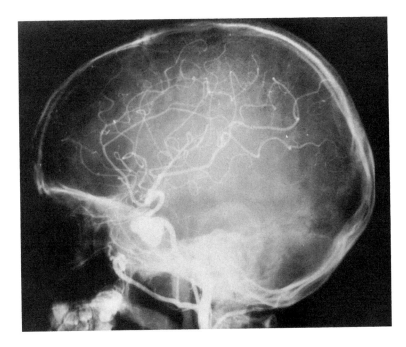

Figure 29–15. Carotid aneurysm in the cavernous sinus secondary to sphenoiditis.

drained. The child made a good recovery with some return of vision in one eye but none in the other.

Intracranial Complications. Intracranial spread of infection from the sinuses may result in subdural empyema, meningitis, cerebritis, or brain abscess. Intracranial extension can occur via the venous system or by direct extension from the sinus. Direct extension is usually through the posterior wall of the frontal sinus that has been affected by osteomyelitis or through immature bone in patients between the ages of 7 and 20 years, when the sinus is maturing. The dura becomes thickened and inflamed, and the extradural empyema results. Bacteria can then penetrate the dura along the vessels traversing the dura, producing subdural empyema, which in turn causes arachnoid inflammation.

Venous spread of infection occurs with progressive thrombophlebitis from the sinus mucosal veins to the cerebral veins. This allows bacteria into the subdural space, resulting in the empyema and the accompanying arachnoid inflammation. The arachnoid is relatively impermeable to bacterial invasion in adults, preventing meningitis. However, in infants the arachnoid is immature, and meningitis can result quite readily. The arachnoid does not prevent thrombophlebitis of the cerebral cortex, and this frequently complicates a subdural empyema, resulting in cerebral edema and infection with accompanying neurologic deficits. When brain tissue is adherent to an area of inflamed dura, brain abscess can result from ischemia or necrosis. Venous occlusion provides the ischemic environment for the growth of anaerobic and microaerophilic organisms. These then invade the cerebrum, resulting in an abscess.

Some form of intracranial extension must be considered in the patient with a suspected sinusitis who develops neurologic deficits, meningeal signs, or signs of elevated intracranial pressure. Conversely, sinus disease must be considered as a source of intracranial infection, even in a child with no prior history of sinus problems.

The most definitive test for the diagnosis of empyema, abscess, or cerebritis is the CT scan. Cerebrospinal fluid (CSF) findings may vary, depending on the location of the disease process. The subdural or parenchymal abscess may yield a sterile CSF culture. Lumbar puncture should be deferred if a space-occupying lesion is suspected, because of the risk of a brain herniation. Plain radiographs will often reveal a sinusitis but not the intracranial problem. Arteriography may show vessel displacement, suggesting intracranial pathology, but the CT scan is the study of choice.[4, 9, 12]

Treatment consists of parenteral antibiotics, drainage via craniotomy, anticonvulsants as needed, and supportive measures. Antibiotics should be effective against anaerobic and microaerophilic streptococci, staphylococci, pneumococci, and gram-negative bacteria. Even with adequate treatment, morbidity and mor-

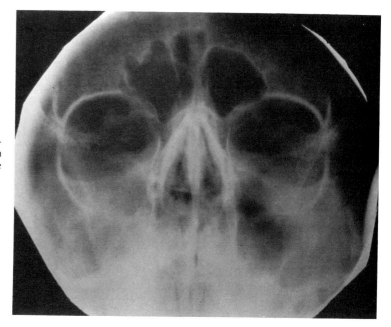

Figure 29–16. Routine sinus radio-graph showing an opaque antrum in a patient with fibrous dysplasia of the antrum.

tality remain high, so early diagnosis is essential to improved survival.[14]

Neoplastic Sinus Disease. In our experience, neoplastic lesions in children involving the ear, nose, and throat almost invariably occur as an acute inflammatory process or what appears to be an acute inflammatory process. However, the neoplasm may become apparent only when the acute inflammation has subsided. In general, the reason for this is uncertain, but possibly the growth is unrecognized until the symptoms and signs of the inflammation direct the attention of the parents or patient to an asymptomatic problem. This certainly holds true for neoplasms involving the paranasal sinuses in the child.

Indeed the neoplasm, by obstructing the ostium of the sinus, may be responsible for the sinus's becoming infected. The symptoms may mimic symptoms of sinusitis, for example, nasal obstruction, persistent rhinorrhea, swelling, and pain about the sinus.

A 14-year-old boy was treated for over a year for sinusitis because of severe pain in the region of the right antrum; standard x-ray views showed an opaque antrum (Fig. 29–16). On two occasions lavage was performed, and each time temporary proptosis was reported during the procedure. The pain persisted in spite of conventional treatment. Subsequent tomography showed a mass in the right antrum (Fig. 29–17). Biopsy by antrostomy was diagnosed as fibrous dysplasia. Resection of this growth along with the involved bone resulted in the complete relief of symptoms.

Thus, if there is anything unusual about the history or findings in patients with what initially appears to be a sinus infection, ultrasonographic studies are helpful in differentiating

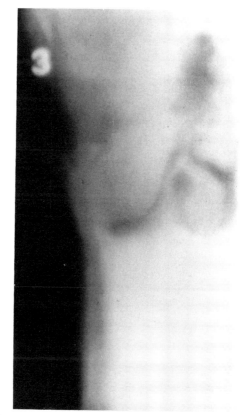

Figure 29–17. Tomogram of the patient in Figure 29–16, showing a mass in the antrum.

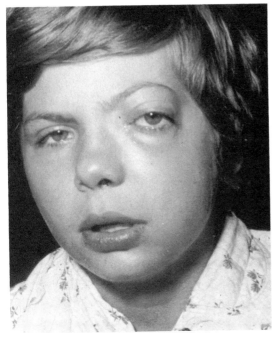

Figure 29–18. Ethmoid lymphosarcoma presenting as ethmoiditis with secondary orbital cellulitis.

fluid from solid tumors but must not be relied on completely. The nuclide studies with gallium or technetium are effective in distinguishing inflammatory changes from tumor masses.[12, 14]

Benign lesions we have encountered that simulated or were associated with sinusitis include fibrous dysplasia; angiofibroma; mucocele; hemorrhatoma; encephalocele in the maxillary sinus, internal nares, or nasopharynx; lymphangioma; ossifying fibroma; antrochoanal polyp; histiocytosis X; and dentigerous cysts. Malignant lesions encountered have been ascribed to rhabdomyosarcoma, chondrosarcoma, lymphosarcoma (Fig. 29–18), reticulum cell sarcoma, and transitional cell carcinoma. The treatment of neoplastic disease of the sinuses is beyond the scope of this chapter, and each tumor must be treated on an individual basis.

References

1. Axelsson A, Runze U: Comparison of subjective and radiological findings during the course of acute maxillary sinusitis. Ann Otol Rhinol Laryngol 92:75, 1983.
2. Brook I, Friedman E: Intracranial complications of sinusitis in children. Ann Otol Rhinol Laryngol 91:41, 1982.
3. Businco L, et al: Clinical and therapeutic aspects of sinusitis in children with bronchial asthma. Int J Pediatr Otorhinolaryngol 3:287, 1981.
4. English G: Sinusitis. Hagerstown, Md., Harper and Row, 1981.
4a. Wald ER, Ciponis D, Ledema-Medina J: Comparative effectiveness of amoxicillin-clavulanate in acute paranasal sinus infections in children. Pediatrics 77:795, 1986.
5. Engquist S, et al: Effects of drainage in the treatment of acute maxillary sinusitis. Acta Otolaryngol 95:153, 1983.
5a. Healy GB: Acute sinusitis in children. N Engl J Med 304:779, 1981.
5b. Siegel JD: Diagnosis and management of acute sinusitis in children. Pediatr Infect Dis 6:95, 1987.
6. Fearon B, Edmonds B, Bird R: Orbital-facial complications in children. Laryngoscope 89:947, 1979.
6a. Reilly JS, Kenna MA, Stool SE, et al: Nasal surgery in children with cystic fibrosis: Complications and risk management. Laryngoscope 95:1491, 1985.
6b. Crockett R, Smith RJH, Catlin FI, et al: Nasal and paranasal sinus surgery in children with cystic fibrosis. Ann Otol Rhinol Laryngol 96:367, 1987.
6c. Gross CW, Lazar RH, Gurucharri MJ: Pediatric functional endonasal sinus surgery. Otolaryngol Clin North Am 22:733, 1989.
7. Frazer J: Chronic sinusitis. In Bluestone D, Stool SE (eds): Pediatric Otolaryngology. Vol 2. Philadelphia, WB Saunders, 1972.
8. Jannert M, et al: Acute sinusitis in children—symptoms, clinical findings and bacteriology related to initial radiographic appearance. Int J Pediatr Otorhinolaryngol 4:139, 1982.
9. Kaufman D, et al: Sinusitis-induced subdural empyema. Neurology 33:123, 1983.
10. Laupus W, Pastore P: Acute sinusitis. In Bluestone D, Stool SE (eds): Pediatric Otolaryngology. Vol 2. Philadelphia, WB Saunders, 1972.
11. Lindahl L, et al: Chronic maxillary sinusitis. Acta Otolaryngol 93:147, 1982.
12. Ostfeld E, et al: Bone scintigraphic diagnosis of acute frontal sinusitis. Acta Otolaryngol 94:557, 1982.
13. Rachelefsky G, et al: Chronic sinusitis in children with respiratory allergy: The role of antimicrobials. J Allergy Clin Immunol 69:382, 1982.
14. Revonta M, Suonpaa J: Diagnosis and follow-up of ultrasonographical sinus changes in children. Int J Ped Otorhinolaryngol 4:301, 1982.
15. Shurin P: Inflammatory diseases of the nose and paranasal sinuses. In Bluestone D, Stool SE (eds): Pediatric Otolaryngology. Vol 1. Philadelphia, WB Saunders, 1983.
15a. Rohr AS, Spector SL, Siegel SC, et al: Correlation between A-mode ultrasound and radiography in the diagnosis of maxillary sinusitis. J Allergy Clin Immunol 78:58, 1986.
15b. Hawkins DB: Advances in sinus disease in pediatrics. Otolaryngol Clin N Am 22:553, 1989.
15c. Shapiro GG, Furukawa CT, Pierson WE: Blinded comparison of maxillary sinus radiography and ultrasound for the diagnosis of sinusitis. J Allergy Clin Immunol 77:59, 1986.
16. Slaven R: Relationship of nasal disease and sinusitis to bronchial asthma. Ann Allergy 49:76, 1982.
17. Sofferman R: Cavernous sinus thrombophlebitis secondary to sphenoid sinusitis. Laryngoscope 93:987, 1983.
18. Su W-Y, et al: Bacteriological study in chronic maxillary sinusitis. Laryngoscope 93:931, 1983.
19. Wald E, et al: Sinusitis and its complications in the pediatric patient. Pediatr Clin North Am 4:77, 1981.

CHAPTER 30

PARANASAL SINUS TRAUMA

Howard W. Smith, MD, DMD

Eiji Yanagisawa, MD, FACS

The sinus cavities of the face are protected by the facial bones, which vary in thickness and form. The purpose of the cavities is to lighten the facial skeleton, provide resonance for the voice, and increase the total mucosal surface, providing secretions to moisten the upper aerodigestive tract. The facial bones surrounding the sinus cavities serve as attachment for various muscles and provide support for the maxillary dentition. These functions relate to the developmental characteristics of the bone, which provides strength where needed in the form of buttress arches. The sinuses surround functioning cavities such as the orbit, the nose, and the mouth. Thus, the facial skeleton is a honeycomb of cavities[1] that is subject to trauma of various types. The facial skeleton functions to protect the skull from trauma coming from the front, whether directly, superiorly, inferiorly, or obliquely.

Trauma to the sinuses varies with respect to the shape of the object, the speed and direction of the object, and whether the skull is at rest or moving. Given our modes of transportation, sinus injury is increasingly complex in an increasing number of cases; however, the magnitude of sinus injury for any given case probably has not changed over the years. Falling objects, interpersonal contact, projectiles, and individual falls have been causes of sinus trauma for thousands of years.

Trauma to the face affects both the overlying soft tissue and the facial bones. Primary consideration has always been devoted to the soft tissue injury and specific facial bone fracture dislocations. Experimental studies have evalu-ated the effect of trauma on the facial skeleton as a whole and have described trauma complexes such as LeFort I, LeFort II, and LeFort III injuries.[2] The effect of trauma on the paranasal sinuses has not been emphasized because concern has been expressed mostly in terms of displacement of certain bones, the external appearance of soft tissue structures, and the major lines of fracture dislocation.

In this chapter the effect of trauma will be considered according to the individual sinuses, the site of trauma, and the direction of the blow.

ETHMOID SINUS TRAUMA

The ethmoid sinuses are readily injured by blows directed to the base of the nose in most directions except from above downward. Trauma at distances from the ethmoid air cells relates to the bones contacted, the size of the object, and the force involved. The ethmoid sinuses are of vital concern for proper functioning of the frontal sinus duct and traction support for the medial canthal tendon.

NASAL BONE TRAUMA

Direct blows to the nose from an anterior to posterior direction may be high or low. With small objects and moderate force low on the nose, the nasal bones are fractured, the septum is buckled, and, unless the object has great force and is sufficiently wide, the ethmoid sinuses are spared.

In direct blows to the nose with considerable force from an anterior to posterior direction at the upper, thicker part of the nose, the force tends to be transmitted backward. There are collapse of the lateral portions of the nasal bone and fracture of the nasal process of the frontal bone (the bony septum), with resulting trauma to the thin ethmoid sinuses, which have no substantial walls (Fig. 30–1). The bordering orbital and nasal cavity walls are collapsed and the ethmoid sinuses flattened backward.[3] The lower portion of the frontal sinus is frequently involved (Fig. 30–2).

Nasal bone trauma from below upward in an anterior to posterior direction tends to crumble the nasal bones upon themselves and collapse the root of the nose. More severe trauma in this direction will collapse the anterior wall of the frontal sinus and impact the solid root of the nose into the frontal sinus, usually sparing the anterior ethmoid air cells, which are protected by the lacrimal crest.

Blows to the nose from above downward in an anterior to posterior direction tend to flatten

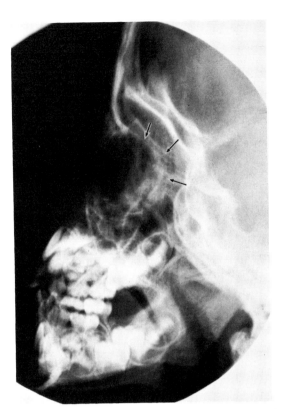

Figure 30–2. Lateral sinus radiograph showing a nasal fracture with ethmoid sinus compression (arrows).

the nasal bones, with considerable trauma to both the thin ends of the nasal bones and the cartilages of the septum. Again, the blow is more shearing in nature and does not compact the ethmoid sinuses.

True lateral trauma to the nose is hard to achieve with objects other than projectiles passing forward of the ethmoid sinuses.

Oblique trauma to the nose is most common. It causes compression detachment of the nasal bone from the nasal process of the maxillary bone on the contact side and hinging superiorly at the frontonasal suture. The opposite effect occurs on the side away from the contact. With increased force, the ethmoid sinuses are compressed by the nasal bones and the underlying perpendicular plate of the ethmoid bone. With an increase in the area of contact and the force applied, there is collapse of both medial rims of the orbit involving the ethmoid sinuses on both sides.

Oblique trauma to the nose from below upward is very similar to the effect of oblique blows on the horizontal plane, except that the frontal sinus is more likely to be involved in addition to the ethmoid sinuses.

Oblique trauma from above tends to produce less severe effects on the ethmoid sinuses; there

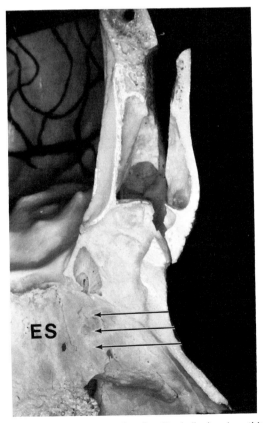

Figure 30–1. Photograph of split skull showing thin ethmoid (ES) posterior to nose (arrows).

is a shearing effect on the nasal bone, with some crushing of the ethmoid sinus distal to the point of contact.

In summary, the ethmoid sinuses are vulnerable in nasal trauma. Obviously, trauma with an impact size approximately equal to the interorbital width (2 to 3 cm) and with sufficient force destroys the sinuses with both forward and lateral transmission of force into the adjacent orbital cavities. It results in detaching and laterally displacing the orbital ligaments and exposing the floor of the anterior cranial fossa through fracture of the thin posterior wall of the frontal sinus. This is a serious injury fraught with cerebral complications and indifferent cosmetic results at best.

FRONTAL BONE BLOWS

Direct trauma to the frontal sinus in an anterior to posterior direction low at the root of the nose tends to collapse the anterior frontal sinus plate posteriorly (Fig. 30–3). The blow has to be forceful to affect ethmoid sinuses. The least force is required in the sagittal area, where the frontal plate is thinnest and where it is poorly supported by the weak walls of the anterior ethmoid air cells (Fig. 30–4). Blows in

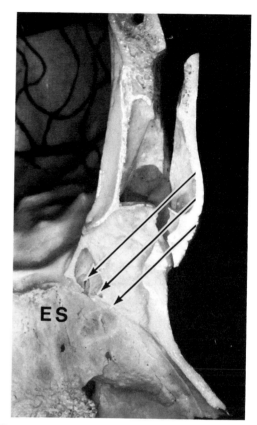

Figure 30–4. Photograph of split skull showing direction of frontal bone blows *(arrows)* to involve ethmoid sinuses *(ES)*.

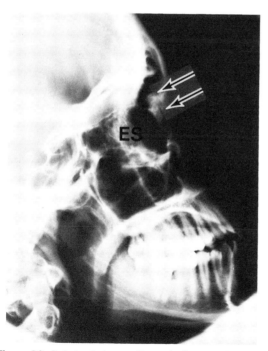

Figure 30–3. Lateral sinus radiograph showing direction of frontal bone blows *(arrows)* toward ethmoid sinuses *(ES)*.

this area have effects similar to those high on the nasal bones. The strong supraorbital ridge resists both fracture and separation, causing a coning of the force directly toward the trigone area of both ethmoid sinuses and the midline anterior cranial fossa.

Direct trauma to the frontal bone, about the level of the eyebrows, will involve the upper portion of the frontal sinus and spare the ethmoid air cells (Fig. 30–5).

Frontal bone trauma from below upward in an anterior to posterior direction tends to copy the effect of direct anterior to posterior trauma on the ethmoid sinus, but to a lesser degree, with the force dissipated into the frontal sinus cavity, a less crushing effect on the middle and posterior ethmoids, and less damage to the lower two thirds of the medial orbital rims. A combined segment of nasal process of the frontal bone and the nasal bones may be carried upward into the frontal sinus after sparing the anterior to posterior lacrimal crests.

Frontal bone trauma from above downward in an anterior to posterior direction is the least disturbing of the direct frontal bone blows in-

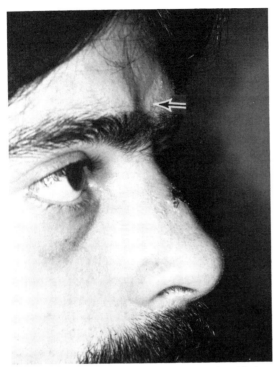

Figure 30–5. Frontal sinus collapse with ethmoid sinus injury *(arrow).*

volving the ethmoid sinuses. The force is transmitted to the bone and tends to hit the nose, causing an inward and downward collapse of the nasal bones. Cracks in the anterior frontal plate with depression occur. The anterior cells of the ethmoid sinus may be collapsed to accommodate the inwardly deflected nasal bones.

Blows to the frontal bone laterally in the region of the zygomatic process tend to collapse the zygoma into the orbit and do not result in ethmoid sinus trauma.

Oblique blows to the frontal bone are most damaging from the upward direction. Depending on the size of the object, the injury can be severe. Objects that are sufficiently small to avoid the shielding offered by the zygoma and the lateral one half of the superior orbital rim can directly encounter the relatively thin superior portion of the medial orbital rim. The force will collapse this portion of the rim, the underlying ethmoid air cells, the frontal sinus floor, and the anterior plate of the frontal sinus on the contact side. The root of the nose moves upward and laterally. The opposite ethmoid sinus may be spared.

MAXILLARY BONE BLOWS

The maxillary bone exposed to trauma consists primarily of the alveolus. Direct blows

from an anterior to posterior direction can be either high or low. High trauma affects the base of the nose and the anterior nasal spine. The force is directed onto a solid structure that is attached to the other facial bones by the thin margins of bone surrounding the maxillary sinus, plus the nasal septum medially and the pterygoid plates posteriorly. The force has a shearing effect, moving the alveolus and roof of the mouth posteriorly as a unit. This causes a horizontal transection of the maxillary sinus (LeFort I fracture) but does not invade the ethmoid sinus area. Blows lower in the alveolus from an anterior to posterior direction have essentially the same effect, plus variable loss of teeth and alveolar arch segmental fractures. This trauma may also cause sagittal splitting of the maxilla.

Greater force distributed over a larger anterior maxillary area, including the frontal process of the maxilla, causes separation of the maxilla from its superior structures along fracture lines that pass through the ethmoid sinuses. A triangular separation that includes the nose (LeFort II fracture) passes through the maxillary sinus higher than the LeFort I. This line of separation crosses the inferior orbital rim to include the root of the nose and then passes through the ethmoid sinuses (Fig. 30–6). This effect is created by anterior force more often directed from below or from above, the former

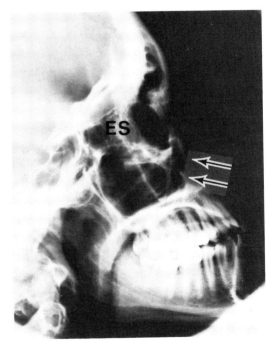

Figure 30–6. Lateral radiograph of skull showing direction of maxillary bone blow to injure ethmoid sinuses *(ES).*

causing impaction rather than simple shearing in the ethmoid sinus cavities (Fig. 30–7). The cribriform plate of the ethmoid bone may be comminuted, exposing the floor of the anterior cranial fossa and causing leakage of cerebrospinal fluid (CSF).

Direct maxillary bone blows from above downward usually cause loss of teeth in segments with areas of avulsion of the alveolus. The ethmoid sinuses are usually spared.

Direct maxillary bone blows from below upward can occur when patients open their mouths in the process of yelling when trauma is anticipated. If the object fits the mouth, there is likely to be a LeFort II injury, with impaction of the middle one third of the face against the base of the skull causing crushing of the ethmoid bones. This collision spares the intercanthal area, as it is cushioned by the ethmoid cells, and does not spread in the same way as blows to the root of the nose. Most of the direct blows to the maxillary bone from below upward occur after the mandible is broken at the condyles and the symphysis, allowing the object to contact the maxillary bone directly at the alveolus. The effect on the ethmoid sinus air cells is the same.

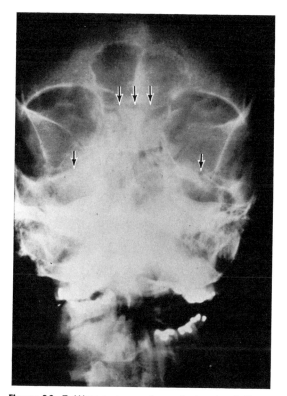

Figure 30–7. Waters view radiograph showing LeFort II facial fracture due to maxillary bone blow with ethmoid sinus injury *(arrows)*.

Lateral maxillary bone blows in the lower portion of the maxilla (alveolus area primarily) effect shearing of the maxilla and cause a LeFort I fracture that avoids the ethmoid sinuses. Higher blows usually encounter the zygoma as the primary site of contact.

Oblique trauma to the maxillary bone is effective in crushing the side of the maxillary bone, especially the nasal process, and collapsing it into the anterior ethmoid air cells. When the force of the trauma is spread over a larger area and the force is sufficient, a LeFort II type of fracture occurs; there is lateral and posterior displacement of the maxilla, causing crushing of the ethmoid air cells on the contact side to a greater extent than on the opposite side.

ZYGOMATIC BONE BLOWS

Blows to the zygoma from an anterior to posterior, lateral, or oblique direction do not cause collapse into the ethmoid area because there is an intervening orbital cavity. One exception is severe trauma to the zygoma in a lateral to medial direction, causing medial collapse of the medial portion of the inferior orbital rim into the ethmoid sinus if the blow was angled upward slightly.

ORBITAL CAVITY BLOWS

Anterior blows to the orbit[4] with objects sufficiently large to cause compression of the cavity contents apply direct pressure on the thin medial wall of the orbital cavity, which is made up in the lower one half by the orbital surface of the ethmoid air cells (Fig. 30–8). These air cells are easily collapsed medially.

Anterior blows to the orbit from above or below tend to be absorbed by either the superior orbital rim or the inferior orbital rim. The superior orbital rim is related medially more to the frontal sinus than the ethmoid, so the ethmoid sinus is less involved, unless the contents of the orbit are compressed.

Inferiorly directed blows from the front also tend to be absorbed by the orbital rim. The thick anterior crest of the lacrimal bone is well anterior to the ethmoid air cells, providing the ethmoid air cells with limited protection.

True lateral blows to the orbit are unrealistic. The oblique blows directed medially to the orbit have direct contact with the ethmoid air cells with only the soft tissue contents of the orbit to intervene. There is a direct soft tissue and a bony cushioning effect of the medial orbital

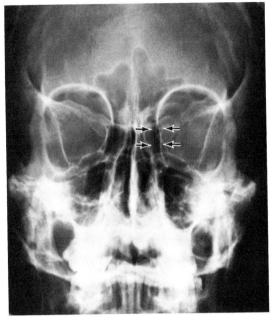

Figure 30–8. Caldwell view radiograph of sinuses showing thin party wall between orbit and ethmoid sinuses *(arrows).*

wall, which collapses to involve the lacrimal, nasal, and frontal bones (Fig. 30–9).

FRONTAL SINUS TRAUMA

Frontal sinus trauma is a serious problem immediately when the posterior wall is involved and cerebrospinal fluid leaks and cerebral herniation occur; delayed consequences include frontal sinus duct obstruction, infection, and mucocele formation. Blows from an anterior to posterior direction in the horizontal plane and from below up are the chief causes of serious injury to the posterior wall of the sinus and the nasofrontal ducts.

NASAL BONE BLOWS

Direct blows to the nasal bones from an anterior to posterior direction may be high or low. With small objects and moderate force, the nasal bones are fractured and collapsed inward, with a breaking of the bony septum and ethmoid sinus involvement. Greater force is required to collapse the floor of the frontal sinus, whether the blow is high or low on the nasal bone (Fig. 30–10). This is so because of the resistance offered by the medial portion of the superior orbital rim as it swings medially and downward to buttress the lacrimal bone. There is, however, little resistance directly beneath the frontonasal suture line where the thin ethmoid air cells meet with the frontal sinus and the orbit. Thus, if sufficient force is transmitted to the nose high up, the fractures are likely to occur at the weak points, namely the

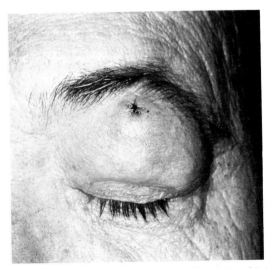

Figure 30–9. Photograph of patient with air in orbital cavity caused by blowing nose following ethmoid sinus injury.

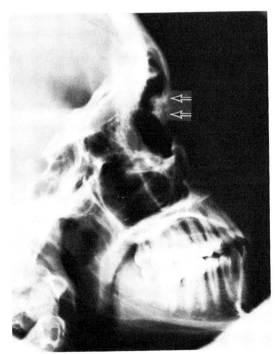

Figure 30–10. Lateral sinus radiograph showing direction of nasal blows causing frontal sinus injury *(arrows).*

thin anterior wall of the frontal sinus superiorly and the nasal frontal ethmoid suture lines laterally (Fig. 30–11).

Nasal bone trauma from below in an anterior to posterior direction tends to collapse the solid section of the nasofrontal bone junction upward and backward through the floor of the frontal sinus.

Anterior to posterior blows to the nose from above downward tend to flatten the nasal bones. Fractures occur below the frontonasal suture line, forcing the nasal bones apart and causing collapse of the ethmoid air cells. This type of blow to the nose may spare the frontal sinus.

Oblique trauma to the nose has the same effect as direct anterior to posterior trauma but tends to involve the frontal sinus more on the side of contact because the object hits directly on the nose. However, as the nose collapses, the force then comes in direct contact with the floor of the frontal sinus, with a shearing effect on the ethmoid sinuses. The nose is driven sideways into the opposite ethmoid sinus and orbital cavity. The magnitude of injury to the frontal sinus is increased if the oblique blow is from below upward and is less when the blow is from above downward.

FRONTAL BONE BLOWS

Direct trauma to the frontal bone from an anterior to posterior direction has an immediate effect on the frontal sinus (Fig. 30–12). Blows high on the forehead may cause a depressed fracture of the skull, with extension of the

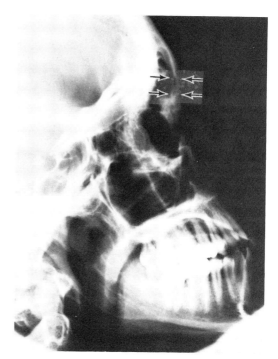

Figure 30–12. Lateral sinus radiograph showing thin anterior frontal sinus wall *(arrows)*.

fractures into the frontal sinuses involving both the anterior and posterior walls of the frontal sinus.[5] Blows slightly lower may cause depression fractures of the skull with some of the force absorbed by the anterior wall of the frontal sinus (Fig. 30–13). Blows even lower begin to

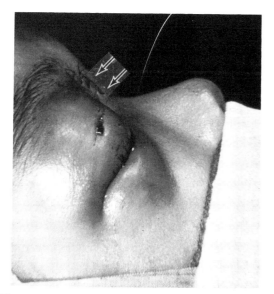

Figure 30–11. Photograph showing collapse of anterior wall of frontal sinus from nasal bone blow *(arrows)*.

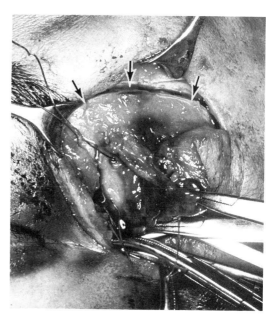

Figure 30–13. Photograph of collapsed anterior frontal sinus wall *(arrows)*.

involve the floor of the frontal sinus in addition to the anterior wall. In all instances, the posterior wall of the sinus is exposed to direct force, causing depressed fractures and involving the frontal lobe of the brain. The smaller the area of contact, the greater the danger of cerebral involvement. Large objects contact over a greater area; the thicker bone offers more resistance and thus protects the posterior wall of the frontal sinus.

Anterior to posterior frontal bone trauma from above downward and that from below upward have much the same effects. Because the force is tangential to the curvature of the bony surface, greater force can be sustained with less damage to the posterior wall of the sinus. Blows from above downward will cause a shearing effect medially on the superior orbital rim and the nose, separating the nasal ethmoid complex from the base of the skull with damage to the nasal frontal ducts.

Lateral and oblique blows to the frontal bone tend to involve one side more than the other, depending on the size of the object. Large objects can cause more damage on the contact side. Small objects tend to concentrate the damage, which often extends to the opposite frontal sinus.

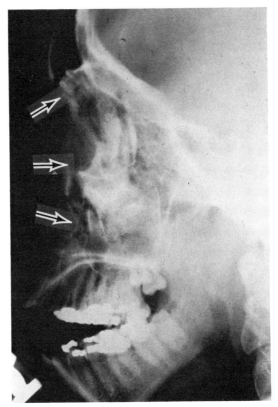

Figure 30–14. Lateral sinus radiograph showing direction of force toward frontal sinus from maxillary bone blow (arrows).

MAXILLARY BONE TRAUMA

Direct blows to the maxilla at the level of the inferior orbital rims contact the facial bones at a very weak point. Small objects tend to penetrate easily, as little resistance is offered by the medial walls of the maxillary sinus and the lower portion of the nose, which is chiefly cartilaginous. The ethmoid sinus, along with the maxillary sinuses and nasal and orbital cavities, absorbs the blow. Larger objects tend to have a wider area of contact, thus involving the maxillary alveolus (anterior nasal spine), the zygomatic bone, and the nasal bones. The path of least resistance is toward the ethmoid sinus and the floor of the frontal sinus (Fig. 30–14). The shearing effect superiorly may be along the frontal ethmoid junction. Laterally, the shearing occurs through the inferior orbital foramen and across the anterior and lateral walls of the maxillary sinus to the pterygoid plates. Medially, the septum and lateral walls of the nasal passages are sheared and the so-called LeFort II fracture occurs. In the majority of these injuries the frontal sinus is spared.

Blows from below upward directed toward this area result in an upward force to the nose and the floor of the frontal sinus (Fig. 30–15). Blows from above downward tend to spare the frontal sinus.

Blows to the maxillary bones at the level of the inferior orbital foramina laterally or obliquely tend to damage the frontal sinus less frequently. However, when the frontal sinus is affected, the site of contact is more likely to be involved, especially if the blow is directed from below upward.

Blows to the maxilla at the level of the alveolus are mostly unrelated to frontal sinus trauma unless the force is great and directed upward with the mouth open or to the undersurface of the mandible. The force directed to the anterior maxilla with the mouth open tends to displace the maxilla upward, impacting the nose against the floor of the frontal sinus (Fig. 30–16). The intensity of this trauma is reduced when the maxillary alveolar structures absorb some of the force. This is true with force directed to the maxilla from below upward indirectly from the site of trauma to the symphysis of the mandible. Often the condyles of the mandible are fractured and the symphysis is split, causing the anterior maxilla to receive

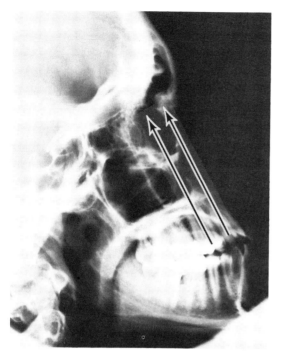

Figure 30–15. Lateral sinus radiograph showing direction of maxillary bone blows affecting floor of frontal sinus *(arrows)*.

the force directly. Great force is required to pass through the mandible and collapse the maxilla against the nose and carry it into the frontal sinus.

ZYGOMATIC BONE TRAUMA

Direct blows to the zygomatic bone either face on, from above down, or from below up in

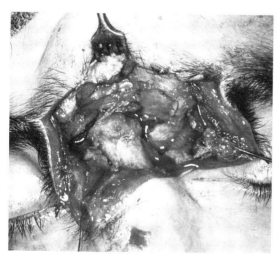

Figure 30–16. Photograph of nasal bones impacted into floor of frontal sinus.

the anterior to posterior direction have no effect on the frontal sinus.

Blows laterally or from an oblique, lateral to medial direction cause separation of the frontozygomatic suture and transmission of the force along the inferior orbital rim; the inferior medial portion of the orbital rim is carried medially and upward into the ethmoid sinus on the side of the injury (Fig. 30–17). Complete collapse of the orbit in severe trauma can cause disruption of the floor of the frontal sinus.

ORBITAL CAVITY BLOWS

Blows directed to the orbital cavity causing a build-up of pressure within the cavity will result in expansion of the medial and inferior walls of the cavity, producing a so-called blowout fracture into either the ethmoid or maxillary sinuses. Less common is the blow-up fracture causing upward collapse of the thin floor of the frontal sinus. Blows to the orbital cavity (other than those in a horizontal, anterior to posterior direction) tend to hit the rim. Those hitting the medial or superior rim likely have the effect of hitting the frontal bone directly and results cannot be attributed to true orbital

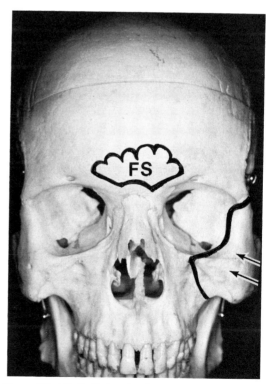

Figure 30–17. Skull showing frontal sinus outlined *(FS)* and zygomatic suture lines *(arrows)*.

cavity trauma. Blows directed to the orbit obliquely tend to have the same effect as direct blows to the nasal bones, frontal bone, or maxillary bone. The object size is important. Small objects tend to traumatize the orbital contents. Objects that are equal in size to or larger than the external orifice of the orbital cavity tend to cause compression and result in lateral expansion of the cavity size by invasion of the adjacent sinuses, with the frontal sinus being least involved.

MAXILLARY SINUS TRAUMA

The large paired maxillary sinuses are subject to direct trauma of their thin walls and to blows affecting all the facial bones.[11]

NASAL BONE TRAUMA

Direct blows to the nose from an anterior to posterior direction may be high or low. With small objects and moderate force low on the nose, the nasal bones are fractured, the cartilaginous portion of the nose collapses, and the force is absorbed by the pyriform aperture of the nose, collapsing the thin maxillary bone forming the piriform rim and anterior medial wall of the maxillary sinus. Larger objects contacting the same area require greater force to cause bilateral collapse. The blows are greatly cushioned by the soft tissue of the nose and the muscles of the face and upper lip. A more likely injury causes the nasal bones to simply collapse and allow force against the alveolus and anterior nasal spine from above; this results in a horizontal linear fracture across all surfaces of the maxillary sinus, plus the nasal septum and pterygoid plates, a LeFort I facial fracture (Figs. 30–18 and 30-19).

Anterior to posterior midline blows to the nose meet greater resistance in the nose itself. Thus force is directed against weaker areas, such as the ethmoid sinuses above. The inferior orbital foramina are involved laterally, with fracture lines passing below the zygomatic bones to affect all walls of the maxillary sinus (except the medial wall). A LeFort II facial fracture results.

Anterior to posterior parasagittal blows to the nose directly from above downward or from below upward tend to displace the nasal bones toward the opposite side and allow force to be directed toward the nasal process of the maxilla, anterior wall of the maxillary sinus, and inferior orbital rim, which subsequently collapses backward (Fig. 30–20).

Lateral and oblique trauma to the nose is much the same as that incurred with parasagittal anterior to posterior force: The nose is collapsed into the maxillary sinus superiorly on the side away from the site of trauma, thus exposing the anterior wall of the maxillary sinus and inferior orbital rim to the object. Thus, the lateral and/ or oblique blow causes a similar crushing effect on the medial superior portion of the maxillary sinus. The strong lacrimal bones tend to resist fragmentation but may be carried along in the direction of the force.

FRONTAL BONE BLOWS

The possibility of direct trauma to the frontal bone on the maxillary sinus is remote with

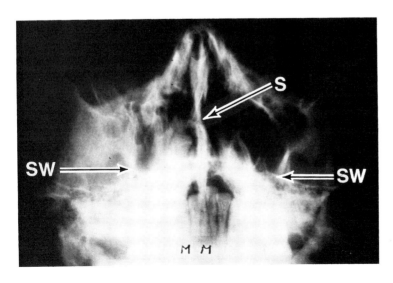

Figure 30–18. Waters view sinus radiograph showing LeFort I fracture. *S*, Septum; *SW*, maxillary sinus wall.

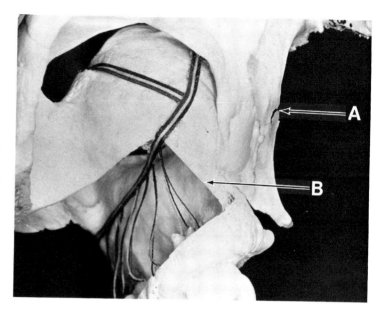

Figure 30–19. Photograph of prepared skull showing thin pterygoid plates and lateral maxillary sinus wall involved in LeFort fractures. *A*, Pterygoid plate; *B*, lateral maxillary sinus wall.

blows from most directions. However, trauma directed from above downward (when the force on the root of the nose is sufficient to collapse the frontal sinus) causes splaying of the ethmoid sinuses and medial orbital walls (Fig. 30–21). The nasal bones are forced downward into the nasal cavity, with collapse of the nasal process of the maxilla and disruption of the anterior superior portion of the maxillary sinus. The force may also create a LeFort II facial fracture (Fig. 30–22).

Parasagittal blows to the frontal bone from above downward are met with some resistance because the frontal bone is thick laterally beyond the superior orbital foramen. This protects the inferior orbital rim and maxillary sinus.

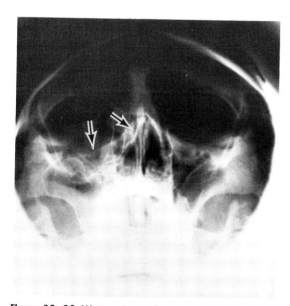

Figure 30–20. Waters view radiograph of sinuses showing effect of parasagittal nasal bone trauma on maxillary sinus *(arrows).*

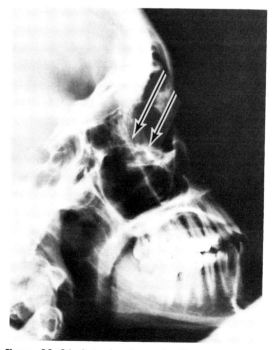

Figure 30–21. Lateral radiograph of sinuses showing direction of frontal sinus blows affecting maxillary sinus *(arrows).*

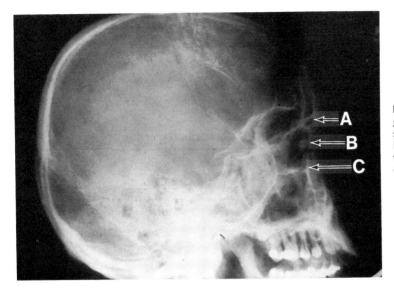

Figure 30–22. Lateral sinus radiograph showing effect of low frontal sinus blow from above downward. *A*, Fracture of lower frontal sinus; *B*, inward displacement of nasal bones; *C*, orbital rim fracture.

MAXILLARY BONE BLOWS

If high, blows to the maxillary bone from an anterior to posterior direction have to be parasagittal to be distinguished from midline trauma directed primarily to the nose and secondarily to the maxillary sinus. Direct trauma over the sinus causes immediate collapse of the anterior maxillary wall, with crushing of the lateral rim of the piriform aperture of the nose (Fig. 30–23). The nasal frontal process of the maxilla is pushed backward into the sinus, and the weak medial section of the inferior orbital rim is pushed backward and downward, carrying the inferior orbital nerve and vessels with a small portion of the anterior floor of the orbit (Fig. 30–24). There may also be inward displacement of the anterior and posterior orbital rims of the lacrimal bone. Force is contained in this area by the strong lateral buttress of the zygomatic bone.

Maxillary bone trauma in the midline directed anteriorly to posteriorly in the region of the anterior nasal spine and alveolar area causes posterior displacement of the alveolus. Fracture lines pass horizontally through all walls of the maxillary sinus, and a LeFort I facial fracture results (Fig. 30–25).

Anterior to posterior blows directed toward the maxilla from below upward tend to collapse the midfacial structures upward. Fracture lines pass through the maxillary sinus obliquely on the anterior surface and horizontally, laterally, and posteriorly, sparing the medial sinus wall

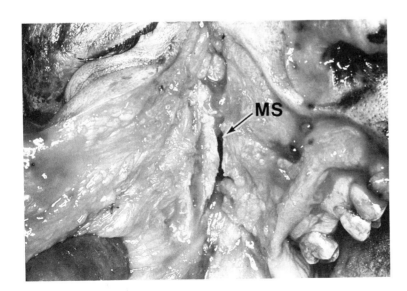

Figure 30–23. Photograph showing direct trauma to maxillary sinus *(MS)*.

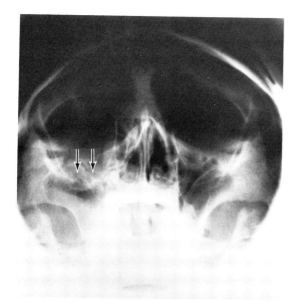

Figure 30–24. Waters view radiograph of sinuses, showing collapse of anterior wall of maxillary sinus *(arrows)*.

ward collapse into the oral cavity, with crushing of the anterior wall of the maxillary sinus laterally (Fig. 30–26). Lateral or oblique blows from above downward cause segmental fractures of the alveolus with a less complete LeFort I facial fracture. Lateral or oblique blows from below may cause a LeFort I type of fracture on the side receiving trauma, with an outward displacement of the zygoma instead of a fracture running through the lateral wall of the maxillary sinus. Another variation is a LeFort II type facial fracture on the side of injury and a LeFort III type facial fracture on the side opposite. This causes considerable disruption of the maxillary sinus on the side incurring injury but minimal involvement of the maxillary sinus on the opposite side.

ZYGOMATIC BONE TRAUMA

The zygomatic bone constitutes the superolateral wall of the maxillary sinus. Any dislocation of the body of the zygoma causes injury to the maxillary sinus.

Direct trauma to the zygomatic bone in an anterior to posterior direction in the horizontal plane will force the bone backward (Fig. 30–27). It tends to hinge on the zygomatic process of the frontal bone. The dislocation usually occurs in the direction of least resistance, which is medially. In addition, the bone may rotate during the process of dislocation (Fig. 30–28). For the maxillary sinus, the net result is that it

to constitute a LeFort II facial fracture. Additionally, the maxillary sinus may be directly entered through segmental fractures of the alveolar process.

Lateral and oblique blows to the maxilla on a horizontal plane tend to have a shearing effect on the maxilla, causing a LeFort I facial fracture. Along the fracture line there may be segmental fractures of the alveolus and down-

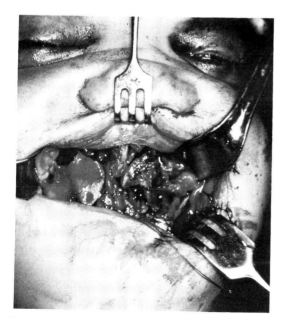

Figure 30–25. Severe facial fractures from a maxillary bone blow.

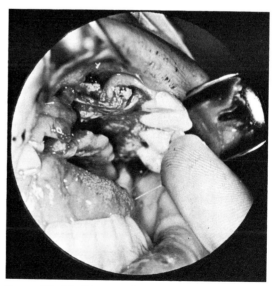

Figure 30–26. Photograph showing oblique blow to maxilla from below upward.

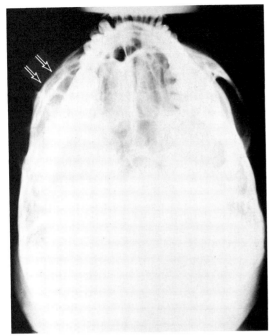

Figure 30–27. Submentovertical radiograph of antero-posterior path of zygoma toward maxillary sinus *(arrows)*.

is made smaller by invasion of either the maxillary process of the zygoma or the zygomatic process of the maxilla, with lowering of the body of the zygoma into the superolateral recess of the maxillary sinus (Fig. 30–29). This invasion can occur with anterior to posterior trauma from either above or below.

Trauma to the zygomatic bone from a lateral to medial direction on the horizontal plane tends to collapse the prominence of the bone by medial displacement along the inferior orbital rim into the zygomatic process of the maxilla. Occasionally, the frontozygomatic suture is disrupted completely, and the whole bone is pushed into the orbital cavity. This is more possible in lateral trauma directed from above downward, whereby the body of the zygoma is forced more into the maxillary sinus than into the orbital cavity. Trauma directed upward from a lateral position tends to allow hinging at the frontozygomatic suture or fracture of the zygomatic process of the frontal bone; the body of the zygoma is directed more toward the orbit, causing an inward and upward movement of the upper lateral portion of the maxillary sinus wall. All zygomatic fractures with dislocation disrupt part of the orbital floor, which constitutes a portion of the roof of the maxillary sinus.

Oblique trauma to the zygomatic bone from a lateral to medial direction causes changes in position of the zygoma and its relation to the maxillary sinus, similar to true lateral trauma

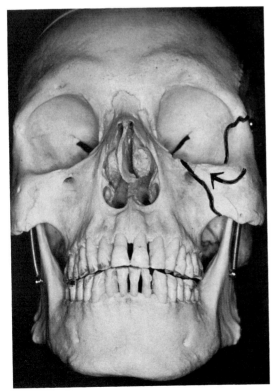

Figure 30–28. Photograph of skull showing zygomatic fracture with rotation displacement *(arrow)*.

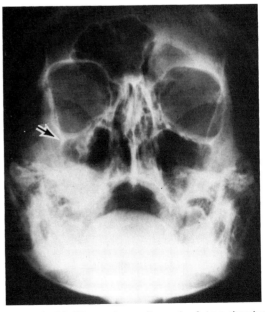

Figure 30–29. Waters view radiograph of sinus showing tripod fracture of zygoma with collapse into the maxillary sinus *(arrow)*.

directed either from above downward or from below upward.

A rare dislocation results from trauma directed obliquely to the zygomatic bone from medial to lateral, causing outward displacement of the zygoma and unroofing the maxillary sinus superiorly and laterally.

BLOWS TO THE ORBITAL CAVITY

Anterior blows to the orbital cavity with objects sufficiently large to cause increased intracavitary pressure result in collapse of the floor of the orbit. This is the roof of the maxillary sinus. The weakest portion of the orbital floor is along the medial surface behind the inferior orbital rim backward toward the inferior orbital fissure medial to the inferior orbital canal. Another area of weakness is lateral to the inferior orbital canal. A collapsed floor of the orbit may include the inferior orbital canal and its contents. The maxillary sinus is directly invaded from above by the herniated contents of the orbital cavity, including orbital fat, inferior rectus muscle, and the thin bone party wall. In some instances, the thin floor may crack in an anterior to posterior direction, spring downward with the ruptured contents, and spring back up again, trapping the inferior rectus muscle in the linear fracture line (Figs. 30–30 and 30–31).

Other blows to the orbital cavity will have

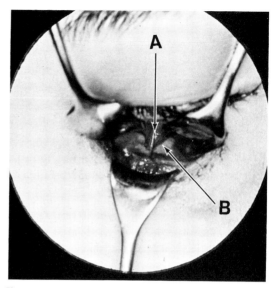

Figure 30–31. Photograph of orbital floor showing inferior rectus muscle trapped in orbital floor fracture. *A*, Inferior rectus muscle; *B*, orbital floor.

similar effects but require greater force to achieve the results obtained by direct anterior to posterior trauma.

SPHENOID SINUS TRAUMA

The sphenoid is the sinus most protected from trauma.[12] Crushing blows to the skull, capable of fracturing its base and passing through the sphenoid sinus, are capable of killing the patient or causing cerebral damage so great that treatment of the sinus injury becomes inconsequential. Fractures of the base of the skull from injuries to the calvarium passing through the sphenoid sinus are less common than those resulting from direct trauma to the sinus.

Trauma to the sphenoid sinus requires a well-aimed blow from a small object. Because the sphenoid sinus varies in size and shape, depending on the extent of pneumatization, the object must traverse the sinus after crushing its anterior wall to deliver significant injury to the other sinus walls, which protect the dura, cerebrospinal fluid, and cerebral contents. Delayed effects, of course, include infection, sinus ostium closure, and mucocele formation.

NASAL BONE TRAUMA

Trauma to the nose in an anterior to posterior direction and in the horizontal plane is in direct

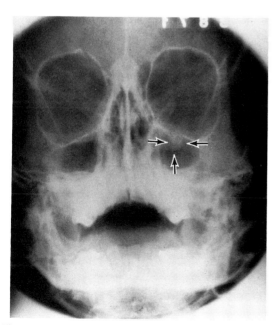

Figure 30–30. Caldwell view radiograph of sinus showing a blow-out fracture of the orbit *(arrows)*.

line with the sphenoid sinus. Blows with small objects contacting the nose high at the base of the nasal bone meet with little resistance once the frontonasal junction has collapsed. The orbital cavity, nasal cavity, and ethmoid sinuses offer little resistance. Inferiorly, farther back the rostrum of the sphenoid and the basisphenoid offer resistance, thus deflecting the force upward into the sphenoid sinus (Fig. 30–32).

Blows to the nasal bones from above downward and below upward, laterally and obliquely, tend to miss the sphenoid sinus.

Blows to the nose in the lower cartilaginous portion, directed slightly upward, have direct access to the sphenoid sinus in a manner similar to that for direct anterior to posterior blows with objects of limited size (Fig. 30–33).

FRONTAL BONE TRAUMA

Trauma to the inferior portion of the frontal bone at the junction of the nasal bone, in the anterior to posterior direction and on a horizontal plane, can affect the sphenoid sinus. Such injury must traverse the cribriform plate of the ethmoid and the frontal lobe skull base. It is less direct than the force from anterior to posterior blows to the nasal bones, which meet less resistance en route to the sphenoid sinus.

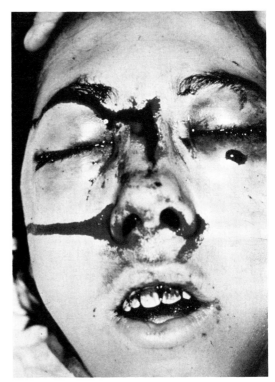

Figure 30–33. Sphenoid sinus injury from a nasal bone blow.

MAXILLARY BONE BLOWS

Objects capable of contacting the hard palate of the maxilla with the mouth open have a direct route to the sphenoid sinus (Fig. 30–34). The distance is even shorter than that through the nasal bone route. The thin palatal bone is easily split in the midline, causing the alveolus to be splayed outward (Fig. 30–35). The thin vomer and the perpendicular plate of ethmoid bone offer minimal resistance. The rostrum of the sphenoid and the sphenoid body direct the object upward into the sphenoid sinus.

ZYGOMATIC BONE TRAUMA

Blows to the zygomatic bone have little or no significant relation to fractures of the sphenoid sinus unless the pneumatization of the sphenoid sinus involves the greater wings of the sphenoid bone.

ORBITAL CAVITY BLOWS

Oblique blows from lateral to medial directed toward the orbit meet only soft tissue

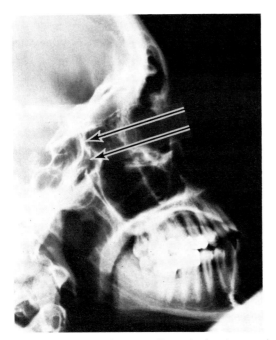

Figure 30–32. Lateral sinus radiograph showing nasal trauma route to sphenoid sinus (arrows).

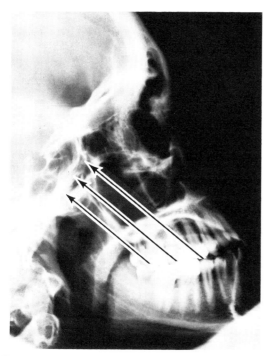

Figure 30–34. Lateral sinus radiograph showing oral route to sphenoid sinus injury *(arrows)*.

resistance en route to the sphenoid sinus. The lamina papyracea of the ethmoid sinuses offers no resistance. The medial superior recess of the maxillary sinus is also surrounded by thin bone offering little or no resistance. A direct blow with an object of limited size is required because the distance is greater than either the transnasal or transpalatal route to the sphenoid sinus.

SINUS OSTIA TRAUMA

FRONTAL

Fractures of the frontal sinus, including injury to the posterior wall with dural tears, CSF leaks, and cerebral herniation, can cause obliteration of the nasal frontal duct. Fractures of the anterior wall of the sinus above the level of the superior orbital rim usually do not obliterate the ducts. Blows to the base of the nose and lower frontal sinus cause backward and downward dislocation, crushing the duct as it passes inferiorly to the ethmoid sinuses and on into the nose (Fig. 30–36). Recognition of duct injury is of great importance in treating frontal sinus injuries.

ETHMOID

The ethmoid sinuses constitute a virtual honeycomb of air cells lateral to the nose and medial to the orbit.[13] They are grouped into anterior cells and posterior cells according to their openings. The anterior cells open into the middle meatus below the middle turbinate, and the posterior air cells open above the middle turbinate. Ethmoid duct obstruction due to trauma can lead to mucocele formation. Because the frontal sinus ducts may not enter the nose directly but drain into the ethmoid air cells, injury to the ethmoid sinus air cells may cause secondary frontal sinus problems.

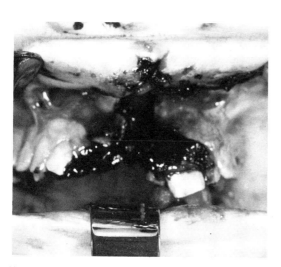

Figure 30–35. Sphenoid sinus trauma via the oral cavity route.

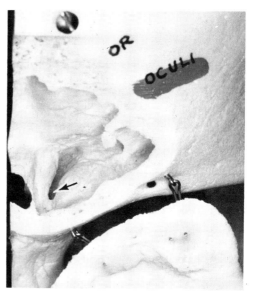

Figure 30–36. Photograph of prepared skull showing location of frontal sinus duct *(arrow)*.

MAXILLARY

The maxillary sinus ostium is located superiorly and medially in the sinus and enters the nose through the narrow ethmoid infundibulum. Its function is directly related to a normally functioning sinus mucosa. A functioning ostium is essential. Its location seems well suited to escape injury in a high percentage of sinus trauma cases.

SPHENOID

The opening in the sphenoid sinus is above and behind the superior nasal concha. It is located on the posterior nasal wall but may also be on the lateral wall, depending on the extent of posterior ethmoid sinus pneumatization. Drainage from the sphenoid sinus, like that of the maxillary sinus, is via ciliary action, as the opening is well above the floor of the sinus.

VISUALIZATION BY COMPUTED TOMOGRAPHY

Conventional radiographs record all structures in the path of the x-ray beam. Those structures nearest to the x-ray film are recorded more clearly; the structures nearer the x-ray tube are less clear. On a conventional x-ray view it is not possible to distinguish all aspects of facial skeletal anatomy lying between the film and the x-ray tube, since portions of the facial skeletal bones overlap. The x-ray film records only varying degrees of density. Density is increased by overlapping bones, producing a white-out on the x-ray film. The tomographic x-ray does not record all the structures on a single film but only portions of each facial bone, depending on the view selected and the level or slice taken. Therefore, it is necessary to have multiple views of the same anatomy all in the same direction but at different levels (slices).

Operators accustomed to the four basic views on conventional plain film, namely Caldwell, Waters, lateral, and submentovertical (base), will need to reorient when viewing computed tomography (CT) scans, since the slices do not present the facial bones in exactly the same direction.[6] Slight distortions caused by positioning errors in the CT scan are more disturbing, since this view may record a different level on the right and left sides.

The vertical view, the basal CT view, and the axial CT view are all in the same direction, but each displays the anatomy in its own way. The conventional submentovertical view is compressed to a composite image. The basal CT view represents a layer or cut with fogging of the structures both proximal and distal to the layer selected. The CT records a thin slice of the anatomy at a selected distance between the tube and the recording mechanism. The recorded data are reconstructed to produce an x-ray film image at each 5-mm slice.

On the *axial CT*, 5-mm-thick slices are obtained along the infraorbital meatal plane, starting at the maxillary alveolar level and proceeding upward through the frontal sinus (Fig. 30–37). From these slices, four are selected for careful study, namely the dentoalveolar (Fig. 30–38), midmaxillary (Fig. 30–39), orbital floor (Fig. 30–40), and midorbital levels (Fig. 30–41).

The *coronal CT* is oriented in a manner similar to a conventional Caldwell radiograph, in which all the facial bones are displayed in layers or slices. The slices are 5 mm apart and start at the surface of the frontal sinus and proceed posteriorly (Fig. 30–42). From this series of slices, levels are selected for study, namely the frontal sinus plane (Fig. 30–43), anterior orbital roof plane (Fig. 30–44), midorbital plane (Fig. 30–45), retrobulbar plane (Fig. 30–46), orbital fissure plane (Fig. 30–47), and choanal plane (Fig. 30–48).

Soft tissue swelling and hematoma tend to

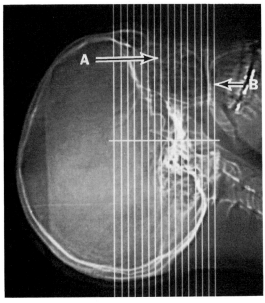

Figure 30–37. Axial CT scan. *A,* Maxillary alveolar plane; *B,* midorbital plane.

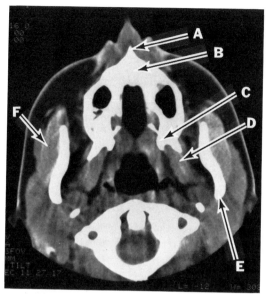

Figure 30–38. Axial CT scan—maxillary alveolar plane. *A*, Anterior nasal spine; *B*, hard palate; *C*, maxillary tuberosity; *D*, medial pterygoid muscle; *E*, vertical ramus of mandible; *F*, masseter muscle.

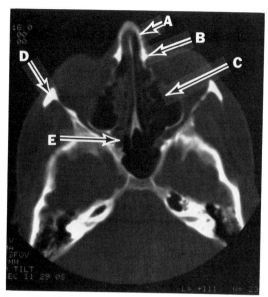

Figure 30–40. Axial CT scan—orbital floor plane. *A*, Nasal bone; *B*, anterior lacrimal crest; *C*, maxillary sinus; *D*, zygoma; *E*, sphenoid sinus.

obscure facial bone anatomy in conventional radiographs, whereas CT clearly shows the soft tissue swelling as well as bony facial skeletal anatomy. The CT is especially helpful in the following ways: separation of facial bone structures from soft tissue; identification of soft tissue elements such as swelling, hematoma, fluid levels, orbital contents, tumors, and foreign bodies; contiguous 5-mm submental analysis of separate facial bones and suture lines, separation of bony fragments, and overlap of bones; and identification of fluid, abnormal linear density, disappearing fragments, subcutaneous and orbital air, and displaced structures.

With these factors, it is possible to trace the

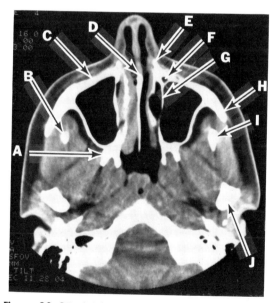

Figure 30–39. Axial CT scan—midmaxillary plane. *A*, Pterygoid process of sphenoid bone; *B*, coronoid process of mandible; *C*, anterior wall of maxillary sinus; *D*, perpendicular plate of ethmoid; *E*, frontal process of maxilla; *F*, bony canal for lacrimal duct; *G*, medial wall of maxillary sinus; *H*, anterior zygomatic arch; *I*, coronoid process of mandible; *J*, condyloid process of mandible.

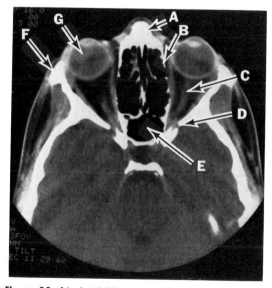

Figure 30–41. Axial CT scan—midorbital plane. *A*, Glabella; *B*, lamina papyracea; *C*, optic nerve; *D*, superior orbital fissure; *E*, sphenoid sinus; *F*, zygoma; *G*, eye globe.

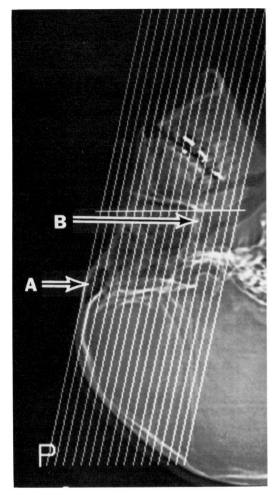

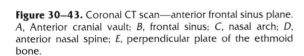

Figure 30–42. Coronal CT scan—plane of cuts. *A*, Frontal sinus; *B*, choana; *P*, plane of cut.

Figure 30–43. Coronal CT scan—anterior frontal sinus plane. *A*, Anterior cranial vault; *B*, frontal sinus; *C*, nasal arch; *D*, anterior nasal spine; *E*, perpendicular plate of the ethmoid bone.

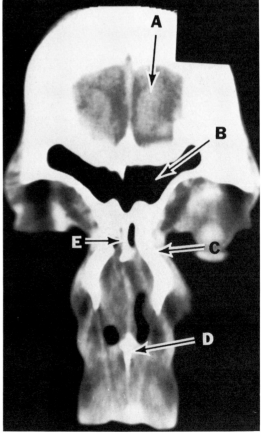

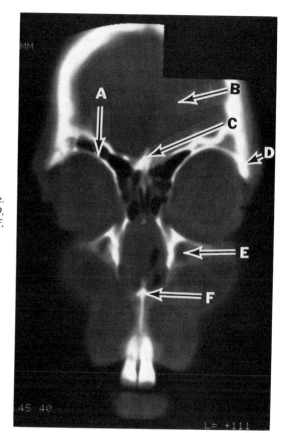

Figure 30–44. Coronal CT scan—anterior orbital roof plane. *A*, Orbital roof; *B*, anterior cranial fossa; *C*, crista galli; *D*, orbital process of the frontal bone; *E*, maxillary sinus; *F*, anterior nasal spine.

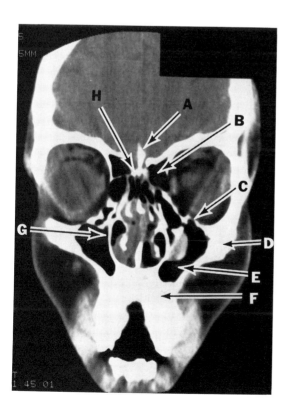

Figure 30–45. Coronal CT scan—midorbital plane. *A*, Crista galli; *B*, ethmoid sinus; *C*, infraorbital canal; *D*, zygoma; *E*, maxillary sinus; *F*, alveolus; *G*, medial wall of the maxillary sinus; *H*, cribriform plate.

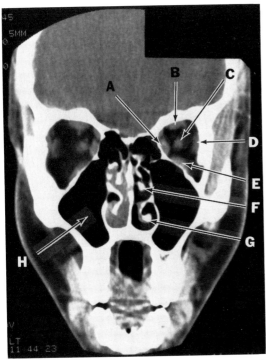

Figure 30–46. Coronal CT scan—retrobulbar plane. *A,* Medial rectus muscle; *B,* superior rectus muscle; *C,* optic nerve; *D,* lateral rectus muscle; *E,* inferior rectus muscle; *F,* middle turbinate; *G,* inferior turbinate; *H,* maxillary sinus.

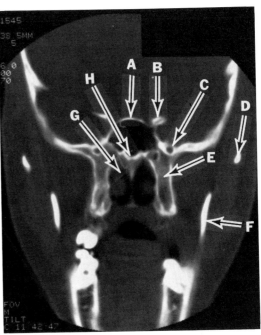

Figure 30–48. Coronal CT scan—choanal plane. *A,* Sphenoidal plane; *B,* lesser wing of sphenoid; *C,* foramen rotundum; *D,* zygoma; *E,* pterygoid process of sphenoid bone; *F,* coronoid process of mandible; *G,* choana; *H,* vomer.

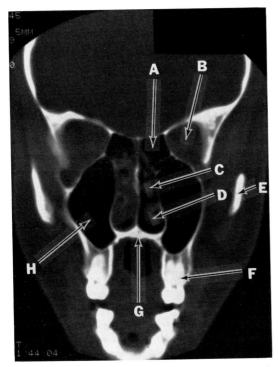

Figure 30–47. Coronal CT scan—orbital fissure plane. *A,* Ethmoid sinus; *B,* posterior orbital cavity; *C,* middle turbinate; *D,* inferior turbinate; *E,* zygoma; *F,* molar tooth; *G,* hard palate; *H,* maxillary sinus.

entire substance of a single bone, such as the zygoma; to analyze its structure completely to determine its articulation with adjacent bones; and to judge its position when displaced. Similar analysis can be made for known possible fracture combinations, such as blow-out orbital fractures, the orbit, LeFort I, LeFort II, LeFort III fractures, sinus walls, and orbital walls.

CT remains the procedure of choice for paranasal sinus and nasal cavity imaging in the diagnosis of facial bone trauma. Three-dimensional reformation of serial 3-mm axial CT slices for facial bone fractures is becoming increasingly helpful in diagnosis for treating facial bone fractures.[7]

Trauma deep to the paranasal sinuses is best displayed by magnetic resonance imaging. CT scans in the nasopharyngeal area require intravenous contrast injection.

Interpretation of CT scans of the facial bones is improved by utilizing the concept of protective struts, pillows, and buttresses. The struts include the nasal septum, nasal bones, orbital floor, and orbital roof.[8] These struts are protected by lateral and medial pillows such as the superior alveolar ridge, the lateral maxillary sinus wall, the orbital wall, the malar eminences, and the orbital processes of the frontal bones.[9] The buttresses of the facial bones *resist backward and upward displacement* and are three in number: the zygomatic process of the temporal bone, the pterygoid processes of the sphenoid bone, and the greater wing of the sphenoid bone. Three buttresses that resist *upward pressure* are the zygomatic process of the frontal bones, the nasal process of the frontal bones, and the roof of the mandibular fossa.[10]

The thin bones of the face that are "on end" show fairly well in routine plain sinus x-ray films. When the bones are fractured, they are displaced and appear to be missing; this is especially true of the LeFort I, II, and III variations, especially LeFort II and III, since these fractures occur along lines of weakness. Various combinations of these three general categories occur. The CT scan is helpful in tracing the position of the major fragments, such as the alveolus, the nasal compound, and the zygomas. These major components provide the building blocks for reconstruction. The process is one of anchoring the zygomas laterally and the nasal compound medially, then "building down" to the occlusion if the mandible is shattered. If the mandible is intact, the process is reversed to "building up" based upon the occlusion.

In either instance, the need for proper occlusion must be met, and the "floating segments" will line up eventually as in a jigsaw puzzle. The multiple fractured sinus areas accompanied by edema and hematoma make the CT scan a must for intelligent evaluation and treatment planning.

RIGID PLATE FIXATION

As with other bones, rigid compression plate reduction and fixation of fractures will promote osteosynthesis, resulting in more rapid primary bone healing. Even when the bones cannot be adequately aligned for compression, plating will allow favorable alignment and fixation of the segments. This is particularly true in areas that are not under functional stresses. The plates also bridge gaps of missing bone better than other techniques, allowing better stability and healing as well as a better facial contour. The use of facial plating may avoid the need for craniofacial suspension wires or head frames, as well as intermaxillary fixation.

The technique is well described in other works. Briefly, it is accomplished using self-tapping or nonself-tapping screws and multihole stainless steel plates. The correct-size plate is chosen (either T-shaped, L-shaped, or straight) and contoured for the area to be reconstructed. Holes are drilled into the broken fragments, the depth is measured, and screws are applied. Technically, miniplates are often easier to apply and more stable in a number of areas in mid-facial fractures. The disadvantage is that many of the plates need to be removed in the future.[14–17]

References

1. Yanagisawa E, Smith HW: Normal radiographic anatomy of the paranasal sinuses. Otolaryngol Clin North Am 6:429, 1973.
2. LeFort R: Etude experimentale sur les fractures de la machoire superieure. Rev Chir Paris 23:208, 360, 479, 1901.
3. Duvall AJ III, Banouetz JD: Nasoethmoidal fractures. Otolaryngol Clin North Am 9:507, 1976.
4. Smith B, Regan WF Jr: Blow-out fracture of orbit: Mechanism and correction of internal orbital fracture. Am J Ophthalmol 44:733, 1957.
5. Work W: Trauma to the frontal sinus. Arch Otolaryngol 59:54, 1954.
6. Dillon WP: Head and Neck Imaging Excluding the Central Nervous System. New York, Raven Press, 1987, pp 329–358.
7. Grossman GB: Magnetic Resonance Imaging and Computed Tomography of the Head and Spine. Baltimore, Williams and Wilkins, 1990, pp 308–346.
8. Mancuso AA, Hanafee WN: Computed Tomography of the Head and Neck. Facial Trauma. 2nd ed. Baltimore, Williams and Wilkins, 1985, pp 43–60.
9. Anderson JE: Grant's Atlas of Anatomy. 7th ed. Baltimore, Williams and Wilkins, 1987, pp 7–8.
10. Dolan KD, Jacoby CG, Smoker WRK: Radiology of Facial Injury. 2nd ed. Philadelphia, Field & Wood Medical Publishers, 1982, pp 12–18.
11. Rowe NL, Killey HC: Fractures of the Facial Skeleton. Baltimore, Williams and Wilkins, 1968.
12. Ritter FN: The surgical anatomy of the nasal sinuses. Otolaryngol Clin North Am 4:3, 1971.
13. McMinn RMH, Hutchings RT, Logan MB: Head and Neck Anatomy. Chicago, Year Book Medical Publishers, 1981.
14. Kellman RM, Schilli W: Plate fixation of fractures of the mid and upper face. Otolaryngol Clin North Am 20:559, 1987.
15. Beals SP, Munro IR: The use of mini-plates in craniomaxillofacial surgery. Plast Reconstr Surg 79:33, 1987.
16. Schilli W, Ewers R, Niederdellman H: Bone fixation with screws and plates in the maxillofacial region. Int J Oral Surg 10:329, 1981.
17. Kellman RM: Methods of rigid fixation for facial fractures. *In* Cummings CW, Fredrickson JM, Harker LA, Krause CJ, Schuller DE (eds): Otolaryngology–Head and Neck Surgery. St. Louis, CV Mosby, 1989, pp 166–191.

CHAPTER 31

ORBITAL COMPLICATIONS OF SINUSITIS

William Lawson, MD, DDS

PATHOGENESIS AND ETIOLOGY

Anatomically, the paranasal sinuses are in intimate contact with the orbit, which is separated only by a thin plate of bone from the frontal sinus superiorly, the ethmoid labyrinth medially, and the maxillary sinus inferiorly. Consequently, acute and chronic inflammatory disease within the sinuses has ready access to the orbit and its adnexa. Orbital extension of infections of the paranasal sinuses may occur through a variety of avenues, which include (1) open suture lines (e.g., ethmoidomaxillary suture line); (2) congenital bony dehiscences in the orbital portion of the maxilla or lamina papyracea of the ethmoid; (3) natural pathways along the anterior and posterior ethmoid blood vessels within the frontoethmoid suture line; (4) necrosis of bone by acute infection or bone erosion from chronic disease; and (5) retrograde thrombophlebitis, or paraphlebitis, or lymphatics (including perineural lymphatics).

The ophthalmic veins are valve-free and course through the orbit, emptying into the cavernous sinus. The superior ophthalmic vein is continuous with the nasofrontal vein, and the inferior ophthalmic vein receives tributaries from the eyelids, lacrimal sac, and orbital muscles. In addition, the venous plexuses of the nasolacrimal duct, turbinates, and sinus linings communicate with the orbital veins.[1] This interconnecting system of veins permits ready access to the orbit and eyelids from infectious processes in the nose and paranasal sinuses.

The developmental anatomy of the paranasal sinuses also influences the orbital extension of disease. The maxillary and ethmoid sinuses are well formed at birth, whereas the sphenoid sinus, although present, does not become clinically significant until 4 or 5 years of age. The frontal sinuses are absent at birth, begin to pneumatize at 6 years, and are not a factor in orbital infections until several years later. These developmental differences are responsible for orbital infections originating from the maxillary sinus in infancy and early childhood, from the ethmoids in later childhood, and from the frontal sinus in adolescence.

Fearon and colleagues considered the frequent upper respiratory infections and increased incidence of sinusitis in children, coupled with the diploic nature of the immature facial bones and the increased vascular and lymphatic channels, as facilitating the spread of infection to the orbit.[2]

Although the complications of sinusitis have been reduced by antibiotics, they continue to occur because of inadequate antimicrobial therapy, impaired host resistance, infection with resistant organisms, and delay or lack of surgical intervention.

Sinusitis is a frequent cause of periorbital and orbital cellulitis; however, trauma, retained foreign bodies, and cutaneous, lacrimal, and dental and postsurgical infections are also etiologic factors. Sinusitis was documented as being responsible for 4 per cent of the 303 cases of Schramm and colleagues,[3] for 64 per cent of the 22 cases of orbital cellulitis reported by Goodwin and colleagues,[4] for 84 per cent of the 104 cases of Watters and colleagues[5] and for 56 per cent of the 165 cases of Rubinstein and

Handler.[6] The occurrence of an antecedent upper respiratory infection appears to be an important predisposing factor and may account for an increased prevalence during the winter months. Gans[7] also noted an increased incidence during periods of influenza episodes. In some cases, there is a history of diving into a swimming pool, which presumably forces contaminated water into the sinuses.[8]

Gamble reported three instances of metastatic infection to the orbit in the preantibiotic era.[9] He also cited osteomyelitis of the neonate as another cause of orbital cellulitis. The converse was reported by Hawkins and Clark.[10] An association between orbital cellulitis and systemic disease has also been established. In addition to occurring in patients with diabetes, leukemia, and immunosuppressive disorders, sino-orbital infections have also been reported with sickle cell anemia,[5, 11] juvenile rheumatoid arthritis,[5] and Wegener's granulomatosis.[8]

In some cases, the infection may be superimposed on an underlying benign or malignant lesion (e.g., polyps, dental cyst, juvenile angiofibroma, lymphoma, sarcoma) within the nose or sinuses.

In a small number of cases, the cause of the infection is an odontogenic sinus infection. A periodontally or pulpally involved maxillary premolar or molar tooth produces an ascending infection that progresses from the antrum into the ethmoid labyrinth, then through the lamina papyracea into the orbit.

However, in the majority of patients with sinogenic orbital infections, nasal and sinus complaints are not prominent. None of the 18 cases with orbital complications reported by Quick and Payne[12] had an antecedent history of sinus disease.

Several workers have noted clinical and bacteriologic differences between patients developing orbital complications following sinusitis and those with sequelae following facial cutaneous infections of injuries. Smith and colleagues[13] and Gellady and colleagues[14] reported the former group to be younger and to have a higher incidence of bacteremia, with *Haemophilus influenzae* the pathogen most commonly isolated.

CLINICAL FEATURES

Orbital complications of inflammatory sinus disease occur in all decades of life; however, they show a predilection for the pediatric age group. The majority of cases involve the eyelids, with only a small number being truly intraorbital.

Fearon and colleagues[2] reported orbital-facial complications in 159 of 6770 patients treated for sinusitis over a 25-year period at the Hospital for Sick Children in Toronto. These include orbital (eyelid) cellulitis in 133, orbital abscess in 17, and cavernous sinus thrombosis in 2 patients.

Schramm and colleagues[3] collected 303 cases of orbital cellulitis from the records of the Children's Hospital and the Eye and Ear Infirmary of Pittsburgh over a 10-year period. The age range was 2 weeks to 66 years; however, 68 per cent of the patients were under 9 years of age, and only 17 per cent were over 15 years of age. Periorbital cellulitis was present in 82 per cent, orbital cellulitis in 4 per cent, subperiosteal abscess in 11 per cent, orbital abscess in 2 per cent, and cavernous sinus thrombosis in 1 per cent of the patients. They found the severity of the orbital disease to increase with increasing age.

On review of 119 patients with inflammatory disease about the eye, Goodwin and colleagues[4] found that in 97 the infection was anterior to the orbital septum (periorbital), and in 22 it was deep to it (orbital cellulitis). In 13 of the latter 22 cases, an abscess was present. The age range of the patients with orbital cellulitis was 5 to 68 years, with a mean of 23 years. Rubinstein and Handler[6] reported that among 165 patients with cellulitis of the eye treated over a 5-year period at the Children's Hospital of Philadelphia, in 142 (86 per cent) it was periorbital and in 23 (14 per cent) it was intraorbital. The age range was 8 days to 17 years, with a median of 3.2 years. Analysis of 190 cases from the Cracow Otolaryngologic Clinic by Gans and colleagues[7] revealed that 130 patients were 2 months to 14 years, 19 were 15 to 20 years, 34 were aged 21 to 50 years and 7 were older than 50 years. In the review by Barkin and colleagues[15] of 71 patients hospitalized at the Children's Hospital of Denver (1972–1976) with periorbital cellulitis, the age range was 10 days to 18 years, with 58 per cent under 4 years. Welsh and Welsh[8] noted that 21 of their 32 cases occurred in patients under 20 years of age, with a random occurrence afterward until 70 years of age. However, in the series of 114 cases reported by Hubert[16] from the Manhattan Eye, Ear, and Throat Hospital (1927–1937), the age range was 2 months to 78 years, with only 24 children between 1 and 10 years involved. This included 31 patients with eyelid edema, 46 with a subperiosteal abscess, 22 with an orbital abscess, 9 with orbital cellulitis, and 4 with cavernous sinus thrombosis.

A left-sided predominance of orbital infections has been noted by Gamble,[9] Schramm and colleagues,[17] and Rubinstein and Handler[6]; however, the opposite was reported by Barkin and colleagues.[15] Bilateral involvement was observed in 6 per cent of the cases of Barkin and colleagues[15] and in 9 per cent of those of Rubinstein and Handler.[6] A male preponderance in the ratio of approximately 2:1 was described by Goodwin and colleagues[4] and Watters and colleagues.[5]

CLASSIFICATION

The classification of the orbital complications of sinusitis into five groups (Fig. 31–1) was originally proposed by Hubert[16] in 1937. He divided orbital infections into eyelid edema, orbital cellulitis, orbital abscess, subperiosteal abscess, and cavernous sinus thrombosis, based on the anatomic location of the inflammation. This system of classification was adopted and popularized by the writing of later workers.[18, 19] Recently, Choi, Lawson, and Urken[20] introduced a new clinical entity termed the *subperiosteal orbital hematoma*, which may represent the earliest stage of orbital extension of sinusitis.

The term *orbital apex syndrome* refers to the complex of clinical features that results from involvement of the neurovascular structures that traverse the superior orbital fissure (superior ophthalmic vein and oculomotor, trochlear, abducens, and ophthalmic nerves) and the optic foramen (optic nerve, ophthalmic artery, sympathetic plexus) by a variety of inflammatory and neoplastic disorders. Clinically, there are multiple ocular signs and symptoms, which include impaired mobility of the eye; anesthesia of the eyelid, cornea, and conjunctiva; optic neuritis; as well as swelling and congestion of the eyelid and conjunctiva and protrusion of the globe (Fig. 31–2). Kronschnabel[21] reported six patients to have orbital inflammatory disease of sinus origin; however, these cases appear to represent a variety of infectious processes.

The anatomic distinction among the various types of orbital infections is important because

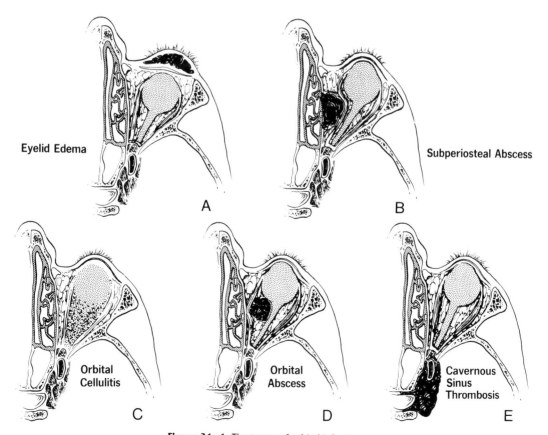

Figure 31–1. The types of orbital infections.

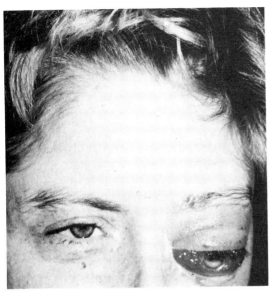

Figure 31–2. Orbital apex syndrome with marked unilateral proptosis, chemosis, and ophthalmoplegia.

it greatly influences the selection and outcome of therapy. Clinically, periorbital (preseptal) infections (e.g., eyelid edema) can be readily differentiated from truly intraorbital infections by the lack of the aforementioned ocular findings. With an orbital (postseptal) infection, both ocular and constitutional symptoms become more prominent. A slow pulse may accompany a high temperature because of the oculocardiac reflex. In the past, surgical exploration was necessary to establish whether the inflammatory process was an orbital abscess, orbital cellulitis, or a subperiosteal abscess. Presently, this information is provided preoperatively by computed tomography (CT) scanning. In patients with cavernous sinus thrombosis, intracranial extension of the infection produces neurologic findings in addition to orbital alterations. The differences in the clinical features, prognosis, and management of each type of infection require their individual consideration.

Eyelid Edema (Periorbital Cellulitis). The periosteum continues from the margins of the orbit into the eyelids as the orbital septum, ending in the tarsal plates. The orbital septum is an important barrier to the spread of infection. Clinically, it has been repeatedly shown to prevent the extension of a periorbital cellulitis into the orbit. This was stressed by Smith and colleagues,[13] who termed periorbital cellulitis a preseptal infection.

Gamble[9] proposed that the eyelid edema resulted from interference with the blood flow from the superior ophthalmic veins into the ethmoid veins by pressure obstruction of the latter by regional inflammation.

Clinically, inflammatory swelling of the eyelids occurs without any abnormality of the orbital contents, such as limitation of extraocular motion, decreased visual acuity, or conjunctival congestion. However, Schramm and colleagues[3] identified a subgroup of patients having periorbital cellulitis with chemosis. Unlike patients with periorbital cellulitis alone, many of these patients failed to improve with antibiotic therapy. Consequently, it is extremely important to force the eyelids apart if they are swollen tightly closed and to evaluate the eye itself.

The segment of the eyelid involved may suggest the sinus of origin. Ethmoid sinusitis may cause edema of the eyelids medially early in the course of the infection and later proceed to involve the entire lid. Frontal or supraorbital ethmoid disease may involve only the upper eyelid. Maxillary sinusitis in infants may produce swelling of the lower eyelid.

In young children, ethmoid sinusitis, which is the most common cause of periorbital cellulitis, characteristically produces diffuse eyelid edema. The inflammatory swelling may totally close the eye and progress to involve the opposite side (Fig. 31–3).

Eyelid edema generally resolves with appropriate antibiotic therapy. Persistent swelling may represent the formation of an eyelid abscess, which will require independent drainage (Figs. 31–4 and 31–5).

Subperiosteal Orbital Hematoma. Although this is a commonly recognized entity in ophthalmology, arising from traumatic, congestive, or spontaneous causes, the role of inflammatory sinus disease in its development is little appreciated. The pathogenesis of the subperiosteal orbital hematoma is (1) traumatic tearing of an orbital vessel; (2) rupture of a subperiosteal vessel secondary to increased venous pressure transmitted by valveless orbital veins from congested sinus mucosa; or (3) erosion of a vessel by orbital extension of an infectious process. It is the orbital equivalent of the intracranial epidural hematoma. Its frequent occurrence in the roof of the orbit may be related to the loose attachment of the periosteum in this area.

Clinically, present are proptosis, generally with displacement of the globe downward; orbital pain; ophthalmoplegia; and decreased visual acuity. In 1988, Choi, Lawson, and Urken[20] reported the occurrence of this entity secondary to ethmoid sinusitis. The patient was a 62-year-old man who presented with right supraorbital

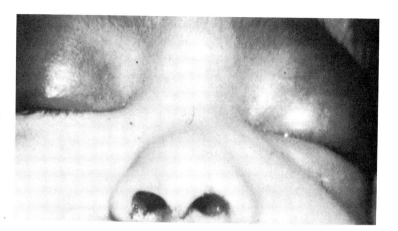

Figure 31–3. Bilateral periorbital cellulitis secondary to acute ethmoiditis in an infant.

headache, periorbital edema, proptosis, chemosis, and ophthalmoplegia. A CT scan revealed clouding of a supraorbital ethmoid cell, with an enhancing mass present along the superior orbital wall (Fig. 31–6). Exploration through an external ethmoidectomy revealed the orbital cavity to be filled with blood. The patient responded promptly to surgical drainage and antibiotic therapy. Review of the literature reveals two definite cases and one other probable case of subperiosteal orbital hematoma secondary to sinusitis. In 1937, Wheeler[22] found a blood-filled "cyst" of the orbital roof on surgical exploration of a patient with frontal sinusitis. In 1978, Harris and colleagues[23] reported a similar case, also secondary to frontal sinusitis. In 1988, Calcaterra and Trapp[24] described a patient who had severe proptosis from a mixed subperiosteal abscess and hematoma that were secondary to ethmoid sinusitis. Analysis of these cases suggests that the subperiosteal orbital hematoma developing from the septic or congestive tearing of a vessel may be the precursor of the subperiosteal abscess.

Management is by surgical drainage and decompression of the orbital hematoma, exenteration of the diseased sinus, and administration of intravenous antibiotics to control the infection.

Subperiosteal Abscess. In this condition, there is a circumscribed collection of pus between the orbital bony wall and its periosteum. The periorbita is loosely attached to the underlying bone and readily separates from it. This may produce displacement of the globe laterally or inferiorly, as well as impairment of ocular motility. Early, there is minimal conjunctival congestion and normal visual acuity; however, with advanced infections, proptosis, ophthalmoplegia, and chemosis become more prominent, and a decrease in vision develops (Figs. 31–7 through 31–9). The abscess may remain

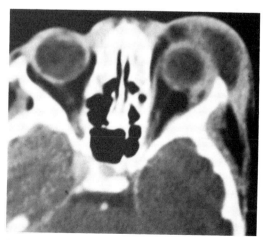

Figure 31–4. Severe periorbital cellulitis secondary to acute unilateral maxillary and ethmoid sinusitis in an 8-year-old child.

Figure 31–5. Computed tomography (CT) scan demonstrating eyelid edema with lid abscess formation. The infection is entirely preseptal; there is no abnormality of the orbital contents.

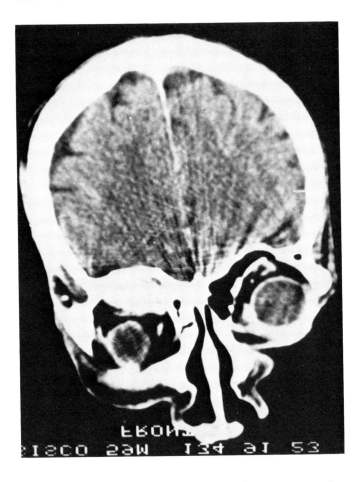

Figure 31–6. CT scan reveals clouding of right supraorbital ethmoid cell associated with a well-defined enhancing mass in the roof of the right orbit.

localized or may penetrate the periorbita to produce an orbital cellulitis or abscess.

Treatment is prompt surgical drainage through an external ethmoidectomy approach, by which the abscess cavity is evacuated, the ethmoid labyrinth is exenterated, and the orbit is drained into the nasal cavity. Sepsis is controlled by appropriate intravenous antibiotics.

Orbital Cellulitis. In this condition, the infection has penetrated the orbital periosteum to involve diffusely the orbital contents. The orbital fat is edematous and contains numerous bacteria and inflammatory cells. Clinically, it is manifested by intense swelling of the eyelids, which may close the eyes. There is also impaired ocular motility, which may range from partial to total ophthalmoplegia, as well as proptosis and conjunctival congestion (chemosis). The latter occurs from obstruction of the ophthalmic veins and may be so intense that prolapse of the bulbar conjunctiva develops.

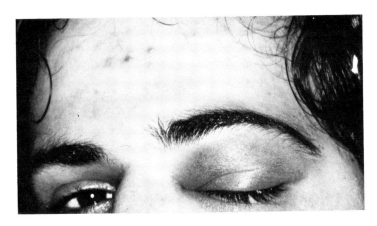

Figure 31–7. An adolescent patient with inflammatory swelling that completely closes the involved eye.

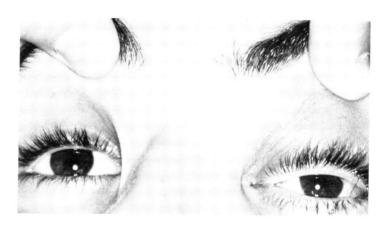

Figure 31–8. Manual forced opening of the eye reveals displacement of the globe outward and downward and slightly impaired ocular motility. Chemosis is absent, and the vision is intact.

Desiccation of the exposed tissues of the proptotic eye carries the risk of necrosis, with globe rupture and panophthalmitis. Continued elevation of the intraocular pressure leads to progressive visual loss and eventually permanent blindness. Constitutional symptoms may be prominent, with fever, malaise, and leukocytosis present.

Treatment is with intravenous antibiotics. The absence of clinical improvement in the ocular findings after adequate medical therapy is suggestive of the formation of an abscess, which requires surgical exploration and drainage and orbital decompression to prevent loss of vision.

Orbital Abscess. With an orbital abscess, a collection of pus is present within the orbital tissues. This may arise from an acute sinus infection penetrating the periosteum or from an orbital cellulitis progressing to suppuration. Clinically, the patient manifests marked prop-

tosis, ophthalmoplegia, and intense congestion and swelling of the eyelids and conjunctiva (chemosis) (Figs. 31–10 and 31–11). The eye is generally pushed outward; however, a lateral, superior, or inferior component to the proptosis may suggest involvement of the ethmoid, maxillary, or frontal sinus, respectively. Rarely, the eye may be displaced inward by a lateral collection of pus.[21] The danger of the continued presence of pus within the orbit under pressure is septic or vascular visual loss.

Intravenous antibiotics are administered, as with all orbital infections. Lack of clinical improvement or the radiologic or ultrasound demonstration of an abscess requires surgical drainage of the orbit.

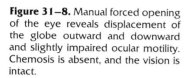

Figure 31–9. Computed tomography (CT) scan revealing the formation of a subperiosteal abscess secondary to ethmoiditis medially as the cause of the exophthalmos.

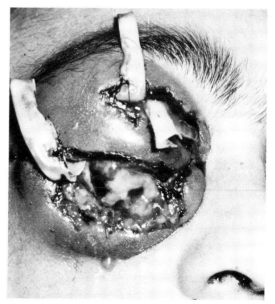

Figure 31–10. Necrotizing orbital infection secondary to ethmoid sinusitis, resulting in destruction of eyelids and globe.

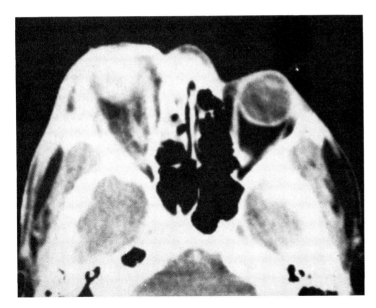

Figure 31–11. CT scan demonstrating orbital abscess formation.

Cavernous Sinus Thrombosis. Progression of an orbital infection posteriorly by retrograde thrombophlebitis of the ophthalmic vein may produce involvement of the cavernous sinus (Fig. 31–12). Clinically, ocular signs now develop in the opposite orbit. This is accompanied by marked constitutional symptoms, as well as signs of intracranial extension. Spiking fevers, malaise, severe headache, meningeal signs, evidence of papilledema, and edema over the mastoid emissary vein appear. Price and colleagues[25] believed that unilateral ocular involvement in association with meningitis or an isolated contralateral oculomotor palsy may represent an early cavernous sinus thrombosis. Ptosis, diplopia, and photophobia have also been cited as premonitory symptoms of cavernous sinus thrombosis.[25, 26] The ophthalmoscopic findings reported include edema of the optic disk, retinal vein congestion, retinal edema and hemorrhage, and central retinal artery thrombosis. Although pupillary, visual, and funduscopic changes occur in patients with cavernous sinus thrombosis, they are not diagnostic because they may be absent and also appear in infections limited to the orbit. In two of the

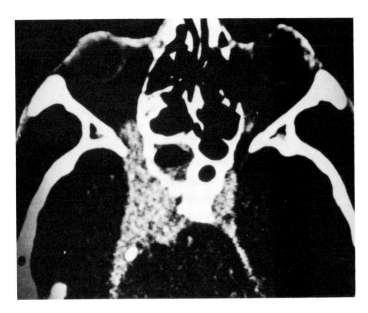

Figure 31–12. CT scan with contrast revealing the presence of an enhancing mass in the cavernous sinus. The ability to demonstrate an infected thrombus radiographically before the clinical development of contralateral orbital signs permits early diagnosis and rapid institution of therapy.

four cases of Price and colleagues,[25] these changes were absent.

Neglected or inadequately treated orbital infections may progress to cavernous sinus thrombosis. Occasionally, the disease may run a fulminant course, especially in the compromised host. This generally involves tissue invasion by an opportunistic mycotic organism. Price and colleagues[25] reported bacterial cavernous sinus thrombosis developing 1 hour after an ethmoidectomy.

On review of 874 reported cases of cavernous sinus thrombosis, Yarington[27] calculated a mortality rate of 80 per cent and a morbidity rate of 75 per cent among the survivors. The disease may prove fatal despite prompt and appropriate antibiotic therapy. Agents that cross the blood-brain barrier well (e.g., penicillin, chloramphenicol) are administered intravenously. The value of treatment with heparin is controversial.

RADIOGRAPHIC EVALUATION

Sinusitis is the most common cause of orbital cellulitis. Its reported radiographic incidence was 47 per cent (27 of 56 cases) by Gellady and colleagues,[14] 65 per cent (121 of 190 cases) by Gans and colleagues,[7] 66 per cent (29 of 44 cases) by Barkin and colleagues,[15] 74 per cent by Schramm et al,[3] 80 per cent (8 of 10 cases) by Zimmerman and Bilaniuk[11] and 84 per cent (77 of 91 cases) by Watters and colleagues.[5] Gellady and colleagues[14] cautioned that the actual incidence of sinusitis may be higher because of difficulties in interpreting sinus radiographs in infants and small children. However, Smith and colleagues[13] found only 4 of 17 children to have radiographic evidence of sinusitis and concluded that it was an uncommon cause of periorbital cellulitis.

The sinuses responsible for orbital infections are, in order of decreasing frequency, the ethmoid, maxillary, and frontal. However, the relative incidence reported reflects the age of the patient population surveyed, with frontal sinusitis prominent in older children and adolescents. Multiple sites of involvement are often observed.

In the 159 pediatric cases reviewed by Fearon and colleagues,[2] the commonest radiographic finding was unilateral involvement of the maxillary and ethmoid sinuses. They considered the periorbital cellulitis observed in children under 1 year of age to represent direct extension of maxillary sinus disease without ethmoid involvement. Among the 24 cases of

Hawkins and Clark,[10] the ethmoids were involved in all, the maxillary sinus in 17, and the frontal sinus in 9. The sites of involvement in the 121 cases of Gans and colleagues[7] were all sinuses (40); maxillary sinus (50); frontal sinus (10); ethmoid labyrinth (8); maxillary and ethmoid sinuses (7); and frontal and ethmoid sinuses (5). Morgan and Morrison[28] observed unilateral pansinusitis to be the most common radiologic finding among 14 patients undergoing surgery for sinus diseases with complications. Among nine cases of orbital cellulitis, Price and colleagues[25] noted pansinusitis in seven patients and maxillary involvement in two others. Barkin and colleagues[15] reported involvement of the ethmoids in 72 per cent of their 29 cases. In addition to the involvement of multiple ipsilateral sinuses, there is often radiographic evidence of bilateral disease. Watters and colleagues[5] noted the presence of unilateral disease in 41 and bilateral disease in 36 of 77 children studied.

Radiographically, plain films generally reveal clouding of the involved sinus or sinuses. The findings are subtler in infants, with only asymmetric aeration of the maxillary or ethmoid sinuses present.[3]

CT is invaluable in evaluating the patient with an orbital complication of sinus disease.[4, 11, 17, 29] Although it is clinically impossible to differentiate periorbital or orbital cellulitis from an abscess, CT scanning with contrast enhancement is capable of localizing an abscess and defining its wall. Gas may be present within an abscess owing to a gas-forming organism or communication with an adjacent sinus.[11] CT scanning also may demonstrate the loss of the normal soft tissue planes between the optic nerve, retrobulbar fat, and rectus muscles, as well as scleral thickening.[11] Based on CT scanning, Zimmerman and Bilaniuk[11] anatomically divided infections within the orbit proper into (1) intraconic—centrally within the muscle cone; (2) extraconic—peripherally between the periosteum and recti; and (3) subperiosteal—between the orbital wall and its periosteum.

In cases with a history of trauma, the CT scan may reveal an unsuspected foreign body (Fig. 31–13). CT scanning also may demonstrate intracranial involvement of the epidural or subdural spaces or cerebral parenchyma. In addition, it provides a modality to monitor the clinical course of a patient with an orbital and intracranial complication.

Ultrasound also has been shown to be a helpful, noninvasive method for detecting an abscess within the orbit. However, it may fail to delineate a lesion at the orbital apex.[25]

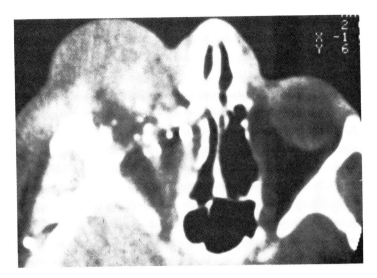

Figure 31–13. CT scan of an orbital abscess secondary to an infection caused by foreign body (metallic pellets) embedded in the ethmoid sinuses.

BACTERIOLOGY

Bacteriologic studies of patients with orbital cellulitis have generally revealed the presence of *Streptococcus pneumoniae, Haemophilus influenzae, Staphylococcus aureus* and β-hemolytic *Streptococcus*. Schramm and colleagues[3] found *H. influenzae* to account for 33 per cent of the positive cultures in children under 4 years of age, but only 5 per cent of those in adults. Rubinstein and Handler[6] reported that 74 per cent of all *Haemophilus* cultures were obtained in children under 3 years of age; 81 per cent of all pneumococcus cultures were found in patients under 2 years; and *S. aureus* and β-hemolytic *Streptococcus* were isolated equally often in children above and below 3 years of age. It has been suggested that the presence of a violaceous discoloration of the eyelid in the absence of trauma is clinically indicative of *Haemophilus* infection.[30]

Among the 14 operated cases reported by Morgan and Morrison,[28] isolated were nonhemolytic *Streptococcus* (4 cases), β-hemolytic *Streptococcus* (2), *Streptococcus pneumoniae* (1), *Staphylococcus aureus* (4), coagulase-negative *Staphylococcus* (2), and diphtheroids (2). No anaerobes were identified.

Watters and colleagues[5] noted bacteremia in 29 per cent of 88 patients whose blood was cultured. It was more frequent in young individuals (under 2 years of age), patients with extensive orbital infections, and those not receiving antibiotics. In 20 of these patients, *Haemophilus* was cultured and in 6, *S. pneu-*

moniae was isolated. Four children had *Haemophilus* meningitis simultaneously.

Barkin and colleagues[15] reported positive blood cultures in 15 per cent of 55 patients studied. *Haemophilus influenzae* was isolated in five; *Streptococcus pneumoniae* in two, and *Staphylococcus aureus* in one patient.

Gellady and colleagues[14] claimed that there were two populations of patients with orbital and periorbital cellulitis. Those 45 patients studied who lacked a history of trauma or a cutaneous focus of infection had a high incidence of positive blood culture results (34 per cent), especially with *Haemophilus* (82 per cent). The 42 patients having a soft tissue infection rarely developed a bacteremia (one case), with a *Staphylococcus aureus* or a β-hemolytic *Streptococcus* isolated from the wound or conjunctiva. Smith and colleagues[13] also identified two such clinical groups of patients with orbital infections, with *Haemophilus* bacteremia commonly found in cases of sinus origin.

In addition to these organisms, gram-negative and anaerobic bacteria have occasionally been isolated.[10, 31]

Whereas Schramm and colleagues[3] considered cultures of eyelid aspirates and eye secretions of little value, Rubinstein and Handler[6] found conjunctival cultures positive in about half the cases in which they were obtained. Barkin and colleagues[15] similarly found seven of nine needle aspirates (78 per cent) and six of nine conjunctival cultures to contain the causative organism. In a study of 26 children with acute ethmoiditis and orbital cellulitis, Haynes and colleagues[31] were able to identify *S. aureus, S. pyogenes, S. pneumoniae,* and *H. influenzae* on nasopharyngeal culture.

TREATMENT

Antibiotic therapy should be administered intravenously and should cover all the organisms cited earlier, including β-lactamase–producing strains. Rubinstein and Handler[6] reported 2 of 38 *Haemophilus* cultures positive for β-lactamase. Schramm and colleagues[3] recommended ampicillin and chloramphenicol in children under 4 years of age and high doses of penicillin in patients over 4 years of age. Barkin and colleagues[15] employed ampicillin and a penicillinase-resistant penicillin in children under 5 years of age, reserving chloramphenicol for cases with a poor response. The newer cephalosporins also would provide effective coverage. Oral antibiotics should be continued for several weeks following cessation of parenteral therapy on discharge from the hospital, as instances of recurrent orbital infections have been reported.[21]

Topical nasal vasoconstrictors and oral decongestants are often used as well. Steroids are valueless in reducing the swelling about the eye and may even be harmful.[21]

SURGICAL THERAPY

The number of cases requiring surgery varies widely and reflects differences in case selection by the reporting institutions. Preseptal infections in children will generally resolve with antibiotic management, except for the occasional case that forms an eyelid abscess and requires incision and drainage. Fearon and colleagues[2] reported resolution of periorbital cellulitis in 133 children without surgery on the orbit. Intraorbital infections are more dangerous, and a relatively large proportion of patients come to surgery for the drainage of an abscess cavity or the offending sinus.

In the series of Gans and colleagues,[7] 27 per cent of the 190 cases required surgery. Surgery was performed in 17 of the 159 cases of Fearon and colleagues.[2] These workers recommended adenotonsillectomy in children developing orbitofacial complications of sinusitis. An antrostomy was also performed in infants, as the maxillary sinus was considered the main focus of infection. Morgan and Morrison[28] reported the operative procedures performed in 14 patients developing complications of sinus disease to be frontal trephine (9 cases), intranasal antrostomy (8), external ethmoidectomy (8), drainage of soft tissue abscess (1), and craniectomy

(1). External drainage procedures were necessary in 7 of the 24 cases of Hawkins and Clark[10] (frontal trephine, 4 cases; external ethmoidectomy, 4; orbital abscess drainage, 1). Six others required intranasal procedures (ethmoidectomy, 4; antrostomy, 2).

Virtually all infections of the frontal sinus that extend into the orbit require drainage through a trephine. If there is concomitant involvement of the ethmoids, one may elect to perform an external frontoethmoidectomy and drain the orbit as well as both sinuses into the nasal cavity. The absence of clinical improvement in the ocular findings after adequate medical therapy is suggestive of the formation of an abscess, which requires surgical exploration and drainage to prevent loss of vision. Blindness generally develops in patients who do not have surgery or in whom it is delayed. Fearon and colleagues[2] reported two cases of blindness occurring in patients with continued orbital inflammation in whom surgical drainage was delayed over 10 days. Surgical drainage is generally accomplished through an external ethmoidectomy performed in the superior medial aspect of the orbit. Some surgeons drain the abscess externally, with a Penrose drain placed through the incision, whereas others favor an external ethmoidectomy providing drainage into the nose. An antrostomy is generally performed because the maxillary sinus is often simultaneously involved.

An effective method of orbital exploration and decompression, reported by Sacks and colleagues[32] for the management of retro-orbital hemorrhage, also can be applied to infectious processes. In their method, the medial wall and floor of the orbit up to the infraorbital canal are removed through an external ethmoidectomy approach, along with the ethmoid labyrinth, permitting expansion of the orbital contents into the ethmoid and nasal cavities. Pressure within the globe can be reduced further by making several radial incisions in the periorbita that permit prolapse of the fat into the surgical cavity.

Although surgery is generally recommended in any patient with clinical, ultrasound, or CT scan evidence of abscess formation, Goodwin and colleagues[4] reported three such patients who improved on antibiotic therapy alone. However, they cautioned that candidates for conservative management should have normal visual acuity and some globe motion and that the patients must repeatedly be re-examined during therapy. After careful review of 303 orbital infections, Schramm and colleagues[3] concluded that surgical drainage of the orbit and involved sinuses should be performed in patients with (1) abscess formation; (2) visual acuity worse than 20/60; (3) progression of disease for more than 24 hours; or (4) lack of resolution on antibiotic therapy for 48 to 72 hours. In addition to surgical therapy for the acute infection when indicated, care must be taken to treat any residual disease in the sinuses.

COMPLICATIONS

The major complications of the orbital extension of sinus disease are blindness and intracranial infection.

Intraorbital infections (subperiosteal hematoma or abscess, orbital cellulitis, orbital abscess) produce an increase in the intraocular pressure, which, in conjunction with the septic process, may lead to blindness from (1) thrombosis of the retinal artery; (2) vasculitis of the vasa vasorum of the optic nerve; (3) a direct effect on the optic nerve; or (4) pressure on the peripapillary plexus. The latter is formed from the short ciliary arteries and provides the blood supply of the laminar and prelaminar areas of the optic nerve. Visual loss may be gradual or sudden. The increased intraocular pressure accompanying orbital suppuration may manifest itself in retinal edema and hemorrhage or evidence of optic neuritis and atrophy. However, blindness may occur without any funduscopic abnormality. Consequently, monitoring of the visual acuity is more important than ophthalmoscopy in following the clinical course of the disease. Visual loss secondary to optic neuritis also may result from acute or chronic sinusitis in the absence of orbital cellulitis. Jarrett and Gutman[33] reported such an occurrence secondary to pansinusitis that resolved on antibiotic therapy. Fearon and colleagues[2] reported a case of sphenoid sinusitis with cephalalgia and bilateral visual loss. I have seen several patients with progressive optic neuritis secondary to an indolent chronic sphenoid sinusitis, in whom vision returned after sphenoid sinusotomy. With acute infections, blindness is usually irreversible; consequently, decreasing vision is an indication for immediate surgical therapy.

Life-threatening intracranial complications may arise from direct extension of the infection from the orbit, via retrograde thrombophlebitis of the ophthalmic veins into the cavernous sinus or through other anatomic routes, such as the optic foramen, superior orbital fissure, and ethmoid canals, where the periorbita continues as the dura. The ethmoid and frontal sinuses are in direct contact with the anterior cranial fossa, and the primary infection may also simultaneously extend intracranially, independent of the orbit.

In some patients with ophthalmoplegia, there may be persistent impairment of extraocular muscle function. The sinus disease that produced the orbital soft tissue infection may concurrently cause osteomyelitis of the surrounding bone. Frontal sinusitis is often accompanied by osteomyelitis, as well as intracranial complications. Fearon and colleagues[2] reported five cases of frontal sinusitis with orbital cellulitis in teenagers, two of whom developed osteomyelitis and intracranial sepsis. Osteomyelitis of the maxilla secondary to sinus disease is virtually limited to infancy.

The mortality and morbidity of orbital infections secondary to sinusitis were fearsome in the preantibiotic era. Hubert[16] reported a fatal outcome in 5 of 31 patients with eyelid edema, in 3 of 22 with orbital abscess, in 6 of 9 with orbital cellulitis, and in 2 of 4 patients with cavernous sinus thrombosis. Gamble[9] reported fatality in 2 of 26 cases of his own, and cited a 17 per cent mortality and a 20 per cent incidence of blindness in the older literature.

Despite the highly favorable impact of antibiotic therapy on these orbital infections, serious sequelae still occur in a significant number of cases. Rubinstein and Handler[6] had only 1 death among their 165 cases. In the 119 cases of Goodwin and colleagues,[4] one patient developed an epidural abscess, another had osteomyelitis of the roof of the orbit, and there were two instances of blindness. The latter patients were operated on 6 and 36 hours after the loss of light perception. Among the 190 orbital complications reported by Gans and colleagues,[7] 15 also developed intracranial complications (encephalomeningitis in 5 and cavernous sinus thrombosis in 10 patients). In this group, two patients died, one had bilateral blindness, and two had abducens paralysis. Among the 175 patients with only orbital involvement, 3 developed blindness, 1 had partial visual loss, 1 had osteomyelitis of the frontal bone, and 1 suffered abducens paralysis. Fearon and colleagues[2] reported two instances of blindness among their 159 cases, but no fatalities. Three of the 24 patients of Hawkins and Clark[10] also had intracranial complications, and osteomyelitis of the maxilla developed in a 1-month-old infant. Among the six cases of orbital abscess reported by Kronschnabel,[21] blindness occurred in two patients and cavernous sinus thrombosis developed in another. Among the 18 cases of Quick and Payne,[12] 2 patients had cavernous sinus thrombosis, 3 had meningitis, 1 had a subdural abscess, 2 developed blindness, and 1 died. In the series of 26 cases of orbital cellulitis secondary to acute ethmoiditis reviewed by Haynes and Cramblett,[31] 1 patient developed meningitis and another had multiple intracranial abscesses. Among the 10 acute orbital infections reported by Zimmerman and Bilaniuk,[11] there were 2 cases of cerebritis, 1 of epidural abscess, 2 patients with osteomyelitis, and 1 instance of endophthalmitis with globe rupture. Morgan and Morrison[28] described 1 instance of blindness in their 11 operated cases (subperiosteal abscess, 8 cases; orbital abscess, 3). One patient also developed cavernous sinus thrombosis. Schramm and colleagues[3] noted a 3 per cent incidence of fatal or permanent sequelae in their 303 cases. Among the seven cases of Jarrett and Gutman,[33] two patients with a subperiosteal abscess had permanent loss of vision; in one it occurred secondary to retinal artery thrombosis, and in the other severe proptosis led to exposure keratitis, corneal ulceration, and endophthalmitis. It cannot be stressed enough that progression of the infection, unresponsiveness to medical therapy, or any evidence of visual loss demands orbital exploration and drainage to prevent disastrous complications.

References

1. Batson OV: Relationship of the eye to the paranasal sinuses. Arch Ophthalmol 16:322, 1936.
2. Fearon B, Edmonds B, Bird R: Orbital-facial complications of sinusitis in children. Laryngoscope 89:947, 1979.
3. Schramm VL, Curtin HD, Kennerdell JS: Evaluation of orbital cellulitis and results of treatment. Laryngoscope 92:732, 1982.
4. Goodwin WJ, Weinshall M, Chandler JR: The role of high resolution computerized tomography and standardized ultrasound in the evaluation of orbital cellulitis. Laryngoscope 92:728, 1982.
5. Watters EC, Wallar PH, Hiles DA, Michaels RH: Acute orbital cellulitis. Arch Ophthalmol 94:785–788, 1976.
6. Rubinstein JB, Handler SD: Orbital and periorbital cellulitis in children. Head Neck Surg 5:15, 1982.
7. Gans H, Sekula J, Wlodyka J: Treatment of the acute orbital complications. Arch Otolaryngol 100:329, 1974.
8. Welsh LW, Welsh JJ: Orbital complications of sinus disease. Laryngoscope 84:848, 1974.
9. Gamble RC: Acute inflammations of the orbit in children. Arch Ophthalmol 10:483, 1933.
10. Hawkins DB, Clark RW: Orbital involvement in acute sinusitis. Clin Pediatr 16:464, 1977.
11. Zimmerman RA, Bilaniuk LT: CT of orbital infection and its cerebral complications. Am J Radiol 134:45, 1980.
12. Quick EA, Payne L: Complicated acute sinusitis. Laryngoscope 82:1248, 1972.
13. Smith TF, O'Day D, Wright PF: Clinical implications of preseptal (periorbital) cellulitis in childhood. Pediatrics 62:1006, 1978.
14. Gellady AM, Shulman ST, Ayoub EM: Periorbital and orbital cellulitis in children. Pediatrics 61:272, 1978.
15. Barkin RM, Todd JK, Amer J: Periorbital cellulitis in children. Pediatrics 62:390, 1978.
16. Hubert L: Orbital infections due to nasal sinusitis. A study of 114 cases. NY J Med 37:1559, 1937.
17. Schramm VL, Myers EN, Kennerdell JS: Orbital complications of acute sinusitis: Evaluation, management, and outcome. Trans Am Acad Ophthalmol Otolaryngol 86:221, 1978.
18. Smith AF, Spencer JF: Orbital complications resulting from lesions of the sinuses. Ann Otol 57:5, 1948.
19. Chandler JR, Langenbrunner DJ, Stevens ER: The pathogenesis of orbital complications in acute sinusitis. Laryngoscope 80:1414, 1970.
20. Choi S, Lawson W, Urken ML: Subperiosteal orbital hematoma: An unusual complication of sinusitis. Arch Otolaryngol 14:1164, 1988.
21. Kronschnabel EF: Orbital apex syndrome due to sinus infection. Laryngoscope 84:353, 1974.
22. Wheeler JM: Orbital cyst without epithelial lining. Arch Ophthalmol 18:356, 1937.
23. Harris GJ, Kay MC, Nilles JJ: Orbital hematoma secondary to frontal sinusitis. Ophthalmology 85:1229, 1978.
24. Calcaterra TC, Trapp TK: Unilateral proptosis. Otolaryngol Clin North Am 21:53, 1988.
25. Price CD, Hameroff SB, Richards RD: Cavernous sinus thrombosis and orbital cellulitis. South Med J 64:1243, 1971.
26. Pascarelli E, Lemlich H: Diplopia and photophobia as premonitory symptoms in cavernous sinus thrombosis. Ann Otol 73:211, 1964.
27. Yarington CT: The prognosis and treatment of cavernous sinus thrombosis. Ann Otol 70:263, 1961.
28. Morgan PR, Morrison WV: Complications of frontal and ethmoid sinusitis. Laryngoscope 90:661, 1980.
29. Goldberg F, Berne AS, Oski FA: Differentiation of orbital cellulitis from preseptal cellulitis by computed tomography. Pediatrics 62:1000, 1978.
30. Londer L, Nelson DL: Orbital cellulitis due to Haemophilus influenzae. Arch Ophthalmol 91:89, 1974.
31. Haynes RE, Cramblett HG: Acute ethmoiditis. Its relationship to orbital cellulitis. Am J Dis Child 114:261, 1967.
32. Sacks SH, Lawson W, Edelstein D, Green RP: Surgical treatment of blindness secondary to intraorbital hemorrhage. Arch Otolaryngol 114:801, 1988.
33. Jarrett WH, Gutman FA: Ocular complications of infection in the paranasal sinuses. Arch Ophthalmol 81:683, 1969.

CHAPTER 32

INTRACRANIAL COMPLICATIONS OF DISEASE OF THE PARANASAL SINUSES

Andrew Blitzer, MD, DDS
Peter W. Carmel, MD, DMedSci

The intracranial complications of sinus disease are perhaps the raison d'etre of a book on paranasal sinus surgery. The inadequate, inappropriate, or poorly timed treatment of sinus disease may have catastrophic consequences.

The total number of cases of sinus disease with intracranial complications has decreased since the advent of antibiotics. The cases of chronic sinusitis with intermittent bouts of acute infection are now the prime offenders. Treatment with antibiotics in inadequate dosage may mask the symptoms associated with intracranial involvement and therefore delay the diagnosis and treatment and increase the severity of complications.

The most common predisposing factor to intracranial complication is altered sinus physiology due to chronic sinusitis. This may be a result of infection, drug abuse, chemical exposure, or trauma. Other predisposing factors include tumors, structural abnormalities such as bony dehiscences in the skull base with or without a meningoencephalocele, immunologic incompetence, or diabetes. Bony abnormalities, such as Paget's disease, osteopetrosis, or fibrous dysplasia, may also make a patient susceptible to an intracranial complication.

The frontal sinus is the sinus most often involved with intracranial complications, followed by the ethmoid, the sphenoid, and the maxillary. All the paranasal sinuses, except the maxillary, have a wall in common with the cranial cavity, which is often very thin bone.[1]

All infections of the central nervous system are secondary complications rather than primary illnesses, and the primary infective site must be treated along with the nervous system infection. Intracranial infection may be associated with sinus disease by three separate mechanisms: (1) penetrating trauma; (2) direct extension along tissue planes; or (3) hematogenous or metastatic spread from sinus or paranasal infection.[2]

A penetrating injury of the skull leaves a potential tract for infection to follow. Such an injury, crossing a sinus before intracranial penetration, may carry with it purulent material if the sinus is infected. A previously sterile sinus may become infected after trauma and secondarily infect the intracranial space. Therapy for a penetrating injury is therefore aimed at removal of nonviable material, thorough debridement, and reconstitution of barriers around the nervous system. The greatest natural barrier is the dura, and the recovery from a missile wound that ruptures this plane is more likely to be complicated by infection than trauma leaving dura intact. In-driven bone fragments must be removed and necrotic brain in the tract aspirated. Lead bullet fragments are removed, generally via the entrance or exit wound. These fragments are inert and may remain if their removal requires violation of specialized cortex. However, jacketed bullets, coated with either copper or nickel, must be removed. These bullets do not fragment on penetrating the skull and are recognized on x-ray films by the waist or crimp that secures the jacket to the lead missile. Jacketed bullets set up electrotonic fields that are damaging to neural tissue.

The dura should be closed in watertight fashion if it is to be a barrier against infection from an adjacent sinus. If dura is missing because of trauma or debridement, it may be reconstituted using pericranium or fascia lata. The damaged mucosa of the opened sinus may be removed and the sinus packed.

Direct extension of sinus infection first produces a focal osteitis, which may proceed to a true osteomyelitis or avascular necrosis of the cranial vault. This, in turn, may cause epidural empyema, and extension through communicating veins may lead to subdural empyema, meningitis, or cerebral abscess.[3] Soft tissues surrounding an infected sinus may also become infected. Ethmoid infection may spread intracranially through the cribriform plate or into the eye via direct extension or through the ophthalmic veins. Sphenoid infections may spread into the adjacent cavernous sinus.

The most common mechanism of intracranial spread of sinus infection is via thrombophlebitis of valveless veins. Mosher and Judd, in 1933, described a complex system of valveless diploic veins (of Breschet) that allowed bacteria to travel via a thrombophlebitic process from the sinus mucosa, through the frontal bone to dural vessels, or into the superior longitudinal sinus or the cavernous sinus.[6] Extension into the subarachnoid space or brain may also occur in this fashion.[7, 8]

OSTEOMYELITIS

Infectious involvement of the cranial vault is a potentially serious event and greatly increases the likelihood of other intracranial complications. The first demonstrated case of osteomyelitis associated with a sinusitis was reported in 1899 by Tilley.[9] In 1913, McKenzie reviewed 43 cases and showed the significance of osteomyelitis as a complication of sinusitis.[10] Osteomyelitis occurs less frequently since the advent of antibiotic therapy but still occurs related to trauma or chronic infection.

When there is infection of the mucosa, a thrombophlebitic process can spread through the haversian system to the periosteum, compromising the arterial supply to the bone. This will lead to an avascular necrosis, resulting in suppuration with the formation of a subperiosteal abscess. *Staphylococcus* is the most common causative organism, followed by aerobic and anaerobic streptococci. It seems to be more common in late childhood or early adulthood, when the diploic system is most extensive.[11-13]

Radiographs are initially not diagnostic, as the bone changes occur slowly. Eventually, a characteristic "moth-eaten" pattern or avascular necrosis appears, owing to decalcification of bone along with sequestration and areas of osteoblastic response.

It is imperative to make an early diagnosis to prevent a locus of infection for further seeding of intracranial structures. With an early diagnosis there is less than a 5 per cent mortality.[1]

Treatment consists of adequate intravenous antibiotic therapy and debridement of the osteomyelitic bone. Because of the avascular nature of the bone and sequestration of the nidus, antibiotics do not penetrate the infected area very well. Bone must be removed to a healthy margin. The sequelae are related mostly to intracranial complications. Reconstruction of the frontal bone must be delayed until there is evidence that the infection has completely remitted (see Chapter 10).

EPIDURAL ABSCESS

Epidural abscess, or empyema, is a collection of purulent material between the cranial vault and the dura and has long been recognized as a complication of sinusitis.[14] In 1909, Gerber reported 52 epidural abscesses in a series of 110 cases of frontal sinusitis, usually with concomitant osteomyelitis of the frontal bone.[16] The incidence of subdural empyema has decreased and now may be more commonly associated with acute exacerbations of chronic disease.

Almost all the cases of epidural abscess are related to the frontal sinus where the dura is loosely adherent to the frontal bone. In the area of the ethmoid and sphenoid, the dura is very adherent to the bone. Dura is resistant to infection, except in the areas of the emissary veins. Often the empyema will be limited to a granulomatous exudate over the dural surface.[1]

Symptoms are usually mild. The local site

may be painful and tender. There may also be headache, low-grade fever, and slight elevation of the white blood cell count and erythrocyte sedimentation rate (ESR). Neurologic deficits are minimal and often entirely absent. These infections are frequently discovered only during investigation of the primary site of illness.[15]

Infection in the epidural space can affect blood flow in the major dural sinuses, which may be compressed by the epidural mass or thrombosed by infection in the sinus wall. Obstruction of a major dural sinus is a leading childhood cause of benign increased intracranial pressure (pseudotumor cerebri). Signs and symptoms are those of increased intracranial pressure. Headache, nausea, vomiting, diplopia, and papilledema may be present. Children with benign increased intracranial pressure often do not appear to be seriously ill despite these symptoms.[3]

Skull radiographs will indicate infection at the primary focus in most cases, and osteomyelitis of the skull may suggest epidural suppuration. Less frequently, changes associated with chronic increased intracranial pressure will be seen. Lumbar puncture pressure may be normal or elevated, and cerebrospinal fluid (CSF) chemical and cellular values are usually normal. Electroencephalogram (EEG) and brain scan results can be abnormal but rarely accurately localize the infected site.

Computed tomography (CT) is currently the preferred method for diagnosing epidural infections. It will reveal enlargement of the epidural space, often with some edema of the underlying brain (Fig. 32–1A). Brain edema may be extensive through both frontal lobes if sagittal sinus thrombosis is present. Neovascular proliferation along the inner abscess surface and within the dura will be revealed as prominent enhancement after intravenous contrast is given[19] (Fig. 32–1B). Instillation of contrast may show a defect in the frontal or ethmoid sinus.[20]

Antibiotic therapy is always required. Some epidural infections will not require surgery; however, if a mass lesion is identified, it should be drained promptly. At operation, removal of all chronically infected granulation tissue should be accomplished, as well as radical removal of infected overlying bone.[16] The dura should not

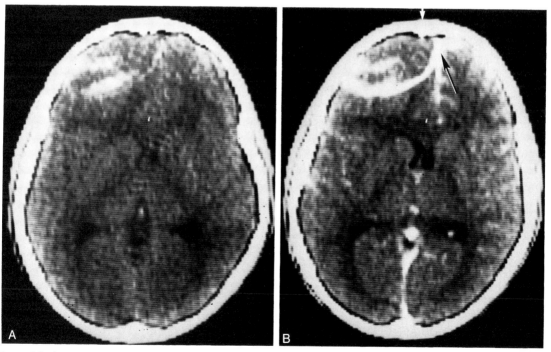

Figure 32–1. A 17-year-old boy with epidural abscess.
  A, Unenhanced axial CT scan. He had been treated at another hospital 2 weeks earlier for a *right* frontal sinusitis. Five days prior to this scan he developed *left* frontal headache. A large mass was seen in the left frontal region, with edema in the adjacent brain. Densities within the mass are hematomas, created when expansion of the abscess tore the bridging veins.
  B, Axial scan following contrast injection. There is marked enhancement of the dura due to the neovascular proliferation. The abscess has pushed the falx from its midline attachment *(arrows)*, allowing the purulent material to cross the midline and collect at the left frontal pole.

be opened to inspect for subdural pus; this should be ascertained by preoperative studies, as the protective dural barrier should not be violated needlessly.[2]

Benign increased intracranial pressure secondary to sinus obstruction is a self-limited process with excellent prognosis. The sinus may recanalize, or venous anastomoses may open.[13] However, chronic papilledema may lead to optic atrophy and visual impairment. Efforts at decreasing the intracranial pressure to protect the optic nerves may include high doses of steroids, repeated lumbar punctures, and decompressive craniectomy.

SUBDURAL ABSCESS

Subdural infection accounts for nearly one fifth of intracranial abscesses.[21] Despite antibiotic therapy, the mortality rate remains close to 40 per cent.[23] Subdural abscess most frequently follows inadequate antibiotic treatment of a prior infection. In adults and older children, subdural empyema is usually associated with otorhinologic infection, whereas in infants it is usually a sequela of poorly treated meningitis with an infected effusion.[3, 24] Subdural abscesses are usually related to frontal sinusitis. Infection spreads from mucoperiosteum via a septic thrombophlebitis of emissary veins to the subdural space. In chronic infections there is often an osteitis leading to necrosis, with direct spread to the epidural and subdural space. Streptococcal organisms (50 per cent anaerobic and microaerophilic) are the most common agents, followed by *Staphylococcus*, with a lower incidence caused by *Pneumococcus*, *Proteus*, *Bacteroides*, and *Aspergillus*.[13, 21, 22]

When paranasal sinus infection is followed by severe headache, alteration of consciousness, fever, meningeal signs, and frontal or orbital swelling, it is clear that the infection has spread beyond the sinus and entered the subdural space. The clinical course may be rapid, often evolving within several hours. Purulent material may spread widely in the subdural space, causing focal or hemispheric neurologic signs.[25] Intracranial pressure is usually elevated, and infants may have fever and an enlarging head.[23] Seizures are not infrequent signs.

The diagnosis must be considered if any or all of the clinical signs and symptoms are present and can best be confirmed with a CT scan with contrast material. Not only will CT scan provide diagnostic information but also it

will help localize loculated portions of the collection.[2, 26] A lumbar puncture will reveal a mildly elevated CSF pressure with increased protein content and an increased white blood cell count with a normal glucose level.

Subdural empyema is treated by early and definitive drainage, coupled with intensive appropriate antibiotic therapy. The purulent cavity must be opened widely and cleaned. Loculated pockets of infected material, usually located along the falx, posterior frontal convexity, and base, must be sought and removed. Adequate drainage may not be possible through bur holes, and wide craniotomy may be necessary.[16] Some surgeons advise irrigation of the space for several days postoperatively via indwelling drains. Systemic steroids will reduce the underlying cerebral edema.[16–18]

There may be cortical vein thrombosis underlying the purulent collection, with extensive venous infarction. Despite adequate surgical evacuation, widespread cortical damage may lead to focal neurologic deficit and persistent seizure activity.[2]

BRAIN ABSCESS

In 1893, Macwen demonstrated that abscess of the brain is a surgically curable disease, with only 1 of his 19 patients succumbing to infection. However, most contemporary reports cite overall mortality rates of 30 to 45 per cent for all forms of therapy, and operative mortality rates of 20 to 40 per cent.[27, 30] Although the introduction of antibiotics has resulted in dramatic improvement in therapy of meningitis and some focal forms of intracranial infection, there has been but slight improvement in treatment of brain abscess.[2] Most brain abscesses were otitic in origin in the preantibiotic era, but rhinogenic abscesses have predominated since.

The incidence of brain abscess is difficult to evaluate but is probably between 2 and 3 per 10,000 general hospital admissions. A preponderance of males is noted in most large series.[30] Brain abscess is rarely found in infants under 1 year of age, but the incidence rises rapidly thereafter, and nearly a third of all cases occur in children.[3, 4] Although the incidence of brain abscesses from otorhinologic sources has fallen markedly since the introduction of antibiotics, they remain the most common cause in most series. In the pediatric age range, however, metastatic abscesses, usually associated with cyanotic heart disease, are now more common.[2, 3, 5]

Most of the brain abscesses secondary to paranasal sinus disease occur in the frontal lobes (Fig. 32–2). Temporal lobe abscesses are less common and are most often otogenic. Temporal lobe abscesses can be related to lateral extension of sphenoid sinusitis, to osteomyelitis of the sphenoid bone secondary to a maxillary sinusitis, or to a widespread subdural abscess.

Abscess formation within the brain starts with an area of cerebritis surrounding an infective focus. Within a few days the center of the area liquefies, becomes necrotic, and is surrounded by edematous, friable brain. Necrotic and edematous regions blend without clear demarcation. Encapsulation of the abscess usually starts at 10 to 14 days. The abscess may extend outward in several directions to form daughter abscesses. In traumatic foreign body wounds,

the abscess often spreads along the penetration tract. Thickening of the abscess wall, liquefaction of the cavity contents, edema of the surrounding brain, and encephalitis contribute to the mass effect of the lesion.[30]

Material from abscess cavities must be immediately cultured, both aerobically and anaerobically. In the preantibiotic era, brain abscess was almost universally attributable to aerobic *Streptococcus* or *Staphylococcus aureus*. In more recent series, anaerobic bacteria have played an increasing role in brain abscess formation, accounting for almost 80 per cent of nontraumatic brain abscesses in some series[3, 27, 30, 32] (see Table 32–1). This is due, in part, to the eradication of many otitic or paranasal sinus infections that might eventually have led to brain abscesses. It also reflects the change in flora caused by use of broad-spectrum antibiotics. A history of pretreatment with broad-spec-

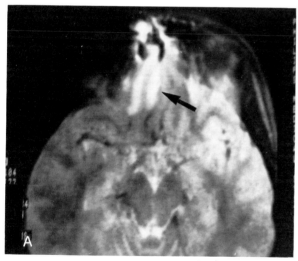

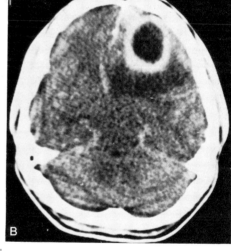

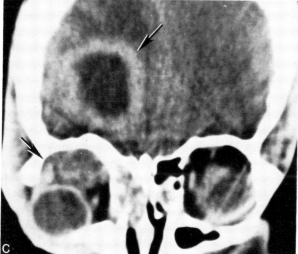

Figure 32–2. *A,* A 30-year-old woman with a frontal sinusitis. An MRI showed evidence of frontal sinusitis with extension via a thrombophlebitic process *(arrow)* into the frontal lobes.

B, Axial enhanced CT scan, showing an intracerebral abscess with edema of the right frontal lobe. Despite the prominent ring enhancement, there was only a poorly formed abscess wall, and the cavity was drained via an indwelling catheter. Some purulent granulation was seen in the subdural space as well.

C, Coronal enhanced CT scan. The intracranial abscess is seen, as well as some enhancement in the subdural space at the convexity laterally. There is a separate abscess cavity seen in the orbit superiorly, depressing the globe downward and laterally.

TABLE 32–1. Infecting Organisms in Brain Abscess

Organism	Percentage
Staphylococcus aureus (coagulase-positive)	26
Anaerobic (microaerobic streptococcus)	18
Bacteroides	7
Hemolytic *Streptococcus*	6
Proteus sp	4
Haemophilus influenzae	3
E. coli	3
Cryptococcus	1
Nocardia	1
Aspergillus	1
Corynebacterium acnes	1
Sterile cultures	19

Data from Idriss and associates[3] and Samson and Clark.[30]

trum antibiotics, usually of insufficient potency and in inadequate dosage, is a common finding in patients with sterile abscesses. An increasing number of cases are related to cocaine abuse (Fig. 32–3).[18a]

The bacterial spectrum in neonates with brain abscesses differs from that in older children and adults. Nearly half of the reported cases in infants of less than 3 months of age have been caused by gram-negative organisms.[24] These organisms include *E. coli, Citrobacter, Proteus,* and *Paracolobactrum.* Brain abscesses in early infancy commonly attain an enormous size because of the expansile skull and large subarachnoid space.[3]

The initial symptoms of brain abscess are more likely to be related to its intracranial mass effect than to the infectious nature of the illness. Lethargy, anorexia, and vomiting are noted, and headache is common. Focal or grand mal seizures may be the first indication of cerebral involvement and may lead to discovery of previously unnoticed neurologic deficits. Fever may be quite mild, and almost half of patients are afebrile on hospital admission, though often giving a history of recent febrile illness. Brain abscesses usually progress rapidly, and the duration of symptoms is often less than a week and seldom more than a month. At initial hospital examination, patients may already be lethargic or comatose, with signs of increased intracranial pressure. Specific neurologic deficits will depend on the area of involvement and may include hemiparesis, sensory impairment, and visual field abnormalities.

Routine blood studies may be normal or may reveal a moderate leukocytosis and elevated erythrocyte sedimentation rate. Skull films often indicate a chronic otorhinologic infection, and occasionally there is evidence of mass effect

or increased intracranial pressure.[27, 30] Slowing of the EEG over the affected hemisphere is present in two thirds of cases but is often not focal.

Many series stress the danger of lumbar puncture in the presence of abscess. If there is indication of increased intracranial pressure or intracranial structure shift, lumbar puncture is contraindicated.[2] The information obtained from the CSF of patients with brain abscess is usually nonspecific and often does not demonstrate the causative organism. There may be risk of fatality due to herniation in obtaining the CSF.

Angiography may be used to define the location of the abscess. Much attention has been devoted to the "ring" sign, a dense circle of vessels surrounding a radiolucent center, which is associated with well-walled abscesses. Unfortunately, this pattern is found in fewer than one third of cerebral abscess angiograms. More typically, signs of midline vessel shift accompanying an avascular mass effect are found, without a surrounding zone of hyperemia.[25] Angiography may not be diagnostic during the early stage of cerebritis or when there are multiple abscesses.[26] Angiography is of increased risk in some children with severe cyanotic heart disease.

Radionuclide brain scanning has proved to be extremely sensitive for cerebral abscesses. Most centers prefer scanning with Tc-99m. Most abscesses larger than 1 cm in diameter produce positive scans. Isotopic scan is particularly helpful in delineating multiple abscesses, which are often not shown by angiography. However, certain regions of the head, covered by either temporal or cervical musculature, are relatively insensitive, and lesions may be missed.

Use of CT scan is clearly a significant advance in the diagnosis and evaluation of therapy of brain abscesses (see Fig. 32–3). Multiple lesions, a noted cause of high mortality in brain abscess, are easily diagnosed by this method. Magnetic resonance imaging (MRI) is quickly becoming the most sensitive tool for evaluating brain pathology. Sinusitis with brain abscess is easily demonstrated (Fig. 32–4). Dosage of steroids, antibiotics, and even mannitol may be adjusted according to observed changes over time.[26] Complex clinical developments during the postoperative course may be clarified by CT scan without resorting to repeated invasive techniques.[19]

Treatment is rapidly initiated with high dosage intravenous antibiotic therapy. Broad-spec-

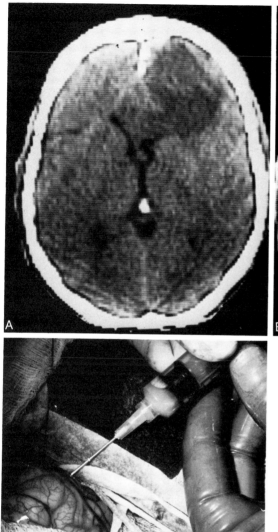

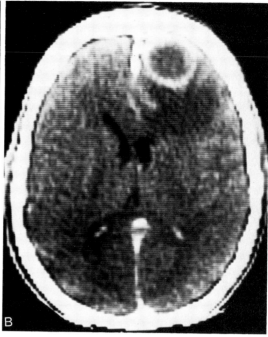

Figure 32–3. A 35-year-old man with chronic sinusitis and known drug abuse. He described several days of headache and was admitted to the hospital following a seizure.

A, Axial CT scan before contrast. There is a large lucent area at the right frontal pole, surrounded by edema. Mass effect has pushed midline structures to the left and partially coapted the right frontal horn of the ventricle.

B, Axial CT scan following contrast injection. There is marked ring enhancement of the abscess wall, surrounded by edema. In this case there was a well-formed abscess wall.

C, Operative photograph. The right frontal lobe is exposed and pushes forward under pressure. Aspiration revealed creamy purulent material, which was cultured, and the abscess was then excised completely.

trum antibiotics that are known to cross the blood-brain barrier are chosen before specific sensitivities are known.[32] Oxacillin and chloramphenicol are frequently used initially. Cephalosporins do not penetrate brain tissue well and are generally to be avoided.

An intracerebral abscess may act as a rapidly expanding intracranial mass around which massive cerebral edema may develop. Secondary midbrain and brain stem compression can lead to coma and death in a very short time. Uncal herniation causing midbrain compression is almost uniformly found in fatal cases of brain abscess. Therapy is therefore aimed at decreasing the intracerebral pressure and mass effect.[2] Dexamethasone is given in large doses, and

osmotic agents, such as urea or mannitol, may reverse the more severe symptoms briefly until definitive therapy can be instituted. Several techniques have been devised for operative treatment of abscesses, and the selection of procedure will depend on the condition of the patient, abscess location, and degree of abscess encapsulation.[27, 30] The clinical condition at the time of operation is a greater factor in determining the result than choice of operative therapy. Decompression of mass effect is the primary goal of surgery.[2, 31]

Aspiration through a bur hole is preferable for abscesses in severely ill patients, for known multiple abscesses, or for those with a thin or poorly developed wall. Catheters may be left

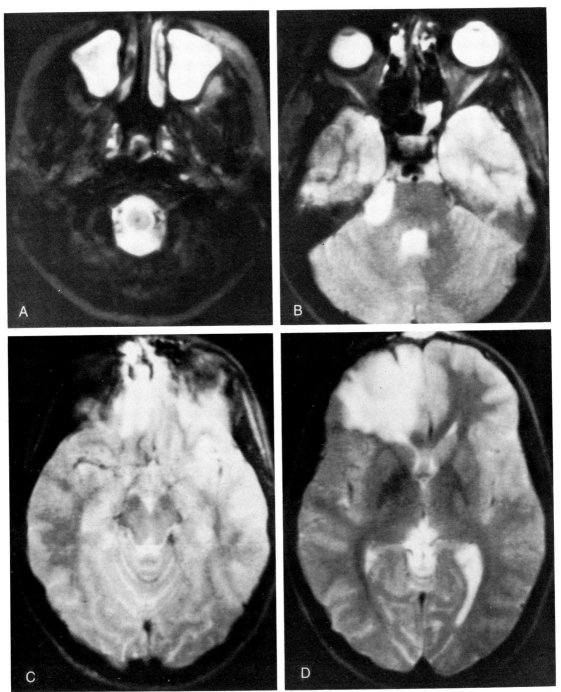

Figure 32–4. Pansinusitis with right frontal lobe abscess. Axial T2-weighted MRI demonstrates high signal within the maxillary sinuses *(A)*, the bilateral ethmoids *(B)*, and the frontal sinuses *(C and D)*, with a right frontal lobe abscess seen in *D.*

in place, allowing further infected material to drain over several days. Irrigation of the cavity with small amounts of saline may help promote drainage. Antibiotic solutions have been used for irrigation, but systemically administered antibiotics will usually achieve adequate levels within the abscess.[32]

Total excision of the abscess achieves immediate decompression of the mass effect and decreases the chance of recurrence due to remaining infected material. However, total excision should be reserved for those well-encapsulated abscesses that have significant mass and that do not underlie a primary cortical area.[2] It should not be employed in patients who are deeply obtunded or moribund. Total excision need not be employed primarily but may be used following a period of treatment with steroids and antibiotics, or even after initial aspiration.[30]

Material from the abscess must be cultured immediately, both aerobically and anaerobically. Antibiotic therapy will be changed according to data obtained from culture, and intravenous antibiotic therapy is generally continued for 2 to 4 weeks after total excision.

Diagnosis of brain abscess can be made with CT scan at the cerebritis stage of abscess evolution. Intraparenchymal regions of cerebritis appear to be more readily curable with antibiotics alone than are well-formed abscesses. Small, formed abscesses may also be treated with antibiotics alone, especially when multiple. Surgical intervention is indicated when the mass effect of the lesion is persistent, progressive, threatening, or resistant to cure by antibiotic therapy.

Anticonvulsants should be given to all patients with supratentorial purulent lesions for at least 2 years following surgery. Seizures are frequently present preoperatively, and the incidence of seizures following surgery is almost 50 per cent. The choice of operative therapy does not appear to alter the incidence of seizures.

High mortality rates for brain abscesses are largely related to two factors. Most significant is late diagnosis. If proper diagnosis is delayed until the patient is obtunded or comatose, mortality rates of 65 to 90 per cent are reported.[19, 26, 27, 29] The second factor is the presence of multiple lesions. Mortality rates of up to 80 per cent have been reported in children with multiple abscesses. Introduction of CT scans has allowed earlier detection of these lesions.[19] A dramatic drop in mortality has already been noted in the first years following introduction

of CT techniques, and mortality rates less than 20 per cent are now generally reported.

MENINGITIS

Meningitis is the most common intracranial complication of sinusitis. It accounted for 70 per cent of the intracranial complications in the series by Courville and Rosenvalt in 1938.[33] Meningitis may also occur as an immediate or delayed complication of facial trauma if there is disruption of the posterior wall of the frontal sinus, ethmoid sinus, or cribriform plate.[34] The traumatic etiology may be iatrogenic and occur at the time of nasal or sinus surgery. Meningitis has also been reported secondary to scuba diving, with spread of organisms along the olfactory perineural spaces.

Hemolytic streptococci were found to be the most frequently identified organism (52 per cent, 121 of 231 cases), followed by Pneumococcus (32 per cent), Haemophilus influenzae (9 per cent), Staphylococcus aureus (3 per cent), and others (3 per cent).[1]

The patients usually have headache, fever, and signs of meningeal irritation. Seizure activity is common. There is often irritability, which may be followed by somnolence, delirium, and then coma.[1, 13] There may be focal neurologic deficits due to involvement of cranial nerves at the skull base or secondary to arteritis and inflammation over the hemispheres. Cerebral edema may be produced, which increases neurologic deficits and which may cause herniation. Late complications of meningitis include hydrocephalus and subdural effusion.

A lumbar puncture will show an increased white blood cell count, increased CSF pressure, and increased protein content. A smear with Gram's stain, culture, and sensitivity testing should be performed on the fluid. An immunoelectrophoresis for a bacterial antigen may be useful when culture results are negative. A CT scan may appear normal but, with contrast, may show enlargement of the cisterns or ventricles.

The treatment should include the appropriate antibiotics, steroids if there is cerebral edema, anticonvulsants for seizure activity, and drainage of the sinus focus. Postinfection sequelae are especially common in children, of whom an estimated 30 per cent will have focal neurologic deficits or mental retardation.[3]

CAVERNOUS SINUS THROMBOSIS

Cavernous sinus thrombosis, first described by Bright in 1831, has been mentioned earlier as a sequela of both epidural and subdural infections. When related to the paranasal sinuses it generally occurs secondary to ethmoid or sphenoid disease. The thrombophlebitis may travel directly to the cavernous sinus or go via the ophthalmic vessels. This process is often a rapidly progressive one in which the sepsis reaches the cavernous sinus by direct extension of the infected thrombus or a shower of septic emboli.[35, 36] The infection may also involve many other venous structures, producing an associated meningitis and extradural, subdural, or cortical abscess.[37] *Staphylococcus* is the predominant organism in cavernous sinus thrombosis, followed by *Streptococcus, Pneumococcus*, and others. Generally, blood culture results are positive, allowing drug sensitivity levels to be determined.

Symptoms begin with fever, headaches, nausea, and vomiting. Orbital symptoms include chemosis, ophthalmoplegia, engorged retinal veins, and papilledema (Fig. 32–5A). As the process extends, it may involve the other eye and produce swelling of the root of the nose and dysesthesia or paresthesia of the eyes, cheek, and forehead.[1] Fever spikes, chills, and tachycardia may appear if generalized septicemia is present. Seizure activity, decreased consciousness, and/or a hemiparesis may occur if widespread cortical vein thrombosis or meningitis develops. Septic emboli can spread to the lungs, muscles, or viscera, and this complication has been reported in almost 40 per cent of cases.[37]

Diagnosis is primarily made on clinical grounds. A lumbar puncture may show a leukocytosis, but culture is usually sterile. CT scan with contrast will often demonstrate both the source of the infection and the cavernous sinus involvement (Fig. 32–5B). Angiography or selective venography may also be useful.

Treatment consists of intravenous antibiotic therapy. Prompt diagnosis and treatment will yield a 70 to 80 per cent survival. There should be a constant evaluation for possible associated intracranial pathology, such as meningitis and subdural or cerebral abscess. Associated complications in the survivors are frequent and reach 75 per cent in some series.[1, 37] The most common sequelae are persistent cranial nerve palsies in 30 per cent and blindness in 15 per cent of patients.[37, 38]

Use of anticoagulants for cavernous sinus thrombosis is still controversial. Some investigators believe they will prevent the propagation of the clot. Others, including Yarington, think

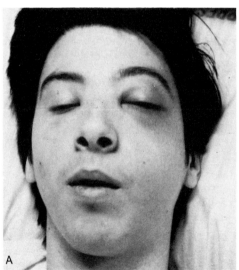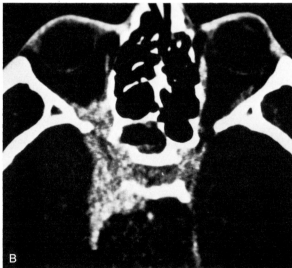

Figure 32–5. An 18-year-old boy with cavernous sinus thrombosis. He complained of left eye pain, followed by diplopia and closing of the eye. There was a total ophthalmoplegia, with sparing of vision.
  A, Note the periorbital swelling, which was red-purple in color.
  B, Axial enhanced CT scan. The left cavernous sinus shows prominent enhancement and is remarkably enlarged. Extensions rostral and caudal to the sinus probably represent thrombosis of major veins draining into the sinus. The patient was treated with antibiotics and anticoagulation, with complete resolution of his symptoms.

that the clot confines the bacterial spread via septic emboli. He reviewed 878 cases and came to the conclusion that anticoagulants should not be used.[37] Some workers also suggested the use of fibrinolysins in cavernous sinus thrombosis to allow destruction of the thrombus.

Pituitary inflammation has also been noted in many of these cases, and steroid therapy might be necessary for adrenal insufficiency. The patients should be evaluated for other possible pituitary deficits.

SUPERIOR LONGITUDINAL SINUS THROMBOSIS

Sagittal sinus thrombosis is usually associated with epidural or subdural abscess and progresses in a manner similar to that of cavernous sinus thrombosis. It starts with a thrombophlebitic process of the diploic veins and extends centrally through the valveless venous system.

Symptoms are related to the location of the thrombus and the region of cortical venous drainage that is obstructed. There may be focal or diffuse motor and sensory deficits, seizures, and changes in the level of consciousness. As venous drainage becomes progressively inadequate, there may be a rapid onset of papilledema, coma, and decorticate posturing. Obstruction of resorption of CSF may lead to hydrocephalus, stupor, and coma.

Unfortunately, the diagnosis is frequently made at autopsy. It can be made premorbidly with a venogram or CT scan with contrast. MRI has added a new dimension of sensitivity to making this diagnosis (Fig. 32–6). Sinus obstruction may be suspected in a pattern of edematous lucency rostral to the point of obstruction.

Treatment consists of appropriate antibiotic, anticoagulant, and anticonvulsant therapy. The prognosis is generally poor and related to the extent of the thrombus.

CEREBROSPINAL FLUID LEAK

This complication is most often associated with trauma or secondary to surgery but may be related to tumor,[39] congenital abnormalities, or conditions leading to hydrocephalus.[40] The diagnosis and management of this condition are discussed in Chapter 25. CT cisternography may often be of value in demonstrating a leak (Fig. 32–7).

PNEUMOCEPHALUS

Pneumocephalus is also usually secondary to trauma or surgery[41, 42] but may occur with certain tumors, infection, and hydrocephalus.[43] There may or may not be related CSF leak. In most cases of traumatic pneumocephalus, the air is resorbed spontaneously. However, a "ball-valve" situation may develop, in which the air is collecting under pressure and compressing

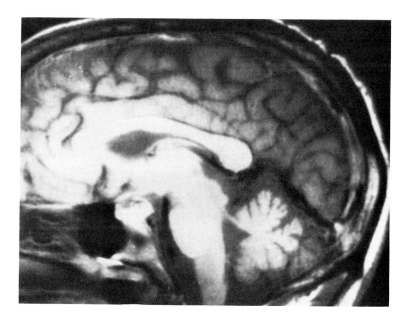

Figure 32–6. Sagittal sinus thrombosis. Sagittal T1-weighted MRI shows increased signal throughout the sagittal sinus owing to subacute clot; compare this with the normal signal void caused by flow within the straight sinus.

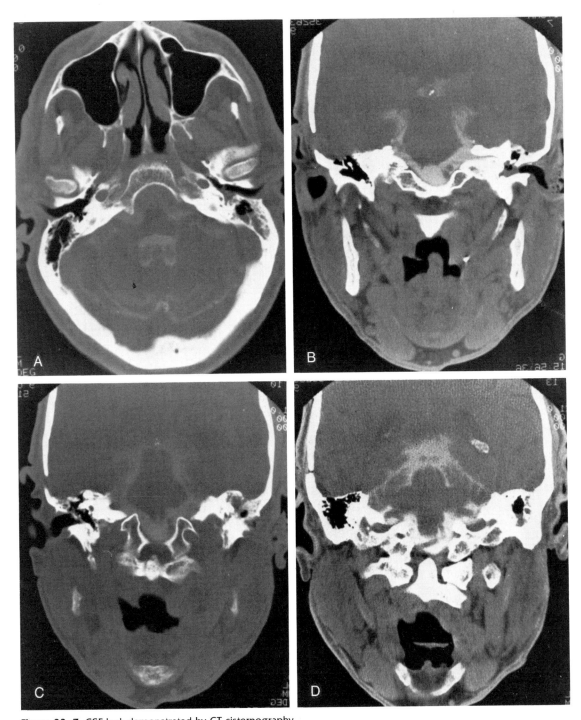

Figure 32–7. CSF leak demonstrated by CT cisternography.

A, Axial CT cisternogram photographed for bone detail demonstrates opacification of the left external auditory canal and mastoid complex, with air-fluid levels present. Note the contrast within the CSF-filled fourth ventricle.

B, C, D, Serial coronal CT scans demonstrate the ossicles bilaterally and show fluid within the middle ear and external auditory canal *(B),* the bony defect superiorly along the left petrous ridge *(C),* and an air-fluid level within the mastoid complex *(D).* Note the contrast surrounding the normal cerebellum and outlining the vertebrobasilar junction in *D*.

the brain. If the air remains, or increases intracranial pressure, surgical treatment to occlude the source may be necessary.[44]

References

1. Fairbanks DNF, Vanderveen TS, Bordley JE: Intracranial complications of sinusitis. In English E (ed): Otolaryngology. New York, Harper and Row, 1983, p 1.
2. Carmel PW: Focal infections of the nervous system. In Rudolph AM (ed): Pediatrics. 17th ed. Norwalk, CT, Appleton-Century-Crofts, 1982, p 61.
3. Idriss ZH, Gutman LT, Kronfol NM: Brain abscesses in infants and children. Clin Pediatr 17:738, 1978.
4. Gellers TM, Donowitz LG: Brain abcess and ethmoid sinusitis presenting as periorbital cellulitis in a two-month-old infant. Pediatr Infect Dis J 6:213, 1987.
5. Moss SD, McLone DG, Arditi M, Yogev R: Pediatric cerebral abscess. Pediatr Neurosci 14:291, 1988.
6. Mosher HP, Judd DK: An analysis of seven cases of osteomyelitis of frontal bone complicating frontal sinusitis. Laryngoscope 43:153, 1933.
7. Yogev R: Suppurative intracranial complications of upper respiratory tract infections. Pediatr Infect Dis J 6:324, 1987.
8. Maniglia AJ, Goodwin WJ, Arnold JE, Ganz E: Intracranial abscess secondary to nasal, sinus, and orbital infections in adults and children. Arch Otolaryngol Head Neck Surg 115:1424, 1989.
9. Tilley H: Fetal case of chronic frontal sinus empyema. Lancet 2:534, 1899.
10. McKenzie D: Osteomyelitis of the frontal bone. J Laryngol Otol 28:6, 1913.
11. Bluestone CD, Steiner RE: Intracranial complications of acute frontal sinusitis. Laryngoscope 43:153, 1933.
12. Bordley JE, Schotberger W: Osteomyelitis of the frontal bone. Laryngoscope 77:1234, 1967.
13. Kaplan RJ: Neurological complications of infections of the head and neck. Otolaryngol Clin North Am 9:729, 1976.
14. Earle J: The Chirurgical Works of Percivall Pott, F.R.S. Philadelphia. James Webster, 1819, p 29.
15. Sellick JA: Epidural abscess and subdural empyema. J Am Osteopath Assoc 89:806, 1989.
16. Galbraith JG, Barr VW: Epidural abscess and subdural empyema. In Thompson RA, Green JR (eds): Advances in Neurology. New York, Raven Press, 1974.
17. Pattisapu JV, Parent AD: Subdural empyemas in children. Pediatr Neurosci 13:251, 1987.
18. Rosenbaum GS, Cunha BA: Subdural empyema complicating frontal and ethmoid sinusitis. Heart Lung 18:199, 1989.
19. Shaw MDM, Russell JA: Value of computed tomography in the diagnosis of intracranial abscess. J Neurol Neurosurg Psychiatry 40:214, 1977.
20. Dietrich K, Feldges A, Nau HE, Lohr E: Epidural abscess following sinusitis—demonstration of communication by epidural contrast medium and coronal computerized tomography. Comput Med Imag Graph 13:351, 1989.
21. Coonrod JD, Dans PE: Subdural empyema. Am J Med 53:85, 1972.
22. Bates J, Clark DR, Chiodini P: Intracranial extension of paranasal sinus aspergillosis. J Laryngol Otol 101:188, 1987.
23. Farmer TW, Wise GR: Subdural empyema in infants, children and adults. Neurology 23:254, 1973.
24. Vogel LC, Ferguson L, Gotoff SP: Citrobacter infection of the central nervous system in early infancy. J Pediatr 93:86, 1978.
25. Wilkins RH, Goree JA: Interhemispheric subdural empyema: Angiographic appearance. J Neurosurg 32:459, 1970.
26. Rosenblum ML, Hoff JT, et al.: Decreased mortality from brain abscesses since advent of computerized tomography. J Neurosurg 49:658, 1978.
27. Beller AJ, Sahar A, Praiss I: Brain abscess; Review of 89 cases over a period of 30 years. J Neurol Neurosurg Psychiatry 36:757, 1973.
28. Rao AN: Brain abscess: A complication of cocaine inhalation. NY State J Med 88:548, 1988.
29. Parker GS, Tami TA, Wilson JF, Fetter TW: Intracranial complications of sinusitis. South Med J 82:563, 1989.
30. Samson DS, Clark K: A current review of brain abscess. Am J Med 54:201, 1973.
31. Johnson DL, Markle BM, Wiedermann BL, Hanahan L: Treatment of intracranial abscesses associated with sinusitis in children and adolescents. J Pediatr 113:15, 1988.
32. Black P, Graybill JR, Charache P: Penetration of brain abscess by systemically administered antibiotics. J Neurosurg 38:705, 1973.
33. Courville CB: Subdural empyema secondary to purulent frontal sinusitis. Arch Otolaryngol 39:211, 1944.
34. Teed RW: Meningitis from sphenoid sinus. Arch Otol 28:589, 1938.
35. Clune JP: Septic thrombosis within the cavernous chamber. Am J Ophthalmol 56:33, 1963.
36. Price CD, Hammeroff SB, Richards RD: Cavernous sinus thrombosis and orbital cellulitis. South Med J 64:1243, 1971.
37. Yarington WT: The prognosis and treatment of cavernous sinus thrombosis. Review of 878 cases in the literature. Ann Otol Rhinol Laryngol 70:263, 1961.
38. DiNubile MJ: Septic thrombosis of the cavernous sinuses. Arch Neurol 45:567, 1988.
39. Brunner H, Spiesman I: Osteoma of the frontal and ethmoid sinuses. Ann Otol Rhinol Laryngol 42:47, 1941.
40. Rajshekar V, Mathai KV, Chandy MJ, Abraham J: Non-traumatic cerebrospinal fluid rhinorrhea: The normal pressure leaks. Acta Neurochir (Wein) 96:114, 1989.
41. Misra BK, Harris P: Tension pneumocephalus following nasal polypectomy. Surg Neurol 28:307, 1987.
42. Komiyama M, Yasui T, Yagura H, Fu Y, Sugata H, Baba M: Magnetic resonance imaging of traumatic pneumocephalus—case report. Neurol Med Chir (Tokyo) 28:677, 1988.
43. Huneidi AH, Afshar F: Chronic spontaneous tension pneumocephalus due to benign frontal sinus osteoma. Br J Neurosurg 3:389, 1989.
44. Steudel WI, Hacker H: Acute intracranial pneumocephalus: Prognosis and management—a retrospective analysis of 101 cases. Neurosurg Rev 12 (Suppl 1):125, 1989.

INDEX

Note: Page numbers in *italics* refer to illustrations; page numbers followed by (t) refer to tables.